Pocket
Companion to
VETERINARY
MEDICINE

D. C. BLOOD

Professor Emeritus
School of Veterinary Science
University of Melbourne
Australia

Baillière Tindall
London Philadelphia Sydney Tokyo Toronto

Baillière Tindall 24–28 Oval Road
W. B. Saunders London NW1 7DX

The Curtis Center
Independence Square West
Philadelphia, PA 19106-3399, USA

Harcourt Brace & Company
55 Horner Avenue
Toronto, Ontario, M8Z 4X6, Canada

Harcourt Brace & Company, Australia
30–52 Smidmore Street
Marrickville
NSW 2204, Australia

Harcourt Brace & Company, Japan
Ichibancho Central Building
22-1 Ichibancho
Chiyoda-ku, Tokyo 102, Japan

A catalogue record for this book is available from the British Library

ISBN 0-7020-1695-0

Typeset by Paston Press Ltd, Loddon, Norfolk
Printed and bound in Great Britain by
Mackays of Chatham PLC, Chatham, Kent

CONTENTS

PART TWO   SPECIAL MEDICINE

LIST OF TABLES

LIST OF ILLUSTRATIONS

PREFACE

Undergraduate and postgraduate students in veterinary medicine may feel over-whelmed on occasion by the large volume of veterinary medical information available to assist in the diagnosis, treatment and control of the diseases of food-producing animals and horses, the species dealt with in *Veterinary Medicine* by Radostits, Blood and Gay.

This Pocket Companion has been produced by condensing the eighth edition of *Veterinary Medicine* so that the clinical sections of the main text would be available for speedy reference in the teaching hospital wards and on the farms of Farm Clinic clients, and for quick revision during the study period leading up to examinations. The objective has been to include only the principal facts, and to omit discussion material. In order to ensure the reader is reminded at all times that the book is only an **aid** to study, and not a treatise on veterinary medicine, all disease descriptions are headed by a VM8 page number, an immediate cross-reference to the eighth edition of *Veterinary Medicine*.

To further enhance the revision purpose of the book, each of the clinical signs listed in Chapter 1, 'Clinical Examination and Making a Diagnosis', is accom-panied by a page number, a cross-reference to a page in the first fourteen chapters, the General Medicine section, of this companion book. Following this revision trail will lead the student, first to a patho-anatomic diagnosis, such as pneumonia, then to a list of possible etiological diagnoses in the last twenty-one chapters, those containing the Special Medicine material.

All of the 1250-plus diseases described in *Veterinary Medicine* are summarized in this book and they can be readily accessed, either via the revision trail or the index, which has also been abbreviated so as to contain only the common, and alternative names of the diseases and the indicants listed in the text. Also, to further facilitate differential diagnosis, each disease description contains a section called diagnosis which includes the names of other diseases with which the subject disease may be confused.

It is anticipated that this book will provide a source of quickly and easily located basic information, making it a worthy companion to *Veterinary Medicine*. It cannot serve as a substitute; the amount of information contained in it is insufficient for a proper understanding of all of the medical diseases of the five animal species, at all stages of their productive lives and reproductive cycles. The major omissions have been in the area of pathogenesis and epidemiology, the sections of veterinary medicine which provide the basics for the understanding of each disease, without which logical, intelligent diagnosis, treatment and control are not possible.

A major problem in the preparation of this volume involved deciding which parts of *Veterinary Medicine* to include and which to omit. Much of the abbreviation has been achieved by a careful balance of text versus tables, and a careful use of sub-headings and other forms of highlighting. The assistance and advice of Drs. Pauline Brightling and Christopher McCaughan in making these decisions is gratefully acknowledged.

1994
Melbourne

HOW TO USE THIS BOOK

The book serves two functions:

♦ Firstly, it is a quick method of revision of individual diseases text for undergraduates. Consult the index, all the diseases in the eighth edition of *Veterinary Medicine* are included, and proceed to the desired summary. Its title includes a page reference (VM8 p. ...) to the identical item in *Veterinary Medicine*.

♦ Secondly it is a simplified manual to assist in the diagnosis of clinical cases. These may be hypothetical cases created for revision purposes, or actual cases. For greater accuracy and a wider listing of diseases in the list of diagnostic possibilities use a computerized diagnostic program, e.g. BOVID, CONSULTANT.

Proceed as follows: identify the most important (critical) sign; the sign on which you want to base your diagnosis. Locate it in Chapter 1. The sign listing will refer you to a page in the General Medicine section where the diseases in which the critical sign occurs frequently will be listed. Then consult the descriptions of these diseases via the index, and select the one that best fits the complete clinical syndrome in the case. These descriptions include cause, epidemiology, clinical signs, the clinical pathology examinations recommended, and the necropsy lesions to be expected, the recommended treatment and control measures.

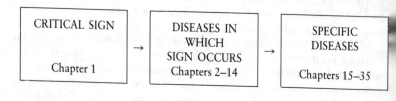

| CRITICAL SIGN

Chapter 1 | → | DISEASES IN
WHICH
SIGN OCCURS
Chapters 2–14 | → | SPECIFIC
DISEASES

Chapters 15–35 |

Cross-references

♦ References to pages in this book are in simple form.
♦ References to pages in the eighth edition of *Veterinary Medicine* are in the form [VM8 p. ...].

NOTE TO THE READER

The editor and publisher of this book have made every effort to ensure that drug dosages quoted are accurate. Readers are, however, advised always to check the product information included with the package of each drug to ensure that additional, valuable information is not neglected.

In the lists of diseases quoted in this book under the heading of Diagnosis it has not been possible, because of the limitations of space, to include all those diseases with which the disease under discussion might be confused. A computer-assisted diagnostic program should be consulted for complete listings.

PART ONE

GENERAL MEDICINE

1

CLINICAL EXAMINATION AND MAKING A DIAGNOSIS

A complete clinical examination, including all the known **indicants** (epidemiological characteristics, clinical signs, clinical pathology and necropsy findings) would be an impractical task in most clinical investigations, because of the time required. In practice, a satisfactory clinical examination includes only those indicants that appear relevant to the particular examination as it proceeds towards the making of a diagnosis.

MAKING A DIAGNOSIS

The standard method of examination of a 'sick' animal, that is when immediate recognition of the diagnosis, for example of a bleeding wound or fractured bone, is not available, is:

1. The **initial cue.** From the client's recounting of the problem the veterinarian selects the critical abnormality.
2. A **plausible hypothesis** is generated by the veterinarian to comply with the observed abnormality. Usually three or four of these are selected, making up a **list of diagnostic possibilities.**
3. **Testing the hypotheses** arranges the diagnostic possibilities in order of probability by:
   (a) asking more critical questions
   (b) conducting laboratory tests, includ-

ing necropsy examinations, radiology, ultrasound, ECG, EMG
   (c) experimentally producing the abnormality
   (d) conducting therapeutic or prophylactic response trials.

In many field investigations in large animal medicine a definitive diagnosis from amongst the diagnostic possibilities is impossible in the time available, or because of the financial or other limitations on the techniques that can be used. As a result it is often necessary to proceed with a short list of diagnoses and to put treatment and preventive programs in place to deal with all of them. The control program then becomes part of the diagnostic process.

CLINICAL EXAMINATION OF THE INDIVIDUAL ANIMAL

STEP 1 LOOKING FOR THE PRINCIPAL SYSTEM INVOLVED AND DEFINING THE ABNORMALITY

Start with taking the disease history, then do a visual check of the patient and an examination of the **vital signs.** You will then:

♦ have an approximate idea of what is the important abnormality (the **initial clue**);

3

- have an idea of the **principal system(s)** involved;
- have a beginning list of **diagnostic possibilities**;
- be in a position to know where to concentrate your **localizing the lesion examination**, the examination aimed at identifying the location and nature of the lesion and its nature, possibly its cause.

The page numbers (p. ...) are cross-references to later entries in this book which describe the sign and refer you to diseases in which the sign is a significant occurrence.

HISTORY-TAKING

Patient data
- Sex
- Age
- Breed

(All important because the disease may be sex-, age-, or breed-related.)
- Parturition status
- Lactation status

(Both may indicate a relationship of the disease to metabolism (p. 510), nutrition (p. 527) or stress (p. 20).)
- Pastured or housed/yarded

(Besides nutritional, metabolic and stress implications there is the additional factor of exposure to poisonous plants (p. 588).)

Present disease history
- Chronology, severity, duration and relative importance of the signs observed by the client

(These assist in establishing the clinical profile of the disease, with the critical signs highlighted.)

VISUAL PATIENT CHECK

Behavior
- Aggressive actions (p. 188)
- Blindness, demeanor indicates (p. 188)
- Chewing movements, continuous (p. 189)
- Coma (see hyporesponsive)
- Compulsive rolling (p. 189)
- Deafness, demeanor indicates (p. 190)
- Exercise tolerance reduced (pp. 131, 155)
- Frenzy (p. 191)
- Head-shaking (p. 192)
- Hyperresponsive to external stimuli (= excitement) (pp. 117, 193)
- Hyporesponsive to external stimuli (= depression, lassitude, somnolence, coma) (pp. 117, 193)
- Imbecility (p. 193)

- Kicking at belly, getting up and lying down, rolling (pp. 59, 60)
- Lassitude (see hyporesponsive)
- Licking, chewing, rubbing of objects or self (p. 189)
- Mania (p. 194)
- Narcolepsy/catalepsy (p. 194)
- Nibbling reaction (p. 194)
- Pawing, flank-watching, repeated rolling (p. 60)
- Restless (pp. 60, 191)
- Somnolence (see hyporesponsive)
- Stretching, sham urination (p. 60)
- Syncope (fainting) (p. 198)

Voice
- Constant bellowing (p. 188)
- Dumbness (voice absent), demeanor indicates (pp. 190, 199)

Breathing
- Coughing, sneezing (p. 154)
- Hyperpnea (p. 154)
- Dyspnea (p. 154)
- Grunting (p. 159)
- Respiratory noise, nasal (p. 159)
- Respiratory noise, laryngopharyngeal (p. 158)
- Abdominal (p. 154)

Eating (mastication, swallowing)
- Food dropped while eating (quidding) (p. 196)
- Cud-dropping (p. 96)
- Eructation missing (p. 96)
- Rumination missing (p. 99)
- Mastication painful (p. 60)
- Mastication slow (p. 60)
- Swallowing difficult (dysphagia) (pp. 63, 190)
- Regurgitation (p. 63)
- Food coughed up (p. 63)
- Vomiting (p. 65)

Defecation
- Frequency increased (p. 57)
- Frequency decreased (p. 57)
- Straining (tenesmus) (p. 64)
- Straining, no feces passed (p. 198)
- Straining with open anus (p. 198)

Urination
- Dribble or small amounts (p. 177)
- Ceased (anuria) (p. 176)
- Dysuria (straining to urinate) (p. 177)

Posture
- Head extended (p. 135)
- Head tilted, deviated, rotated (p. 192)

- Opisthotonus, (head dorsiflexed) (p. 195)
- Orthotonus (head held forward) (p. 195)
- Back arched (p. 215)
- Back down-arched (p. 157)
- Elbows abducted (pp. 155, 217)
- Stance rigid (pp. 197, 220)
- Standing preferred (p. 220)
- Rising difficult (p. 147)
- Recumbency (lying down most of time) (pp. 197, 220)
- Crossed limbs (pp. 190, 219)
- Limb rested (p. 219)
- Limb weight shifted (p. 219)
- Limbs splayed (p. 219)
- Scapula protrudes above top-line (p. 220)
- Shoulder displaced laterally
- Fetlock(s) knuckling (p. 191)

Gait
- Stiff (p. 198)
- Stumbling (p. 198)
- Cerebellar ataxia (p. 189)
- Sensorimotor ataxia (p. 197)
- Sensory ataxia (p. 197)
- Dysmetria (p. 190)
- Hypermetria (p. 193)
- Incoordinated/exaggerated (p. 193)
- Jerky limb action (p. 219)
- Drifting sideways gait (p. 190)
- Leaning gait (p. 194)
- Falls to one side (p. 191)
- Falls easily (p. 191)
- Weak limb syndrome (p. 199)
- Hoof dragged along ground (p. 192)
- Walks on hoof dorsum (p. 192)
- Sway test positive (p. 198)
- Lameness (p. 218)
- Lameness shifting (p. 219)

Progression
- Aimless wandering (pp. 188, 199)
- Compulsive walking (pp. 189, 192)
- Head-pressing (p. 192)
- Circling (p. 189)

Body weight
- Low (less than normal) (pp. 157, 216)
- Very low (emaciation) (p. 216)

Conformation
- Dwarfism (p. 216)
- Giantism (p. 216)
- Asymmetrical (p. 216)

Skin and hair coat
- Dehydrated (p. 57)
- Alopecia (p. 231)

- Hypotrichosis (p. 231)
- Skin missing (p. 230)

Vital signs

Temperature
- Fever (p. 17)
- Hyperthermia (p. 15)
- Hypothermia (p. 16)

Species	Normal °C	Critical °C
Horse	38.0	39.0
Cattle	38.5	39.5
Sheep	39.0	40.0
Goat	39.5	40.5
Pig	39.0	40.0

Respiration
- Rate (per minute)
- Hyperpnea (p. 154)
- Dyspnea (p. 154)

Species	Normal range
Horse	8–10
Cattle	10–30
Sheep	10–20
Goat	25–35
Pig	10–20

Heart
- Heart or pulse rate (per minute)
  - Tachycardia
  - Bradycardia
  - Rhythm irregular (p. 129)
  - Amplitude, small or wide (p. 132)

Species	Normal range
Horse	30–40
Colt <1 year	70–80
Cattle	60–80
Calf <3 months	100–120
Sheep and goats	70–90
Pig	60–100

Mucosae
- Pallor (p. 144)
- Capillary refill slow (p. 143)
- Cyanosis (p. 154)
- Hemorrhages (p. 143)
- Jaundice (p. 117)

Ruminal sounds (ruminants only)
- Absent (none in 2 minutes) or reduced (p. 98)
- Excessive/continuous (p. 98)

Large intestinal sounds (horses only)
- Absent (none in 2 minutes) or reduced (p. 59)
- Excessive/continuous (p. 59)

STEP 2   IDENTIFYING THE LOCATION AND NATURE OF LESION

This examination will be concentrated on the system(s) identified in the previous examination. You are looking for additional signs to confirm your suspicion about the system involved and, additionally, to locate the lesion within the system and its nature. The signs you might encounter in the standard physical examination are set out below on an anatomical (regional) basis, and in a pattern in which you are likely to conduct a physical examination. You are then directed to another section of the book where the specific diseases are listed in which the identified signs occur.

REGIONAL EXAMINATION

Head and neck

Eye

Eyelids
♦ Swollen (p. 231)
♦ Snapping shut during convulsion (p. 191)
♦ Closed (blepharospasm) (p. 231)
♦ Paralyzed (p. 191)
♦ Third eyelid prolapse (p. 198)
♦ Eye discharge (p. 231)
Conjunctiva
♦ Inflamed (p. 230)
♦ Mass (p. 230)
Cornea
♦ Opacity (p. 230)
♦ Vascularized (p. 230)
♦ Ulcerated (p. 230)
Sclera
♦ Pallor (p. 144)
♦ Jaundice (p. 117)
♦ Cyanosis (p. 154)
Eyeball
♦ Microphthalmia
♦ Absent (anophthalmia)
♦ Fused or cyclopian (p. 217)
♦ Protruding (exophthalmos) (p. 191)
♦ Nystagmus (p. 194)
♦ Deviation (strabismus, squint) (p. 190)
♦ Hypopyon (p. 231)
♦ Hyphaema (pp. 143, 193)
♦ Unpigmented iris
♦ Growths on iris
♦ Opaque lens
♦ Lens absent
♦ Pupil dilated, not reducible (p. 196)
♦ Pupil constricted (p. 196)
♦ Retinal degeneration
♦ Retinal tumor mass
♦ Retinal hemorrhage

♦ Pupillary light reflex absent (p. 197)
♦ Menace reflex absent (p. 194)
♦ Corneal reflex absent (p. 190)
♦ Palpebral reflex absent (p. 195)

Ear
♦ Swollen (p. 231)
♦ Drooping (paralyzed – not swollen) (p. 190)
♦ Exudate (p. 231)
♦ Gangrenous (p. 231)

Head
♦ Cranium domed (p. 216)
♦ Cranial meningocele (p. 220)
♦ Cyclopian defect (p. 217)
♦ Horn, mass at base (p. 231)
♦ Horn(s) absent (p. 231)
♦ Head-shaking (p. 192)
♦ Head-bobbing (p. 189)

Mouth/pharynx
♦ Mucosal erosions, vesicles, etc. (p. 60)
♦ Mucosa absent (p. 60)
♦ Gum swollen (p. 59)
♦ Foreign body (p. 59)
♦ Palate cleft (p. 66)
♦ Pharynx foreign body (p. 70)
♦ Saliva drooling, excessive (p. 63)

Tongue
♦ Shrunken or swollen (p. 65)
♦ Paralyzed (p. 198)
♦ Papillae small (p. 65)

Teeth
♦ Eruption retarded (p. 64)
♦ Malpositioned (p. 64)
♦ Enamel/dentine defective (p. 64)
♦ Discolored (brown, pink) (p. 64)
♦ Worn/lost prematurely (p. 64)

Jaw
♦ Jaw bones swollen
♦ Chewing movements (p. 189)
♦ Chewing/licking objects (p. 189)
♦ Jaw-champing (p. 193)
♦ Teeth-grinding (p. 99)
♦ Clenched shut (trismus) (p. 199)
♦ Jaw dropped (p. 193)
♦ Submandibular edema (p. 130)
♦ Salivary glands swollen (p. 163)

Lips, muzzle
- Cleft lip (hare lip) (p. 66)
- Lip paralysis (p. 191)
- Muzzle dry
- Muzzle erosion, scabs, sloughs (pp. 60, 66)
- Muzzle skin missing (p. 60)

Nasal cavities, nostrils
- Nostril dilation (p. 158)
- Mucosal congestion (p. 158)
- Mucosal erosions, ulcers, etc. (p. 158)
- Polyp, nodule (p. 158)
- Discharge (froth, food, pus) (p. 155)
- Epistaxis (p. 155)
- Foreign body in passage (p. 155)
- Nasal breath volume decreased (p. 155)
- Foul-smelling breath (p. 155)

Neck
- Rigid (p. 194)
- Flaccid paralysis (p. 195)
- Deformed (p. 220)
- Throat swollen (p. 221)
- Throat painful (p. 221)
- Thyroid enlarged
- Jugular inlet abnormality (p. 132)
- Jugular vein distended (p. 132)
- Jugular pulse excessive (p. 132)
- Brisket swollen (p. 130)

Abdomen

External appearance
- Distended (pp. 56, 94, 197)
- Distended (asymmetric) (pp. 56, 94)
- Gaunt (shrunken) (p. 56)
- Asymmetrical distension (p. 56)

Abdomen though body wall
- Intestine sounds exaggerated (p. 59)
- Intestine sounds diminished, absent (p. 59)
- Splashing on ballottement right side (p. 99)
- Splashing on ballottement left side (p. 99)
- Ping on percussion, right side (p. 97)
- Ping on percussion, left side (p. 97)
- Pain elicited on percussion (pp. 60, 97)
- Mass palpable (pp. 56, 97)
- Viscus, firm/distended palpable (p. 99)
- Liver enlarged (pp. 60, 118)
- Liver painful (pp. 60, 97, 118)

Paracentesis abdominis fluid
- Contains blood (p. 61)
- Cloudy (p. 61)

Rumen (ruminants only)
- Rumen distended (p. 98)
- Rumen empty/collapsed (p. 98)
- Rumen small (p. 98)
- Rumen doughy/firm (impacted) (p. 98)
- Tympanitic (p. 98)
- Splashing on percussion over rumen (p. 99)
- Rumen movements but sounds muffled (p. 98)
- Rumen movements and sounds absent (p. 98)
- Rumen movements absent, sounds tinkle (p. 98)
- Rumen movements, both sounds absent (p. 98)
- Rumen movements, sounds increased (p. 98)

Rectum, anus
- Anus absent (p. 57)
- Anus constricted (p. 57)
- Anus dilated (paralyzed) (pp. 57, 188)
- Anal reflex absent (p. 188)
- Rectal prolapse (p. 89)
- Rectum constricted (p. 61)
- Rectal obstruction (p. 61)
- Rectum wall thickened (p. 63)
- Rectum impacted with feces

Abdomen per rectum
- Adhesions in (pp. 56, 94)
- Mass in (p. 56)
- Displaced viscus (p. 99)
- Distended intestine (loops) (pp. 59, 96)
- Distended abomasum (p. 94)
- Distended rumen (p. 98)
- Impacted abomasum (p. 94)
- Impacted intestine (p. 59)
- Impacted rumen (p. 98)
- Tight mesenteric band (p. 56)
- Enlarged, displaced spleen (horse) (p. 81)

Feces
- Absent (p. 58)
- Scanty (volume decreased) (p. 58)
- Profuse (volume increased) (p. 58)
- Watery (pp. 58, 96)
- Pasty (p. 96)
- Diarrhea (p. 58)
- Dry, hard (p. 58)
- Constipation (p. 58)
- Abnormal color (black, yellow, white) (pp. 58, 117)
- Contain fresh blood (hematochezia) (pp. 58, 96)
- Contain digested blood (melena) (p. 58)
- Contain mucus/fibrin (pp. 58, 96)
- Contain undigested seeds, grain, pips (p. 58)
- Foul odor (pp. 58, 96)

Stomach tube passage

- Obstructed (p. 63)
- Fluid reflux (p. 63)

Rumen contents abnormal

- Frothy (p. 97)
- Fetid (p. 97)

Thorax

Respiratory system

- Double respiratory movement (p. 158)
- Pain on percussion (p. 159)
- Loud tracheal sounds (p. 156)
- Lung breath sounds absent (p. 156)
- Lung breath sounds crackling (p. 156)
- Lung breath sounds loud (p. 156)
- Lung breath sounds wheezing (p. 156)
- Peristaltic sounds (p. 156)
- Pleural friction or fluid sounds (p. 156)

Paracentesis thoracis fluid

- Blood stained (p. 159)
- Cloudy (p. 159)

Cardiovascular system

- Apex beat enlarged or displaced (p. 129)
- Bleeding tendency (p. 117)
- Cardiac thrill (p. 130)
- Heart murmurs (p. 131)
- Heart sounds irregular (p. 129)
- Heart sounds loud (p. 131)
- Heart sounds muffled (p. 131)
- Pericardial friction or fluid sound (p. 132)

Urinary system

- Bladder distended or painful (p. 176)
- Bladder wall thickened (p. 176)
- Kidney enlarged, painful (p. 178)
- Urine discolored (p. 177)
- Urine cloudy (p. 179)

Nervous system

Paralysis/paresis

- Flaccid, generalized (p. 195)
- Tetanic (spastic) (p. 198)
- Thoracic and pelvic limbs (p. 195)
- Pelvic limbs only (p. 195)
- Single limb only
- Tail paralysis (p. 198)
- Larynx paralysis (p. 193)
- Slap test positive (p. 197)
- Pharynx paralysis (p. 196)
- Horner's syndrome (p. 192)
- Facial nerve paralysis (p. 191)

- Jaw paralysis (p. 193)
- Trismus (p. 199)
- Muscle atrophy, neurogenic (p. 194)
- Anus reflex absent (p. 188)
- Paresis, spastic intermittent (p. 197)
- Proprioceptive defect (p. 196)

Limb reflexes

- Patellar reflex absent (p. 196)
- Withdrawal reflex absent (p. 199)

Involuntary movement

- Tremor, intention (p. 199)
- Tremor (pp. 198, 199)
- Convulsions (p. 190)
- Myoclonus (p. 194)
- Jaw-champing (p. 193...)

Musculoskeletal system

Limbs

- Contracture, rigidity (p. 219)
- Deformity (p. 216)

Limb joints, bursae, tendon sheaths

- Joints hot and/or painful (p. 218)
- Joint pain (p. 218)
- Joint enlarged (p. 218)
- Joint fixation (rigid) (p. 218)
- Joint hypermobility (p. 218)
- Joint creaking/crepitus (p. 218)
- Bursa inflamed (p. 216)
- Tendon sheath inflamed (p. 221)

Limb bones

- Pain in (p. 216)
- Deformity, absence (p. 216)
- Soft (p. 216)
- Easily fractured (p. 217)
- Discharging sinus (p. 216)

Hooves

- Pain in (p. 217)
- Deformity (p. 217)
- Interdigital skin lesion (p. 218)
- Coronet vesicles, erosions, scabs (p. 216)
- Coronet skin missing (p. 216)
- Hoof sloughing (p. 217)
- Sole under-run, ulcer, thin, puncture (p. 218)

Muscle masses

- Pain in (p. 219)
- Small (atrophied) (p. 219)
- Large (hypertrophied) (p. 219)
- Asymmetric (p. 219)

- Enlarged, swollen, hard, painful (p. 219)
- Rigidity, contracture (p. 219)

Skull
- Cranium domed (p. 216)
- Meningocele (p. 219)
- Probatocephaly (p. 220)
- Craniofacial deformity (p. 220)
- Jaw deformity (p. 89)
- Cleft palate (p. 66)
- Hare lip (p. 66)

Trunk
- Spinal column rigid (p. 220)
- Spinal column deformed (p. 220)
- Back pain elicited (p. 215)
- Brisket swollen (p. 216)
- Ventral abdominal wall fluid swelling (p. 215)
- Ventral abdominal wall sunken (uni- or bilateral) (p. 215)
- Umbilical area swollen (p. 221)
- Umbilicus drips pus or urine (p. 186)
- Inguinal area swollen (p. 218)
- Perineum swollen (p. 220)

Pelvis
- Sacroiliac mobile, crepitus (p. 220)
- Bones deformed (p. 216)

Tail
- Absent, deformed (p. 220)
- Held in air (p. 220)
- Stiff, rigid (p. 220)
- Paralyzed, anaesthetized (p. 220)
- Tail head elevated, hair loss (p. 220)
- Tip cellulitis (p. 220)
- Tip alopecia (p. 220)

Lymph nodes and vessels
- Nodes enlarged generally (p. 143)
- Nodes enlarged locally (p. 143)
- Vessels thickened (p. 143)

Skin and hair coat

Hair coat
- Hair absent, partial or complete (p. 231)
- Hair coat sparse (p. 231)
- Hypopigmented (p. 231)
- Fibers broken off (p. 231)
- Curly (p. 231)
- Singed (p. 231)

Skin
- Anesthesia (p. 188)
- Hyperesthesia (p. 192)
- Paresthesia (p. 196)
- Pruritus (p. 234)
- Panniculus reflex (p. 196)
- Perineal reflex (p. 196)
- Anal reflex (p. 188)
- Thick, wrinkled (p. 234)
- Scaly (dandruff) (p. 234)
- Sebaceous exudate (p. 231)
- Hyperelastic, fragile (p. 231)
- Tents easily (p. 234)
- Hypopigmented (pp. 230, 234)
- Sweating excessively (hyperhidrosis) (p. 234)
- Sweating deficient (anhidrosis) (pp. 230, 234)
- Discrete lesions (crusts, epithelial masses, excoriations, fissures, gangrene, necrosis, nodules, plaques, pustules, scabs, sinuses, suppuration, ulcers, vesicles, wheals) (p. 231)
- Absent (p. 230)
- Lesions only white areas back and sides (pp. 118, 234)

Subcutaneous tissues

- Edema extensive (anasarca) (pp. 117, 130, 234)
- Inflammatory edema (p. 234)
- Emphysema (p. 234)
- Hemorrhage (p. 234)
- Suppuration (phlegmon) (p. 231)
- Nodules, masses (p. 231)
- Cords connecting nodes (p. 230)

Horns

- Absent (p. 231)
- Mass at base (p. 231)

Female reproductive tract

Ovary
- Small, inactive
- Cystic
- Gross enlargement

Uterus
- Prolapsed
- Ruptured
- Distended
- Contents abnormal
- Deformed
- Mass in wall

Vagina
- Deformed
- Discharge
- Mucosal erosion, pustules, vesicles, granular lesion, necrosis, mass

♦ Torsion of
♦ Prolapse

Vulva
♦ Swollen
♦ Discharge
♦ Mucosal erosions, pustules, vesicles, necrosis, mass

Placenta
♦ Retained
♦ Discrete lesions

Miscellaneous female infertility
♦ Estrus abnormal
♦ Conception failure
♦ Abortion
♦ Birth premature
♦ Gestation prolonged
♦ Stillbirth
♦ Dystokia

Male genital tract

Testicle
♦ Retained (cryptorchid)
♦ Inflamed (orchitis)

Penis
♦ Epithelial mass
♦ Erosions, pustules
♦ Swelling
♦ Deviation
♦ Paralysis

Prepuce
♦ Discharge
♦ Erosions, pustules
♦ Enlargement

♦ Distension
♦ Prolapse

Miscellaneous male infertility
♦ Libido loss
♦ Sperm numbers low
♦ Impregnation failure

Mammary glands

Udder
♦ Small (p. 251)
♦ Enlarged (p. 250)
♦ Edematous (p. 250)
♦ Hard, may or may not be painful (p. 251)
♦ Flaccid (p. 250)
♦ Gangrene (p. 250)
♦ Hard masses in (p. 251)
♦ Drops away from abdominal wall (p. 250)

Teats
♦ Swollen, painful (p. 250)
♦ Edematous (p. 250)
♦ Sphincter blocked (p. 250)
♦ Slack, udder full (p. 250)
♦ Sore at tip (p. 250)
♦ Discrete skin lesions (p. 250)
♦ Skin reddened laterally (p. 250)

Milk
♦ Yield nil (p. 250)
♦ Yield drops suddenly (p. 250)
♦ Pink, brown or contains blood clots (p. 249)
♦ Orange, thick (p. 249)
♦ Watery (p. 249)
♦ Watery with flakes (p. 249)
♦ Clotted (p. 249)
♦ Purulent (p. 249)

STEP 3   ESTABLISHING THE SPECIFIC CAUSE

Having, it is to be hoped, developed some idea of the nature of the cause, elicit further relevant historical information about feeding, breeding and general management, if necessary conduct a search of the environment looking for a poisonous plant, an abrasive floor in a barn, a lack of ventilation, and so on, and/or collect specimens of feed, soil, water, and clinical pathological or necropsy specimens to identify the presence of a toxin, a nutritional deficiency, an inherited enzymic defect.

Disease history

♦ Number affected
♦ Course:
  • Congenital
  • Sudden death ≤1 hour
  • Chronic ≥2 weeks

♦ Exercise-enhanced
♦ Cohabits with other species
♦ Morbidity, case fatality, culling rates
♦ Prior treatment, prophylactic and control measures
♦ Introductions to group
♦ Previous disease

Nutritional history

♦ Mostly milk replacer
♦ Excess fiber
♦ Inadequate fiber
♦ Excess carbohydrate
♦ Inadequate carbohydrate
♦ Inadequate protein
♦ Excess protein
♦ Inadequate minerals (p. 527)
♦ Excess minerals (p. 571)
♦ Inadequate vitamins (p. 548)
♦ Excess vitamins
♦ Inadequate water (p. 32)
♦ Excess water (p. 147)
♦ Access to poisonous plants (p. 588)

Production history

♦ Milk yield reduced (p. 33)
♦ Growth rate slowed, weight lost (p. 33)
♦ Wool yield reduced (p. 33)
♦ Racing performance poor (p. 34)

Climate history

♦ Wet-weather-related diseases (p. 555)
♦ Cold-related diseases (p. 16)
♦ Heat-related disease (p. 15)

General management history

♦ Breeding management related to reproductive efficiency and to inherited defects (p. 627)

♦ Husbandry competence and stress-related disease (p. . . . .)

Examination of the environment

Outdoor environment
♦ Topography, soil type
♦ Stocking rate (population density)
♦ Pasture, supplementary feeding
♦ Water supply
♦ Waste disposal

Indoor environment
♦ Sanitation, hygiene
♦ Ventilation
♦ Floor space per animal
♦ Floor quality
♦ Bedding
♦ Floor plan

Clinical pathology

Consult the specific recommendations under the heading of 'Clinical Pathology' in each disease. The most benefit that these examinations can provide is to establish the class of the cause, i.e. whether it is an infectious disease, a nutritional deficiency, a poisoning, an inherited defect and so on, and to narrow the list of diagnostic possibilities. It is often sufficient to make a strongly favored provisional diagnosis. Finalizing the definitive diagnosis in production and racing animals is the province of:
♦ Exploratory surgery
♦ Chemical analysis of feed materials or body tissues
♦ Necropsy examination
each of which is also detailed under relevant headings in the descriptions of individual diseases.

EXAMINATION OF THE HERD

When the problem to be examined relates to a herd or flock of animals some additional aspects need to be included in the examination. The basic clinical examination of some individual animals is still the critical feature, but supplementary considerations need to be addressed as follows.

Step 1: define the abnormality as a clinical syndrome or as a production fault including volume, composition or quality of production, including failure to reach targets or standards in each area.

Step 2: define the pattern of occurrence in terms of age group, lactation status, genetic group, geographical location, nutrition, physical exercise severity and location, pattern of occurrence in time, prophylactic or therapeutic medication regimen. This may require the examination of a number of animals to establish the morbidity rate, and examinations at intervals to measure the change in it.

Step 3: identify the specific cause by laboratory analysis, experimental production or treatment response. An initial step of identifying a group of pathogens, e.g. intestinal parasites, without identifying the specific helminth, may be adequate for the occasion.

The prior existence of complete records provides an excellent basis for making a herd diagnosis. A complete herd or flock health program should utilize its data to constantly monitor production and disease parameters. It is of particular value when the problem is a self-limiting one, e.g. the development of a herd immunity.

2

GENERAL SYSTEMIC STATES

Systemic states affect the body as a whole and, between them, contribute to the effects of most diseases.

TOXEMIA [VM8 p. 38]

Toxemia is a systemic state following injury to body cells, and activation of body defense mechanisms, caused by toxins deriving from infectious agents and damaged tissues.

Etiology

Antigenic toxins
From infectious agents, especially bacteria, they include:
♦ **Exotoxins** released into surrounding tissues by living bacteria, e.g. botulinus, tetanus toxins.
♦ **Endotoxins** are lipopolysaccharides released mostly when cell walls of gram-negative bacteria break down. **Endotoxemia** results from bodily invasion by these bacteria in coliform septicemia, or from increased absorption of toxic amines produced in the gut by the bacteria, and normally excreted in the feces, when the toxins regurgitate into the small intestine in bowel obstruction, or when gut wall is ischemic or otherwise damaged, or fecal material enters the peritoneal cavity.
♦ **Enterotoxins** produced by enterotoxigenic *Escherichia coli* and cause hypersecretory diarrhea in neonates

Metabolic toxins
♦ Toxic products, including urea, from normal body metabolic processes accumulate when excretory processes in liver or feces, or detoxification in plasma or liver, are disrupted
♦ Abnormal metabolism, e.g. in ketosis,

rumen overload, produces excessive toxic ketone bodies and lactic acid

Clinical findings

General signs are as follows. Space-occupying signs occur in local infections (p. 19)

Acute – toxic or septic shock
♦ Short course, up to several days
♦ Mucosal pallor or congestion, prolonged capillary refill, hemorrhages in some
♦ Hypothermia (hyperthermia initially), cool extremities
♦ Tachycardia, small-amplitude pulse, low blood pressure
♦ Diarrhea usually
♦ Oliguria
♦ Hemorrhagic tendency
♦ Muscle weakness, recumbency
♦ Depression, anorexia

Subacute – chronic toxemia
♦ Moderate to long course, weeks to months
♦ Depression, lethargy, separation from group, inappetence
♦ Weight loss, failure to grow or produce, emaciation
♦ Constipation
♦ Tachycardia, small amplitude pulse, reduced intensity heart sounds
♦ Low grade fever, hypothermia terminally
♦ Terminal recumbency, coma or convulsions

Clinical pathology

♦ Hypoglycemia
♦ Elevated blood non-protein nitrogen level
♦ Elevated total serum protein, especially globulin level
♦ Aplastic anemia
♦ Albuminuria
♦ Hemoconcentration in acute endotoxemia
♦ Leukopenia in acute endotoxemia. Leukocytosis may occur in chronic endotoxemia

Necropsy findings

♦ Initiating lesion, e.g. coliform mastitis, intestinal obstruction, coliform septicemia
♦ Parenchymal degeneration liver, kidney, myocardium, adrenals

Diagnosis

Endotoxemia is a common secondary diagnosis in other primary diseases, e.g. thromboembolic colic in horses. **Idiopathic toxemia** is a primary diagnosis in cases presenting the indefinite syndrome described above and lacking specific signs suggesting involvement of specific organs, e.g. chronic peritonitis, chronic suppurative metritis.

Treatment

♦ Elimination of primary cause if possible
♦ Non-specific broad-spectrum antimicrobial cover
♦ High dose rates of fluids and electrolytes (p. 22), usually including glucose, in endotoxic shock
♦ Anti-inflammatory agents, including corticosteroids and non-steroidal substances, are standard therapy in cases of endotoxic shock

PUERPERAL TOXEMIA
(PARTURITION SYNDROME) [VM8 p. 44]

A serious and common problem in the recently calved cow.

Etiology

Usually a combination of two or more of the following diseases:
♦ Acetonemia (p. 519)
♦ Abomasal displacement, left (p. 109) or right (p. 110)
♦ Fat cow syndrome/pregnancy toxemia (p. 521)

♦ Mastitis, peracute or acute (p. 252)
♦ Septic metritis (p. 44)
♦ Peritonitis, especially acute diffuse form (p. 91)
♦ Non-paretic, parturient hypocalcemia (p. 510)
♦ Simple indigestion (p. 99) in cows switched to high-energy diets at parturition

Clinical findings

♦ Anorexia
♦ Milk yield seriously reduced
♦ Ruminal movements infrequent
♦ Defecation infrequent
♦ Temperature high normal range
♦ Depressed, lethargic

BOVINE POSTPARTUM SEPTIC
METRITIS [VM8 p. 44]

Etiology

♦ Uterine involution incomplete
♦ Infection of uterine contents by mixed infection, e.g.
  Actinomyces (Corynebacterium) pyogenes
  Escherichia coli
  Staphylococcus spp.
  Streptococcus spp.
  Pseudomonas aerogenes
  Proteus spp.
  Clostridium spp. occasionally

Epidemiology

♦ In first week (usually 2–4 days) after calving
♦ Placenta retention and attempted manual removal of placenta also common precursors. Retention prevalence high in dystocia, abortion, multiple births
♦ All ages susceptible; commonest in mature dairy cows
Other possible risk factors include:
♦ Old age
♦ Long gestation length
♦ Hormone-induced parturition
♦ Fetal anasarca
♦ Uterine prolapse
♦ Fetotomy
♦ Prior placentitis
♦ Vitamin E and selenium nutritional deficiency
♦ Vitamin A nutritional deficiency

Importance is due to serious loss of milk yield in all cases, cessation of lactation in some cows, death in a few. Unexplained high prevalence in some herds at some times.

Clinical findings

♦ Complete anorexia
♦ Milk yield seriously reduced
♦ Mild fever, 39.5 to 41°C
♦ Heart rate elevated 90–120/min
♦ Respiratory rate elevated to 60–70/min
♦ Ruminal movements depressed or absent
♦ Foul-smelling diarrhea common
♦ Dehydration
♦ Placenta retained in many cases, often not visible externally
♦ Profuse, dark brown to red, foul-smelling exudate, containing shreds of necrotic placenta discharging from vulva in many; may not be detectable without manual examination
♦ If uterus palpable through cervix, placenta adhered to caruncles and may be difficult to detach
♦ Distended, flaccid uterus palpable per rectum, especially in cases where placenta retained but cervix closed
♦ Tenesmus, especially after manual examination per vagina
♦ Course 10–14 days until all necrotic placenta discharged. May be followed by thick purulent vulvar discharge for weeks

Clinical pathology

♦ Leukon shows leukopenia, neutropenia, degenerative left shift
♦ Secondary ketosis, especially fat cows
♦ Irreversible liver damage, indicated by elevated blood levels of liver enzymes, especially in overweight cows
♦ Mixed bacterial infection on culture of uterine exudate

Necropsy findings

♦ Uterus distended, flaccid, contains several liters dark brown, foul-smelling, turbid liquid containing shreds of placenta
♦ Uterine mucosa necrotic, hemorrhagic. Uterine wall thick, edematous
♦ Serosal surface of uterus may carry shreds of fibrin
♦ Enlarged, fatty liver commonly
♦ Mild degeneration of myocardium and renal parenchyma

Diagnosis

Differentiation from other diseases contributing to parturition syndrome (see above) may be difficult. Deciding which is the precipitating disease when several are present often means that a combined diagnosis is necessary, and several diseases may need to be treated at the one time.

Treatment

♦ Parenteral antibiotic or other antibacterial drug at full therapeutic doses daily for several days until signs relieved
♦ Parenteral fluids and electrolytes in large doses required by severely toxic cases
♦ Intrauterine antibacterial medication plus manual removal of placenta and fluid, possibly aided by uterine siphon, commonly practised, but benefit debated. Forceful removal of placenta universally forbidden
♦ Medication with oxytocin, ergonovine, estrogens or prostaglandins to restore uterine tone and promote uterine involution also used but advantage unlikely
♦ Treatment should be effective in 10–12 days; good response is recovery in 5–7 days. Treated cows should be checked at 5–6 weeks for signs of pyometra or chronic endometritis, and for suitability for commencement of a breeding program

ABNORMALITIES OF BODY TEMPERATURE

HYPERTHERMIA [VM8 p. 48]

Elevation of body temperature induced by physical causes of excessive heat production, or absorption, or inadequate loss. Moderate level referred to as heat stress; severe hyperthermia referred to as heat stroke.

Etiology

♦ High environmental temperature usually associated with
♦ High humidity
♦ Especially in animals treated with ataractic drugs
♦ Dehydration
♦ Severe muscular exertion

♦ Malignant hyperthermia in pigs
♦ Poisons including iodine, levamisole, dinitrophenols, and the mycotoxins citrinin, ergotamine, tunicamycin in Claviceps purpurea and Acremonium coenophialum, the causes of epidemic hyperthermia
♦ Cattle with bovine hereditary syndactyly
♦ Neurogenic hyperthermia due to lesions in hypothalamus

Epidemiology

Exposure to high environmental temperature and humidity, especially in some circumstances:

♦ Animals acclimatized to cool climate suddenly moved to hot climate
♦ Unaccustomed exertion, e.g. endurance rides, bulls fighting
♦ Close confinement with inadequate ventilation, e.g. ship or rail transport

Importance
Epidemic hyperthermia in cattle herds grazing fungus-infested pasture can cause major losses of milk production in large numbers of cattle. Malignant hyperthermia can cause heavy mortality in transported pigs of the right genetic makeup. Losses of sheep during ship transport bedevil international trade in live sheep destined for meat markets.

Clinical findings

♦ Temperature elevation: >42°C (107°F) up to 43.5°C (110°F)
♦ Heart rate increased, pulse large amplitude initially, very weak and fast terminally
♦ Dyspnea: respirations terminally shallow and irregular
♦ Increased sweating and salivation initially; sweating ceases terminally
♦ Restless initially, subsequently dull, with stumbling gait, tendency to lie down, seeking of shade and water, immersion, splashing. Terminally collapse, recumbency, convulsions, coma and death

With prolonged, clinically tolerable hyperthermia, abortion, embryonic mortality, anestrus, infertility and reduced litter size in sows are recorded. Experimental hyperthermia can cause congenital defects in exposed fetuses.

Clinical pathology

No significant changes reported.

Necropsy findings

Poorly defined changes of vasodilation, rapid rigor mortis, putrefaction.

Diagnosis

Environmental data and environment search important in detection of cause. Body temperature in serious cases exceed those usually encountered (41°C–106°F) in septicemia or toxemia. Mucosal petechiae and positive blood culture suggest septicemia or bacteremia.

Treatment

♦ Cold applications by hosing or spraying and brisk wind draft, immersion, cold water enemas, ice packs
♦ If animal activity is contributing to heat stress a tranquilizer will reduce severity of hyperthermia, but care needed because of complicating hypotension and heat gain
♦ Provide plenty of drinking water, forced ventilation, reduce overcrowding
♦ Parenteral fluids containing glucose during convalescence

HYPOTHERMIA (Cold stress) [VM8 p. 49]

Etiology

♦ Exposure to cold air temperatures without adequate compensatory heat production or retention in the body to maintain homeothermy is the principal cause, most commonly in neonates. In lambs and, to a lesser extent piglets, hypothermic deaths can occur in outbreaks because of the circumstances in which they are husbanded
♦ Sporadic cases occur where there is inadequate muscle tone response, e.g. in hypocalcemic states, during anesthesia, sedation, shock, dehydration as in the 'cold cow syndrome', and in the terminal stages of many diseases
♦ Induced hypothermia has some significance in human surgery as an alternative to conventional anesthesia. Normal thermostatic mechanisms have to be overpowered by anesthesia before temperature depression is achieved

Epidemiology

Occurs principally in cold environmental temperatures especially when:

♦ Heat loss exacerbated by rain, strong wind, lack of shelter from wind (windbreaks)
♦ Reduced heat absorption in cloudy weather compared with high exposure to sun
♦ Animals lose their insulating cover, e.g. recently shorn sheep subject to post-shearing mortality, thin animals lacking fat cover
♦ Animals acclimatized to hot weather moved to cold environment
♦ Neonates, especially piglets; lambs to a lesser extent, because of weakness due to birth injury or hypoxia, to poor mothering because of dam characteristics including age and breed, or multiple births, from small birth weight, or from environmental circumstances, including poor feed supplies for dams, lack of protection from weather

Clinical findings

♦ Hypothermia: temperature <37°C
♦ Weakness, staggering gait, recumbency, loss of sucking drive, strong inclination to huddle
♦ Depression, lethargy, coma

Clinical pathology

Reduced blood sugar and insulin levels are standard findings.

Necropsy findings

There are no specific necropsy lesions of hypothermia. Hypothermic neonates, exposed also to starvation, have negligible perirenal adipose deposits and empty alimentary tracts, often extensive subcutaneous hemorrhages if there has been birth injury, and edema of the distal parts of limbs.

Diagnosis

The history of the case, examination of the environment, and negative clinical and necropsy findings identify the disease. Apportioning blame to low environmental temperature, management procedures or inadequate nutrition, and terminal hypoglycemia is often difficult.

Treatment and prevention

♦ Most cases of hypothermia could be prevented if animals were housed in cold, wet weather. The economic demands of modern farming preclude this system of husbandry in many circumstances
♦ Neonatal hypothermia losses can be reduced by a control program that detects cases early by close surveillance, then resuscitation in an incubator. Many farmer-designed devices, made from common farm materials and warmed by an electrical fan-driven heater, are used successfully
♦ Cases in neonates selected for treatment on basis of low body temperature (37–39°C in lambs)
♦ Total immersion of lamb in warm (38°C) water for 30 minutes restores body temperature, but is labor-intensive and requires complete drying immediately afterwards
♦ Parenteral alimentation with warm glucose–saline solutions is not practicable when the number of animals affected is large. Feeding milk (50 ml/kg) by stomach tube is a practical solution
♦ Prior drying of wet coat enhances heat intake
♦ Twin and triplet lambs and calves need special attention because of low birth weight and inadequate mothering

FEVER (PYREXIA) [VM8 p. 51]

The systemic state combining hyperthermia and toxemia in the patient, caused by substances circulating in the blood.

Etiology

Septic fever caused by bacteria, viruses, protozoa or fungi as:
♦ Local infection in abscess, cellulitis, empyema
♦ Intermittent systemic infection, e.g. in bacteremia
♦ Consistently systemic, e.g. septicemia

Aseptic fever including:
♦ Chemical fever caused by intake of chemical substance, e.g. foreign protein injection, ingestion of dinitrophenol
♦ Surgical fever caused by damage to tissue
♦ Tissue necrosis after injection of necrotizing substance, intravascular hemolysis, infarction, neoplasm
♦ Immune reactions, e.g. anaphylaxis, angioedema

Clinical findings

♦ Dullness, depression, disinclination to move

♦ Moderate temperature elevation, up to 41°C (106°F), may be intermittent (peaks for 2–3 days between normal periods) or biphasic (2 peaks)
♦ Pulse rate increased, amplitude and strength diminished
♦ Hyperpnea
♦ Oliguria, often with albuminuria
♦ Thirst, anorexia, constipation
♦ Muscle weakness, recumbency
♦ Weight loss in long-standing cases
In most cases there are additional signs induced by the specific infection, e.g. peritonitis, pneumonia, mastitis, or a necrotic or neoplastic lesion.

Clinical pathology

There are no changes specific only to fever.

Necropsy findings

The lesions are those of toxemia plus those of hyperthermia.

Diagnosis

A diagnosis of 'fever of unknown origin' is made when there are no signs visible which indicate its origin.

Treatment

♦ Identify and treat primary disease; usually control of infection, possibly removal of necrotic material in aseptic fever
♦ Non-specific treatment with antiinflammatories or antipyretics provided the primary infection is under control
♦ Fever of any duration is commonly accompanied by dehydration, requiring treatment with fluids and electrolytes

SEPTICEMIA–BACTEREMIA, VIREMIA [VM8 p. 54]

The systemic state manifested by patients with large numbers of bacteria, viruses or protozoa in the bloodstream.

Etiology

The commoner septicemias include:
♦ **All species:** anthrax, leptospirosis, pasteurellosis, salmonellosis, Rift Valley fever
♦ **Cattle:** bovine virus diarrhea, bovine malignant catarrh
♦ **Sheep:** bluetongue
♦ **Pigs:** hog cholera, swine fever
♦ **Horses:** African horse sickness
Special causes of septicemia include immunosuppression (p. 37) with resulting septicemia caused by normally non-invasive organisms.
Bacteremia is the periodic, temporary presence of a few bacteria in the blood, usually originating from a permanently infected focus of inflammation, e.g. chronic metritis, arthritis, lung abscess. The cause is whatever infection is present in the chronic local lesion.

Clinical findings

Septicemia (bacteremia is symptomless)
♦ Sudden onset
♦ Dullness, depression, disinclination to move
♦ Moderate temperature elevation, up to 41°C (106°F), may be intermittent (peaks for 2–3 days between normal periods) or biphasic (2 peaks)
♦ Pulse rate increased, amplitude and strength diminished
♦ Hyperpnea
♦ Oliguria, often with albuminuria
♦ Thirst, anorexia, constipation, sometimes vomiting, diarrhea
♦ Muscle weakness, recumbency, weight loss
♦ In some cases mucosal hemorrhages, lymph node enlargement, splenomegaly. Hemorrhagic diathesis in some
♦ Signs referable to localization in joints, heart valves, meninges or eyes in cases surviving more than a few days

Clinical pathology

♦ Isolation of the causative agent by blood culture or animal inoculation
♦ Leukocytosis in bacterial infections, leukopenia in viral infections
♦ Presence of fibrin degradation products in blood. Decline in platelet count and prothrombin and fibrinogen values due to consumption coagulopathy

Necropsy findings

Lesions of toxemia and hyperthermia plus petechiae in subserosal, submucosal sites, and embolic lesions in many organs.

Diagnosis

Many of the signs and lesions of septicemia are mirrored by **bacteremia**, except that it is characterized by intermittent appearances of bacteria in the blood, usually due to minor escapes from local lesions and for brief periods only, and it does not produce clinical signs. Implantation of the vagrant microorganisms in other organs can result in embolism and the development of further local infections.

Treatment

♦ Urgent treatment, usually parenterally, with specifically targeted or broad spectrum antibacterial agents
♦ Specific antitoxins or antisera are still used in some specific infections
♦ Non-steroidal anti-inflammatory agents are now used in many cases
♦ Because most of the septicemias are infectious diseases, treatment programs may need to be accompanied by strict hygienic measures

LOCALIZED INFECTIONS [VM8 p. 55]

Local aggregations of pus, usually as abscesses, are described elsewhere under the headings of pharyngeal, retroperitoneal, hepatic, splenic, pulmonary, brain, spinal cord and subcutaneous abscesses. Larger aggregations are recorded in empyema, pleurisy, peritonitis, osteomyelitis, navel infection. Other miscellaneous localizations are recorded here.

Etiology

♦ Common skin contaminants e.g. *Actinomyces pyogenes, Fusobacterium necrophorum*, streptococci, staphylococci
♦ Specific infections with *Corynebacterium pseudotuberculosis, Rhodococcus equi, Streptococcus equi, Actinobacillus mallei, Pseudomonas pseudomallei, Mycobacterium phlei* and other atypical mycobacteria
♦ Accidental, sometimes neglectful, penetration of skin or mucosa by injections or incisions, e.g. on tail-docking, castration
♦ Metastatic implantation from another body source, e.g. lymphadenitis

Clinical findings

♦ Signs of toxemia including fever, depression, anorexia, weight loss
♦ Posture and gait abnormalities due to local pain
♦ Local swelling and edema
♦ Palpable internal masses
♦ Radiologically visible masses
Specific local infections include:
♦ Inguinal abscess in horses after castration
♦ Tail abscess after docking or tail-chewing in lambs and pigs
♦ Tail tip cellulitis in feedlot cattle (p. 677)

♦ Urachal abscess as a sequel to omphalophlebitis (p. 48)
♦ Perirectal abscess in horses after rectal examination
♦ Postinjection cellulitis due to accidental infection or use of escharotic material
♦ Traumatic injury
♦ Pituitary abscess

Clinical pathology

♦ Leukocytosis and left shift in acute lesions. Chronic encapsulated lesions may cause no abnormality. Less chronic lesions cause lymphocytosis, monocytosis, sometimes anemia due to bone marrow depression
♦ Needle aspiration of a locatable mass plus culture of aspirate may identify infection and best treatment

Necropsy findings

The lesion is usually readily located and identified in a patient so severely affected as to die or be euthanized.

Diagnosis

Local swellings due to herniae, diverticulae, hematomas and aneurysms are the usual causes of misdiagnosis, and sometimes of accidental fatalities when they are opened in error.

Treatment

♦ Surgical drainage and irrigation
♦ Local, parenteral if necessary, treatment with antibacterial agents
♦ Aspiration of infected material and replacement with antibacterial agent
♦ Hot fomentation, hydrotherapy, appli-

cation of rubifacients are widely used to encourage abscesses to point and rupture
♦ Systemic treatment of inaccessible lesions

may cause conversion to a chronic lesion unless antibacterial therapy is intensive and prolonged

PAIN [VM8 p. 57]

Etiology

Cutaneous pain
♦ Burning, freezing, cutting, crushing, inflammation, foreign body penetration or compression

Visceral pain
♦ Serous surface inflammation
♦ Viscera distension
♦ Stretching of mesentery, mediastinum
♦ Tissue swelling by inflammation, edema, especially brain and peripheral nerves
♦ Compression, e.g. peripheral nerves, dorsal nerve roots

Somatic (musculoskeletal) pain
♦ Muscle tears, hematomas, inflammation, ischemia, spasm
♦ Bones – osteomyelitis, fracture, arthritis, joint dislocation, ligament and tendon sprain

Clinical findings

♦ Anorexia, sham drinking, anxious expression, restlessness
♦ Moaning, grunting, teeth-grinding
♦ Tachycardia
♦ Polypnea
♦ Pupillary dilation
♦ Hyperthermia
♦ Sweating
♦ In musculoskeletal pain – lameness, shuffling gait, limb carrying, weight shifting at rest
♦ In visceral pain – crouching, pawing, flank-watching, stretching, rolling, lying down
♦ Eliciting pain by pressure, percussion, active or passive movement of a limb, stimulating a cough
♦ Painful defecation, urination, coughing

Diagnosis

Other causes of restlessness and anxiety include **paresthesia**, as in snakebite, photosensitive dermatitis. Abnormalities of gait and posture are also caused by non-painful lesions of musculoskeletal and nervous systems.

Treatment

Suitable **analgesics** for use in large animals include:
♦ **Salicylates:** 100 mg/kg × 12 hours orally for moderate pain. Cattle 35 mg/kg × 6 hours I/V, **horse** 25 mg/kg × 4 hours I/V
♦ **Phenylbutazone:** horse 4.4 mg/kg daily × 5 days, oral or I/V. Dose repeated twice the first day. Cattle, orally 10–20 mg/kg loading dose, then 2.5–5.0 mg/kg daily × 5 days. Prolonged use subject to toxic effects. Not recommended for use in food-producing animals
♦ **Xylazine** may be used alone 0.5 mg/kg I/V, or in combination with butorphanol or dipyrone
♦ **Flunixin meglumine:** 1.1 mg/kg orally or parenterally
♦ **Butorphanol:** 0.025 mg/kg I/V
♦ **Detomidine:** 20–40 μg/kg
♦ Many older drugs, e.g. chloral hydrate, pethidine, pentazocine are moderately effective and may have the advantage of a much lower cost

Supportive treatment includes hot fomentations and hosing, and the provision of appropriate bedding or slings.

STRESS [VM8 p. 60]

Etiology

A poorly defined systemic state caused by the long-term application of stressors. Stressors are internal or external stimuli which excite hypothalamic neurones to release corticotropin-releasing hormones at greater than normal rates. For example:
♦ Prolonged transport including long standing, compression, injury, lack of feed and water, high temperature and humidity

◆ Climate, especially cold, wet, windy weather, or sudden change
◆ Crowding stimulating aggression, boredom, cannibalism
◆ Absence of bedding
◆ Absence of housing as shelter
◆ Diet – lack of energy, bulk, fiber, water
◆ Harassment by noise, human intervention, other animals
◆ Separation from group in animals used to flocking or herding
◆ Excessive physical effort, e.g. endurance ride, fighting between bulls, boars, capture of wild animals
◆ Pain as in equine colic, laminitis

Clinical findings

A poorly defined and inadequately substantiated pattern of signs and pathogeneses includes:

◆ Poor productivity, especially in milk production and fertility in cows, relative to available nutritional resources
◆ Inefficiency of milk let-down by cows
◆ Increased susceptibility to infection
◆ Possibly hypocalcemia, hypomagnesemia, ketonemia
◆ Gastric or abomasal ulcer

Clinical pathology

High blood levels of cortisol and ACTH are definitive.

Necropsy findings

None listed.

Diagnosis

The observed signs of stress are easily attributed to other causes, including a simple physiological response to environmental stimuli, without the need for a separate diagnosis.

Treatment

Avoidance of environmental stress is an integral part of animal agriculture but is at present largely limited by financial considerations. Increasing awareness by the community generally of the need to promote the welfare of animals will undoubtedly cause greater consideration to be given to management systems that minimize stress to the animals.

SUDDEN DEATH [VM8 p. 64]

Animals observed to die without prior signs being observed, or animals which are observed closely at least once each day and are found dead are included in this category.

Etiology

Single animals
◆ Spontaneous internal hemorrhage. **Cows** – cardiac tamponade. **Horses** – ruptured aorta, inherited aortic aneurysm, atrium or verminous mesenteric aneurysm, exercise-induced pulmonary hemorrhage.
◆ Acute heart failure in horses, often exercise-induced. Calves – inherited cardiomyopathy
◆ Adverse drug reactions e.g. anaphylactoid reactions, commonly to penicillin in horses
◆ Peracute endotoxemia after rupture of stomach (horse), abomasum (cattle), colon (mares after foaling)
◆ Fulminating septicemia, especially in neonates, and most commonly in foals

◆ Snakebite, but very few cases recorded except in very young
◆ Accidental trauma to brain via skull or atlanto-occipital joint by collision, fighting, pulling back on halter, or sadistic injury
◆ Iatrogenic deaths due to intravenous injection of toxic solution, e.g. calcium or magnesium solutions to cows, ivermectin, procaine penicillin suspensions, too bulky saline solutions in patients with pulmonary edema, potassium iodide in mistake for sodium iodide. Intra-arterial injections in mistake for intravenous ones, e.g. of penicillin, phenothiazine-derived tranquillizers
◆ Many cases are undiagnosed

Group deaths
These agents may cause single deaths but are commonly group causes:
◆ Lightning stroke, electrocution
◆ Nutritional deficiencies – selenium, vitamin E, copper (falling disease). Peracute hypomagnesemia
◆ Poisons, especially cyanogenetic glyco-

sides, nitrite, fluoroacetate, monensin and other ionophores, especially in horses, organophosphatic compounds, usually as insecticides, peracute lead poisoning
◆ Poisonous plants: those containing cardiac glycosides, tunicamycin, fluoroacetate, and *Phalaris* spp., the hemlocks (*Cicuta* and *Oenanthe* spp.), and many others
◆ Peracute cases of some septicemias, e.g. anthrax, blackleg, hemorrhagic septicemia, peracute pneumonic pasteurellosis, enterotoxemia in cattle and sheep; mulberry heart disease and edema disease in pigs. Colitis-X in horses
◆ Bloat in cattle
◆ Acute carbohydrate engorgement in ruminants
◆ Acute bovine pulmonary emphysema and edema

Special examination of sudden deaths

More than usual care required, especially in group deaths, because cases may involve litigation or insurance assessments. Procedure should include:
◆ Detailed contemporary records
◆ History of change of feed, possible exposure to poison, any medication
◆ Check environment for toxins, source of electricity. Special attention to personal welfare during examination
◆ Check cadavers for evidence of bleeding from orifices, foam from nostrils, struggling, bloat, mucosal pallor, singe marks on feet, trauma, especially center of forehead, gunshot wound. Bodies found in water need to be examined at necropsy for evidence of water inhalation
◆ Arrange for or perform careful necropsy on typical cadavers, with two sets of samples for pathology and toxicological examination, preferably sealed and warranted, one set for the opposition in the case of litigation

DISTURBANCES OF BODY FLUIDS, ELECTROLYTES, AND ACID–BASE BALANCE [VM8 p. 66]

The disturbances described singly in the next section rarely occur singly in nature. Usually they occur in combinations in clinical cases, and principally in diseases of the alimentary tract, e.g. dehydration is usually accompanied by an electrolyte deficit, and often by acidosis or alkalosis.

Although these disturbances occur only as auxiliaries to standard diagnoses they do add to the complexity of the symptomatology and are often sufficiently important to make the difference between life and death for the patient.

Clinical signs, clinical pathology and necropsy signs of fluid and electrolyte disturbances are not sufficiently definitive to make their clinical diagnosis possible, and the frequent use of expensive blood gas analysis equipment to detect the abnormalities, and then to monitor the changes in what are often rapidly changing parameters, is possible only in large veterinary hospitals. The purpose of describing the individual disturbances is to itemize the problems that can occur. What happens and what needs to be done in field cases is described in a sub-

sequent section on **Naturally occurring combined abnormalities** (p. 26).

Clinical, biochemical and biophysical parameters used in a complete assessment of electrolyte and fluid status of patients, but not dealt with here are:
◆ History and clinical findings, indicating the nature of the disease
◆ Packed cell volume (PCV) (or total serum protein)
◆ Total and differential leukocyte counts
◆ Blood pH, blood gases, serum electrolytes
◆ Anion and osmolal gaps
◆ Arterial blood pressure
◆ Central venous blood pressure

DEHYDRATION [VM8 p. 66]

Etiology

Decreased water intake
◆ Water deprivation
◆ Intake reduced because of toxemia, stomatitis, esophageal obstruction

Excessive fluid loss in
♦ Diarrhea the common cause
♦ Loss to the exterior by vomiting, polyuria, excessive sweating
♦ Internal loss in intestinal obstruction, acute carbohydrate engorgement, abomasal dilation and torsion

Clinical findings

Severity of the dehydration and type of electrolyte imbalance varies with type of dehydration.

Due to tissue fluid loss
♦ Loss of skin elasticity; wrinkled, shrunken appearance, skin tents easily, subsides slowly
♦ Mucosal dryness
♦ Eyeballs recede into sockets
♦ Thinness, weight loss, reduced milk yield, emaciation, weakness
♦ Feces dry, scant in water deprivation
♦ Urine flow decreased, except polyuria
♦ Hyperthermia, moderate, of dehydration
♦ Increase in voluntary water intake unless toxemia reduces thirst

Due to reduced blood volume
♦ Mental depression, anorexia

Clinical pathology

♦ Hemoconcentration (elevated PCV, total serum solids)
♦ Reduced circulating blood volume
♦ Increased plasma osmolality
♦ Increased plasma sodium concentration in water deprivation
♦ Acidosis
♦ Moderate increase in blood NPN

♦ Urine concentrated, specific gravity increased

Diagnosis

The difficulty of diagnosis of dehydration is that it is usually a relatively subtle and subsidiary complaint, overshadowed by a more clinically demonstrable syndrome. Its importance is that neglect of its treatment will delay convalescence and possibly contribute to the death of the patient. (See also the syndrome of water deprivation.)

Treatment

Severity of dehydration usually estimated clinically in terms of body weight loss, hence fluid replacement need, by clinical signs and clinical pathology findings (Table 2.1). Electrolyte replacement and acid–base adjustment may also be necessary.

HYPONATREMIA [VM8 p. 68]

Etiology

♦ Water excretion in urine increased to compensate for loss of tissue fluid osmolality
♦ Hypovolemia causes hypotension, peripheral circulatory failure, renal failure
♦ Excess loss with fluid in enteritis
♦ Dehydration of hyponatremia is usually isotonic because fluid is lost at the same time as the sodium

Clinical findings

Mental depression, muscular weakness, hypothermia, marked dehydration, polyuria.

Table 2.1 Degrees of severity of dehydration and guidelines for assessment (VM8 p. 68)

Body weight loss (%)	Sunken eyes, shrunken face	Skin fold test persists for (seconds)	PCV (%)	Total serum solids (g/l)	Fluid required to replace volume deficit (ml/kg body weight)
4–6	Barely detectable	—	40–45	70–80	20–25
6–8	++	2–4	50	80–90	30–50
8–10	+++	6–10	55	90–100	50–80
10–12	++++	20–45	60	120	80–120

Clinical pathology

♦ Plasma sodium level reduced
♦ Increased volume of low specific gravity urine

Diagnosis

Hyponatremia produces a syndrome too indistinctive to be differentiated from other metabolic defects. Diagnosis is usually laboratory based.

Treatment

See Table 2.2.

HYPOCHLOREMIA [VM8 p. 70]

Etiology

An increased net loss of chloride from body tissues occurs as a result of hypersecretion from the stomach or abomasum into the lumen, due to the distension of the abomasum or intestine when they are obstructed, and failure to reabsorb it in the small intestine, for the same reason.

Clinical findings

♦ Lethargy, anorexia, weight loss
♦ Mild polydipsia, polyuria
♦ Hypochloremia can contribute to a fatal outcome in cases of right abomasal torsion and displacement, and intestinal obstruction

Clinical pathology

♦ Metabolic alkalosis
♦ Low blood levels of chloride, sodium and potassium
♦ High blood levels of non-protein nitrogen

Diagnosis

Hypochloremia contributes to the symptomatology in bowel obstructions but is not usually diagnosed as a separate entity.

Treatment

See Table 2.2.

HYPOKALEMIA [VM8 p. 70]

Etiology

♦ Loss into gut lumen via abomasal stasis and fluid accumulation, intestinal obstruction, enteritis
♦ Renal excretion as compensatory mechanism in patients with alkalosis
♦ Prolonged administration of mineralocorticoids
♦ Prolonged administration of potassium-free solutions to dehydrated, diarrheic patients

Clinical findings

♦ Muscle tremor, weakness, recumbency
♦ Mental depression, coma
♦ Cardiac arrhythmia

Clinical pathology

♦ Low blood levels of potassium and chloride. Care needed in interpreting blood potassium levels because they may not accurately reflect the levels in tissues
♦ Metabolic alkalosis

Diagnosis

Hypokalemia contributes to the syndrome in cases of abomasal distension. It is unlikely to be diagnosed as a separate entity.

Treatment

Normal saline solutions are usually adequate to treat cases with hypokalemic alkalosis. High potassium content solutions are required only in extreme cases. See also Table 2.2.

HYPOCALCEMIA [VM8 p. 72]

See parturient paresis.

ACIDOSIS [VM8 p. 72]

Etiology

♦ Excessive loss of bicarbonate ion in severe enteritis in adults and diarrhea in neonates
♦ Acute intestinal obstruction in horses
♦ Excessive exogenous acid absorption in carbohydrate engorgement in ruminants
♦ Excessive administration of acidifying preparations in cases of alkalosis
♦ In cases of cardiac or pulmonary disease

Table 2.2 Summary of disturbances of body water, electrolytes and acid–base balance in some common diseases of cattle and horses, and suggested fluid therapy (VM8 p. 80)

Disease	Major abnormalities and deficits	Fluid and electrolyte requirements
Neonatal calf diarrhea (including piglets and lambs)	*Metabolic acidosis*, low plasma bicarbonate, severe dehydration, loss of sodium, hyperkalemia when acidosis severe	Equal mixtures of isotonic saline and isotonic sodium bicarbonate with 5% dextrose. Balanced electrolytes too. Intravenously and orally
D-Lactic acidosis (carbohydrate engorgement of ruminants)	*Metabolic acidosis*, low plasma bicarbonate, severe dehydration	Sodium bicarbonate initially followed by balanced electrolytes. Intravenously
Acute diffuse peritonitis	*Dehydration*. Slight metabolic alkalosis due to paralytic ileus	Balanced electrolyte solutions in large quantities intravenously for hydration and maintenance
Right-side dilatation/abomasal torsion of cattle, abomasal impaction (dietary or vagal nerve injury)	*Metabolic alkalosis*, marked hypochloremia, hypokalemia, severe dehydration	Balanced electrolyte solutions or high potassium and chloride acidifying solution intravenously. May give acidifying solutions orally. Can also use mixture of 2 liters of isotonic saline (0.9%), 1 liter isotonic potassium chloride (1.1%) and 1 liter isotonic dextrose (5%)
Peracute coliform mastitis	*Severe dehydration*, mild electrolyte deficits including mild hypocalcemia. Acidosis if diarrhea present	Balanced electrolyte solutions intravenously in large quantities for hydration, and maintenance for 24–48 hours (100–150 ml/kg body weight/24 h)
Acute diarrhea in the horse (enteric salmonellosis, colitis-X)	*Severe dehydration*, marked hyponatremia, *metabolic acidosis*. Hypokalemia occurs following bicarbonate therapy	Hypertonic sodium bicarbonate (5%) 3–5 liters (500 kg body weight) followed by high sodium, high potassium alkalinizing solution to correct hypokalemia following bicarbonate therapy all by the intravenous route
Acute grain engorgement in the horse	*Metabolic acidosis*, *dehydration* and shock	Hypertonic sodium bicarbonate (5%) 3–5 liters (500 kg body weight) followed by balanced electrolytes intravenously
Water and electrolyte deprivation. Esophageal obstruction in horse	Moderate dehydration	Balanced electrolytes intravenously. When obstruction relieved, provide electrolyte solution orally
Acute intestinal obstruction	*Metabolic acidosis* or alkalosis dependent on level of obstruction. Severe dehydration in horse, moderate in cow	Isotonic sodium bicarbonate initially, 3–5 liters (500 kg body weight) followed by balanced electrolytes intravenously. Horses may develop hypokalemia following bicarbonate therapy and must be given potassium chloride

with carbon dioxide retention, e.g. pneumonia, emphysema, congestive heart failure
♦ In cases of renal insufficiency in which acid excretion is impeded

Clinical findings

♦ Mental depression, loss of sucking drive in neonates
♦ Muscle weakness, lethargy, recumbency, coma
♦ Respiratory rate and depth increased
♦ Tachycardia, decreased pulse amplitude and blood pressure. Combined with hyperkalemia, acidosis can cause sudden death due to heart block

Clinical pathology

♦ Low blood bicarbonate
♦ Blood pH variable, often within normal range 7.0–7.8

Diagnosis

Acidosis is a serious and common complication of many animal disease but it is unlikely to be a primary diagnosis. Its diagnosis depends entirely on laboratory blood gas analysis.

Treatment

Isotonic solutions of sodium bicarbonate as set out in Table 2.2.

ALKALOSIS [VM8 p. 74]

Etiology

♦ Overdosing with bicarbonate, e.g. in treatment of lactic acidosis
♦ Excessive loss of acid as in gastric dilation, abomasal dilation and volvulus. Hypochloremia, hypokalemia are common accompaniments
♦ Excess CO_2 excretion by hyperventilation

Clinical findings

♦ Slow, shallow respiratory movements initially. May be hyperpnea, dyspnea terminally
♦ Muscle tremor, tetany, clonic–tonic convulsions in some

Clinical pathology

♦ Low blood levels of chlorine, potassium usually
♦ High plasma bicarbonate

Diagnosis

Laboratory blood gas analysis provides the only satisfactory means of diagnosis of this important subsyndrome.

Treatment

Acidifying solutions used in the treatment of alkalosis usually contain isotonic potassium and isotonic sodium solutions (see Table 2.3).

NATURALLY OCCURRING
COMBINED ABNORMALITIES OF
FLUID, ELECTROLYTE AND ACID–
BASE BALANCE [VM8 p. 74]

Some of the serious diseases in which abnormalities of body fluids and electrolytes are important secondary problems are set out in Table 2.2 showing the metabolic abnormalities and indications for therapy, and Table 2.4, which shows laboratory findings likely to be found in some of the diseases. With respect to the latter table it is necessary to realize that it tests only a range of possible results, and that blood levels of the electrolytes can change dramatically in a short time in a single case. Besides the obvious losses that can be assessed approximately by clinical examination and medical and management history of the case, it is also necessary to take into account the effects of the compensatory mechanisms operated by the respiratory, circulatory and urinary systems, and the homeostatic effects of the biochemical buffering systems. It is not practicable to make assessments of all of those mechanisms in a clinical environment. Instead it is expedient to assess the principal parameters and recommend reparative therapies.

Fluid and electrolyte therapy

In practice, fluid and electrolyte therapy is based on broad principles, case experience and simple clinical and clinical pathology assessments. Theoretically (and in major hospital practice) more sophisticated techniques, described in detail in *Veterinary Medicine*, are used. Descriptions of the fluid and electrolyte disturbances, and recommended

Table 2.3 Composition (mmol/l) and indications for use of electrolyte solutions used in fluid therapy (VM8 p. 82)

Solutions	Na$^+$	K$^+$	Cl$^-$	Mg^{2+}	Ca^{2+}	HCO$_3^-$	Lactate or acetate	Dextrose	Major indications
0.9% Sodium chloride (isotonic saline)	155		155						Expanded circulating blood volume
1.3% Sodium bicarbonate (isotonic)	155					156			Acidosis
1.3% Sodium bicarbonate in 5% dextrose	155					156		5%	Acidosis
5% Sodium bicarbonate (hypertonic)	600					600			Severe acidosis
Equal mixture of isotonic saline and isotonic sodium bicarbonate	155		78			78			Acidosis and dehydration
Balanced electrolyte solution (i.e. McSherry's solution)	138	12	100	5	3		50 (acetate)		Acidosis, alkalosis, electrolyte losses and dehydration
Lactated Ringer's solution	130	4	111		3		28 (lactate)		Acidosis
High sodium, alkalinizing solution. Lactated Ringer's solution plus sodium bicarbonate (5 g/l)	190	4	111			60	27 (lactate)		Acidosis and hyponatremia
High sodium, high potassium, alkalinizing solution. Lactated Ringer's solution plus 1 g/l potassium chloride and 5 g/l sodium bicarbonate	190	18	125			60	27 (lactate)		Acidosis, hyponatremia, hypokalemia
High-potassium acidifying solution. Isotonic saline plus 2.5 g potassium chloride/l	154	35	189						Alkalosis, hypochloremia, hypokalemia
Mixture of: 1 l isotonic potassium chloride (1.1%), 2 l isotonic saline (0.9%) and 1 l dextrose 5%									Metabolic alkalosis in cattle with abomasal disease

Table 2.4 Representative laboratory values (mean ± SD) in body water and electrolyte disturbances (VM8 p. 77)

Clinical pathology	Acute diarrhea in horse	Acute diarrhea in calf	Metabolic alkalosis due to abomasal dilatation impaction/torsion in cattle	Acute intestinal obstruction	Acute carbohydrate engorgement in ruminants
Packed cell volume (%)	60 ± 7	45.3 ± 7.0	42 ± 6	64 ± 5	45 ± 6
Total serum solids	10 ± 2	8.6 ± 1.5	8.2 ± 1.5	11.5 ± 1.5	8.5 ± 1.8
Blood pH (venous)	7.10 ± 0.15	7.08 ± 0.12	7.49 ± 0.15	7.15 ± 0.04	7.10 ± 0.05
Plasma bicarbonate (mmol/l)	12 ± 3	13.7 ± 4.2	35.4 ± 5.7	18 ± 6	12.5 ± 3.5
Partial pressure of carbon dioxide (mm Hg)	45 ± 8	46.8 ± 6.4	46.4 ± 7.5	48 ± 6	40 ± 6
Serum sodium (mmol/l)	126 ± 3	138 ± 9.4	138.5 ± 5.4	135 ± 5	132 ± 4
Serum chloride (mmol/l)	99 ± 3	101.4 ± 7.5	88.6 ± 12.8	98 ± 4	93 ± 3
Serum potassium (mmol/l)	3.0 ± 1.2	7.4 ± 1.6	3.4 ± 0.6	3.8 ± 0.6	5.0 ± 2.5
Blood urea nitrogen (mg/dl)	60 ± 30	50.1 ± 30.5	40 ± 15	65 ± 35	55 ± 25

treatments are also dealt with in the sections on individual diseases.

Estimate of the needs for replacement therapy

To estimate the electrolyte deficit it is necessary to be able to measure the patient's:

♦ Serum electrolyte values
♦ Specific electrolyte deficit in mEq/liter
♦ Size of the extracellular fluid space as a percentage of the total body weight. This varies between cases and between electrolytes, and a range of approximate constant values is used

Composition and volume of fluids

♦ If the patient's electrolyte deficit can be accurately estimated, a specific regimen for the fluids to be used is then possible. Compositions and recommended uses of commercially available fluids are in Table 2.3
♦ For general use, and in the absence of clinical pathology data, solutions containing sodium, potassium chloride and calcium at concentrations equal to those in normal extracellular fluid are used. Lactate or acetate may also be included when the treatment of acidosis is a target; their metabolic end-product is bicarbonate. Many also contain glucose. They are adequate for the treatment of dehydration and moderate acidosis or alkalosis
♦ For severe acidosis or alkalosis, and for specific electrolyte deficits, solutions listed in Table 2.3 should be used
♦ The volumes of fluid required need to take into account the immediate deficit and the maintenance requirement over the period of treatment, including a factor to compensate for continuing losses. It is usual to begin with a high **hydration therapy** dose rate and continue with a lower **maintenance** dose rate. Sample estimates are included in Table 2.5

Route of administration

♦ Intravenous injection is the preferred parenteral route because of diffusion difficulties from tissue sites in hypovolemic patients. Difficulties include phlebitis when the injection is carried out over a long period, pulmonary edema in patients with cardiopulmonary problems and when the infusion rate is too rapid. In farm animals the need for continuous supervision of the patient raises difficulties
♦ Oral fluid therapy is highly practicable for single ruminant patients on farms, provided there are no absorption problems, especially stasis or inflammation. Estimated daily requirements are given at intervals appropriate to the case. Calves are usually dosed at 2–4 hour intervals. Powdered preparations, suitable for dissolving in water on the farm, are commercially available
♦ Oral fluid administration to horses with diarrhea is not successful and often exacerbates the diarrhea

Parenteral nutrition

Total hyperalimentation by the intravenous infusion of electrolyte solutions which also contain protein hydrolysates, glucose and lipid emulsions to patients, especially neonates, who are not able to take nourishment by mouth, can be carried out but is limited by its high cost and practical considerations related to the fluid's hypertonicity.

Table 2.5 Examples of amounts of fluid required for hydration and maintenance therapy (VM8 p. 83)

Animal	Degree of dehydration (% of body weight)	Fluid required for hydration	maintenance (liters)
Mature horse (500 kg)	8	40	25–50
	12	60	25–50
Newborn calf (50 kg)	8	4	2.5–5
	12	6	2.5–5
Mature cow (700 kg)	8	56	35–70
	12	84	35–70

DISTURBANCES OF APPETITE, FOOD INTAKE, AND NUTRITIONAL STATUS [VM8 p. 86]

Hunger and appetite are subjective sensations attributable only to humans. Anorexia, inappetence, hyperorexia are similarly inappropriate, but widely used expressions in discussions about animals.

POLYPHAGIA [VM8 p. 86]

♦ Overeating is common to all animal species and to all individual animals in inadequately supervised management systems. Individual animals which are more gluttonous than their herd-mates are more susceptible to overeating diseases, e.g. grain engorgement in ruminants, and to most poisonings
♦ Diseases in which polyphagia may be a sign include intestinal malabsorption, internal parasitism in which feed aversion is not evident. Deficiency of pancreatic enzymes, hypothyroidism, diabetes mellitus and chronic gastritis, in which polyphagia might be anticipated are rare in farm animals

ANOPHAGIA OR APHAGIA [VM8 p. 87]

Causes include:
♦ Painful conditions of the mouth or pharynx. Pharyngeal and esophageal diseases are more likely to provoke attempts to eat followed by coughing rejection or vomiting of feed
♦ Toxemia, fever, hyperthermia
♦ Nutritional deficiency of cobalt, thiamin in monogastric species, possibly zinc
♦ Pain, excitement, estrus activity, fear, fatigue, very bad weather, especially high wind, driving rain, sudden confinement of animals accustomed to free range
♦ Heavy trichostrongylid infestations in ruminants
♦ Feed aversion, most commonly attributed to poisons, e.g. monensin, fungal toxins in grain rations fed to pigs, or to some poisonous plants in pastures used for ruminants

Reduced feed intake is damaging in all animals but especially in late pregnant or recently calved, high-producing cows, and in late pregnant ewes and goat does, in which pregnancy toxemia and fat cow disease can be highly fatal outcomes.

Therapeutic measures are recommended in some quarters but are unlikely to make significant contributions unless the specific cause is removed, and highly palatable feed provided. They include:
♦ Stimulants, e.g. strychnine, parasympathomimetic drugs
♦ Injections of insulin aimed at causing hypoglycemia
♦ Thiamin orally or parenterally in high doses
♦ Rumen flora transplant from a normal animal (10–20 liters in cattle)

Substitution therapy by short-term parenteral administration of solutions containing electrolytes and an energy source, usually glucose, is standard practice (see Table 2.2). Oral administration of propylene glycol or glycerine, as in the treatment of ruminant ketosis is recommended in those species. Parenteral alimentation is not a viable form of therapy.

PICA OR ALLOTRIOPHAGIA [VM8 p. 87]

Ingestion of materials other than normal feed for the species. Includes licking, chewing (without necessarily swallowing), drinking.
Causes include:
♦ Dietary deficiency of bulk, possibly fiber, in herbivores. Salt deficiency and unknown dietary factors are commonly blamed
♦ Boredom in closely confined animals accustomed to free range
♦ Possibly as a result of overcrowding, e.g. tail-biting in pigs
♦ Disturbances of consciousness, e.g. nervous acetonemia, rabies
Bad sequels include:
♦ Botulism
♦ Lead poisoning
♦ Foreign bodies in alimentary tract, especially in oropharynx
♦ Sand or fiber impactions in alimentary tract
♦ Foreign-body perforations of stomach or reticulum
♦ Grazing time reduced
Types of allotriophagia:
♦ Osteophagia – bone-chewing
♦ Infantophagia – eating of young. May be sow hysteria
♦ Coprophagia – eating of feces
♦ Wool-eating in sheep
♦ Bark-eating – in horses
♦ Carrion-eating
♦ Coat-licking

◆ Earth-eating
◆ Urine-drinking, may be mixed with silage effluent
◆ Cannibalism, including tail-biting and ear sucking in pigs

STARVATION [VM8 p. 88]

Etiology

Complete deprivation of feed as in drought, flood, bushfire or human intervention.

Clinical findings

◆ Hunger
◆ Increased muscle power, endurance
◆ Weight loss (up to 60%), especially subcutis fat
◆ Skin tenting increased
◆ Hyperlipemia in late pregnant pony mares
◆ Dramatic fall in milk yield
◆ Fecal output declines to zero at day 4 in horses
◆ Water intake declines but urine output maintained
◆ Recumbency due to hypocalcemia in sheep
◆ Bradycardia, pulse amplitude and blood pressure reduced
◆ Weakness, staggery gait, recumbency terminally

Clinical pathology

◆ Hypoglycemia
◆ Hyperlipidemia
◆ Blood urea nitrogen and urine total nitrogen levels greatly increased terminally

Necropsy findings

◆ Body fat lacking
◆ Skeletal muscles, especially non-postural ones reduced in mass to as low as 30% of normal
◆ Gut contents greatly decreased in volume, rumen contents mostly water
◆ General tissues atrophy

Diagnosis

◆ History and examination of environment usually identify problem
◆ Malicious deprivation may be difficult to comprehend

Treatment

◆ Small amounts of highly digestible carbohydrate and protein nutrients orally because ability of tissues to metabolize nutrients may be severely reduced. Parenteral glucose may be passed in urine
◆ Avoid lipids which may exacerbate ketosis
◆ See special diets in next section (p. 32)

INANITION (MALNUTRITION) [VM8 p. 88]

The diet is inadequate in total and all components are reduced; there is no specific deficiency of one or more components. The condition is compatible with life.

Etiology

◆ Drought, overstocking, end-of-winter shortage of feed stores
◆ Livestock kept outdoors in winter months in very cold climate and fed poor quality roughage without grain supplement
◆ Young calves fed milk replacer containing large amounts of non-milk protein and carbohydrate
◆ Beef calves sucking heifers with low milk yield
◆ **Hobby farm malnutrition** imposed by owner because of ignorance of nutritional needs, especially of young ruminants

Clinical findings

See also thin sow syndrome, weaner ill-thrift.
◆ Mental depression
◆ Weight loss
◆ Decline in temperature, heart and respiratory rates
◆ Anasarca, especially intermandibular edema
◆ Anestrus
◆ Weakness, recumbency, refusal to eat palatable feed. Recumbency, die quietly. Heavy mortality rate. Some deaths due to abomasal impaction

Calves – additional signs

◆ Young calves fed poor quality milk replacer usually have bad diarrhea
◆ Calves on cows with little milk suck hard, bellow a lot, then eat dry feed, drink urine

and surface water. Sternal recumbency and die quietly

Clinical pathology

No changes in moderate cases. Terminally in bad cases same as starvation.

Necropsy findings

♦ Severe reduction muscle mass
♦ Depot fat deficient, serous atrophy of fat in calves

Diagnosis

History and environment examination indicate malnutrition. Response to supplementary feeding confirms, except for poor response in terminal cases.

Treatment

♦ Shelter from weather important, indoors if possible
♦ Severely debilitated animals may need intravenous alimentation with balanced electrolyte solutions containing glucose, amino acids or protein hydrolysates until ingestion of feed, or drinking of milk capable of sustaining nutritional requirement. Long-standing cases, especially neonates, may need high quality care beyond economically rational point
♦ Ingested feed needs to be palatable, nutritionally high quality, small amounts frequently. Legume hay plus ground grain plus mineral and vitamin supplement best for adults. For horses less fiber, added molasses and grain or bran mash used. Milk, milk powder, eggs not recommended for herbivores because of absence of appropriate enzymes for digestion
♦ Stomach tube alimentation for horse unable to eat. Daily administration in 2 to 3 equal amounts of:
  • Electrolyte mixture 210 g (sodium chloride 10 g, sodium bicarbonate 15 g, potassium chloride 75 g, potassium phosphate 60 g, calcium chloride 45 g, magnesium oxide 24 g)
  • Water 21 liters
  • Dextrose 300 g, increasing to 900 g in 7 days
  • Dehydrated cottage cheese 300 g up to 900 g by day 7

THIRST [VM8 p. 90]

Thirst, the subjective sensation of the need to imbibe fluid, is manifested in farm animals by **polydipsia**, or **allotriophagia** in the form of drinking abnormal fluids, especially urine.

Etiology

Increased thirst or fluid intake occurs in:
♦ Cellular dehydration from fluid loss in diarrhea, vomiting, sweating, polyuria
♦ Dietary deficiency of salt in milking cows
♦ Dry oropharynx due to water deprivation
♦ In thin sow syndrome
♦ Diabetes insipidus

Clinical findings

Partial water deprivation
♦ Restless, loitering around water supply aggressive, licking inanimate objects
♦ Decreased milk yield, weight loss

Complete water deprivation for periods exceeding 96 hours in ruminants
♦ Sunken eyes, hollow abdomen, skin tenting
♦ Tremor, excitement, frothing at mouth, gait stiff, uncoordinated, recumbency
♦ Terminally cattle become very excited, frenzied, damage fences, gates, watering facilities
♦ Recovered pregnant cows may abort decomposed calves, suffer dystokia and fatal metritis for variable period after incident

Clinical pathology

♦ Increased serum osmolality; elevated serum levels urea, sodium, total protein
♦ Hemoconcentration; increased PCV
♦ Increased blood levels creatinine kinase, SGOT
♦ Urine specific gravity increased

Necropsy findings

♦ Tissues dehydrated
♦ Fat deposits liquefied
♦ Fetal death, liquefaction, abortion

Diagnosis

The diagnosis is easily missed unless the history is taken carefully. Look for recent movement of cattle to new paddock, especially recently weaned calves, or change of water supply, e.g. from fresh to brackish, from pond to artesian or deep well. Examination of the environment is also often crucial in diagnosis.

Treatment

Replacement therapy with balanced electrolyte fluids, parenterally if possible, slowly in small amounts to avoid water intoxication and polioencephalomalacia.

SHORTFALLS IN PERFORMANCE [VM8 p. 90]

Diagnosed by comparing herd or individual performance with industry standard or peers in similar environments. In dairy cows index could be:

♦ Milk (or butterfat) production per cow per lactation (liters/hectare, or liters/cow)
♦ Mean intercalving interval (as index of reproductive efficiency)
♦ Percent calving survival to 1 year old
♦ Longevity (% mortality/year or average age of cows in herd + culling rate per year)
♦ Culling rate (needs to differentiate from culling due to illness or poor productivity versus sale as productive animal)
♦ Acceptability of product at sale (e.g. milk bulk cell count, poor quality, low solids not fat, low butter fat)

Standards are not quoted here because they vary so much between geographical areas and financial investment in the enterprise, from which appropriate income must be earned. Possible causes of **poor performance** in the absence of clinical signs or identifiable disease include:

♦ **Nutrition** inadequate in calories, protein, minerals, vitamins or water
♦ **Inheritance** of feed conversion efficiency, reproductive fertility
♦ **Housing** and the protection it provides from environmental stress
♦ **Managerial expertise,** e.g. efficiency of heat detection, body weight assessment
♦ **Disease wastage** by clinical and subclinical diseases

Investigation of these parameters requires a knowledge of farming practices as well as animal disease. Some recognized disease entities belonging to these managerial diseases include ill-thrift of sheep, poor performance syndrome of racehorses, thin sow syndrome, summer slump of dairy cows, low butter fat syndrome, weak calf syndrome

WEIGHT LOSS OR FAILURE TO GAIN WEIGHT (ILL-THRIFT) [VM8 p. 91]

Weight loss in the presence of ample feed and good appetite.

Nutritional causes

♦ Poor weight estimation, leading to inadequate feed
♦ Hobby farm malnutrition (ignorance of the real nutritional needs of animals)
♦ Poor feed, e.g. half-filled grain, mature hay
♦ Group feeding with domination by some members
♦ Underestimation of nutritional needs to balance production out-goes
♦ Trace element deficiency in diet
♦ Poor dentition for grazing pasture
♦ Interference with grazing by insect worry, estrus, separation from weaned young, inclement weather

Bodily loss of protein and carbohydrate

♦ Glycosuria, proteinuria in nephrosis, diabetes mellitus
♦ Protein enteropathy
♦ Proteinuria in nephritis, nephrosis
♦ Heavy worm or external parasite burden

Faulty digestion, absorption and metabolism

♦ Diarrhea
♦ Villous atrophy
♦ Parasitic lesions, e.g. granuloma, verminous arteritis
♦ Abnormal physical gut movements, e.g. vagus indigestion, grass sickness
♦ Inadequate metabolism of absorbed nutrients, e.g. in hepatic insufficiency
♦ Neoplasm in any organ likely to increase needed supply of feed

♦ Chronic disease; toxemia causes anorexia, poor enzymatic activity
♦ Specific effects of some poisons include off-feed effects, food refusal, mostly associated with mycotoxicoses
♦ Poor oxygenation of tissues, e.g. in congestive heart failure

POOR RACING PERFORMANCE IN HORSES [VM8 p. 93]

Well-performed horses lose their supremacy without intervention by a discernible disease or lameness, the classic **loss-of-form** condition, and not including horses which, because of poor conformation, temperament or heart size, never have done well.

Causes detectable by simple clinical and laboratory examination

♦ Internal parasite infestation
♦ Anemia
♦ Subacute hepatic injury
♦ Myocarditis and ECG abnormality
♦ Respiratory virus, with poorly defined signs including:
    Poor training gallop performance
    Prolonged dyspnea (blowing) after fast work
    Not quite finishing feed
    Transient mild fever
    Dandruffy coat
    Slight ocular, nasal discharge
    Enlarged submandibular lymph nodes
    Intermittent cough
    Small-volume, foul-smelling feces

    Stiffness after exercise
♦ Endocarditis
♦ Chronic bronchitis, obstructive respiratory disease
♦ Subclinical osteodystrophia fibrosa
♦ Hyponatremia, hypochloremia, hypokalemia
♦ Poor sweating efficiency
♦ 'Going sour' change in temperament

Causes detectable only in specialist equine sports medicine units

♦ Musculoskeletal lesions, e.g. stress-related lesions such as sclerosis of radial fossa of third carpal bone, chronic sacroiliac damage, post-exercise myopathy
♦ Cardiac problems such as exercise-induced cardiac arrhythmia, detectable only by telemetry
♦ Respiratory problems detectable by videotaped recordings of endoscopic examination during high-speed exercise on a treadmill
♦ Inadequate conditioning

PHYSICAL EXERCISE AND EXHAUSTION [VM8 p. 95]

Etiology

♦ Prolonged competitive exercise in horses, e.g. marathon and endurance rides
♦ Prolonged fighting by boars, bulls, stallions and rams

Clinical findings

♦ Depression, lethargy, restlessness
♦ Dehydration, hyperthermia
♦ Hyperpnea or dyspnea
♦ Tachycardia
♦ Mucosae pale or cyanotic, slow capillary refill
♦ Muscle tremor
♦ Abdominal pain in some
♦ Relaxed anal sphincter

♦ Slow return to normal respiratory and cardiac rates
Supplementary syndromes include:
♦ **Heat exhaustion** in physically stressed, overweight horses during hot weather. Signs include:
    • Muscle weakness, tremor and stumbling gait
    • Recumbency
    • Dyspnea
    • Convulsions
    • Marked hyperthermia (42°C, 107.5°F).
♦ Rhabdomyolysis in severe cases. Signs include:
    • Restlessness
    • Myoglobinuria
    • Recumbency
    • Exacerbation of signs if patient transported long distances for treatment

♦ Synchronous diaphragmatic flutter may also occur at this time

Clinical pathology

Standard exhaustion cases:
♦ Hypoglycemia
♦ Hyperproteinaemia, PCV increase
♦ Reduction in plasma Ca, Mg, Na, K
♦ Modest rises in blood lactate, LDH and CPK
♦ Elevation of BUN
♦ Neutrophilic leukosis with shift to left
In **rhabdomyolysis** additional grossly increased serum levels of CPK and SGOT

Diagnosis

Exhaustion after racing is indicated by the history. Fighting is usually observed and affected animals have lacerations, kick, and bite wounds.

Treatment

♦ For dehydration and electrolyte deficiencies by infusion of balanced polyonic solutions (Table 4)
♦ Inclusion of calcium if diaphragmatic flutter present
♦ Slow intravenous infusion to avoid cardiac overload and pulmonary edema
♦ 20–30 liter total infusion usual

Prevention

♦ Experienced veterinary attention during these events to watch for listed damaging clinical changes
♦ Drinking permitted during the race. Should be at intervals of no longer than one hour
♦ Oral saline drenches containing sodium, potassium, calcium, magnesium are standard prophylaxis
♦ Intravenous injections provide more precise replenishments
♦ Pre-competition training
♦ Pre-competition clinical and laboratory examination to detect potential errors

ALLERGY AND ANAPHYLAXIS [VM8 p. 99]

Tissue hypersensitivity due to enhanced immune responsiveness includes disease states:
♦ Allergy (see Chapter 33)
♦ Anaphylaxis, a severe reaction with a sudden onset
♦ Anaphylactic shock, a more severe still, life-threatening state
Other immediate hypersensitivity reactions include:
♦ Pulmonary disease, e.g. chronic obstructive respiratory disease of horses
♦ Dermatological disease, e.g. Queensland itch
♦ Cardiovascular disease e.g. purpura hemorrhagica, alloimmune hemolytic anemia of neonates

♦ Repeated intravenous injections of glandular extracts
♦ Repeated injections of vaccines, e.g *Brucella abortus* strain 19, *Pasteurella multocida* and *P. hemolytica* vaccines and antisera. Some reactions are anaphylactoid and occur in animals with no history of previous exposure
♦ Repeated injections of antibiotics, e.g. penicillin
♦ Rarely after first injections of pharmaceuticals, e.g. a sulfonamide or antibiotic or test agent, e.g. bromsulfalein
Sporadic cases occur in:
♦ Severe reactions in cows with milk allergy at drying off
♦ Cattle in which *Hypoderma* spp. larvae are killed in subcutaneous sites

ANAPHYLAXIS AND
ANAPHYLACTIC SHOCK [VM8 p. 100]

Etiology

Most cases after injection of a biological product:
♦ Repeated blood transfusions from the same donor

Clinical findings

Similar syndrome in horses and cattle. Pigs and sheep less commonly affected but a syndrome similar though less well defined.

In all species clinical signs commence up to 20 minutes after injection of reagin. Death in a few moments in some cases.

- Anxiety, distress
- Profuse salivation in some
- Bloat in some
- Diarrhea in some
- Tachycardia
- Hyperthermia in some, up to 42.5°C
- Collapse
- Sudden, severe dyspnea
- Increased breath sounds, crackling on auscultation
- Hiccough
- Wild paddling convulsions
- Nystagmus
- Cyanosis
- Rhinitis with nasal discharge
- Urticaria, angioedema, erection of hair
- Generalized sweating
- Cough
- Fine nasal froth
- Laminitis in some
- Death in few minutes, or recovery in 2, up to 24 hours if pulmonary edema marked

Clinical pathology

Poorly defined because of brief course.
- Blood histamine levels elevated in some cases only
- PCV elevated
- Plasma potassium levels elevated
- Neutropenia

Necropsy findings

- Severe pulmonary edema and engorgement, emphysema in some
- Gut wall edema and hyperemia in horses and protracted cases in calves
- Subcutaneous edema
- Laminitis in some

AMYLOIDOSIS [VM8 p. 103]

Very rare disease in farm animals.

Etiology

- Repeated injections antigenic material in serum-producing horses
- Long-standing, suppurative diseases
- Repeated infections in immunodeficient patients
- Severe strongyliasis in horses
- Many cases unexplained

Diagnosis

- Characteristic syndrome
- History of injection. Occurs rarely afte ingestion
- Acute bacterial pneumonia includes toxe mia but virus pneumonia may resembl anaphylaxis

Treatment

- Must be immediate
- Epinephrine 4–8 mg I/M or S/C. In emerg ency one fifth dose I/V very slowly
- Antihistamines too unreliable because his tamine often not the mediator of the reac tion
- Suspect animal can be tested for hyper sensitivity before an injection but many false negatives because cutaneous and pul monary sensitivity not necessarily related

OTHER HYPERSENSITIVITY
REACTIONS [VM8 p. 102]

Cell-mediated delayed hypersensitivity pro duce localized, mild syndromes:
- **Allergic rhinitis** after inhalation of reagin as in summer snuffles in cattle
- Sudden diarrhea accompanied by urticaria or angioedema or bloat
- **Eczema** after cutaneous contact. On lower limbs when reagin is in pasture; mostly local swelling, itching, sebaceous exudate behind pastern and on heel bulbs. Middle of back, down sides when sensitivity is to insect bites

Signs transient, respond to antihistamines, but may persist for long periods if sensitizing agent persists in environment. Corticosteroids, systemically or locally recommended for persistent cases. Patients improve when kept housed.

Clinical findings

- **Cutaneous amyloidosis** Hard, painless, chronic skin plaques mostly sides of neck and trunk in horses
- **Nasal amyloidosis** causes dyspnea in horses
- **Renal amyloidosis** in cattle – kidney enlargement, dense proteinuria, profuse diarrhea, anorexia, emaciation, anasarca, recumbency, coma, uremia. Deposits also in spleen and liver

♦ **Corpora amylacea**. Small, round concretions of amyloid in mammary tissue in cows. Inert, may cause teat canal blockage

Clinical pathology

♦ Hyperglobulinemia; globulin levels elevated, albumin depressed
♦ Hypocalcemia in cattle
♦ Blood urea and creatinine levels elevated
♦ Dense proteinuria
♦ Low urine specific gravity
♦ Bromsulfalein clearance times may be increased
♦ Biopsy of cutaneous plaques provides accurate diagnosis

Necropsy findings

♦ Affected organs swollen, waxy appearance, diffuse or circumscribed deposits
♦ Deposits stain with aqueous iodine, congo red

Diagnosis

Renal amyloidosis resembles chronic pyelonephritis, nephrosis.

Treatment

No effective treatment. Course is long and disposal not urgent.

IMMUNE DEFICIENCY DISORDERS [VM8 p. 104]

Etiology

Primary
Congenital, permanent defects in neonates:
♦ Combined immunodeficiency of Arab foals (CID)
♦ Agammaglobulinemia, standardbred and thoroughbred horses
♦ Selective deficiency of one or more globulins e.g. of IgM in Arabs and quarterhorses
♦ Lethal trait A46 (inherited parakeratosis), a T-lymphocyte deficiency of cattle
♦ Selective IgG2 deficiency of Red Danish cattle
♦ Chediak–Higashi syndrome of several species. A defect of neutrophil and monocyte phagocytic activity; not a real immunodeficiency

Secondary
Patient with normal immune processes at birth loses immunoefficiency, usually temporarily, because of effects of **immunosuppressors**.
♦ FPT, failure of passive transfer of antibodies in colostrum
♦ Virus infections, e.g. equine herpesvirus infection in neonatal foals, rinderpest, bovine virus diarrhea, hog cholera, causing lymphatic tissue suppression
♦ Bacterial infections, e.g. *Mycoplasma* spp., *Mycobacterium paratuberculosis*
♦ Physiological stresses, e.g. birth causing immunosuppression in fetus and in dam, e.g. periparturient rise of worm infestation
♦ Plant toxins, e.g. ptaquiloside in bracken, mycotoxins, e.g. T2 mycotoxin, industrial chemicals, e.g. tetrachlorethylene extracted soybean meal, atomic irradiation
♦ Environmental pollutants, e.g. polychlorinated biphenyls (possibly)
♦ Glucocorticoids
♦ Nutritional deficiency of zinc, and possibly many other nutrients
♦ Possibly cold and heat stress

Clinical findings

♦ Repeated or continuous infections, especially in young during first 6 weeks of age, which respond poorly to treatment
♦ Increased susceptibility to low-grade pathogens and infectious agents not usually encountered in immunocompetent animals
♦ Usually innocuous, attenuated vaccines cause illness
♦ Persistent leukopenia, lymphopenia or neutropenia, sometimes with thrombocytopenia

Clinical pathology

♦ Changes in ratios of classes of immunoglobulins (IgG, IgA, IgG(T), IgM)
♦ Numbers of lymphocytes
♦ T-lymphocyte function
♦ Changes in serum levels of complement

Necropsy findings

♦ Hypoplasia of lymph nodes and thymus
♦ Depletion of lymphocytes and absence of germinal centres in lymphoid tissue

♦ Lesions of incidental infectious disease with minimal infiltration by inflammatory cells

Diagnosis

Easily missed unless a group affected with poorly pathogenic infections, especially neonates.

Treatment

No effective, long-term treatment for primary disease. Secondary immunodeficiencies may recover spontaneously when suppressor removed but recovery rate not high because of death due to infection, in many cases with organisms not susceptible to standard antibacterial agents.

3

DISEASES OF THE NEWBORN

Diseases of animals born alive at term during their first month of life need to be viewed in the context of perinatal disease, disease of the offspring just before, during and immediately after parturition.

PERINATAL DISEASE [VM8 p. 107]

Includes:
- **Fetal disease** – diseases during intrauterine life, fetal death, mummification, goiter, developmental defects. Prolonged gestation, premature birth, abortion, stillbirth. Minimal gestational age for viable birth:
  - Foal – 300 days
  - Calf – 240 days
  - Lamb – 138 days
  - Piglet – 108 days
- **Parturient disease** – disease developing during parturition, e.g. fetal hypoxia, soft tissue bruising
- **Postnatal disease:**
  - Early postnatal disease (within 48 hours of birth), e.g. hypothermia, starvation
  - Delayed postnatal disease (2–7 days of age), e.g. congenital defects, omphalophlebitis, septicemia related to hypogammaglobulinemia
  - Late postnatal disease (1–4 weeks), e.g. late onset enteric and respiratory disease

Lambs

Well-managed flocks average <10% mortality; 35% not uncommon; higher in flocks with specific problems
- Mostly perinatal disease due to physical causes, exposure to bad weather (hypothermia), dam mismothering, insufficient milk (hypoglycemia)

- Indicators include low birth weight lambs, too high birth weight causing dystocia, poor body condition or overweight ewes, inexperienced maiden ewes
- Stillbirths in overweight single lambs causing fetal hypoxia and fatal dystokia
- Infectious abortion
- Predation and predation injury
- Poor mothering, especially merinos or dams with multiple lambs

Dairy calves

Well-managed herds with no problems average mortality of 2–4%. With poor management can be 20%, with a major disease problem in some years losses can be as high as 60%. Important risk factors are:
- Deficiency of colostrum intake
- Poor accommodation in housed herds
- Quality of care by minders
- Presence of highly pathogenic *Escherichia coli* serotypes

Beef calves

Accurate perinatal figures not common; most data relate to birth-to-weaning mortality; 3–7% the usual range. Risk factors include:
- Birth size
- Dystokia index in dam; heifers much higher
- Hypothermia in cold climates

♦ Scours and pneumonia the common diseases
♦ Inherited congenital defects in closely bred stud cattle in most breeds

Piglets

Non-infectious causes are the big risks up till weaning. Pre-weaning losses average 12–19% of pigs born alive. Important risk factors:
♦ Crushing
♦ Starvation, insufficient teats, milk, poor mothering
♦ Congenital abnormalities, e.g. splayleg, gut atresia, cardiac defects
♦ Infectious disease
♦ Stillbirths, piglets dying during the birth process

Restraining losses depends on management including:
♦ Batch farrowing to ensure close surveillance
♦ Farrowing crates to reduce crushing
♦ Selection of sows for mothering ability
♦ Cross-farrowing to equalize varied birth weights
♦ Artificial rearing, with added gammaglobulin, to reduce enteric disease
♦ Avoid too big litters and low birth weights
♦ Avoid hypothermia

Foals

Mortality usually less than 2%. Risk factors include:
♦ Multiple births: less than 50% of twins survive
♦ Immaturity due to premature birth
♦ Congenital defect

♦ Birth injury
♦ Maladjustment syndrome
♦ Enteric infections
♦ Septicemia

Close surveillance and intensive care for newborn foals can greatly reduce their mortality

SPECIAL INVESTIGATION OF ANY NEONATAL DEATHS (ILLNESS)

History

♦ Duration of pregnancy – are births at term
♦ Serological. Dam, newborn (precolostral also if possible)
♦ Age of onset, age of death
♦ Prevalence in age, family and management groups, including dam parity groups
♦ Litter size
♦ Health of littermates
♦ Environment quality including weather, housing, care by staff, especially colostrum intake

Clinical examination

♦ What is abnormality
♦ Characteristic clinical signs

Necropsy examination

♦ Estimate gestational age from body weight, crown–rump length
♦ Time of death relative to parturition
♦ Did neonate drink?
♦ Any birth injury
♦ Specimens for lab examine; abortus, placenta.

CONGENITAL DEFECTS [VM8 p. 112]

Etiology

Virus infections

♦ Hog cholera virus – natural infection and vaccine strains
♦ Bluetongue virus – natural infections and vaccine strains
♦ Bovine virus diarrhea virus – natural and experimental infections with non-cytopathic biotypes
♦ Border disease virus
♦ Akabane virus
♦ Cache Valley virus
♦ Unidentified virus causing congenital tremor of pigs

Elemental and industrial poisons

♦ Parbendazole, cambendazole
♦ Methallibure
♦ Apholate
♦ Organophosphatic compounds, possibly

Poisonous plants

♦ Veratrum californicum
♦ Lupinus spp.
♦ Astragalus and Oxytropis spp.
♦ Nicotiana spp.
♦ Conium maculatum
♦ Leucaena leucocephala

Inherited defects

A very large number of inherited defects is dealt with in Chapter 34.

Nutritional deficiencies
♦ Iodine
♦ Copper
♦ Manganese
♦ Cobalt
♦ Vitamin A
♦ Vitamin D

Physical agents
♦ Beta or gamma irradiation, severe exposure
♦ Hyperthermia, experimentally only

Pathogenesis

Disruptive events, including genetic influences, viral infections and poisons, during a pregnancy may cause:
♦ Chromosomal aberration, genetic mutations in unattached zygotes
♦ Early fetal death or abortion at blastula or gastrula stage
♦ Embryonic death or malformation in attached embryo undergoing organogenesis. Early insults cause more defects. Organs affected are those undergoing major change at the time. At fetal growth period insults cause fetal death leading to abortion, mummification or stillbirths, or weak neonates, destined to die. Animals with congenital defects are the survivors

Congenital defects, depending on the locus of effect of the noxious agent, may cause:
♦ Local defects in morphogenesis causing structural malformations
♦ Deformities in parts of the body that have already undergone tissue differentiation
♦ Enzyme deficiencies e.g. citrullinemia and the abiotrophies

Clinical findings

Details of each congenital defect are listed under the heading of each causative agent. General principles include:
♦ Half the neonates with congenital defects are stillborn and may escape the diagnostic net
♦ Congenital defects of the nervous and musculoskeletal systems are readily visible and may achieve a distorted importance in statistical data
♦ Defects present at birth may be more often identified than those that develop subsequently, e.g. the abiotrophies, the lysosomal storage diseases
♦ Many patients have more than one defect

Clinical pathology

Tests for individual nutritional deficiencies and poisonings are dealt with under their several headings.
♦ In suspected viral teratogens precolostral blood samples from the patient may indicate intra-uterine infection by the presence of specific antibodies. After drinking colostrum a positive titre may have been attained by passive absorption
♦ High blood levels of gammaglobulins in precolostral patients suggest antenatal infection without identifying the specific agent
♦ Blood samples for attempted isolation of unknown viruses, or subsequent check for antibodies when a new agent is isolated, are standard practice

Necropsy findings

The need is for complete necropsy examinations of suspect patients. This includes careful histopathological examination of suspected organs, and the use of special stains where necessary.

Diagnosis

A patho-anatomic diagnosis is usually not difficult using a standard clinical and necropsy examination. Specific etiological diagnoses are more difficult because most congenital defects can be caused by a variety of pathogens. Deciding which of the possibles is the specific cause can be an expensive exercise and is not undertaken unless a number of animals or a large area is involved. A major difficulty is that the defect is not observed until a long time after the noxious influence, often a fleeting one, was applied.

A detailed examination of a congenital defect incident must include:
♦ Pedigree analysis
♦ Nutritional history of dams, including changes in feed sources
♦ Disease history of dams
♦ History of drugs used in treatment of dams
♦ Movement of dams to other localities during pregnancy
♦ Season of year when teratogen operated
♦ History of animals, especially sires, introduced to herd

INTRA-UTERINE GROWTH RETARDATION [VM8 p. 117]

Failure to attain normal stature, distinct from failure to gain weight.

Etiology

♦ Dwarfism in cattle
♦ **Runting** in piglets

Runting
Small stature at birth and subsequent failure to grow at same rate as litter mates. Crown-to-rump measurement less than normal, slighter build, relatively larger head than nor-mal, domed forehead. Have a low metabolic rate and reduced skeletal muscle respiratory enzyme activity. Core body temperature depressed and lesser response to cold. Mortality higher than normals but can be raised with proper care.

NEONATAL NEOPLASIA [VM8 p. 117]

Rare. Recorded in sporadic bovine leukosis. Sporadic cases of lymphosarcoma (foal), melanoma (foals, piglets), myeloid leukosis (piglet), hemangiosarcoma and lipoma in calves.

PERINATAL DISEASES CAUSED BY PHYSICAL AND ENVIRONMENTAL INFLUENCES [VM8 p. 118]

PRENATAL DISEASE

Modern perinatology, especially with foals, commences with examination of the fetus and its environment in utero by abdomino-centesis, ECG, and ultrasound, in order to establish the viability of the fetus, to detect abnormalities, and to predict future viability. The procedures involved are unlikely to come into everyday clinical use.

Prediction of early foaling, and the consequent high mortality rate, is an important prophylactic measure. Tests used include:
♦ Plasma progestogen levels are of some value in thoroughbreds
♦ Milk calcium concentrations fall dramatically just before birth

PREMATURE FOALS [VM8 p. 118]

Foals born from 300–320 day pregnancies can survive with adequate care.

Etiology

♦ Hypoadrenal corticalism is basic cause
♦ Additional dysfunctions may include pulmonary immaturity, leading to hypoxia.

Clinical findings

♦ Low birth weight
♦ Muscle weakness, recumbent, poor righting reflex
♦ Weak suck reflex
♦ Dyspnea
♦ Short, silky hair coat, pliant ears, soft lips
♦ Excessive passive limb mobility
♦ Very sloping pastern
♦ Incomplete tarsal and carpal ossification, lung immaturity radiologically

Clinical pathology

♦ Neutropenia, lymphopenia with narrow neutrophil to lymphocyte ratio. Poor-risk foals continue with this leukon
♦ Low blood glucose, low plasma cortisol
♦ Blood pH <7.25

Necropsy findings

♦ Placental pathology present including placentitis and large areas villous atrophy
♦ Long umbilical cords may be associated with fetal death or malformation
♦ Placental weight and surface area are likely to be other important criteria

IMMATURE FOALS [VM8 p. 118]

Full-term foals with all the above signs of prematurity.

DYSMATURE FOALS [VM8 p. 118]

Full-term foals with signs of immaturity and evidence of placental dysfunction or intra-uterine deprivation.

PARTURIENT INJURY AND
INTRAPARTUM DEATH [VM8 p. 119]

Injury during birth may result in death of the fetus. Intrapartum death may result from other causes.

Etiology

Intrapartum death

♦ Impaired fetal circulation and fetal hypoxia due to compression of umbilical cord between fetus and dam
♦ Fetal hypoxia due to prolonged birth process
♦ Injury to fetus by compression when fetus too large or dam's pelvis too narrow. Overfat dams, over-sized fetuses, immature, small dams
♦ Assisted birth with excessive traction may cause injury including limb dislocations, epiphyseal detachments, vertebral fracture, chest compression and rib fracture, intracranial hemorrhage

Parturient injury

♦ Non-fatal injury due to compression or excessive traction
♦ Fetal hypoxia may be a major factor in the development of weak calf syndrome
♦ Occlusion of the umbilicus or placental dysfunction during the second stage of labour in a mare can result in the foal being born in an advanced state of hypoxia, and is likely to be stillborn when delivered
♦ Hypovolemia caused by premature cutting of the umbilical cord in thoroughbred horses leads to hypoxia and the neonatal adjustment syndrome

Clinical findings

♦ Recumbency, weakness, poor sucking vigor, early death
♦ In prolonged gestation the head, especially the tongue, and limbs may be edematous, especially calves
♦ Hypoxic foals may be profoundly dyspneic at birth, and respiratory failure may occur at any time.

Clinical pathology and necropsy findings

Findings of trauma, shock, and multiple injuries in neonate and history of difficult birth usually confirm the diagnosis. Care

needed to differentiate from alloimmune hemolytic anemia in foals, and peracute septicemias in all species.

Treatment

♦ Warm environment, fluid and electrolyte therapy for shock, parenteral alimentation to replace lost intake of nourishment. Bone fractures, dislocations may need surgical treatment
♦ In foals avoidance of acidosis, following the collapse of blood flow regulation, is an essential part of treatment (200 ml of a 5% sodium bicarbonate solution I/V). A supply of oxygen and an oxygen delivery system are essential. Because respiratory failure is likely to occur at any time suitable resuscitation treatments need to be on hand
♦ Resuscitation system includes clearing the airway, artificial respiration by machine or manually via blowing in one nostril with the other closed off
♦ Failure of a dyspneic foal to respond to resuscitation therapy may be due to permanent lung problem, e.g. atelectasis
♦ Proper surveillance of parturition so as to avoid prolongation of the process can prevent fetal hypoxia

NEONATAL HYPOTHERMIA AND
HYPOGLYCEMIA [VM8 p. 120]

See also sections on hypothermia and baby pig disease.

Etiology

♦ Inadequate heating and bedding in housing, especially for piglets
♦ Lack of shelter, e.g. windbreaks, shelter sheds for lambs born outside in cold, wet weather
♦ Poor maternal nutrition due to underfeeding or specific nutritional deficiency reduces: fetal size, brown fat reserves, mammary size, colostrogenesis, milk flow jeopardizing energy supply, resistance to infection
♦ A poor mother–offspring bond may be maternal (usually genetic, e.g. highly strung Merinos, or inexperience as in primipara) or offspring (birth trauma a common cause). Harassment at parturition, separation from the group, young getting lost in long grass can disrupt bonding process. Worst form is sow hysteria

Clinical findings

♦ Tremor, weakness, lethargy, recumbency, coma
♦ Shrunken appearance
♦ Hypothermia

Clinical pathology

♦ Hypoglycemia
♦ Dehydration

Necropsy findings

♦ Empty gut
♦ Gelatinous brown fat depots
♦ Dehydration

Diagnosis

♦ Resembles neonatal septicemia, e.g. *Histophilus ovis* but fever rather than hypothermia
♦ Identification of cause e.g. mismothering hypoglycemia versus evaporative hypothermia depends on climate history and examination of environment for evidence of shelter provision

Treatment

♦ Glucose 2 g/kg Bwt (20% solution I/peritoneal)
♦ Thorough drying, exposure to hot dry air in a box or by a fan heater (40°C/104°F). Avoid hyperthermia
♦ Need good artificial rearing program or supervised return to dam on recovery
♦ **Prevention** requires correct timing for lambing or proper provision of shelter, e.g. shed lambing. Ewes shorn before lambing more likely to seek shelter than those in full wool

INDUCTION OF PREMATURE
PARTURITION (VM8 p. 122)

Cows

Induction of parturition in cows by the injection of corticosteroids during the last 6 weeks of pregnancy is now a widely used **management tool**:
♦ In areas where exact timing of lactation to fit pasture growth is financially rewarding
♦ Concentrate calving to permit maximum surveillance and minimize losses during calving
♦ Reduce calf size and minimize dystokia in heifers
♦ Synchronize calving and facilitate milk fever prevention with vitamin D analogs

Problems relate mostly to small size and viability of calves, poor colostrum antibody transfer and a higher than normal prevalence of mismothering. Retained placenta may also be a problem in some herds.

Mares

Induction by the injection of oxytocin is used in individual mares as a matter of management convenience. Unless the mare is pregnant more than 320 days, has substantial mammary development, and a good supply of colostrum, weak, injured foals, highly susceptible to infection, may result.

Piglets

Large-scale induction by a single injection on day 112–114 of cloprostenol (a prostaglandin analog) is very successful.

Ewes

An uncommon practice; dexamethazone or flumethasone used.

NEONATAL INFECTION [VM8 p. 124]

Etiology

All species – common infections
  Corynebacterium pyogenes
  Sphaerophorus necrophorus
  Streptococcus faecalis
  S. zooepidemicus
  Micrococcus spp.
  Pasteurella spp.

Calves – common infections
♦ Bacteremia and septicemia:
  Escherichia coli
  Listeria monocytogenes
  Pasteurella spp.
  Salmonella spp.
  Streptococcus spp.
♦ Enteritis:
  E. coli (enterotoxigenic serotypes)
  Salmonella spp.
  Rotavirus
  Coronavirus

Cryptosporidium parvum
Clostridium perfringens, types A B C
Rarely infectious bovine rhinotracheitis
and bovine virus diarrhea viruses

Calves – less common infections
Pseudomonas aeruginosa
Streptococcus pyogenes
Streptococcus faecalis
Streptococcus zooepidemicus
Pneumococcus spp.
◗ Enteritis due to:
Providentia stuarti
Chlamydia spp.
Actinobacillus equuli

Lambs – common infections
◗ Septicemia:
Escherichia coli
Listeria monocytogenes
◗ Bacteremia with arthritis:
Streptococcus spp.
Micrococcus spp.
Erysipelothrix insidiosa
◗ Umbilicus gas gangrene:
Clostridium septicum
Clostridium oedematiens
◗ Lamb dysentery:
Clostridium perfringens type B

Lambs – less common infections
◗ Tick pyemia:
Staphylococcus aureus
◗ Enteritis:
Escherichia coli
Rotavirus
◗ Pneumonia:
Salmonella abortusovis

Piglets – common infections
◗ Septicemia with joint, endocardium, and
meninges localization:
Streptococcus suis type 1
Streptococcus equisimilis
Streptococcus zooepidemicus
◗ Septicemia and arthritis:
Erysipelothrix insidiosa
◗ Septicemia:
Listeria monocytogenes
◗ Bacteremia, septicemia and enteritis:
Escherichia coli
Transmissible gastroenteritis virus
Swine pox virus
Vomiting and wasting disease virus
◗ Enteritis:
Clostridium perfringens
Rotavirus
Coccidia spp.

Foals – common infections
◗ Septicemia with localization in joints, etc.:
Escherichia coli
Actinobacillus equuli
Klebsiella pneumoniae
Streptococcus spp. (α hemolytic)
Streptococcus zooepidemicus
Rhodococcus equi
Salmonella typhimurium
◗ Septicemia:
Listeria monocytogenes
◗ Enteritis:
Clostridium perfringens
Rotavirus

Foals – less common infections
Enterobacter cloacae
Staphylococcus aureus
Pasteurella multocida
Pseudomonas aeruginosa
Serratia marcescens

Epidemiology

Source and route of infection
◗ Main source is enteric plus respiratory tract
flora of dam contaminating the environment
◗ Contamination of environment by other
neonates
◗ Also environment generally. Most neonatal infections are acquired externally
after birth
◗ Invasion portals include ingestion and
inhalation plus **umbilicus** by contact or
sucking by another calf
◗ Some infections acquired in utero, e.g.
Actinobacillus equuli, Salmonella abortivoequina, usually causing abortion, stillbirths and some neonates with septicemia
with localizations in joints, etc.

Risk factors
◗ Accumulation of infection in continuous
throughput housing and high stocking rate
at pasture
◗ Greater susceptibility in young to Escherichia coli, Clostridium perfringens types B
and C

Colostral considerations
◗ The immune system of newborn farm animals is anatomically complete, but functionally ineffective at birth and for the first
30 days of life. It is capable of producing
antibodies, even in the fetus; use is made of
this in the diagnosis of intra-uterine infections

♦ Farm animal neonates do not receive maternal antibodies transplacentally and are at grave risk if colostrum supply or antibody content are diminished

♦ Maternal antibodies (as IgG, IgA, IgM) are concentrated in colostrum by secretory activity of the mammary epithelium

♦ The antibodies are transferred passively across the neonatal intestinal epithelium during the first few hours of life and reach the circulation via the lymphatics

♦ Unabsorbed or re-excreted antibody exerts a protective effect against infection in the bowel

♦ Efficiency of passive immunity generated by ingestion of colostrum governed by **immunoglobulin mass** ingested by the neonate. The mass is dependent on **concentration** of immunoglobulins in the colostrum, and the **volume** of colostrum ingested

♦ Concentration of immunoglobulins in colostrum is much greater at the first milking of the lactation than at any other time. Factors that reduce colostral immunoglobulin levels are:
• Cows with leaky teats
• Cows pre-milked to relieve udder congestion
• Short dry periods (<30 days)
• Premature births
• Some breeds, e.g. American Holsteins. Amongst horses Arabians have the highest colostral immunoglobulin levels, thoroughbreds the lowest.
• Young cows, compared to mature cows
• The volume of colostrum that a neonate has to ingest in the first 24 hours varies with its immunoglobulin content. For Holstein calves 2.4 liters is recommended, preferably fed at the first feeding. For weak calves assistance will be required, e.g. helping the calf to suck the cow, nipple bottle or esophageal tube feeding. Dairy calves need assistance often, beef calves rarely. Lambs and piglets also achieve adequate intakes in most natural circumstances. Factors reducing colostrum intake include:
• Poor mothering by dam
• Bad udder, teat conformation
• Neonates weakened by birth trauma, hypothermia
• Husbandry systems that harass the neonate and dam
• The efficiency of absorption of ingested immunoglobulin is seriously influenced by the time lapse between birth and ingestion. Efficiency is much reduced by 8 hours and stopped by 24-36 hours.

Clinical findings

Septicemia

In infections with virulent, toxicogenic organisms fever, depression, mucosal petechiation, weakness, dehydration, acidosis recumbency, coma and death after a course often as short as 24 hours. Case mortality rate of the order of 75%.

Bacteremia

Depression, fever, toxemia, anorexia, often with heart murmur (endocarditis), pus in the anterior chamber of the eye (hypopyon, panophthalmitis), meningitis (pain, rigidity, convulsions), or arthritis (lameness and swollen joints). Course prolonged, several weeks. Survival rate high but some patients have continuing infirmity.

Clinical pathology

In horse practice, laboratory examination is used extensively to predict potential susceptibility of normal foals, and status of sick ones.

♦ Blood culture is the critical test, because it also helps to identify the specific cause and direct the treatment

♦ Variable leukon. Leukocytosis to leukopenia. High band neutrophil forms with toxic changes

♦ Hypoglycemia, hypoxia and acidosis are usual

♦ Serology of **precolostral serum** if intrauterine infection suspected

♦ Level of immunoglobulins in **postcolostral sera** as indicator of efficiency of **passive immunity transfer**. Early estimates at 12–18 hours allow time for prophylaxis in an individual case. Sampling can be much later when a herd check of husbandry procedures is the objective. Test kits are commercially available as latex agglutination, zinc sulphate turbidity, sodium sulphite precipitation test and a refractometer test

♦ **Specific gravity of colostrum** indicates immunoglobulin content and a good guide in mares to serum immunoglobulin levels likely to be attained in the foals. A similar but less efficient relationship applies to cattle

Necropsy findings

Lesions of toxemia and hyperthermia plus:
♦ Subserosal and submucosal hemorrhages

Embolic foci in many locations

Arthritis, endocarditis, meningitis, panophthalmitis in cases of longer duration

Diagnosis

Hypothermia and hypoglycemia cause similar syndromes to terminal septicemias in neonates. Bacteremias cause clinically recognizable syndromes but their significance, in terms of the need for a herd approach to prevention, is easy to miss.

Treatment

♦ Establish a specific antibacterial therapy, based if possible on a sensitivity test of the causative agent
♦ Mass medication not possible, individual injections and supportive fluids and electrolytes essential
♦ Blood transfusions (10–20 ml/kg I/V), or plasma (half dose rate) for calves provides antibodies. Plasma dose for foals 20 ml/kg I/V.

Prevention

♦ **Standard hygiene** includes cleanliness of the environment, quarantine of nursery if disease occurs, disinfection and clamping of navel, removal from the parturition unit as soon as possible after establishment of the dam–neonate bond
♦ A **nursery policy** of continuous throughput is most dangerous for infection; batch birthing and an all-in all-out policy, with cleaning and disinfection between batches recommended
♦ **Supervised parturition**, without unnecessary harassment, to minimize prolonged births, exposure to cold, or high temperatures, and minimize hypoxia, hypoglycemia, hypothermia (or hyperthermia) and birth injury
♦ **Colostrum intake** must be adequate (10% of birth weight in first 24 hours). If necessary in dairy herds milk colostrum and administer by nipple bottle or esophageal tube within first 4 hours of birth, either as a single feed or 12-hourly feeds; leave the calf on the cow for 24 hours. Force-feeding is

not used in beef herds other than for injured calves which cannot suck normally
♦ Newborn calves bought into veal units can be **tested for blood levels of immunoglobulins**. Those with low levels can be placed under special surveillance or prophylactic antibiotic cover or culled. A safer policy is to avoid buying calves not guaranteed to have been adequately colostrumed
♦ Newborn lambs for rearing units have the same problems, especially those from multiple births. Lambs require 200 ml/kg colostrum during first 18 hours
♦ **Stored colostrum** has the advantage that colostrum with a high immunoglobulin content can be selected and used to supplement normal supply. Storage can be refrigeration for 7 days or freezing
♦ **Cross-species colostrum**, usually bovine, is used for goat kids, piglets and foals but absorbed immunoglobulins have short half-life and a hemolytic anemia occurs in some lambs fed bovine colostrum
♦ Piglets have a special need for **supplemental heat** for the first 10 days, and to have their needle teeth clipped. Porcine immunoglobulin (10 g/kg then 2 g/kg daily for 10 days) a valuable support mechanism in problem herds and in the smaller piglets in large litters
♦ **Passive immunity** has disappeared in most animals by 6 months of age. The decline is fastest early so that effective immunity is likely to be lost by one month in foals and 2 months in calves
♦ Active immunization of neonates by **vaccination** is not practiced before 2 months of age because of the inadequate response of an immature immune system
♦ Increasing the colostral content of immunoglobulins by **vaccination of the dam** during pregnancy has some currency in the prophylaxis of neonatal diarrhea due to *Escherichia coli* infections in piglets and calves
♦ A common recommendation is to avoid **moving late-pregnant females** to new, distant locations to avoid exposing their offspring to infectious agents of which they have had no previous experience. The practice of calving females away from the home farm is also a common practice, and is not associated with obvious errors of immunity

PRINCIPLES OF PROVIDING CRITICAL CARE TO THE NEWBORN [VM8 p. 137]

Procedures devised principally for the care of valuable foals with life-threatening diseases include:
♦ The foal to be kept in a highly sanitary environment, entailing separation from the mare
♦ Maintain the environmental temperature and avoid hypothermia
♦ Appropriate bedding, e.g. air mattress, to avoid pressure sores; massage, grooming, turning
♦ Systemic supportive care provided until foal capable of independent survival. Includes fluids and electrolytes, immunoglobulins, alimentation with glucose, possibly protein hydrolysates or amino acids, plasma in foals with hypovolemia

♦ Frequent, complete physical and chemical monitoring of all body systems
♦ Ensure adequate passive immunity
 Foals in which the specific cause of illness is known can be supported beyond the specific treatment by this program. When the diagnosis is still uncertain the program offers a substantial alternative to a dedicated antibacterial regimen.
 Intensive care systems requiring expensive equipment and 24-hour attendance by skilled nursing personnel are beyond the resources of most practices. An alternative is a seasonal hospital unit by an independent organization to provide the service for a number of neighboring practices.

OMPHALITIS, OMPHALOPHLEBITIS AND URACHITIS IN NEWBORN FARM ANIMALS (NAVEL-ILL) [VM8 p. 140]

Etiology

Mixed infections with *Escherichia coli*, *Proteus* spp., *Staphylococcus* spp., *Actinomyces* (*Corynebacterium*) *pyogenes*

Epidemiology

Mostly sporadic cases. Enzootic in some herds or flocks where bedding or camping grounds are contaminated, or where hygiene at assisted births is inadequate.

Clinical findings

Omphalitis
♦ Signs commence 2–5 days after birth
♦ Umbilicus swollen, hot, painful, may drain via fistula
♦ Fever, depression, anorexia

Omphalophlebitis
♦ In older calves (1–3 months old)
♦ Mild fever
♦ Anorexia, lethargic
♦ Unthrifty due to chronic toxemia
♦ Umbilicus may or may not be enlarged
♦ Palpation or ultrasound examination may detect liver abscess

Omphaloarteritis
♦ Same age group and signs as omphalophlebitis except any abscesses are caudal to the umbilicus

Urachitis
♦ Same age group and signs of toxemia as omphalophlebitis
♦ Umbilicus normal or enlarged
♦ Cystitis with frequent, painful urination. Urine discharged at umbilicus or urethra or both
♦ Large abscess may be palpable posterior to umbilicus
♦ Contrast radiography reveals fistula connection to bladder

Clinical pathology

♦ Leukocytosis with shift to left
♦ Pyuria in urachal infection

Diagnosis

Distinctive syndromes except in older animals when umbilicus normal. Young patients with endocarditis, meningitis, arthritis and other embolic diseases resulting from bacteremia should be considered as candidates for an umbilical diagnosis.

Treatment

♦ Systemic, broad-spectrum antibiotic treatment needs to be continued for several weeks

♦ Surgical excision of thick-walled abscesses may be necessary
♦ Prevention depends on sanitary environment in the birthing area and application of residual disinfectants such as iodine tincture

4

PRACTICAL ANTIMICROBIAL THERAPEUTICS

This chapter discusses the principles of usage of antimicrobial therapeutic agents so as to avoid repeating them a number of times in the subsequent chapters.

SELECTION OF AN
ANTIMICROBIAL TREATMENT

Theoretical considerations

Successful antimicrobial therapy consists of maintaining at the site of infection a concentration of the drug that will result in the death or control of the infectious agent, without damaging the host. To achieve this it is necessary to know:
* The location of the infection
* The identity of the infection, established by culture
* The minimal inhibitory concentration of the relevant drugs

It would then be possible to select from amongst these drugs the preferred one on the basis of the drug's ability to:
* be active against the organism at the site of infection. The sample needs to be taken at or close to the site, and the specific sensitivity of the organism in the sample needs to be tested. Consideration of antimicrobial sensitivity of isolates is imperative in the light of increased resistance resulting from wide exposure of organisms to the antibiotics
* be administered in such a way as to maintain an effective inhibitory or lethal concentration
* be within the bounds of financial practicability

In the case of the acutely ill individual animal it is not possible to use all of the above criteria in the selection of an antimicrobial drug because of the need to commence treatment immediately. It is preferable to submit specimens from the patient for laboratory examination so that the interim choice of drug can be ratified or changed subsequently. In the case of an outbreak of disease in a group of animals examination of samples for causative microorganisms, and testing them for antibacterial sensitivity are essential steps before large-scale treatments begin. They are also advisable in single animal cases where the additional cost can be justified because a large capital investment is involved.

Practical applications

The alternative procedure to the complete laboratory examination for selecting an antimicrobial treatment is **selection on the basis of a complete clinical examination**. For example, a clinical diagnosis of strangles, or gangrenous staphylococcal mastitis can be quite accurate, and treatment needs to be instituted immediately if the animal or, in the case of mastitis, the gland is to be saved.

When there is a **group of possible diagnoses** the recommended alternatives include:
* Treatment of the two, or three, most likely infections
* Use of a broad-spectrum single drug or combination with **validation of the choice** based on response

Collection of samples for diagnosis

* Collect samples from acutely ill patients. Necropsy specimens from a fresh cadaver are best

- Samples taken from the expected locus of infection, e.g. rectal mucosal biopsy rather than feces for Johne's disease, tracheal aspirates for lung disease in preference to nasal swabs
- In a group problem sample a number of patients

Antimicrobial sensitivity tests

Sensitivity testing is unnecessary in most infections where sensitivity of the causative microbe is well established and not likely to vary. It is desirable for organisms whose sensitivity does vary or is susceptible to change by continued treatment by one or a group of antibacterial agents. Recommended applications of sensitivity testing include:

- **Simple disk tests** are approximate only because they take no account of the degree of sensitivity of the organism. It may be classed as insensitive to a drug but in fact be sensitive at a greater dose rate than that mirrored in the disk
- **Tube dilution tests** are an exact method for determining dose levels at which an organism is susceptible to each drug, but are laborious and expensive
- **Kirby–Bauer disks** give an indication of the minimal inhibitory concentration of each drug for the particular microorganism but have serious limitations in veterinary work and the results achieved with them should be considered with care. As in all sensitivity testing it is possible to get an excellent response to a clinical diagnosis when the laboratory sensitivity test indicates resistance of the infection to the drug
- **Sensitivity testing of subcultures** is much preferred to tests conducted on original platings because of the risks of interpretation in a mixed culture. Tests on original platings are condoned when:
  - Pure culture infections are likely, e.g. bovine mastitis
  - Speed is important and follow-ups on subcultures will be available

ANTIBIOTIC DOSAGE: THE RECOMMENDED DOSE

- Recommended, label doses of antibiotics are often too low and the time intervals between doses too long. They are **minimum** doses
- Dose rates should be 3–5 times the minimal inhibitory concentration for the causative organism
- Unnecessary overdosing should be avoided

because of potential toxicity with some drugs, the probability that resistance to the antibiotic will develop, the cost and the extended withdrawal time, an important consideration in farm animals

- Increased dose rates are necessary where the causative organism has only partial sensitivity, where there is necrotic tissue and a long diffusion path, or where mustering and handling problems require a single dose regimen
- Suitable doses for specific infections have been arrived at by the best possible method, clinical response trials, and are included, where necessary, in the sections on individual disease

ROUTES OF ADMINISTRATION

Each route has advantages and disadvantages.

Intravenous injection

Advantages

- Immediacy. Blood and tissue levels are attained quickly
- Blood and tissue levels are higher than with any other route. This is useful in:
  - Infections with moderately susceptible organisms
  - Chronic infections surrounded by necrotic tissue or abscess wall
  - Reducing the chance of development of stepwise resistant mutant organisms
  - Administration of low concentration, high volume antibacterials, e.g. sulfonamides

Disadvantages

- Chances of a toxic reaction are increased
- Accidental intravenous use of an intramuscular drug preparation
- Treatments must be given slowly
- Perivascular accidental lesions may follow use of an irritant solution

Intramuscular injection

Peak blood concentrations vary widely depending on formulation; the average is 30 minutes to 2 hours. Intramuscular injection is the most popular injection method in large animals but has some disadvantages:

- Encourages scar tissue formation, bad in meat producers
- In meat animals recommended injection in neck where scar most easily trimmed
- Bioavailability of injection varies with site.

Best in neck, moderate in shoulder and gluteal muscles, least in dewlap
♦ Drug residue persists longest at injection site; recommend no more than 20 ml at one site
♦ Severe reactions in some horses, especially oil-based formulations, rules site out in particular patients
♦ Irritant solutions in neck cause reining problems in horses; malpractice in some countries; preferred site is intramuscular between forelimbs
♦ Accidental intravascular injection can be fatal; avoided by withdrawal of syringe plunger

Intraperitoneal injection

Favored in:
♦ Feedlot animals close to marketing to avoid local reaction
♦ Pigs used for bulky injections
♦ Cases of peritonitis; in cattle injection at midpoint right paralumbar fossa
♦ Horses with peritonitis; injection via paracentesis cannula at ventral midpoint of abdomen (linea alba)
♦ For injections likely to cause respiratory distress by intravenous route, e.g. toxemic patients, tetracyclines

Subcutaneous injection

Unpopular alternative to intramuscular injection in large animals. Used mostly in very small animals, e.g. piglets.
♦ Deposition in fat depot impairs absorption
♦ Irritant formulations cause swelling, possibly sterile abscess

Oral dosing

Used extensively in pre-ruminants, foals and piglets. Popular for repeat treatments by farmers. Best route for enteric infections but long-term ingestion can cause villous atrophy in calves.
♦ Blood levels much less than after injection; requires 2–5 times injection dose. Due to destruction in rumen; varies between antibiotics
♦ Absorption efficiency varies with volume and nature of ingesta, gut motility
♦ Benzyl penicillin is destroyed in stomach
♦ Aminoglycosides and polymixin drugs not absorbed from gut
♦ Administration of antibiotics in glucose–electrolyte–glycine solution probably increases absorption

♦ Administration in milk of some drugs (e.g. oxytetracycline, chloramphenicol, trimethoprim) binds the drug and reduces absorption
♦ In ruminants, disrupts ruminal flora causing depression, anorexia, ruminal stasis, custard-like feces with much undigested fibre; requires gut repopulation by cud transfer
♦ In horses over 3 months old, commonest with tetracycline, lincomycin, can cause persistent debilitating, sometimes fatal, diarrhea
♦ Blood levels variable and delayed (12–18 hours)

Mass medication by ingestion
Prolonged (>2 weeks) oral medication (especially tetracyclines, chloramphenicol) in all species may cause superinfection with yeasts, *Pseudomonas* or *Staphylococcus* spp. causing persistent, severe diarrhea.

Pigs
Popular in water or feed for treatment, prophylaxis pigs:
♦ Preferred regimen is initial injection treatment of sick pigs, plus mass medication for subsequent treatments and prophylaxis for rest of group
♦ Sick pigs more likely to drink, so water preferred. Also home mixing quicker and easier with water
♦ In automatic watering systems, header tank isolated and medicated or turned off and special small drinking drums with nipple drinkers substituted
♦ Drug needed in one day water supply = total body weight of pig group × mg/kg dose rate of antibiotic
♦ Fresh mixture daily because of drug deterioration in water
♦ Medicate group for 5 days

Cattle
Unreliable and difficult in water so usually supplied in feed:
♦ Rate of supplementation determined on basis of amount of feed being fed so system best suited to feedlot. Cattle at pasture can be fed a daily supplement ration containing daily dose of antibiotic

Miscellaneous other routes of antibiotic administration

Popular alternative routes, aimed at providing closer proximity of drug to organism, include:

Intra-articular
Intramammary
Intrapleural
Subconjunctival
Intratracheal
Intra-uterine
In most cases supplementation by parenteral
injection provides better antibiotic cover for
all local tissues. Mastitis therapy is character-
ised by almost universal intramammary
therapy.

DRUG DISTRIBUTION

Oral absorption

Most antibiotics and sulfonamides are ab-
sorbed from the alimentary tract, with vary-
ing degrees of efficiency. Exceptions are:
   Aminoglycosides
   Benzyl penicillin
   Methicillin
   Phthalylsulfathiazole
   Phthalylsulfacetamide
   Sulfaguanidine
   Succinyl sulfathiazole

Distribution in body compartments

♦ The rate of diffusion of antibiotics from the
   vascular system to tissue fluids, and into
   cells is governed by many factors and details of these in large animals are complex
   and not subject to generalization
♦ Most antibiotics diffuse freely in extracellular fluid
♦ Sulfonamides, tetracyclines and chloram-
   phenicols are unique in that they can enter
   cells
♦ Barriers to diffusion from blood to cerebrospinal fluid and brain, to serous cavities,
   synovial fluid, eye, placenta and fetus have
   limited significance because the barriers are
   breached when they are inflamed

Excretion

♦ Excretion of most antibacterial agents is
   via urine
♦ Excretion via the bile (an enterohepatic
   cycle) occurs with penicillins, tetracyclines
   and possibly erythromycin

DURATION OF TREATMENT

♦ Generally treatment needs to be for 3–5
   days or for 1 or 2 days after signs disappear

♦ Chronic disease with localization 2–3
   weeks

DRUG COMBINATIONS

Fixed dose antibiotic combinations are declining in popularity because of alternative
ways of obtaining a broad spectrum of antibacterial activity for mixed infections, or a
synergistic effect for the control of single
organism infections. Whether synergism
occurs and its degree is obscure in most
situations and use of combinations for this
purpose is unwarranted.
♦ Mixtures of bactericidal drugs give indifferent results
♦ Mixtures of bacteriostatic drugs also give
   indifferent results
♦ Mixtures of bactericidal and bacteriostatic
   effects may result in antagonism
♦ Fixed dose combinations are frowned on;
   recommended procedure is the full dose for
   each of the components of the combination, given separately at separate sites
♦ Some well-known synergistic combinations are:
   • Penicillin–streptomycin for sheep foot-
      rot, mycotic dermatitis
   • Carbenicillin–gentamicin for *Pseudomo-
      nas aeruginosa*, *Klebsiella* and *Proteus*
      spp. infections
   • Tylosin–oxytetracycline for *Pasteurella*
      spp. infections
   • Trimethoprim–sulfonamides for a var-
      iety of infections
♦ The availability of genuine broad spectrum
   antibiotics, e.g. ampicillin or amoxycillin,
   and trimethoprim potentiated sulfonamides has reduced the need for combinations. Combinations usually have the
   advantage of a lesser price tag, and in most
   comparisons are less toxic than the single
   drugs

ADDITIONAL FACTORS
DETERMINING THE SELECTION
OF AN ANTIMICROBIAL AGENT
FOR THERAPY

Cost
Primary cost differences are tangible. The
need for revisits with some drugs may bias
veterinarians against them

Toxicity
Especially at:
♦ High dose rates
♦ Long course
♦ Extra-label use

Freedom from adverse reactions

Bactericidal versus bacteriostatic drugs (Table 4.1)

Bacteriostatic drugs have advantages including better diffusibility into cells but are contraindicated in circumstances where:

♦ The microbial population is overwhelming, e.g. septicemia
♦ Normal body defenses are impaired as in bracken poisoning
♦ Localization, e.g. in joints, is likely
♦ Infection is with a capsulated organism, e.g. *Rhodococcus equi*, *Klebsiella* spp. with antiphagocytic activity

Packaging to prevent deterioration of drug

Includes instructions on preservation of reconstituted preparations and how long they should be kept

Poor response to treatment

Selection of an antibacterial drug in many clinical situations is an educated guess. How to make a second choice depends on the following:

♦ A 3 day test period is standard practice
♦ Change to a completely different class of drug

Table 4.1 Mode of action of antimicrobial drugs [VM8 p. 151]

Group 1: bactericidal	Group 2: bacteriostatic
Penicillins	All sulfonamides
Benzylpenicillin	Tetracycline
Methicillin	Macrolides
Cloxacillin	Erythromycin
Ampicillin	Oleandomycin
Amoxycillin	Spiramycin
Carbenicillin	Tylosin
etc.	Carbomycin
Aminoglycosides	Chloramphenicol
Streptomycin	Lincomycin
Kanamycin	Trimethoprim
Neomycin	
Gentamicin	
Paromomycin	
Polymyxins	
Cephalosporins	
Vancomycin	
Bacitracin	
Novobiocin	
Nitrofurans	

♦ Continue with same treatment but at a higher dose, more frequent intervals, different route, e.g. I/V instead of oral
♦ Supplement the treatment with local treatment, e.g. into a joint
♦ Surgical drainage or excision where much necrotic tissue present or other circumstance where diffusion path is long
♦ Ensure that supplementary treatment, e.g for dehydration, is performed
♦ In the best of all possible circumstances change to the drug indicated by the sensitivity and culture test initiated when the case was first seen

Withdrawal requirements

Residues of antibacterial treatments in animal tissues and excretions are forbidden because they:

♦ Are a public health hazard
♦ Damage industrial food processes
♦ Violate local and international laws
♦ The public's insistence on wholesome food

Veterinarians are legally responsible for warning farmers to withdraw animals from sale and to withhold milk from cows treated with antibiotics for the duration of legally specified

♦ **withdrawal times** for meat animals
♦ **withholding time** for milk

specified on the label of the drug used. These times include the time needed for the excretion and metabolism of the drug and in the case of repeated dosing with aminoglycosides, a **washout period** to permit removal of deposits from some tissues.

When a veterinarian uses an antibacterial other than as specified on the label, an **extra-label** use, such as by:

♦ Larger dose rate
♦ At shorter intervals
♦ For a longer period
♦ By a different route of administration
♦ Or for an unspecified disease

or when the necessary information is neither advertised nor available, there is a risk of the animal or product being condemned when offered for sale and the veterinarian becoming liable to a claim for redress by the farmer.

To ensure that the patient's tissues and products are clear of violative residues, and to avoid the inevitable informed guesswork in unusual situations, field tests are available to circumvent the high costs and delays of full laboratory assays. The tests are accurate in detecting penicillins but many are unreliable for other antibacterials and give many false positives because of natural inhibitory substances in tissues.

Antibiotic residues in milk commonly originate from:

- Extended usage
- Excessive doses
- Forgetting to record treatment
- Prolonged clearance time of the drug or formulation used
- Failure to identify and mark treated animals
- Contamination of milking equipment
- Non-compliance with instructions by farmer
- Products used other than as specified on label
- Failure of veterinarian to advise farmer of withdrawal or withholding time
- Withholding of milk from treated quarter only when contamination of other quarters will have occurred
- Purchase of cows not known to have been treated
- Use of long-acting dry period treatments in lactating cows
- Milking dry cows

Antibiotic residues in red meat, cull cows and bob calves especially; fat cattle are largely disease-free in the period just before sale. Most common causes:

- Failure to observe the withdrawal period
- Use of an unapproved drug
- Use of an approved drug in an unapproved manner, usually excessive dosage
- Feeding milk or colostrum from a treated cow to a calf
- Intramuscular injection, less commonly oral (especially boluses given to calves), and intramammary infusions
- Early calving or short dry period after administration of dry period treatment

Principal violative drugs in red meat are:
streptomycin
penicillin
oxytetracycline
gentamicin
sulfamethazine
neomycin

Antibiotic residues in pig meat are as for red meat plus the more serious source of antibiotic inclusions in feeds. Sulfonamides are a major source of error. Common errors are:

- Failure to observe withdrawal requirements
- Carryover from treated to untreated feed in the mill or on the farm
- Continuous, cutaneous contamination with polluted feces or urine; coprophagy may also contribute
- Contamination of water system as a result of mass medication via drinking water

5

DISEASES OF THE ALIMENTARY TRACT – I

CLINICAL INDICANTS

The principal clinical signs and clinicopathological findings on which diagnoses of alimentary tract disease are based include the following.

Abdomen, adhesions in

Clinical findings Thin, strong threads or sheets of tissue connecting viscera to each other or peritoneum; mainly vertical, often forming a jumbled mass of tough fibrous tissue. Can be confused with **tight mesenteric bands** in equine colic.

Occurs in Chronic peritonitis.

Abdomen distension

Clinical findings Abdominal volume significantly increased above normal.

Occurs in:
♦ Gut distension (see below)
♦ Chronic peritonitis
♦ Ascites

Abdomen distension, asymmetric

Clinical findings Unilateral distension, occurs significantly only in ruminants.

Occurs in:
♦ Left distension – rumen tympany
♦ Right upper – colon and/or cecum distension
♦ Right lower – abomasum distension

Abdomen gaunt

Clinical findings Abdominal volume significantly less than normal.

Occurs in:
♦ Chronic enteritis, e.g. Johne's disease
♦ Starvation

Abdomen, mass in

Clinical findings Mass palpable per rectum, rarely through abdominal wall. (See also impacted viscus.)

Occurs in:
♦ Fat necrosis
♦ Intussusception
♦ Phytobezoar
♦ Neoplasm
♦ Mesenteric, retroperitoneal abscess

Abdomen pain

See Pain, abdominal, this section.

Abdomen, tight mesenteric bands in

Clinical findings Thin edge of mesentery stretched tight, palpable rectally extending more or less vertically in posterior abdomen; usually associated with a heavy section of intestine distended with fluid or impacted with ingesta.

Occurs in:
♦ Intestinal obstruction, horse
♦ Impaction, large intestine, horse

Anus dilated

Occurs in   Cauda equina lesion.

Anus missing

Occurs as   Congenital atresia.

Anus constricted

Occurs in   Inherited constriction rectum–vagina, cattle, pigs.

Back down-arched

See Pain, abdominal – spontaneous, this section.

Ballottement

See gut distension.

Body weight low

Clinical findings   Weight loss, failure to gain weight, emaciation. Caused by most of the abnormalities in this list, e.g. faulty prehension, mastication, swallowing, digestion, absorption.

N.B. Probably the commonest cause of emaciation in farm animals, singly and in groups, and often the last to be considered as a diagnostic possibility.

Constipation

Includes **scant feces** of cattle.

Clinical signs include:
♦ Decreased frequency of defecation
♦ Decreased water content and volume of feces; **scant feces** in cattle are very small amounts (200–300 ml), pasty (ketchup consistency) and over-digested
♦ Firmer than normal consistency
♦ Prolonged alimentary tract transit time
♦ Full rectum in some

Causes include:
♦ Peritonitis, e.g. traumatic reticuloperitonitis of cattle causing pain on straining
♦ Pyloric achalasia, spasm. Diseases causing decreased outflow from stomachs
♦ Vagus indigestion (scant feces)
♦ Large intestine impaction in horses
♦ Debility of old age
♦ Deficient diet bulk, usually fiber lack
♦ Chronic dehydration
♦ Partial obstruction large intestine
♦ Painful condition of anus

♦ Paralytic ileus
♦ Grass sickness
♦ Chronic zinc poisoning in cattle
♦ Rectum paralysis due to cauda equina neuritis
♦ Late pregnancy cattle

Coughing up food

See Swallowing faults, this section.

Cud dropping

See Mastication faults, this section.

Defecation frequency increased

Clinical findings   Diarrhea.

Occurs in:
♦ Enteritis
♦ Intestinal hypermotility
♦ Diet with high water content

Defecation frequency decreased

Clinical findings:
♦ Constipation
♦ Gut motility diminished

Occurs in:
♦ Low digestibility diet
♦ Late pregnancy
♦ Rumen indigestion
♦ Intestine obstruction
♦ Paralytic ileus
♦ Intestine impaction
♦ Peritonitis
♦ Rectum paralysis
♦ Cauda equina neuritis

Defecation straining

See Tenesmus, this section.

Dehydration-shock

An important feature of alimentary tract disease in which vomiting and diarrhea are important signs. Also in acute obstructions in pigs and horses where accumulation of saliva and gut secretions causes distension and reflex hypersecretion of fluids into the gut lumen. Except for obstructions at the pylorus and upper duodenum, hypersecretion not such a serious factor in ruminant intestinal obstruction.

Diarrhea

Clinical findings:
♦ Increased frequency of defecation
♦ Increased fecal water content and volume
♦ Thinner consistency of feces
♦ Decreased alimentary tract transit time
♦ Dehydration

Causes include:
♦ Enteritis
♦ Secretory enteropathy, e.g. colibacillosis
♦ Malabsorption due to
  • Villous atrophy
  • Hypocuprosis due to excessive molybdenum intake
  • Lactose intolerance in foals
♦ Carbohydrate engorgement in ruminants
♦ Undifferentiated diarrhea in horses
♦ Neurogenic, e.g. excitement
♦ Some cases of ileal hypertrophy, ileitis–diverticulitis–adenomatosis
♦ Abomasum or stomach ulcer
♦ Tumor, e.g. intestine adenocarcinoma
♦ Portal vein hypertension as in:
  • Congestive heart failure, end stages
  • Hepatic fibrosis
♦ Endotoxic mastitis, cattle

Digestion tests failure

Tests used mostly in horses:
♦ Tests of gastric, small intestinal, pancreatic function – starch digestion test
♦ Lactose digestion in foal – lactose digestion test
♦ Test for radioactive material in feces after I/V injection to test for protein-losing enteropathy

Endoscopic abnormality

Limited use of fiberoptic gastroendoscopy in sedated horses for observation of lesions in esophagus, stomach

Feces, abnormality of

Volume increased in:
♦ Diarrhea generally
♦ Reduced bowel absorption – malabsorption syndrome
  • D-Xylose absorption test
  • Oral glucose absorption test
  • Feces bulky
♦ Enteritis

Volume decreased in:
♦ Constipation generally
♦ Intestine impaction
♦ Intestine obstruction
♦ Paralytic ileus
♦ Vagus indigestion

Feces absent:
♦ Intestinal obstruction
♦ Paralytic ileus
♦ Intestine impaction
♦ Rectum stricture
♦ Rectum impaction
♦ Rectum obstruction
♦ Anus atresia
♦ Intestine segment atresia

Feces dry, hard:
♦ Constipation
♦ Intestine impaction

Feces soft, watery:
♦ Diarrhea
♦ Enteritis
♦ Malabsorption syndrome

Feces contain excess mucus:
♦ Enteritis

Feces contain undigested seeds:
♦ Carbohydrate indigestion

Feces contain blood:
♦ Digested blood in:
  • Pharyngeal laceration, rarely
  • Gastric, abomasal ulcer
  • Enteritis especially salmonellosis, coccidiosis
  • Abomasal ulcer, gastric ulcer, enteritis
♦ Undigested blood in lower bowel hemorrhage, e.g.
  • Rarely in intestinal obstruction, e.g. thromboembolic colic
  • Mesenteric vessel occlusion, e.g. mesentery torsion in horse

Feces color abnormal consistent with medication and diet:
♦ Pale on milk diet
♦ Pale in very rare circumstance of complete absence bile pigments

Feces abnormal odor:
♦ Putrescent in severe enteritis, usually accompanied by high mucus content

Flank-watching

See Pain, abdominal, this section.

Food dropped, not prehended

Clinical findings Patient is hungry and attempts to feed but is either very slow taking it in or fails to do so due to difficulty in:
♦ Moving feed into mouth with tongue
♦ Grasping feed with teeth
♦ Biting off pasture with teeth or dental pad

Occurs in:
♦ Tongue paralysis
♦ Masseter muscle paralysis
♦ Tongue swollen
♦ Tongue shrunken
♦ Malapposition incisor teeth with teeth or dental pad
  due to:
  • Inherited displaced molars
  • Inherited mandibular prognathism
  • Inherited congenital osteopetrosis
♦ Rickets
♦ Absence of some incisor teeth
♦ Pain in mouth due to:
  • Stomatitis, glossitis
  • Oral foreign body
  • Decayed teeth, fluorosis
♦ Congenital defects tongue, lips
♦ Inherited smooth tongue

Foreign body

♦ Mouth (see stomatitis)
♦ Pharynx (see pharynx obstruction)
♦ Ruminant forestomachs (see traumatic reticuloperitonitis, traumatic hepatitis, traumatic splenitis, abomasitis)
♦ Intestine (see intestinal obstruction)

Gums swollen

See Stomatitis, this section.

Intestine distension

Clinical findings:
♦ Distension of abdomen in some cases
♦ Distended loops of intestine palpable per rectum
♦ Ping on percussion of abdomen over viscus distended with gas
♦ Fluid sloshing signs on ballottement or shaking of abdomen

Occurs in:
♦ Intestine tympany, horses, pigs
♦ Obstruction, impaction of large intestine of pig
♦ Meconium retention in some foals
♦ Small intestine obstruction of horse
♦ Cecum–colon distension/volvulus

Intestine impacted

Clinical findings:
♦ Impacted loops intestine palpable per rectum
♦ Intestinal sounds reduced
♦ Feces dry, formed
♦ Subacute abdominal pain

Occurs in:
♦ Impaction large intestine horse
♦ Meconium retention foal

Intestinal sounds increased

Clinical findings:
♦ Increased frequency and intensity of intestinal sounds
♦ Decreased sojourn of ingesta in gut, including diarrhea
♦ Pain, usually in bouts, severe, synchronous with periods of hypermotility
♦ Vomiting if hypermotility sufficiently intense

Occurs in:
♦ Spasmodic colic
♦ Enteritis
♦ Distension of gut, e.g. early stages acute intestine obstruction, long term in chronic dilation, e.g. vagus indigestion, colic due to gut constriction by adhesions

Intestinal sounds reduced/absent

Clinical findings:
♦ Decreased frequency and intensity of intestinal sounds
♦ Increased alimentary tract sojourn, overdigestion
♦ Persistent dull pain due to chronic, mild distension
♦ Decreased food intake

Occurs in:
♦ Debility
♦ Old age
♦ Impaired prehension, mastication
♦ High fiber diet
♦ Intestine impaction
♦ Peritonitis
♦ Paralytic ileus

Kicking at belly

See Pain, abdominal, this section.

Liver enlargement

Clinical findings:
Liver palpable behind costal arch

Occurs in:
♦ Hepatitis
♦ Neoplasia
♦ Amyloidosis

Liver painful

Clinical findings:
Pain on percussion over caudal right ribs

Occurs in:
♦ Liver abscess
♦ Caudal vena caval syndrome
♦ Infectious necrotic hepatitis
♦ Cholangiohepatitis

Mastication painful

Clinical findings:
♦ Slow jaw movements interrupted by pauses
♦ Dropping feed while eating, e.g. quidding, cud dropping
♦ Expression of pain while chewing
♦ Salivation and refusal to chew
♦ Much undigested feed in feces

Occurs in:
♦ Stomatitis, glossitis
♦ Oral foreign body
♦ Decayed teeth

Mastication slow

Clinical findings:
♦ Slow chewing
♦ Pausing for long periods while chewing

Occurs in:
♦ Paralysis in jaw muscles
♦ Teeth malpositioned
♦ Mental disturbance as in
  • Encephalomalacia
  • Hepatic encephalopathy

Mouth/muzzle, mucosal erosions

Clinical findings:
♦ Shallow, initially small, discrete (later contiguous, large) mucosal discontinuities
♦ Commonest on lingual mucosa, mouth commissures
♦ Inappetence
♦ Salivation

Occurs in stomatitis.

Mouth/muzzle mucosa absent

Clinical findings:
♦ Section of mucosa with clean cut edge, missing
♦ Tissue below is healthy
♦ No inflammation
♦ Usually contiguous with section of skin

Occurs in Epitheliogenesis imperfecta.

Pain, abdominal – elicited

Clinical findings Pain grunt elicited by firm percussion over site of affected abdominal organ

Occurs in:
♦ Traumatic reticuloperitonitis
♦ Abomasal ulcer
♦ Peritonitis

Pain, abdominal – spontaneous

Clinical findings:
♦ Pain caused by disease of the abdominal viscera is similar irrespective of organ involved
  Horse – acute:
♦ Pawing, vigorous, persistent
♦ Flank-watching, sometimes nipping at flank
♦ Rolling, repeatedly
  Subacute:
♦ Bouts of flank-watching, kicking at belly, lying down without much rolling, stretching, sham urinating, walking backwards, dog-sitting posture, lying on back, compulsive walking
♦ Excessive pawing
♦ In **peritonitis** also pain, rigidity on palpation abdominal wall

Occurs in:
  Horse – acute:
♦ Intestinal obstruction, e.g. volvulus
♦ Spasmodic colic, paralytic ileus
♦ Gastric dilation
♦ Enteritis, e.g. salmonellosis
  Subacute:
♦ Thromboembolic colic
♦ Peritonitis
♦ Impaction large intestine

Ileum hypertrophy
Cattle (see Chapter 6)

Paracentesis, abdominal

Best indicator of peritoneal status.
   Technique: Full aseptic site preparation. Local anesthesia. **Horse:** midline, halfway between xiphoid and umbilicus. Incision through into linear alba. Sterile blunt pointed cannula thrust through incision. May need to suck with syringe. Two samples, one in anti-coagulant. **Cattle:** more difficult to locate best site. Either caudal to xiphoid and right (4–10 cm) of midline; or left of midline 3–4 cm medial and 5–7 cm cranial of entrance foramen for left mammary vein.
   Normal fluid 1–5 ml crystal clear, straw colored, watery consistency.
   Potential errors
♦ Features change quickly, repeated samples recommended
♦ Localized abnormalities may not affect all fluid
♦ Needs to be considered in light of clinical signs, history
   Abnormalities (Tables 5.1 and 5.2) detectable:
♦ Turbidity, indicates leukocytes, possibly fibrin
♦ Green color indicates chlorophyll and plant material and leakage from gut
♦ Orange–green indicates bile pigment and leakage from biliary system
♦ Pink to red indicates hemoglobin and leakage from vascular system
♦ Red–brown indicates gut wall necrosis
♦ Particles indicate fibrin or gut contents
♦ High specific gravity indicates plasma leakage as in peritonitis or gut wall infarction
♦ Free fluid flow suggests bladder rupture, ascites, acute diffuse peritonitis, very chronic peritonitis
♦ Blood commonly from rupture of skin vessel or spleen during collection, or suggests rupture of spleen, bladder, uterus, or severe congestive heart failure, hemorrhagic disease, e.g. warfarin poisoning
♦ High leukocyte count requires differential staining; polymorphs indicate peritonitis, monocytes indicate chronic peritonitis, mesothelial cells with mitotic figures suggest neoplasm, erythrocytes suggest hemoperitoneum
♦ Packed cell volume of peritoneal fluid <5% suggests gut wall infarction, >20% suggests hemorrhage into cavity
♦ Green color and containing motile protozoa indicates sample is from gut lumen, especially if sharp needle used instead of blunt cannula. Also indicated by absence of mesothelial cells.

Pawing

See Pain, abdominal, this section.

Ping on abdomen percussion

Clinical findings Clear, sharp, high-pitched sound elicited by sharp, localized tap or finger flick over a tightly gas-distended abdominal viscus.

Occurs in:
♦ Abomasum displacement
♦ Amomasum distension
♦ Abomasum torsion
♦ Intestinal obstruction
♦ Cecum–colon distension

Quidding

See Mastication faults, this section.

Radiographic and ultrasound abnormality

Limited information and uncommon method of examination, partly because of lack of availability of equipment at the clinical location, partly because of size and lack of controllability of patient, partly due to cost.
   Some use in foals, piglets, calves and small ruminants, for abnormalities of swallowing at the esophagus, abdomen for intestine abnormalities.

Rectum constricted

Occurs in:
♦ Acquired rectal constriction in pigs
♦ Inherited anovaginal stricture in cattle

Rectum impacted

See Rectum obstructed, this section.

Rectum obstructed

Clinical findings:
♦ Rectal examination blocked by closure
♦ Feces impacted
♦ Moderate abdominal pain

Occurs in:
♦ Strangulation by pedunculated lipoma
♦ Rectal stricture in pigs

Table 5.1 Guidelines for the classification and interpretation of bovine peritoneal fluid [VM8 p. 167]

Classification of fluid	Physical appearance	Total protein g/dl	Specific gravity	Total RBC × 10⁶/μl	Total WBC × 10⁶/μl	Differential WBC count	Bacteria	Particulate matter (plant fiber)	Interpretation
Normal	Amber, crystal clear 1–5 ml per sample	0.1–3.1 (1.6) Does not clot	1.005–1.015	Few from puncture of capillaries during sampling	0.3–5.3	Polymorpho-nuclear and mononuclear cells, ratio 1:1	None	None	Increased amounts in late gestation, congestive heart failure
Moderate inflammation	Amber to pink, slightly turbid	2.8–7.3 (4.5) May clot	1.016–1.025	0.1–0.2	2.7–40.7 (8.7)	Non-toxic neutrophils, 50–90% macrophages may predominate in chronic peritonitis	None	None	Early stages of strangulation, destruction of intestine; traumatic reticulo-peritonitis; ruptured bladder; chronic peritonitis
Severe inflammation	Serosanguineous, turbid, viscous 10–20 ml per sample	3.1–5.8 (4.2) Commonly clots	1.026–1.040	0.3–0.5	2.0–31.1 (8.0)	Segmented neutrophils, 70–90%. Presence of (toxic) degenerate neutrophils containing bacteria	Usually present	May be present	Advanced stages of strangulation, obstruction; acute diffuse peritonitis; perforation of abomasal ulcer; rupture of uterus, stomachs or intestine

♦ Inherited anovaginal stricture cows
♦ Rectum paralysis

Rectum wall thickened

Occurs in:
♦ Johne's disease
♦ Coccidiosis

Regurgitation

Clinical findings:
♦ Largely effortless, backward flowing of ingesta from esophagus characterized by:
  • Large volume
  • Odorless
  • Neutral pH
  • Regurgitus undigested
♦ May be accompanied by:
  • Coughing up feed
  • Aspiration pneumonia
  • Laryngeal spasm and asphyxia
  • Bronchial spasm and reflex cardiac and respiratory arrest

Occurs in:
♦ Physical blockage of esophagus by foreign body, etc.
♦ Spasm of esophagus
♦ Paralysis of esophagus, megaesophagus

Rolling

See pain, abdominal, this section.

Salivary gland swollen

Clinical findings:
♦ Parotid or submaxillary salivary gland swollen, sometimes unilaterally
♦ May be pain on palpation, painful mastication

Occurs in:
♦ Parotitis
♦ Salivary duct atresia/obstruction

Saliva drooling

Clinical findings:
♦ Drooling of saliva, often in long strings, distinct from frothing at mouth
♦ Minimal lip smacking movements

Occurs in:
♦ Stomatitis
♦ Pharynx obstruction
♦ Swallowing fault (see below)
♦ Poisons
  • Andromeda, Oleander spp.
  • Pennisetum clandestinum possibly with fungus Myrothecium spp.
  • Slaframine in Rhizoctonia leguminicola, ergot alkaloids in Acremonium coenophialum, Claviceps purpurea
  • Iodine
  • Methiocarb
♦ Watery mouth of lambs
♦ Sweating sickness

Shock

See dehydration, this section.

Stomach tube passing obstructed – in esophagus obstruction

Stomach tube fluid reflux

Occurs in:
♦ Gastric dilation
♦ Upper intestine obstruction

Stretching–sham urination

See pain, abdominal.

Swallowing difficult (dysphagia)

Clinical findings:
♦ Forceful attempts to swallow
♦ Initial extension, followed by forceful flexion of head
♦ Violent supporting contractions neck and abdominal muscles followed by onward passage of bolus

Occurs in Obstruction in pharynx or esophagus caused by
  • Pharyngitis
  • Esophagitis
  • Esophagus dilation
  • Esophagus diverticulum
  • Esophagus spasm at mucosal erosion
  • Cardia achalasia, very rarely

Table 5.2 Guidelines for the classification and interpretation of adult equine peritoneal fluid [VM8 p. 168]

Classification of fluid	Physical appearance	Total protein g/dl	Specific gravity	Total RBC $\times 10^6/\mu l$	Total WBC $\times 10^6/\mu l$
Normal	Pale yellow, crystal clear	0.5–1.5 Does not clot	1.000–1.015	None	0.5–5.0
Suspected inflammation	Slightly cloudy, yellow	1.6–2.5 Usually does not clot	1.016–1.020	0.05–0.1	5.0–15.0
Moderate inflammation	Yellow-pink turbid, viscous	2.6–4.0 May clot	1.021–1.025	1.0–0.2	15.0–60.0 Segmented neutrophils, 70–80%, few toxic neutrophils
Severe inflammation	Pink to sero-sanguineous, turbid, thick viscous	4.7–7.0 Commonly clots	Greater than 1.025	0.3–0.6	Greater than 60.0

Teeth discolored

Occurs in   teeth, congenital defects

Teeth enamel, dentine defective

Occurs in   Teeth, congenital defects

Teeth grinding

See pain, abdominal, this section.

Teeth malpositioned

Occurs in   Teeth, congenital defects

Teeth premature loss

Clinical findings:
♦ Weight loss
♦ Dropping feed while eating

Occurs in:
♦ Periodontal disease
♦ Osteodystrophy

Teeth retarded eruption

Occurs   in   Nutritional   deficiency   of calcium

Tenesmus

Clinical findings:
♦ Straining as if to defecate in cattle, rare in horses
♦ Straining at defecation and afterwards, as if it causes pain

Occurs in:
♦ Inflammation lower bowel, e.g. proctitis, colitis, as in coccidiosis
♦ Inflammation lower reproductive tract, e.g. vaginitis, retained placenta
♦ Estrogen overdose, e.g. *Fusarium* spp. poisoning, excessive medication
♦ Poisoning, methiocarb, 4-aminopyridine
♦ Spinal cord (cauda equina neuritis) lesion, spinal cord abscess

Differential WBC count	Bacteria	Particulate matter (plant fiber)	Interpretation
Polymorpho-nuclear and mononuclear cells, ratio 1:1	None	None	Increased in late gestation, congestive heart failure
Segmented neutrophils, 50–60%; mesothelial cells	None	None	Modified transudate
May be present	None	Early stages of strangulation, obstruction, uterine torsion, colonic torsion	
Segmented neutrophils, 70–90%; toxic or degenerate neutrophils containing bacteria	Commonly present	May be present	Infarction of intestine; perforation or rupture of viscus

♦ Rectal paralysis, e.g. rabies
♦ Constipation in sows

Tongue papillae small

Occurs in   Congenital defects
Causes difficult prehension

Tongue shrunken/swollen

Occurs in   Stomatitis

Vomiting

Clinical findings:
♦ Rare in farm animals especially horses in which it is usually terminal
♦ Acid vomitus differentiated from alkaline regurgitus from esophagus
♦ Alkaline with bile vomit from duodenum in pigs
Clinical signs include:
♦ **Projectile vomiting** of large volumes of fluid due to reverse peristalsis due to over-filling of stomach(s) in horses, ruminants
♦ **True vomiting** due to gastric mucosal irri-

tation includes expulsion small amounts pasty, porridge-like material and pro-longed, repeated **retching movements** composed of:
• Extension of head
• Contractions of abdominal wall
• Contractions of neck muscles
♦ Fluid and electrolyte loss
♦ Asphyxia due to acute laryngeal spasm
♦ Aspiration pneumonia
♦ Stomach rupture a terminal event in vomiting horses

Occurs in:
♦ foreign body in esophagus (retching movements only)
♦ *Horses* – terminally in acute gastric dilation
♦ *Cattle:*
• End stage milk fever
• Arsenic poisoning
• Poisonous plants *Eupatorium rugosum, Geigeria* spp., *Hymenoxis* spp., *Andromeda* spp., *Nerium oleander, Conium maculatum*
• Overloading rumen in lavage
• Passage of large bore stomach tube

- Cud-dropping
♦ *Pigs* – part of many diseases in young pigs, especially:
  - Transmissible gastroenteritis

- Vomiting and wasting disease
- Acute chemical poisonings e.g. phosphorus
- Poisoning by *Fusarium* spp. fungus

DISEASES OF BUCCAL CAVITY AND ASSOCIATED ORGANS

MUZZLE CONGENITAL DEFECTS
[VM8 p. 171]

Harelip, single or dual, some contiguous with cleft palate.

MUZZLE DERMATITIS [VM8 p. 171]

Cattle
♦ Photosensitisation
♦ Bovine malignant catarrh
♦ Bovine papular stomatitis
♦ Rinderpest
♦ Peste de petits ruminants
♦ Bovine virus diarrhea

Sheep
♦ Ecthyma
♦ Bluetongue

Pigs
♦ Swine vesicular disease
♦ Vesicular exanthema of swine
♦ Foot and mouth disease
♦ Vesicular lesions caused by poisoning with furanocoumarins in fungi

STOMATITIS [VM8 p. 171]

Includes **glossitis**, **palatitis**, and **gingivitis**

Etiology

Physical causes:
♦ Drenching or balling gun injury
♦ Foreign body injury
♦ Teeth malocclusion
♦ Plant materials including bristles, spines, awns

Chemical agents:
♦ Irritant drugs e.g. chloral hydrate
♦ Rubifacients licked from skin
♦ Irritant chemicals mistaken for medicines
♦ Part of systemic poisoning, e.g. bracken, *Heraclum* spp., furazolidone, fungi (*Stachybotris, Fusarium* spp., mushrooms, toadstools)

♦ Part of uremia syndrome in horses
Infectious agents:

Cattle
♦ Oral necrobacillosis (*Fusobacterium necrophorum*)
♦ Glossal ulcer in Actinobacillus lignieresi infection
♦ Granulomatous gingival ulcers in Actinomyces bovis infection
♦ Vesicular lesions in foot and mouth disease and vesicular stomatitis and furanocoumarin poisoning
♦ Proliferative lesions in papular stomatitis, papillomatosis, rarely rhinosporidiosis
♦ Oral mucosal necrosis in bovine sweating sickness
♦ Miscellaneous injuries and causes, some with secondary infection e.g. *Mucor, Monilia* spp., and extending to cellulitis or phlegmon
♦ Idiopathic necrosis of tongue tip in feedlot steers

Sheep
♦ Granulomatous lesions in some cases of ecthyma in young lambs; also in sheep pox, ulcerative dermatosis, coital exanthema
♦ Erosive lesions in bluetongue, peste de petits ruminants, rinderpest
♦ Rarely vesicular lesions in foot and mouth disease

Horses
♦ Vesicular stomatitis
♦ Occasional lesion in equine herpesvirus infections
♦ Rare lingual abscess due to Actinobacillus spp.

Pigs
♦ Vesicles in swine vesicular disease, vesicular exanthema of swine, foot and mouth disease, vesicular stomatitis

Clinical findings

Oral mucosal lesions may be erosions, ulcers, granulomas, vesicles or diffuse catarrhal when due to chemical burn
- Secondary lesions include micro-abscesses (usually containing *Actinomyces pyogenes*) in tongue, local cellulitis causing swelling of face or throat, or infection in pharyngeal lymph nodes
- Reduced feed intake
- Slow mastication
- Chewing movements, lip-smacking
- Salivation, frothy small amounts or drooling stringy depending on whether patient swallows; may contain mucosal shreds
- Fetid odor in mouth with secondary bacterial invasion
- Sham drinking
- Patient resents manipulation of mouth
- Toxemia when systemic disease or secondary cellulitis present
- Similar lesions on other parts of body in systemic infections
- Shrinking of tongue due to fibrous contraction, sloughing of tongue tip sequels in some. These, and tongue tip loss due to predator bite, cause faulty mastication with green saliva leaking from commissures, staining face; the so-called **tobacco-chewers**

Clinical pathology

Bacterial or viral isolations attempted but difficult to isolate pathogens from swabs of live material.

Necropsy findings

Performed only in cases when attempting to identify systemic primary disease.

Diagnosis

Differentiation of diseases causing stomatitis critical to the identification of highly infectious viral diseases discussed in foot-and-mouth disease.
    Diseases characterized by hypersalivation include:
- Poisoning by:
  - Slaframine
  - Ergot alkaloids
  - Plants, e.g. Andromeda, Oleander, Pennisetum spp.
- Oral foreign body
- Pharyngeal paralysis, obstruction
- Pharyngitis
- Esophagus paralysis, obstruction
- Esophagitis
- Sweating sickness
- Watery mouth of lambs

Treatment

Superficial lesions heal very rapidly and need no treatment. More serious cases need consideration of:
- Isolate and feed and water from separate utensils when infectious disease suspected
- Non-specific remedy for local lesions is frequent application of mild, antiseptic collutory, e.g.
  - 2% copper sulfate solution
  - 2% suspension borax
  - 1% suspension of a sulfonamide in glycerine
- For extensive cellulitis use oral or parenteral injection broad spectrum antibacterial
- Long-standing ulcers respond to curettage or cautery with silver nitrate stick or iodine tincture
- Ensure teeth not causing laceration
- Supportive treatment includes –
  - Soft palatable feed
  - Intravenous fluids or complete alimentation
  - Anti-inflammatories to ease discomfort and enhance feed intake

DISEASES OF TEETH

Congenital teeth defects [VM8 p. 174]
- Inherited malocclusion
- Red–brown staining due to inherited porphyrinuria
- Defective enamel formation on all teeth, teeth are pink, plus joint hypermobility in bovine osteogenesis imperfecta; also in horses
- Retarded eruption as in nutritional deficiency calcium

Dental fluorosis

Enamel hypoplasia [VM8 p. 174]
- Due to helminthiasis in sheep

Periodontal disease [VM8 p. 174]

Premature wear and loss of incisors in high percentage of mature sheep in isolated locations.

Etiology

♦ Cause unknown. Mineral nutrition appears not to be involved
♦ *Bacteroides gingivalis* common inhabitant in plaque on teeth
♦ Possibly related to spiny grass seeds and sand in rough environment in Scotland and New Zealand where disease common

Clinical findings:

♦ Little weight loss initially then secondary starvation even though feed supply good
♦ Loss of incisors at 3.5–6.5 years old necessitating early culling. Normals have full mouths at 7 years
♦ Gums red, edematous, bleeding at first, then recede, form pockets between teeth and gum
♦ Crowns lengthen, teeth loose, periodontitis
♦ Incisors and molars damaged and worn

Clinical pathology

Bacteriological identification of *Bacteroides gingivalis, Fusobacterium* spp. and spirochetes

Diagnosis

Resembles:
♦ Nutritional deficiency of calcium
♦ An enzootic occurrence of excessive wear of molars without molar involvement also in New Zealand; no periodontitis nor shedding
♦ Dentigerous cysts occur in sheep

Treatment, control

♦ Glued-on prosthetic incisors have been used
♦ Prophylactic antibiotics have no effect
♦ Cutting incisor teeth to prevent loss also tried but not approved

PAROTITIS [VM8 p. 175]

Inflammation of salivary glands.

Etiology

♦ Sporadic cases only, avitaminosis A may predispose
♦ Localization blood-borne infection
♦ Invasion up salivary duct from stomatitis
♦ Grass awn in duct
♦ Irritation by salivary calculus
♦ Penetrating wounds from exterior o mouth cavity

Clinical findings:

♦ Diffuse enlargement, pain, warmth o gland. Sometimes edema
♦ May interfere with, prevent or slow down mastication and swallowing
♦ Abnormal, stiff head carriage and movement
♦ Painful, passive head movement. Patient resents manipulation

Clinical pathology

Culture of discharge to aid in selection of antibiotic to be used.

Diagnosis

Resembles:
♦ Local lymphadenitis
♦ Throat abscess
♦ Metastases in lymph node from squamous cell carcinoma from eye cancer or mandible lymphoma
♦ Acute pharyngeal phlegmon is much more severe with fever, toxemia, obstruction to swallowing and breathing, diffuse swelling, a short course and a high case fatality rate

Treatment

♦ Systemic sulfonamides or broad spectrum antibiotic
♦ Drainage of abscess may be necessary, but care needed because of proximity large blood vessels
♦ Persistent fistula may be a sequel

DISEASES OF THE PHARYNX AND ESOPHAGUS

PHARYNGITIS [VM8 p. 176]

Etiology

Physical causes
♦ Drenching or balling gun, or endotracheal tube injury
♦ Accidental ingestion caustic, irritant substances
♦ Foreign bodies, grass, cereal awns, wire, pieces of bone, gelatin capsules lodged in pharynx or suprapharyngeal diverticulum pigs

Infectious causes in cattle
♦ Oral necrobacillosis
♦ Actinobacillosis, as a granuloma
♦ Infectious bovine rhinotracheitis

Horse
♦ Strangles
♦ Anthrax
♦ Equine viral rhinopneumonitis
♦ Parainfluenza virus infection
♦ Equine influenza
♦ Equine viral arteritis
♦ Adenovirus and rhinovirus infections
♦ Chronic follicular pharyngitis

Pig
♦ Anthrax
♦ Aujeszky's disease, some outbreaks

Clinical findings

♦ Reluctant to eat, swallow
♦ Swallowing causes pain, may cough up feed
♦ Passive opening of mouth resented
♦ External pharyngeal compression causes pain, cough
♦ Throat may be swollen
♦ Painful cough
♦ Nasal discharge, may be bloody or contain feed
♦ Nasal regurgitation when swallowing attempted
♦ Head extended
♦ Saliva drools
♦ Frequent, tentative jaw movements
♦ Retropharyngeal and parotid lymph nodes may be swollen

♦ Endoscopic examination reveals exact type and location of lesions
♦ Guttural pouch empyema a possible sequel
♦ Aspiration pneumonia a sequel in severe cases with dysphagia

Traumatic pharyngitis of cattle
♦ Through the mouth can see lacerations, diphtheritic membranes
♦ Palpation detects diverticulae in pharynx wall filled with ingesta

Equine chronic follicular pharyngitis
♦ Granular, nodular mucosa with white tips on hyperplastic lymphoid follicles
♦ Bad cases have a soft lymphoid mass hanging from pharyngeal roof
♦ Racing performance appears not to be affected unless secondary bacterial infection follows

Clinical pathology
♦ Nasal or oral swabs may identify causative bacteria in purulent cases
♦ *Moraxella* spp. and *Streptococcus zooepidemicus* common isolates

Necropsy findings

♦ In severe cases there will be edema, hemorrhage, abscessation or cellulitis and a foul-smelling exudate from mural lesions

Diagnosis

Resembles:
♦ Chronic pharyngitis with secondary bacterial infection accompanied by purulent nasal discharge, cough persistently, especially during exercise, are dyspneic and tire easily
♦ **Idiopathic pharyngeal phlegmon**, intermandibular cellulitis, is a severe, often fatal, necrosis of pharynx wall, caused by *Fusobacterium necrophorum*, with an acute onset, high fever, tachycardia, dyspnea, severe toxemia, and diffuse swelling of the throat

Treatment

♦ Systemic antibiotic or sulfonamides, intensive in pharyngeal phlegmon

- Treatment in electuary or topical spray in horses
- Electrical or chemical cautery in pharyngeal lymphoid hyperplasia

PHARYNGEAL OBSTRUCTION
[VM8 p. 177]

Etiology

- Foreign body, e.g. corn cob, piece of wire
- Tissue swelling – **cattle**
  - Retropharyngeal lymphadenopathy or abscess e.g. tuberculosis, actinobacillosis, leucosis
  - fibrous or mucoid polyp
- Tissue swelling – **horse**
  - Retropharyngeal lymph node hyperplasia and lymphoid granuloma as part of chronic follicular pharyngitis
  - Retropharyngeal abscess, cellulitis
  - Retropharyngeal lymphadenitis of strangles
  - Pharyngeal cysts, e.g. remnants of thyroglossal duct
- Dermoid cysts
- Goitrous thyroids
- Tissue swelling – **pig**
  - Diffuse lymphoid enlargement pharynx wall, soft palate
  - Food, foreign body impaction in suprapharyngeal diverticulum of pig

Clinical findings

- Drinks all right
- Hungry, but attempts to eat end in coughing up food
- Esophagus not dilated
- No nasal regurgitation
- Loud snoring respiration
- Inspiration prolonged with abdominal effort
- Loud inspiratory stertor on tracheal auscultation
- Manual palpation may locate lesion
- Endoscopic examination reveals lesion
- Chronic cases low feed intake, secondary starvation
- Lymph node rupture liberates pus. May develop inhalation pneumonia

Horses – additional signs

- Nasal discharge
- Halitosis
- Tongue laceration

Clinical pathology

- Tuberculin test
- Bacteriological examination pharyngeal swab
- Radiography for metallic foreign body

Necropsy findings

Foreign body or swollen tissue filling of pharynx.

Diagnosis

Resembles:

- Tuberculosis, actinobacillosis, strangles
- Pharyngitis
- Pharyngeal paralysis
- Esophageal obstruction
- Nasal obstruction

Treatment

- Parenteral antibacterial for acute infectious process
- Chronic abscess needs surgical drainage, some temporary reduction after treatment with iodides
- Foreign body removed through mouth

PHARYNGEAL PARALYSIS [VM8 p. 178]

Etiology

Peripheral nerve injury

- Injury to glossopharyngeal, recurrent laryngeal nerves
- Guttural pouch infection, horses
- Throat trauma
- Possibly cud-dropping

Part of specific disease

- Rabies and other encephalitides
- Botulism
- African horse sickness
- Idiopathic disease in horses

Clinical findings

- Attempts to swallow followed by coughing up of feed, nasal regurgitation
- Saliva drools
- No swallowing reflex when pharynx compressed
- Endoscopic examination reveals defect
- Dehydration, emaciation

♦ Aspiration pneumonia in some
♦ Usually irreversible, fatal
♦ **cud-dropping** – patient normal except that regurgitated boluses dropped from mouth as flattened disks of fibrous material. Transient for few days

Clinical pathology and necropsy findings

No specific findings.

Diagnosis

Resembles:
♦ Pharyngeal obstruction
♦ Esophageal paralysis, obstruction

Treatment

♦ No effective treatment
♦ Nasal tube or intravenous alimentation until diagnosis confirmed

ESOPHAGITIS [VM8 p. 179]

Etiology

♦ Chemically irritant substance dosed, drunk, eaten
♦ Foreign body laceration
♦ Forceful thrusting with probang or stomach tube
♦ Death of Hypoderma lineata larvae

Clinical findings

♦ Saliva drools
♦ Pain at swallowing attempts
♦ Coughing up feed, nasal regurgitation
♦ Palpation cervical esophagus causes pain
♦ Endoscopy reveals lesion

With perforation
♦ local pain, swelling, crepitus, compression of esophagus, severe toxemia
♦ Local cellulitis may rupture to exterior
♦ Fistula may develop
♦ Rupture of thoracic esophagus may cause fatal pleurisy, pyemia

Sequel
♦ Fistula, chronic stenosis

Clinical pathology

Leukocytosis and left shift with accompanying cellulitis.

Necropsy findings

No specific findings other than gross esophagitis.

Diagnosis

Resembles:
♦ Pharyngitis
♦ Esophageal obstruction

Treatment

♦ Withhold feed 2–3 days
♦ Parenteral alimentation
♦ Antibiotic cover to combat possible perforation
♦ Recommence feeding with gruel or moist feed

ESOPHAGEAL OBSTRUCTION [VM8 p. 180]

Etiology

Ingested material
♦ Turnips, potatoes, oranges, peaches, apples
♦ Gelatin capsules in horses
♦ Gorging on dry feed, bedding, e.g. bran, shavings, chopped hay
♦ Foreign body, e.g. part of stomach tube
♦ Phytobezoar

External compression
♦ Tuberculous, neoplastic lymph nodes in mediastinum
♦ Abscess in mediastinum, cervical fascia
♦ Local swelling after injury
♦ Persistent right aortic arch
♦ Esophageal paralysis, diverticulum, megaesophagus
♦ Congenital muscle hypertrophy, ectasia, stenosis, double esophagus
♦ Stomach carcinoma
♦ Esophageal hiatus hernia
♦ Cicatricial contraction, mucosal granuloma after esophagitis
♦ Thymoma

Clinical findings

Acute obstruction – choke in cattle
♦ Usually high cervical obstruction
♦ Sudden cessation feed intake
♦ Anxious, restless
♦ Forceful swallowing attempts
♦ Saliva drools

- Nasal regurgitation
- Cough
- Severe bloat in most
- Ruminal movements continuous, sounds loud
- Systolic murmur (relieved when bloat relieved)
- Esophageal tube will not pass
- Solid mass palpable from exterior in most cervical obstructions
- Spontaneous passage of obstruction usual within hours
- Obstructions persisting for a week cause pressure necrosis, subsequent stenosis

Acute obstruction – choke in horses

- May be at any level in esophagus
- Impacted dry feed just palpable as small cylinder
- Patient difficult to restrain because of anxiety
- Forceful swallowing or retching causes horse to panic, extend neck, paw wildly, resist nasal intubation
- Nasal regurgitation
- Profuse sweating, tachycardia
- May spontaneously relax and pass obstruction. Much less likely than in cattle. Gelatin capsules tend to persist 3–4 days

Sequels in either species

- Aspiration pneumonia
- Esophageal stenosis
- Death from dehydration, starvation

Chronic obstruction in cattle

- Persistent mild bloat for long periods
- Rumen hypermotility
- Swallowing may require second movement when feed bolus reaches obstruction
- Dilated esophagus palpable
- Water and stomach tube often pass, but food obstructs
- Projectile regurgitation
- Patient may refuse solid feed

Chronic obstruction horse

- Persistent coughing at eating, nasal regurgitation
- Weight loss

Clinical pathology

Radiographic examination, contrast radiography, endoscopy are valuable aids.

Diagnosis

Resembles:

- Esophageal paralysis, e.g. megaesophagus
- Esophagitis
- Colic
- Chronic bloat due to ruminal atony
- Cleft palate

Treatment

- Remove all access to water or feed till obstruction cleared
- Sedation may be necessary before examination possible. May relieve spasm
- Attempts to push obstruction not very successful. Undue force likely to perforate wall.
- In cattle, manual removal of object in first part of esophagus possible, or pass wire loop over it and pull, or cutting object into pieces with a probang with a cutting wire loop
- Horses with packed dry feed in esophagus treated with lavage. Repeated irrigation/siphoning with 0.5 l warm water, avoiding overfilling and aspiration into lungs
- Waiting several hours for spontaneous recovery recommended. Cattle will need trocarization with trocar sewn in place. Beyond this, necrosis of mucosa, subsequent stenosis probable
- Esophagotomy, possibly gastrotomy for cardial obstruction, the end choice. Fistula a common sequel
- Limited access for horses to bran mashes and water after obstruction removed

DISEASES OF THE NON-RUMINANT STOMACH AND INTESTINES

EQUINE COLIC [VM8 p. 183]

Diseases of the alimentary tract of the horse are characterized by abdominal pain, and in some cases abnormalities of gut sounds, on rectal examination, and in the peritoneal fluid obtained by paracentesis, some of which respond to medical treatment but others which terminate fatally without surgical intervention.

Findings and procedures applicable to all cases of colic are included in this section. Those applicable to individual types of colic, and therefore important in their differential diagnosis are set out in Table 5.3. The principles of pathogenesis in colic which play a part in the clinical syndrome, and which need to be addressed in treatment are:

- Abdominal pain
- Endotoxemia
- Dehydration
- Shock

Etiology

Each type of colic has its own special cause. Those causes fall within the following general groups:

- Gut distension
- Gut hypermotility
- Gut wall ischemia and infarction
- Peritoneal inflammation
- Peritoneal stretching

Epidemiology

Occurrence
- Universal
- Highest incidence in pastured horses where parasite control inadequate
- In stabled horses where feed insufficiently digestible, or too much

Animal risk factors
- **Age** See in Table 5.3
- **Breed** Special susceptibilities in American miniature horses (colon impaction, enteroliths), Arabians (enteroliths), heavy breeds (large bowel displacements)
- **Physical activity** Wild galloping in play, mating activity by stallions
- **Previous attacks** peritoneal adhesions, gross feeding, gut hypermotility due to excitement

Environmental risk factors
- **Diet** Indigestible roughage; feeds suitable for cattle but not horses, tough meadow hay, sorghum
- Overfeeding, especially ponies
- Parasite, especially *Strongylus* spp., control inadequate

Importance
- The most serious medical disease of horses in developed countries
- Wastage due mostly to deaths, some to interference with competitive sporting activities, and costs of treatment
- Case fatality rates in medical colic very low, surgical colics 10%

Clinical findings

Pain
- Continuous or episodic between quiet periods
- Severity varies from mild, controllable by alternative activity, e.g. walking, to severe, uncontrollable by even potent analgesic
- Chronic cases have mild to moderate attacks at intervals of days or weeks

Behavior
- Pawing ground
- Kicking at belly
- Restless walking
- Frequent getting up and lying down, rolling
- Looking or nipping at flank
- Sham drinking
- Anorexia

Posture
- Straddling as if to urinate, protrusion of penis without urinating
- Sitting on haunches like a dog
- Lying on back

Defecation
- Usually ceases except in cases of enteritis
- Feces firm, dry except in enteritis or colitis

Abdominal size increase
- Unusual except with severe gas accumulation

Vomiting
- Rare, suggests impending gastric rupture

Table 5.3 Differentiation of equine colics (for general signs, see p. 73). Signs listed here are those pathognomonic to each form of the disease

	History	Syndrome	Clinical pathology	Treatment response
Gastric dilation (Over-eating) [VM8 p. 199]	Over-eating or drinking, after racing, surgery. Reflex from tension on gastrocolic ligament from distended intestine. Pyloric obstruction. Gastric torsion, windsucking	*Average case* – Severe colic, dehydration, vomiting, nasogastric reflux. *Severe case* – Dyspnea, cough, abdominal distension, gas in reflux, tympany on percussion. Severe colic. *Chronic case* – repeated mild episodes	Gastric fluid pH2. Intestinal fluid pH7 +	Periodic nasogastric intubation till reflux stops. Parenteral fluid replacement
Gastric dilation (Grain engorgement) [VM8 p. 199]	Access to unlimited grain, gross feeder in group of horses getting trough feed. Intake > 10g/kg B.wt of grain	Moderate colic, foul smelling gas on intubation. Severe dehydration. Severe laminitis in some. No vomiting. Nasogastric lavage refluxes little grain	Gastric fluid pH about 2 Acidosis	Repeated gastric lavage. Oral lubricant. *Gastrotomy* – stomach filled by sour doughy mass
Gastric impaction [VM8 p. 200]	Diet of mature grass, alfalfa hay, corn, sorghum, ensilage. Insufficient water, old age, poor dentition	Subacute colic, dog-sitting posture, sham drinking. Minor nasogastric tube reflux, nasal regurgitation; feces small. Volume, dry hard	Nil	Oil or fluid by tube mostly ineffective. Laparotomy. Intestines are empty. Stomach filled with fiber mass
Gastric ulcer of foals [VM8 p. 200]	Foals 1–6 months old. Stress. Access to roughage inadequate, or at too early an age	Mild, intermittent colic, teeth grinding. Slobbering, lying on back for long periods. Pain on palpation at paracostal site. Fluid reflux on intubation. May be blood stained. Secondary anemia; perforation. Causes fatal peritonitis	Endoscope, contrast radiography. Leukocytosis and abdominocentesis fluid inflammatory with perforation	Surgical repair effective if undertaken early. Cimetidine, ranitidine widely used. Alkalinizing agents orally
Paroximal enteritis (Duodenitis) [VM8 p. 193]	No risk factors identified	Mild to severe colic, fever, no intestinal sounds, bad mucosal refill and color. Large volume gastric reflux through nasogastric tube, may be blood stained, relieves colic. Rectally	High PCV, dehydration	Repeated gastric decompression. Exploratory surgery. Duodenojejunostomy or duodenocecostomy effective

Condition	Risk factors / epidemiology	Clinical signs	Diagnosis	Outcome / Treatment
Small intestine torsion [VM8 p. 203]	No specific risk factors. Possibly peak occurrence in horses with nematode infestations. High prevalence in 2–6 month foals	Severe colic, rapid onset, development. Dehydration. Distended intestine loops after 8–12 hours. Loops after 8–12 hours on rectal examination gut sounds, defecation cease. Rectum sticky to touch, empty. Heart rate exceeds 100/min. Nasogastric tube reflux. Death at 48 hrs, may vomit, due to endotoxemia or intestine rupture	Blood stained paracentesis fluid	Necrotic, infarcted loop of small intestine on laparotomy. Resection effective if early; paralytic ileus a risk sequel
Small intestine intussusception (Ileum into Cecum) [VM8 p. 203]	No specific risk factors. [VM8 p. 203] Occurs all ages. see also Large intestine intussusception	Acute, subacute or chronic colic all occur depending on degree of involvement of blood supply. As for torsion in acute cases	As for torsion in acute cases	Surgery the essential outcome
Small intestine strangulated inguinal hernia [VM8 p. 203]	In adult entire males related to mating activity. Also congenital or soon after birth in congenital hernia	Severe colic, distended loops on rectal exam hours after strangulatiuon. Tight mesenteric band to inguinal canal. Scrotum swollen	As for torsion in acute cases	Surgery obligatory
Small intestine strangulated diaphragm hernia [VM8 p. 204]	Often subsequent to fall or abdomen-compressing injury. Also congenital. Signs several weeks after birth	Severe colic. Gut sounds as resonance on percussion in chest. Persistent walking backwards. Lateral recumbency persistently, opposite side to hernia	As for torsion plus radiology or ultrasonography	Surgical repair effective. Most cases confirmed at exploratory laparotomy
Small intestine strangulation through epiploic foramen [VM8 p. 204]	In older horses. Some in yearlings	Mild to severe depending on completeness of strangulation and blood supply occlusion. Mild cases often become suddenly worse as strangulation completed. No distended intestine loops palpable. Fatal portal vein rupture possible sequel	As for acute torsion	Diagnosis not possible without laparotomy. Resection required
Small intestine intra-mural hematoma [VM8 p. 204]	No risk factors identified	Mild to severe colic depending on degree of luminal occlusion. May progress from mild to severe	In severe case as for acute torsion	Diagnosis possible only on laparotomy. Resection required therapy

Table 5.3 (cont'd)

	History	Syndrome	Clinical pathology	Treatment response
Small intestine ileum diverticulum [VM8 p. 204]	No risk factors identified	Bouts of mild to moderate colic over period of years	Nil	Responds to antispasmodics. Diagnosed only on exploratory surgery
Small intestine strangulation in mesenteric tear (Gastrosplenic ligament defect, behind ventral ligament of bladder, through tear in broad ligament of uterus.) [VM8 p. 205]	No risks factors identified	As for epiploic foramen incarceration	As for acute torsion	Diagnosed at exploratory surgery
Small intestine impaction of duodenum [VM8 p. 204]	Chewed wood, kernels of cracked corn, massive accumulations of ascarids in yearlings	Severe, acute colic without endotoxemia, no vascular compromise. Nasogastric reflux. No abnormality rectally	Elevation of PCV. Paracentesis fluid normal	Lesions inaccessible for surgery but can confirm diagnosis
Small intestine idiopathic muscular hypertrophy [VM8 p. 205]	In horses more than 5 years, up to 18 years old	Mild chronic or intermittent colic, reduced appetite, weight loss. Weeks or months. Thickened ileum palpable rectally at cecal base. Thick-walled distended loops of intestine, mostly ileum, also jejunum. No vascular compromise	Nil	Confirmable by exploratory surgery. Treatment impracticable
Small intestine constricting adhesions [VM8 p. 202]	Prevalent in heavily parasitized horses, or subsequent to infection of lymph nodes as in strangles, or Meckel's diverticulum	Mild, chronic or intermittent colic. Adhesions or tight mesenteric bands palpable rectally in some. Very similar to chronic intussusception. Loud bode	Possibly inflammatory fluid on paracentesis	Surgery makes diagnosis confirmable. Rarely resection possible

Condition				
Small intestine ileocecal valve impaction [VM8 p. 205]	Feeding low-grade finely chopped indigestible roughage	Subacute pain 24 hrs, followed by severe acute colic. No vascular compromise. Dehydration without endotoxemia. Gut sounds increased early, absent later. Impacted ileum palpable. Small intestine dilated. Large bowel empty. Profuse nasogastric reflux after 24 hours	Paracentesis fluid normal. High PCV	Lesion inaccessible. Repair possible by jejunocecostomy. Fatal unless surgically repaired
Paralytic ileus [VM8 p. 204]	After extensive surgery. Also part of acute peritonitis, gut wall ischemia or infarction	Functional gut stasis; identical colic signs to acute intestinal obstruction	Dehydration	Cisapride effective preventive in post-operative cases, not in peritonitis or ischemia
Large intestine intussusceptions [VM8 p. 205]	Predisposed by miscellaneous intramural lesions	Variable syndrome depending on degree of occlusion and compromisation of blood supply. Palpable mass in right dorsal abdomen	Variable depending on lesion and syndrome. Dehydration $\pm$ endotoxemia	Surgical bypass operations satisfactory in most, provided infarction limited
Ileum–Cecum intussusception [VM8 p. 205]	Young horses <3 yrs	Severe colic with dehydration and endotoxemia or chronic weight loss, anorexia, depression, small amounts normal feces, intermittent, post-prandial colic for weeks. Distended ileum, hypertrophy of wall	As for large intestine	As for large intestine
Cecum–Cecum and Cecum–Colon [VM8 p. 205]	Most common in small horses and ponies	Acute colic or chronic wasting with scant, soft diarrhea. Rectally palpable lesion in anterior, ventral abdomen	As for large intestine	As for large intestine
Small colon intussusception [VM8 p. 205]	No risk ractors identified	Moderate colic, no feces passed, caudal end of intussception just inside anus or protruding	Nil	Surgery the only possible solution

Table 5.3 (cont'd)

	History	Syndrome	Clinical pathology	Treatment response
Left colon dorsal displacement [VM8 p. 205]	Prolonged starvation before surgery predisposes. Reduction of starvation period from 24 to 12 hours reduces occurrence	(Nephrosplenic ligament entrapment). Moderate to severe colic, gut sounds present but reduced, vital signs little change. Spleen medially displaced. Pain in left dorsal anterior abdomen. Pelvic flexure missing from left, lower abdomen. Nasogastric reflux in some. Persists several days	Nil	Poor response to standard analgesics, High success rate for rolling procedure. Recommended only if diagnosis positive
Right colon displacement [VM8 p. 206]	No risk factor identified	(Right colon displaced to diaphragm, between right body wall and cecum) Severe colic, abdominal distension. Gas distended colon horizontal. Palpable rectally	Nil	Surgical correction
Mural neoplasia of colon [VM8 p. 206]	Aged horses	Intermittent moderate colic. Severe weight loss. May also cause distended loops and incarceration	Nil	Nil
Mural hematoma small colon [VM8 p. 206]	Nil	(Also constriction of lumen by external neoplasm) Variable colic continuous or intermittent mild to severe colic. Rectally palpable impaction oral to lesion	Variable minor variation	Diagnosable and correctable only by surgical intervention
Lipoma strangulation rectum, small colon [VM8 p. 206]	Aged horses, >12 yrs. Sudden onset, often during exercise	Moderate–severe colic. No toxemia or dehydration. Vital signs good. Rectal palpation, lumen cones down to impenetrable orifice	Nil	Surgical excision of lipoma pedicle relieves

Enteroliths, phytobezoars fecaliths [VM8 p. 205]	Adult (>10 years) horses. Commonest ponies and American miniature horses. Enteroliths common some areas e.g. Northern California. Linear foreign bodies e.g. halters. Nibbled plastic or rubber coating from fence wire	intermittent mild–moderate colic. Vital signs good. Pain may be during exercise. During attack no feces passed, may be distension of abdomen. Not readily palpable rectally	AM	Nil
Equine myenteric ganglionitis [VM8 p. 206]	Nil	Pseudo-obstruction. Recurrent small colon impaction	Nil	Nil
'Irritable colon' [VM8 p. 206]	Nil	Partial constriction right dorsal colon intermittently. Recurrent moderate colic with scant, hard dry feces, gas distended colon	Nil	Surgical bypass effective
Spasmodic colic [VM8 p. 207]	Predisposed by excitable temperament, strongyle infestation. Precipated by thunderstorms, preparation for show, racing, cold drinks	Moderate colic intermittently in brief attacks. Loud borborygmi. Spontaneous recovery in 1–2 hours. Negative rectal exam	Nil	Depomidine, xylazine, butorphanol effective
Intestinal tympany [VM8 p. 208]	Primary tympany on ingestion large quantities fermentable lush green feed	Secondary to and part of some intestinal obstructions, especially adhesions. Abdominal distension, severe colic, rectal examination finds distended loops of bowel	Nil	Oral mineral oil, turpentine (15–30 ml). Trocarization of dorsal cecal sac
Thromboembolic colic [VM8 p. 209]	Strongylus spp. larval damage to blood vessels or gut wall	Moderate colic 3–4 days. No defecation, gut stasis, no sounds. Rectally tight bands mesentery palpable and saggy distended bowel loops. Endotoxemia severe. Hemorrhage into mesentery or gut lumen causes anemia in few. Mesenteric arteries thickened, lumpy	Rarely anemia, hypoalbuminemia	No successful treatment because of multiple infarcts

79

Table 5.3 (cont'd)

	History	Syndrome	Clinical pathology	Treatment response
Large intestine impaction [VM8 p. 210]	Low-grade indigestible roughage. Too long intervals between feeds. Inadequate mastication due to poor dental care. Horses starved too long before surgery. Indigestible seeds. Inadequate water. Indigestible seeds. Horses accustomed to pasture, put into boxes, palatable bedding. American miniature horses susceptible. Amitraz administration, banned in horses. Late pregnant mares susceptible to spontaneous impaction. Meconium retention, in colt foals mostly	Moderate colic 3 to 4 days. Vital signs normal, no endotoxemia or serious dehydration. Anorexia. Hard fecal balls with thick mucus infrequently or no defecation in enterolith obstruction. Sham drinking in meconium retention, relentless, debilitating straining to defecate a consistent sign. Meconium masses digitally palpable in rectum. Rectal in adults – impacted mass palpable in pelvic flexure, ventral colons, small colon in right dorsal flank, cecum from right flank to center floor of abdomen	Nil	Respond well to oral lubricant (mineral oil, for severe cases dioctyl sodium sulfo-succinate). Surgery obligatory for enteroliths etc. or persistent feed impactions. Cecal rupture in some, especially pregnant mares. Impactions not corrected medically after 72 hrs and 3 treatments, surgical intervention an option
Sand colic [VM8 p. 212]	Horses on pasture on sandy soil. Feed contaminated by dust storm	Severe to mild colic bouts intermittently over days, chronic diarrhea, weight loss. Distended cecum and colon rectally, rarely rock hard. Much sand in feces. Gut sounds characteristically 'gritty'	Nil. Paracentesis may perforate gut and show sand. Visible radiologically	Psyllium (hydrophilic mucilloid hemicellulose) orally in warm water, better than oral mineral oil repeated daily. Surgical intervention necessary in some

Pulse rate
40–100+

Respiratory rate
18–40 usually, 80 in extreme cases.

Oral mucosa
- Pale, dry, clammy in shocked or dehydrated patients
- Red to purple, congested with slow capillary refill (2–8 seconds) indicates endotoxemia

Abdomen auscultation
- Continuous borborygmi in spasmodic colic
- Complete cessation in paralytic ileus
- Frequent monitoring desirable to detect sudden change
- Critical site is right flank for abnormalities of ileo-cecal valve function
- Combined **auscultation and percussion** for detection gas cap
- Abdominal **ballottement** for detecting pain of peritonitis

Rectal palpation
- Obligatory in all colic cases except ponies, foals, and horses which strain badly
- Abnormalities:
  - Masses of impacted feces or ingesta
  - Gas/fluid distension loops of intestine
  - Tight stretch mesenteric bands
  - Saggy bowel loops of thromboembolic colic
  - Sloppy feces of enteritis
  - Splenic displacement
  - Lumpy enlargement of anterior mesenteric artery

Nasogastric intubation
Looking for gastric or intestinal distension evidenced by fluid reflux.

Paracentesis abdominis
For evidence of inflammation or ischemic damage to gut wall.

Terminal stages
- Most remain standing
- Sobbing dyspnea
- Gross muscle tremor
- Profuse sweating
- Delirious, staggering, aimless wandering
- Severe dehydration
- Impalpable pulse, tachycardia

Course
Can be as brief as 24 hours in complete obstruction of small intestine to a week in large bowel impaction.

Clinical pathology

Diagnostic
- hematology:
  - Leukocytosis of acute local peritonitis
  - Leukopenia of endotoxemia or acute diffuse peritonitis
- gastric fluid pH:
  - Acid with primary gastric dilation
  - Alkaline, bile-stained in intestinal obstruction
- **paracentesis abdominis fluid** Blood-staining, large volume, high protein and white cell count (>5000/ml) indicate gut wall devitalization.

Prognostic
- High PCV (>45%), high serum protein (>7.5 g/dl) or lactate (>10 mg/dl) indicate dehydration
- Abnormal electrolyte levels indicate acidosis or alkalosis
- Indicators also identify necessary support treatment with fluids, electrolytes
- Best indicators of **endotoxemia** are thrombocytopenia, prolonged thrombin times, elevated levels fibrinogen degeneration products

Radiography useful mostly in foals but can detect enteroliths, sand accumulations in adults.

Ultrasound can detect increased peritoneal fluid volume, gas/fluid filled bowel loops, tissue masses, gut displacement.

Colic Monitoring Protocol for horses kept under observation for better diagnosis or prognosis. Hourly intervals for suspected acute intestinal obstruction – 4 hourly for impactions; 1–2 days for chronic adhesion colic.

Check:
- **pain** – severity, frequency increases
- **defecation** – amount, consistency
- **urination** – check some is passed
- **pulse** – rate increase, amplitude decline indicate dehydration, shock
- **mucosal color, capillary refill time** – cyanosis, CRT >2 seconds indicate endotoxemia, shock
- **temperature** – hyperthermia best clinical indicator of peritonitis
- **dyspnea** – in absence severe pain indicates terminal endotoxemia

♦ **gut sounds** decline indicates development of paralytic ileus; ping on percussion indicates gas accumulation
♦ **rectal exam** – development of gas/fluid filled bowel loops suggests obstruction. Empty, sticky mucosa rectum indicates complete intestinal obstruction, administered oil without feces indicates incomplete obstruction
♦ **nasogastric intubation** – reflux indicates developing gastric or intestinal distension
♦ **paracentesis** – fluid accumulation suggests gut wall devitalisation
♦ **hematology** – increase of 5% in an hour indicates severe fluid loss
♦ **response to analgesic** – declines in worsening disease situation. Flunixin contraindicated until diagnosis made
♦ **reaction to exercise** – willingness to walk, interest in surroundings, less rolling indicate improvement.

Necropsy findings

For individual colics see Table 5.3. General lesions:
♦ Paralytic ileus
♦ **Ischemic necrosis/infarction** in many obstructive colics
♦ Diffuse mucosal degeneration in obstructive colics

Diagnosis

Colic resembles other diseases, e.g.:
♦ Laminitis
♦ myositis
♦ pleuritis
♦ hepatitis
♦ lactation tetany of mares
♦ tetanus
♦ obstructive urolithiasis
♦ bladder rupture in foals
♦ colon, ileum atresia
♦ gastric ulcer in foals
♦ acute peritonitis
♦ uterine distension, e.g. due to imperforate hymen, palpable rectally
♦ ovarian pain during estrus; pain on ovarian palpation
♦ spermatic cord torsion testicle swollen, painful, spermatic cord linked tightly to inguinal canal
♦ snakebite
♦ acute enteritis, e.g. colitis-X
♦ Proximal (anterior) enteritis (**duodenitis– proximal enteritis**) fever, mild to severe colic, bad mucosal color, slow capillary refill, heart rate >100/min, no intestinal

motility, profuse, sometimes blood-tinge reflux through nasogastric tube, par relieved by gastric emptying but recurs an stomach may rupture; responds to admi istration of analgesic, preferably flunixir repeat gastric decompression, duodenoje junostomy in intractable cases

Differentiation between types of colic – refe to Table 5.3.

Treatment

Medical and surgical treatments availabl Many cases treated medically then proceed t surgery (see 'Exploratory surgery' below Medical treatment includes analgesia, ant spasmodics, lubrication or purgation, an fluid and electrolyte replacements and co rection.

Analgesia
♦ Acetylpromazine much used but contrair dicated
♦ Older drugs hyoscine (Rx Buscopan), peth idine, pentazocine, chloral hydrate, dipyr one still used because of low cost
♦ Detomidine (20 μg/kg mild cases, 40 μg/k severe cases)
♦ Xylazine (Rx Rompun, 0.5 mg/kg I/V)
♦ Either of these alone or combined wit butorphanol (0.025 mg/kg I/V). All last 4 –120 minutes
♦ Flunixin meglumine (1.1 mg/kg I/V) lasts hours but masks deterioration. Best used diagnosis accurate and either the cause i medical or surgery is planned
♦ If these analgesics are ineffective perform either surgery or euthanasia

Lubrication or purgation
♦ Anthraquinone purgatives not recom mended, but used where lubrication no available
♦ Cholinergic drugs may have use as follow up after lubrication but unpopular because of transient effect
♦ Mineral oil by nasogastric tube most used
♦ Dioctyl sodium sulfosuccinate (DOSS) fo severe impactions
♦ All impactions profit by hydration before lubrication. Obligatory with DOSS

Antispasmodics
Atropine, dipyrone, myspamol unpopular. Decrease natural motility and other side effects.

Fluids and electrolytes

Surgical colics mostly hypovolemic. Impactions improve after hydration program, See Chapter 2 for dose rates and fluid compositions.

Antibacterials

Broad-spectrum antibiotic recommended if peritoneal cavity invasion possible through devitalized gut wall.

Exploratory surgery

Indicated when any of the following indicators present, but **if there is doubt, then operate:**

♦ Severe, persistent colic without identifiable cause for more than 48 hours
♦ Recurrent attacks of colic
♦ Efficient analgesic fails to provide relief for 20 minutes
♦ Rectally palpable lesion known to be susceptible only to surgery
♦ Intractable large bowel impaction not relieved by medical means after 4 days
♦ Persistent reflux of more than 2 liters, especially bile-stained, alkaline, fluid through nasogastric tube
♦ Severe abdominal distension
♦ Peritoneal fluid blood-tinged, high protein, high leucocyte count
♦ Rapid worsening of previously moderate pain and vital signs during 2–4 hours

Because of difficulty identifying lesion, decision on abdominal surgery more urgent in:
♦ Small horses and foals
♦ Horses with lesions in anterior abdomen

General recommendations about care of colic cases

♦ If indicators positive, early surgery
♦ After long transport if surgery not urgent, delay 12 hours
♦ Intensive pre-surgery hydration therapy if possible
♦ Monitor clinical and clinical pathology indicators regularly until case concluded
♦ Maintain contact with owner for approval for exploratory surgery or euthanasia

Prevention

♦ Rasp teeth at least annually; facilitates mastication
♦ Avoid indigestible roughage, especially old or debilitated horses
♦ Avoid finely chopped roughage. Fine chaffing often used to facilitate digestion of poorly digestible hay.

♦ Feed gluttonous feeders separately, when group husbandry practiced
♦ Muzzle horses after surgery to prevent eating of bedding
♦ Strict helminth control program (ivermectin every 2 months)

GASTRITIS (INFLAMMATION OF THE MONOGASTRIC STOMACH, ABOMASTIS) [VM8 p. 212]

Etiology

Ruminants

♦ Gross overeating in calves
♦ Foreign materials, rarely
♦ Elemental poisons arsenic, lead, mercury, copper, phosphorus
♦ Mycotoxins, e.g. of *Fusarium, Stachybotris* spp.
♦ Lactic acid formed by rumen fermentation
♦ Viruses of rinderpest, bovine virus diarrhea, bovine malignant catarrh
♦ Rarely extension from oral necrobacillosis, hemorrhagic enterotoxemia (*Clostridium perfringens* A, B, C), as part of enteric lesion in colibacillosis, *Mucor* and Aspergillus spp. fungal infection of existing abomasal ulcers
♦ *Trichostrongylus, Ostertagia, Haemonchus* spp. infestations; migrating larval paramphistomes

Pigs

♦ Foreign bodies
♦ Frosted feeds
♦ Elemental and zootoxins (as above)
♦ Gastric mucosal hyperemia and mural infarction in erysipelas, salmonellosis, swine dysentery, acute colibacillosis (in weaned pigs), swine fever, African swine fever, swine influenza
♦ Secondary infection of existing lesions by fungi
♦ Infestation with *Hyostrongylus rubidus, Ascarops strongylina, Physocephalus sexalatus*

Horses

♦ Foreign bodies (as above)
♦ Poisons (as above)
♦ Rarely. Possibly *Clostridium perfringens*
♦ Massive infestation with Gasterophilus spp.
♦ *Habronema* spp. infestation causes granulomatous and ulcerative lesions

Clinical findings

Acute gastritis – refers mostly to pigs

- Vomiting, forceful, with retching, repeated
- Vomitus small amount, contains mucus, sometimes blood
- Feed intake reduced
- Water intake increased, sham drinking, licking cold objects
- Breath rank
- Abdominal pain
- Feces pasty and soft to diarrheic
- Excessive vomiting accompanied by dehydration, alkalotic tetany, hyperpnea

Chronic gastritis
- Appetite reduced, depraved
- Sporadic vomiting, mostly after feeding
- Viscid mucus in vomitus
- Weight loss to emaciation

Abomasal foreign body
- Anorexia
- Abomasum distension
- Chronic abdominal pain
- Feces scant, pasty, melenic often

Clinical pathology

Samples of vomitus, feces for examination for toxins, infectious agents, internal parasites.

Necropsy findings

- Lesions vary from diffuse catarrhal gastritis to severe hemorrhagic gastritis in acute cases to ulcerative lesions with thickened walls in chronic cases
- Erosive lesions in mucosal diseases
- Thickening and edema of wall in parasitic disease
- Rugal tips and pyloric region most affected in chemical gastritis
- Venous infarction of septicemia and viremia is characterized by extensive submucosal hemorrhages resembling hemorrhagic gastritis

Diagnosis

- Gastric dilation similar but vomitus more profuse and projectile
- Esophageal obstruction – vomitus odorless, not high acidity
- Intestinal obstruction – vomitus alkaline, more likely to contain bile pigments, fecal material

Treatment

- Treat primary disease
- Withhold feed
- Gastric sedatives (magnesium hydroxide o carbonate, kaolin, pectin, charcoal) ever 2–3 hours
- Attempts to evacuate poisons should us bland agents, e.g. mineral oil
- Fluid and electrolyte replacement
- In convalescence bran mashes for adul herbivores, gruels for pigs and calves

GASTRIC ULCER [VM8 p. 214]

Of horses and pigs; for cattle see under abo masum ulcer.

Etiology

Horses
- Sequel to infestation with Gasterophilus Habronema spp.
- Many cases idiopathic. See Table 5.3 fo disease in foals

Pigs
- Esophagogastric ulcer a major disease o pigs
- In association with hepatic dystrophy in vitamin E deficient pigs
- Fungus *Rhizopus microspora* a common secondary infection

Clinical findings

Uncomplicated ulcer
- Mild, intermittent abdominal pain
- Reduced feed intake
- Constipation or diarrhea

Hemorrhagic ulcer
- Sudden death with mucosal pallor
- Melena, mucosal pallor, weakness, scanty, pasty feces

Perforating ulcer
- Stomach rupture causes sudden death due to acute diffuse peritonitis, profound endotoxemia
- Leakage cause acute local peritonitis, anorexia, intermittent fever and diarrhea

With consequential splenic abscess (horse)
- Fever, anorexia, pain on palpation in left flank

Clinical pathology

- Tests on feces for blood not usually necessary
- Leukocytosis with left shift if peritoneal leakage occurs
- Leukocytosis and left shift in splenic involvement
- Abdominal paracentesis will detect peritonitis

Necropsy findings

- Ulcer very evident; may be hemorrhagic, infected with fungal growth
- May be acute diffuse or acute or chronic local peritonitis, or adhesions stomach to spleen, suppurative splenitis

Diagnosis

Resembles squamous cell carcinoma of stomach wall.

Treatment

- Alkalinizing agents, e.g. magnesium hydroxide, carbonate or trisilicate useful but treatment needs to be frequent over long period
- Cimetidine, preferably ranitidine, effective in horses
- Hemorrhagic cases need blood transfusion, parenteral coagulants

ACUTE GASTRIC DILATATION/ TORSION IN PIGS [VM8 p. 216]

Clinical findings

- Related to intense excitement and activity by sow during eating of sloppy feed
- Death 6–24 hours later

Necropsy findings

- Enormous distension
- Hemorrhagic contents, gas
- Rotation 90–360°
- Displaced spleen

Diagnosis

- Similar distension in **intestinal reflux** due to intestinal obstruction; intestine and stomach distended with fluid. Projectile vomiting relieves temporarily

INTESTINE OBSTRUCTION IN PIGS [VM8 p. 216]

Etiology

- Torsion of coiled colon in adults
- Small colon obstruction due to eating barley chaff bedding by young pigs
- Heavy lactose feeding causes dilation/ atony

Clinical findings

- Abdomen distension
- No feces passed
- Complete anorexia
- Death in 3–6 days

IMPACTION OF THE LARGE INTESTINE OF PIGS [VM8 p. 216]

Etiology

- Sows fed wholly on grain and getting little exercise develop impaction of the colon–rectum
- Similar lesions in pigs overcrowded on sandy, gravelly outdoor yards
- Coiled colon obstruction in young weaned pigs
- Presumed inherited megacolon of fattening pigs

Clinical findings

Posterior paresis.

MECONIUM RETENTION IN PIGS [VM8 p. 216]

Clinical findings

- Anorexia, dullness, recumbency
- Scanty, hard, mucus-covered feces. Weakness, recumbency

RECTUM PARALYSIS IN PIGS [VM8 p. 216]

Etiology

In late pregnant sows.

Clinical findings

- Straining without defecation
- Anus and rectum ballooned
- Spontaneous recovery after parturition

ENTERITIS (INCLUDES
MALABSORPTION, ENTEROPATHY,
DIARRHEA) [VM8 p. 217]

Etiology

Listed below are the diseases in which diarrhea, whether caused by enteritis or malabsorption, is the principal sign, and in which a cause and effect relationship is established between the nominated cause and the clinical syndrome. Duodenitis is dealt with as a cause of equine colic.

Cattle
+ Enterotoxigenic *Escherichia coli*
+ *Salmonella* spp.
+ *Clostridium perfringens* types B and C
+ *Mycobacterium paratuberculosis*
+ *Proteus* spp., *Pseudomonas* spp.
+ *Candida* spp.
+ Rotavirus, Coronavirus, Winter dysentery coronavirus
+ Bovine virus diarrhea (mucosal disease)
+ Rinderpest
+ *Ostertagia* spp.
+ *Eimeria* spp., *Cryptosporidium* spp.
+ Poisoning by arsenic, fluorine, copper, mercury, sodium chloride, molybdenum, nitrate
+ Poisonous plants, mycotoxins
+ Molybdenum-induced secondary nutritional deficiency of copper
+ Overfeeding, simple indigestion
+ Inferior milk replacers
+ Intestinal disaccharidase deficiency
+ Congestive heart failure
+ Toxemia of coliform mastitis

Sheep and goats
+ Enterotoxigenic *E. coli*
+ *Clostridium perfringens* type B, *C. perfringens* type D
+ *Salmonella* spp.
+ *Mycobacterium paratuberculosis*
+ Rotavirus, Coronavirus
+ *Nematodirus* spp., *Ostertagia* spp.
+ *Eimeria* spp., *Cryptosporidium* spp.

Pigs
+ Enterotoxigenic *E. coli*
+ *Salmonella* spp,
+ *Clostridium perfringens* type C
+ *Treponema hyodysenteriae* (swine dysentery)
+ Transmissible gastroenteritis virus, rotavirus, coronavirus
+ *Isospora* spp.
+ *Ascaris lumbricoides*, *Trichuris suis*

+ Nutritional deficiency of iron
+ Proliferative hemorrhagic enteropathy

Horses
+ *Salmonella* spp.
+ *Actinobacillus equuli*, *Corynebacterium equi*
+ *Clostridium perfringens* type A, *C. cadaveris* (equine clostridiosis)
+ Rotavirus, coronavirus, adenovirus
+ *Ehrlichia risticii* (Potomac horse fever)
+ *Aspergillus fumigatus*
+ *Strongylus*, *Trichonema*, *Ascaris* spp.
+ Sand colic
+ Stress-induced
+ Dioctyl, phenylbutazone poisoning
+ Lymphosarcoma
+ Colitis-X
+ Granulomatous enteritis
+ Tetracycline-induced diarrhea
+ Foal-heat diarrhea

Clinical findings

+ DIARRHEA, often malodorous
+ Dysentery in some cases
+ Mucofibrinous casts in feces rarely
+ Variable smudge patterns on perineum
+ Straining, followed by rectum prolapse, in some
+ Dehydration
+ Abdominal pain in horses, occasionally calves; often severe
+ Pain on abdominal palpation in young animals
+ Rectal flatus occasionally in horses
+ Fluid rushing sounds on auscultation of abdomen in early stages of enteritis; silence other than tinkling gas movement sounds in paralytic ileus
+ Tachycardia, sometimes bradycardia, arrhythmia
+ Toxemia
+ Fever

Sequels include
+ Intussusception
+ Rectum prolapse
+ Weight loss
+ Anasarca due to hypoproteinemia

Clinical pathology

+ **Feces** – examination for causative agent; fecal leukocytes and epithelial cells as indicators of inflammation
+ **Blood** – common findings include hemoconcentration, acidosis, hyponatremia, hypochloremia, hypokalemia but results

vary widely between cases; laboratory analysis necessary for best results, especially in horses

Digestion tests necessary to confirm malabsorption tests

Intestinal biopsy necessary for confirmation chronic lesions

Serum electrophoresis, radioactive albumin excretion tests necessary for confirmation of protein-losing enteropathy diagnosis

Necropsy findings

The intestinal contents provide as much information as the mucosal lining, which may look grossly normal in a calf that has died of enterotoxigenic colibacillosis in which the suggestive lesion is an intestine filled with non-inflammatory fluid

In acute enteritis lesions include:

- Mucosal hyperemia, edema, hemorrhage, with foul-smelling contents, or
- Fibrinous inflammation, or
- Necrosis and ulceration, with epithelial shreds, fibrinous casts, frank blood.
- Mesenteric lymph nodes enlarged, edematous, congested

Chronic enteritis – thick, edematous intestine wall

Diagnosis

- Differentiation of the causes of enteritis depends on a primary separation into:
  - Inflammatory lesion due to infectious, toxic agents
  - Hypersecretion diarrhea
  - Malabsorption diarrhea due, for example, to villous atrophy
  - Osmotic diarrhea due, for example, to indigestible feeds, in disaccharidase deficiency
  - Intestinal hypermotility due, for example, to stress
- Fecal, intestinal composition, give some diagnostic assistance:
  - in **small intestinal disease,** voluminous, liquid, contain little fecal material.
  - in **large intestinal disease,** small in volume, porridge-like, often much mucus, with much fecal material.
  - in **dietary diarrhea** bulky, soft, odorless
- A large part of the examination of a herd problem of diarrhea is concerned with examination of environment, and careful taking of the history relative to access to nutritional needs and poisons, and to helminth prophylaxis

- Many diseases with other predominant clinical signs, e.g. buccal mucosal erosions, congestive heart failure, have diarrhea as a prominent sign
- A necropsy of an untreated early case of the disease, complemented by a blood culture is the best insurance of an accurate diagnosis

Treatment

Specific treatment for causative agent e.g. anthelmintic, is paramount. Secondary treatments include:

- Change of diet in dietary diarrhea
- Reduction of feed intake, where possible, during peak of enteritis; supplementation with fluid and electrolytes
- Oral fluid and electrolyte therapy suitable except in horses
- **Antibacterials** are used routinely in cases of enteritis suspected to be caused by bacteria. Controversy exists about validity of this procedure. Oral medication is satisfactory but parenteral administration also recommended where systemic invasion is suspected
- **Mass medication** in drinking water common practice when numbers of animals affected and prophylaxis in contact animals seems wise
- **Fluids and electrolytes** best supplied as directed by laboratory tests. Guidelines include:
  - Severe (10%) dehydration administer standard isotonic electrolyte solutions intravenously over a 4–6 hour period to –
500 kg horse	50 l
75 kg foal	7.5 l
45 kg calf	4.5 l
- For severe acidosis use 5–7 ml/kg (100 ml/min) 5% hypertonic sodium bicarbonate solution
- Maintenance by isotonic electrolyte solutions 100–150 ml/kg over 24 hours
- Horses may have severe hyponatremia (weakness and gross tremor). Hypertonic sodium bicarbonate used for acidosis will repair this but additional potassium may also be needed.
- Preruminant calves accept oral treatment (see colibacillosis)
- **Intestinal protectants-absorbents** have little identifiable advantage
- **Motility-reducing treatments** – opiates and anticholinergic drugs reduce gut motility and have proponents for use in diarrhea but no real; evidence of any value. They may reduce abdominal pain

♦ **Anti-secretory drugs** including chlorpromazine, atropine, prostaglandin inhibitors are used but balance of support is for use of supplementary fluids and electrolytes.

INTESTINAL HYPERMOTILITY
[VM8 p. 227]

Includes:
♦ Equine spasmodic colic
♦ Nutritional deficiency of copper, and dietary excess of molybdenum (peat scours, teart pasture)
♦ Change to lush pasture
♦ Dietary diarrhea in neonates

DIETARY DIARRHEA OF CALVES
[VM8 p. 227]

Etiology

♦ Inferior quality milk replacers in calves <3 weeks old
  • Heat-denatured skim milk powder
  • Excessive quantities non-milk carbohydrates, proteins
  • Excessive use soybean, fish proteins
♦ Cross-species milk use has some problems. Cows' milk and products may cause diarrhea in lambs, piglets, foals
♦ Excessive dilution of replacers cause fluid feces
♦ Feeding excessive volumes of whole milk does not usually cause diarrhea but may predispose to enteric infection. Excessive milk production by the dam is commonly credited with causing transitory diarrhea
♦ **Foal heat diarrhea** occurs but is imperfectly understood

Clinical findings

Beef calves, nursing
♦ Bright and alert, good appetite
♦ Light yellow, sloppy, foul-smelling feces smudge perineum
♦ Spontaneous recovery common

Dairy calves, artificially overfed
♦ Dull, anorexia
♦ Voluminous, foul-smelling feces, much mucus
♦ Distended abdomen
♦ Respond to volume limitation, oral fluid therapy

Dairy calves on inferior quality milk replacer
♦ Chronic diarrhea
♦ Weight loss
♦ Many have alopecia
♦ Weak, recumbent
♦ Drink well, bright, alert
♦ Depraved appetite, eat bedding
♦ Poor response to treatment
♦ Death from starvation at 2–4 weeks
♦ Secondary colibacillosis and salmonellosis
Chronic diarrhea due to dietary error is n[ot?] quickly fatal; weight loss, weakness, depraved appetite.

Clinical pathology

♦ Monitoring of fluid and electrolyte status may be of value in guiding support treatment
♦ Bacterial check advisable for secondary invaders

Necropsy findings

Emaciation, dehydration, serous atrophy of body fat.

Diagnosis

Resembles – enteritis

Treatment

Dairy calves, hand-fed
♦ Substitute oral electrolyte solution for milk for 24 hours
♦ Prophylactic fluids and antibacterials in high risk situations
♦ Review replacer management and quality
♦ Prevention
  • Whole milk for first 3 weeks
  • Use only replacers containing milk products

Beef calves on dams
Keep under observation for appearance toxemia, recumbency, then full antibacterial fluid and electrolyte therapy.

Foals with foal heat diarrhea
♦ Muzzle for 12 hours, strip mare
♦ Oral electrolytes, antibiotic and antidiarrheal for 24 hours

NTESTINAL OR DUODENAL
JLCERATION [VM8 p. 229]

Etiology

- Sporadic as part of enteritis due to virus and bacterial infection. Lesions mostly in terminal ileum, cecum, colon
- Occasional perforation cattle, horse causing subacute peritonitis
- Phenylbutazone poisoning in ponies

DIVERTICULITIS AND ILEITIS OF
PIGS (PROLIFERATIVE ILEITIS)
[VM8 p. 229]

Etiology

- Cause unknown

Clinical findings

- Piglets up to 3 months old have acute disease
- Sudden onset anorexia, thirst
- Dull, recumbent
- Death in 24–36 hours
- Pigs up to 8 months have chronic peritonitis

Necropsy findings

- Diffuse peritonitis
- Thickening, ulceration, perforation terminal ileum

RECTAL PROLAPSE [VM8 p. 230]

Etiology

- Enteritis with profuse diarrhea, straining
- Spinal cord abscess (cauda equina neuritis)
- Engorgement of pelvic organs
- Estrogen poisoning
- Rabies

RECTAL STRICTURE [VM8 p. 230]

Etiology

- Inherited rectal stricture of Jersey cattle
- 2–3 month old feeder pigs. Cause unknown; possibly inherited; possibly sequel to enterocolitis with ulcerative proctitis and annular cicatrisation

Clinical findings

- Abdominal distension
- Anorexia, weight loss
- Pasty to watery feces
- Palpable stricture
- Correctable surgically

CONGENITAL DEFECTS OF THE ALIMENTARY TRACT

CONGENITAL HARELIP AND
CLEFT PALATE [VM8 p. 231]

Harelip uni- or bilateral, involving only lip, or to nostril, causes dysphagia. Combined with cleft palate or alone. **Cleft palate** causes nasal regurgitation of fluid, risk of aspiration pneumonia. Sporadic, inherited or Veratrum californicum poisoning

CONGENITAL ATRESIA OF THE
SALIVARY DUCT [VM8 p. 231]

Distension then atrophy of gland. Duct may be distended.

AGNATHIA AND MICROGNATHIA
[VM8 p. 231]

- Mandibles partially or completely absent
- Inherited or sporadic

PERSISTENCE OF THE RIGHT
AORTIC ARCH [VM8 p. 231]

Esophageal occlusion, dysphagia, nasal regurgitation, chronic bloat.

CHOANAL ATRESIA [VM8 p. 231]

- Bucconasal membrane persists, bi- or unilateral
- Nasal breathing difficult or impossible
- Incompatible with life

CONGENITAL ATRESIA OF THE
INTESTINE AND ANUS [VM8
p. 231]

Etiology

- Sporadic idiopathic or inherited, especially of colon in Overoo horses

♦ Suspected cause by fetal manipulation during pregnancy diagnosis discredited

Clinical findings

♦ No feces passed
♦ Abdominal distension
♦ Non-passage of rectal sound
♦ Death at day 7–19.
♦ **Small intestine defect** associated with fetal abdominal distension and dystokia.
♦ **Anal atresia** may be surgically salvageable. Intestine repair unrewarding (30–50% recovery) because of nerve supply defects and multiple atresia sites

Anal constriction [VM8 p. 232]
Included with vaginal constriction combined with rectovaginal or recto-urethral fistula as inherited defect in Jersey cows.

Multiple organ defects [VM8 p. 231]
Gut and urinary tract combinations or accompanying pancreas, gall bladder defects cause fatal outcomes.

NEOPLASMS OF THE ALIMENTARY TRACT

MOUTH [VM8 p. 232]

♦ Papillomas
♦ Bracken poisoning
♦ Sporadic squamous cell carcinomas in aged animals

PHARYNX AND ESOPHAGUS [VM8 p. 232]

♦ Papillomas
♦ Enzootic idiopathic, malignant tumors in adult cattle in South Africa and Scotland; persistent moderate tympany, or dysphagia

STOMACH AND RUMEN [VM8 p. 232]

♦ Sporadic gastric squamous cell carcinoma in horse and cattle

Horse Anorexia, weight loss, anemia, dysphagia when lower esophagus involved, colic and diarrhea rarely. May perforate, peritonitis following. Metastases to abdominal (palpable rectally), thoracic cavities, with large fluid effusion.

Cattle:
♦ Ruminal tumors cause chronic bloat
♦ Lymphosarcoma of abomasal wall cause chronic diarrhea, melena, pyloric obstruction, rectally palpable masses

INTESTINES [VM8 p. 233]

Rare; causes chronic diarrhea, or colic, or chronic abdominal distension in horses, cattle, sheep.
♦ **Intestinal wall lymphosarcoma** of horses causes chronic diarrhea, weight loss, poor oral glucose absorption test, masses palpable rectally, fluid effusions in body cavities, sometimes colic. Examination paracentesis fluid – mitotic figures in cell nuclei
♦ **Enzootic intestinal carcinoma** recorded in pastured sheep in many countries, mostly in abattoir material; sometimes related to use of herbicides
♦ Most **perianal tumors** are anogenital papillomas

DISEASES OF PERITONEUM

PERITONITIS [VM8 p. 233]

Etiology

All species
♦ Traumatic penetration abdominal wall by stake wound
♦ Faulty asepsis at injection, trocarisation, surgery
♦ Infarcted gut segment leakage
♦ Spread from subperitoneal infection in spleen, liver, umbilicus

Cattle
♦ Traumatic reticuloperitonitis
♦ Leaking abomasal ulcer
♦ Abomasum rupture after torsion

- Rumenitis followed by rupture
- Liver abscess due to black disease
- Vagina rupture, intercourse, sadism
- Semen deposition in peritoneum
- Chemical peritonitis; injection hypertonic solution
- Intraperitoneal injection non-sterile solution
- Intestine transection by compression against pelvis during parturition
- Uterine rupture during parturition, relief of dystokia
- Rectum spontaneous rupture during parturition
- Part of specific disease, e.g. tuberculosis, sporadic bovine encephalomyelitis

Horse
- Colon, dorsal cecal sac, rupture at foaling
- Cecum rupture anesthetised foal during gastric endoscopy
- Cecum stasis/dilation/perforation after administration non-steroidal inflammatories
- Rectum tear during manual examination
- Extension from retroperitoneal infection e.g. Streptococcus equi, Rhodococcus equi with Strongylus spp. infestation
- Gastric erosion/ulceration by *Habronema*, *Gasterophilus* spp.
- Cecal perforation due to *Anoplocephala perfoliata*
- Spontaneous gastric rupture
- Actinomyces equuli infection

Pig
- Regional ileitis
- Glassers disease

Sheep
- Abscess due to Oesophagostomum spp. larvae
- *Mycoplasma* spp. serositis-arthritis

Goats
- *Mycoplasma* spp. serositis/arthritis

Clinical findings

Acute–subacute peritonitis
- Toxemia, fever
- Partial or complete anorexia
- Spontaneous abdominal pain, as in colic, especially horses; arched back, reluctant to move in cattle
- Grunting respiration
- Pain on external palpation, percussion (grunt test in cattle), rectal palpation
- Fecal output reduced, usually absent; rectum dry and tacky, contains dry fecal balls covered with mucus or scant, pasty, sticky, malodorous. Early diarrhea in some
- Alimentary tract stasis; rumen stasis, no gut sounds in horses
- Adhesions palpable per rectum

Peracute diffuse peritonitis
- Sudden onset after parturition, gut rupture
- Profound toxemia, hypothermia
- Depression, recumbency
- Complete anorexia
- Very high heart rate, imperceptible pulse
- Death in 4–48 hours; sooner in horses than cattle

Chronic peritonitis
Cattle
- Chronic toxemia, wasting
- Intermittent bouts of pain accompanied by distended gut loops on palpation, increased gut sounds
- Abdominal distension due to exudate accumulation in a few, usually segregated in sac, e.g. omental bursa. Careful paracentesis may reveal it
- Adhesions palpable per rectum in some

Horse
- Ill-thrift for weeks; severe weight loss
- Intermittent mild–moderate colic
- Gut sounds diminished
- Subcutaneous edema of ventral abdominal wall
- Secondary pleurisy in some
- Inflammatory fluid on paracentesis

Clinical pathology

- Leukocytosis with left shift in acute–chronic cases
- Leukopenia with toxic granulation of neutrophils in peracute cases
- Cases with walled-off lesions may have normal hemograms
- Peritoneal fluid by paracentesis (Tables 5.1 and 5.2) a positive indicator of severity and cause of peritonitis. Failure to obtain sample does not rule out peritonitis as diagnosis
- Radiography limited to very young animals. Standing reticular radiography used in traumatic reticuloperitonitis

Necropsy findings

♦ Hemorrhage, exudation, fibrin deposits, pus accumulation, most evident in ventral abdomen. Bad odor due to *Fusobacterium necrophorum* and *Actinomyces pyogenes* in cattle
♦ Adhesions and walled-off pockets of pus in chronic cases

Diagnosis

Cattle

♦ Acute local peritonitis resembles:
  • Intestinal obstruction
  • Splenic, hepatic abscess
  • Abomasal displacement, right or left
  • Postpartum metritis
  • Acetonemia
♦ Acute diffuse peritonitis resembles:
  • Parturient paresis (milk fever)
  • Peracute coliform mastitis
  • Carbohydrate engorgement
  • Abomasal ulcer perforation
  • Postpartum septic metritis
  • Uterus rupture
♦ Chronic peritonitis
  • Vagus indigestion
  • Fat necrosis mesentery, omentum
  • Persistent leakage abomasal or intestinal lesion
  • Ascites
  • Bladder rupture

Horses

♦ Intestinal obstruction colic
♦ Internal abdominal (retroperitoneal) abscess
♦ Intra-abdominal neoplasm

Treatment

♦ Specific treatments are listed under specific diseases, e.g. intestine rupture, traumatic reticuloperitonitis
♦ In undifferentiated cases a parenteral, broad spectrum antibacterial drug is standard. Recovery from acute phase good unless gut rupture and massive endotoxemia. Sequel of adhesive gut constriction uncommon
♦ Intraperitoneal injection limited in value because of probability of local sequestration in masses of fibrin. Should always be complemented by intravenous, subcutaneous or intramuscular injection
♦ Drainage of large volumes of fluid in chronic cases

♦ Peritoneal lavage is attempted but results are not rewarding

RECTAL TEARS [VM8 p. 238]

Etiology

♦ Damage during rectal examination the commonest cause
♦ Misdirected penis during mating
♦ During parturition especially dystokia

Clinical findings

Mucosa-only tears

♦ Tear can be felt to happen
♦ No signs but infection of wall occurs

Retroperitoneal tears

♦ Local cellulitis in pelvic fascia
♦ Fever, toxemia for 7–10 days
♦ Mild abdominal pain
♦ Then sudden onset acute diffuse peritonitis
♦ Endotoxic shock
♦ Death in 24–36 hours

Peritoneal tears

♦ Acute diffuse peritonitis within an hour
♦ Endotoxic shock
♦ Death within 24–36 hours

Treatment

♦ Reduce peristalsis with atropine for 3 days
♦ Empty feces from rectum
♦ Pack rectum with medicated gauze sponges and retain with anal purse string suture
♦ Broad spectrum antimicrobial cover for 3 days
♦ Minimal bulk in feed; pellets, no hay
♦ Suture of tears via anus if possible
♦ Suture via laparotomy, if necessary with a colostomy

RETROPERITONEAL ABSCESS [VM8 p. 239]

Includes:

♦ Internal abdominal abscess
♦ Chronic peritonitis
♦ Infected verminous aneurysm
♦ Omental bursitis

Etiology

♦ Post-strangles localisation
♦ Erosion through gastric mucosal lesion e.g.

Gasterophilus, Habronema spp. or squamous cell carcinoma, or gastric ulcer
Sequel to rectal tear

Clinical findings

Chronic leakage causes recurrent attacks of peritonitis
Chronic or, rarely, intermittent colic
Anorexia, weight loss
Intermittent, low grade fever
Anemia
Abdomen distended with fluid, rarely
Involvement of pelvic fascia causes constipation, straining at defecation, pain during rectal examination
Palpable enlargements, especially in pelvis and posterior abdomen
Ultrasonographic imaging of abscess is possible

Clinical pathology

♦ Neutrophilia with left shift in acute infections
♦ Abdominocentesis fluid cultured but often negative when abscesses present

Diagnosis

Resembles:
♦ *Abdominal neoplasm*
♦ Splenic abscess
♦ Liver abscess
♦ Pelvis fascia abscess

Treatment

♦ Broad spectrum antibacterial over a period of at least 2 weeks preferably several months. Usual 3 day treatment produces temporary response and relapse
♦ Surgical excision attempted in some of the many poor responses to medical treatment. Rarely successful because of extensive adhesions

ABDOMINAL FAT NECROSIS
(LIPOMATOSIS) [VM8 p. 240]

Etiology

♦ Cause unknown but possibles include:
♦ Inherited
  • High incidence in some herds attributed to ingestion
  • Acremonium coenophialum infested tall fescue grass
  • Sharp incidence increase of sporadic cases with advancing age

Clinical findings

♦ Large, hard masses necrotic fat palpable rectally in cattle, may cause intermittent external compression, and obstruction of intestine, pylorus causing:
  • Intermittent abdominal pain
  • Passage small amounts pasty feces

Treatment

Nil, salvage recommended.

Pedunculated lipoma [VM8 p. 240]
♦ Can knot around loop of intestine anywhere from pylorus to rectum
♦ Causes sudden onset of severe colic in horses older than 12 years
♦ Can cause palpable constriction of lower colon
♦ Urgent surgical excision mandatory

6 DISEASES OF THE ALIMENTARY TRACT – II

CLINICAL INDICANTS

The principal clinical syndrome, signs and clinicopathological findings on which diagnoses of alimentary tract disease in ruminants are based include the following.

BASIC SYNDROME – PRIMARY GASTROINTESTINAL DYSFUNCTION IN RUMINANTS

The syndrome which indicates that primary gastrointestinal dysfunction is present includes the following clinical and clinical pathology findings, in the absence of evidence of disease in another system:
♦ Partial or complete anorexia
♦ Failure to regurgitate and chew the cud
♦ Abdominal distension, possibly symmetrical, most commonly of the left abdomen or gaunt and empty
♦ Ruminal contents may feel abnormal through left paralumbar fossa – doughy, gassy, liquid
♦ Ruminal movements indicate hypermotility, hypomotility or atony
♦ Spontaneous abdominal pain indicated by:
  • **Acute colic** – kicking at belly, stretching
  • **Subacute pain** – humping of back, reluctant to move
♦ Induced abdominal pain on deep palpation, e.g. in peritonitis
♦ Rarely, dropping regurgitated cuds
♦ Normal temperature, heart rate, respirations, except in cases of:
  • Peritonitis – fever or subnormal temperature, toxemic shock in some cases
  • Carbohydrate engorgement – dehydration, acidosis
  • Abomasal torsion – dehydration, alkalosis
♦ Feces scant, possibly absent for as long as 48 hours, pasty (over-digested), foul-smelling, except in:
  • Carbohydrate engorgement – increased in amount, sweet–sour smelling, may contain undigested material

The following clinical and clinical pathological abnormalities occur commonly in alimentary tract dysfunction in ruminants, in addition to the signs listed at the beginning of the previous chapter. Consulting the cause of each of these indicators will lead the diagnostic process towards the identification of the specific cause of the disease.

Abdomen distension

Occurs in:
♦ Rumen distension due to:
  • Ruminal tympany
  • Vagus indigestion
♦ Abomasal dilation/torsion, impaction
♦ Intestinal obstruction, paralytic ileus
♦ Ascites
♦ Chronic peritonitis
♦ Hydrops amnii
♦ Pneumoperitoneum

Abdomen distension with asymmetry

See Fig. 6.1.

Abdomen, pain

See pain, abdominal, this section.

Abomasum distended, impacted

♦ Large, tense, distended viscus in lower right abdomen – in abomasal torsion
♦ Firm, distended viscus in lower right abdomen. Most cases of abomasal impaction occur in late pregnancy and are not palpable because of the uterus

Adhesions in abdomen

Tight bands of adhesion in peritonitis.

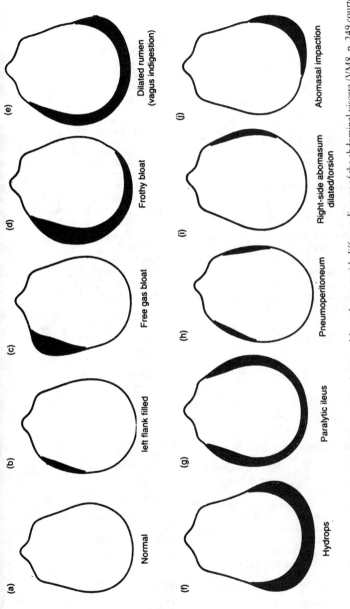

Figure 6.1 Silhouettes of the contour of the abdomen of cattle, viewed from the rear, with different diseases of the abdominal viscera (VM8, p. 249 courtesy of the authors and the editor of *Bovine Practitioner*).

(a) Normal
(b) left flank filled
(c) Free gas bloat
(d) Frothy bloat
(e) Dilated rumen (vagus indigestion)
(f) Hydrops
(g) Paralytic ileus
(h) Pneumoperitoneum
(i) Right-side abomasum dilated/torsion
(j) Abomasal impaction

Cud-dropping

Clinical findings Coughing up a compressed cud of undigested fiber.

Occurs in Pharyngeal paralysis.

Eructation diminished

Belching is a reflex act in response to gas accumulation in the rumen. Reduction causes ruminal tympany.

Causes:
+ Ruminal contents frothy
+ Esophageal cardia below fluid level as in lateral recumbency
+ Neurological deficit in reflex
+ Peritonitis
+ Esophageal obstruction

Feces color abnormal

+ Pale with milk diet
+ Color darker with slowing of rate of passage, lighter when rate increased
+ Black–green in patients producing much bile pigments e.g. in hemolytic anemia; pale olive green in patients with bile duct obstruction

Feces contain blood

+ Dark brown to black, tarry (**melena**) in hemorrhage in abomasum and upper small intestine
+ Red from large intestinal hemorrhage
+ Streaked with clotted blood (**hematochezia**) in rectal hemorrhage

Feces contain mucus/fibrin

+ Sheets of **mucus** on dry balls of manure indicate overlong sojourn in the gut
+ A plug of tenacious **mucus** as the sole contents of the rectum indicates functional obstruction, e.g. paralytic ileus
+ Large quantities clear, watery **mucus** common in enteritis
+ **Fibrin** in shreds or long strands, or coagulated into an **intestinal cast**, indicative of enteritis

Fecal odor foul

Offensive odor when there is:
+ Putrefaction of products of inflammation
+ Putrefaction of protein in rumen when, for example, milk products fed to adults or esophageal reflex fails in calves drinking milk

Feces pasty

Much variation occurs naturally, depending on feed composition
+ Pasty (homogenous, sloppy, containing much undigested fiber) in left abomasal displacement
+ Sticky and tenacious in vagus indigestion, chronic peritonitis

Feces volume decreased

Scant feces for several days in:
+ Traumatic reticuloperitonitis
+ Vagus indigestion
+ Omasal impaction
+ Abomasal impaction
+ Abomasal displacement, left and right
+ Abomasal torsion
+ Abomasal ulcer
+ Peritonitis
+ Paralytic ileus
+ Idiopathic intestinal tympany
+ Severe toxemia
+ Abdominal fat necrosis

No feces passed in any of the above plus:
+ Intestinal obstruction by phytobezoar, trichobezoar, enterolith
+ Intussusception
+ Coiled colon torsion
+ Mesenteric root torsion
+ Cecal torsion

Feces watery

Occurs in:
+ Enteritis
+ Dietary diarrhea

Feed intake reduced or absent

An early and sensitive indicator of alimentary dysfunction, but occurs in diseases of most systems; not a specific indicator of alimentary tract dysfunction

Intestine distended

+ Long, distended, mobile organ with blind end in right upper abdomen – in cecal torsion
+ Small loops distended small intestine in intestinal strangulation
+ Distended loops of intestine suspended by

tight cord-like mesentery in mesenteric torsion
♦ Dilated loop of intestine in fixed position – intestinal incarceration

Laparoscopic examination

A flexible fiberoptic colonoscope is being used.

Laparotomy examination

Surgical exploration of the abdomen is an essential part of a clinical examination for surgical conditions of the gut, e.g. carbohydrate engorgement, abomasal displacement, intestinal torsion and intussusception, mesenteric torsion, cecal dilation/torsion, whether the diagnosis is final or only tentative. Diseases in which laparotomy is almost always tentative are: chronic reticuloperitonitis, atypical abomasal displacements, intussusception, intestinal incarceration.

Liver painful on percussion over right caudal ribs

Occurs in:
♦ Liver abscess
♦ Cholangiohepatitis
♦ Hepatitis

Mass in abdomen

Small, floating, hard-to-find, cylindrical mass in intussusception.

Pain, abdominal – elicited

Clinical findings:
♦ Pain grunt elicited by applying deep percussion or pressure to abdomen, preferably at end of respiration
♦ Most positive grunt findings are in anterior abdomen – **anterior abdominal pain**

Occurs in:
♦ Traumatic reticuloperitonitis
♦ Traumatic splenitis
♦ Leaking abomasal ulcer
♦ Liver abscess with right side percussion

Pain, abdominal – spontaneous

Clinical findings:
Acute
♦ Bouts of down-arching of back, kicking at belly, lying down, rarely rolling, bellowing

Subacute
♦ Permanent posture back arched upward
♦ Grunt on walking, lying down
♦ Spontaneous grunting with each respiration, exacerbated when recumbent
♦ Grunt on deep palpation abdomen
♦ Disinclination to walk
♦ Teeth grinding

Occurs in:
Acute
♦ Intestinal obstruction
♦ Poisoning by *Pennisetum clandestinum*, *Andromeda* spp., *Nerium oleander*, *Cicuta* spp.
Subacute
♦ Traumatic reticuloperitonitis
♦ Abomasal ulcer
♦ Peritonitis generally

Ping on percussion right abdomen

Occurs in:
♦ Right abomasal dilation/torsion
♦ Cecal dilation/torsion
♦ Coiled colon torsion
♦ Patient with tenesmus (colon, rectum filled with air)
♦ Intestinal idiopathic tympany e.g. in puerperal cow
♦ Mesenteric root torsion, calf
♦ Intussusception
♦ Pneumoperitoneum

Ping on percussion over rumen

Occurs in:
♦ Left abomasal displacement
♦ Empty rumen, rarely
♦ Pneumoperitoneum

Rumen contents abnormal

Abnormal rumen contents by stomach tube, trocar, vomitus, rumenotomy include:
♦ Milky-gray color in carbohydrate engorgement, blackish-green in prolonged stasis with putrefaction
♦ Watery consistency in abomasal reflux and in ruminal floral inactivity
♦ Frothy in primary frothy bloat and vagus indigestion
♦ Moldy, rotting odor in protein putrefaction, sour odor in carbohydrate engorgement
♦ Normal pH of 6.2–7.2 elevated to 8–10 in protein putrefaction, depressed to <5 in carbohydrate engorgement
♦ Normal motile protozoal numbers in

ruminal fluid (5–7 per low power micro-scopic field) absent in carbohydrate engorgement.

Rumen distension

Clinical signs include:
- Distension left side mostly but can be on lower right also (Fig. 6.1)
- Ruminal movements absent in indigestion, carbohydrate engorgement, or increased in vagus indigestion, early bloat
- Ruminal percussion gives tympanitic (free gas bloat) or dull (frothy bloat) sound
- Relief by trocarization (free gas bloat) or froth exudes (frothy bloat)
- Relief by stomach tube in free gas bloat (gas emission) or abomasal reflux (fluid emission)
- Relief by sitting up a recumbent cow
- Distended L-shaped rumen with ventral sac extending into lower right abdomen on rectal – vagus indigestion
- Cardiac systolic murmur in many

Occurs in:
- Primary bloat (pasture, feedlot)
- Esophageal obstruction
- Vagus indigestion
- Pyloric or upper duodenal obstruction, e.g. by phytobezoar, with fluid reflux
- Lateral recumbency
- Carbohydrate engorgement
- Simple indigestion

Rumen doughy, firm, impacted

Clinical findings:
- Rumen firm, doughy, modest overfilling in left flank
- Hypomotility

Occurs in:
- Simple indigestion (impaction)
- Peritonitis
- Dehydration
- Diet indigestible, e.g. tree loppings

Rumen empty, collapsed

Occurs in:
- Starvation, voluntary or involuntary

Rumen movements present, sounds absent

Occurs in:
- Left abomasal displacement
- Frothy bloat
- Vagus indigestion

Rumen movements, sounds both absent/diminished

Clinical findings:
- Most severe diseases of the ruminant fore-stomachs, abomasum and intestines
- Hypomotility – movements less than 1 every 2 minutes
- Atony – no ruminal movements

Occurs in:
- Simple indigestion
- Carbohydrate engorgement
- Peritonitis
- Traumatic reticuloperitonitis
- Lead poisoning
- As part of most severe diseases in which a systemic reaction occurs

Rumen movements, sounds increased

Clinical findings:
- Ruminal cycles more than 2 per minute
- Ruminal sounds exaggerated or decreased (frothy bloat)

Occurs in:
- Early stages of bloat
- Vagus indigestion

Rumen movements absent, tinkling sounds only

Occurs in Starvation.

Rumen small

Small size rumen in left abomasal displacement.

Rumen sounds muffled

Clinical findings Rumen sounds muffled but normal frequency.

Occurs in:
- Left abomasal displacement
- Ascites

Rumen sounds tympanitic, resilient on percussion

Occurs in:
- Bloat
- Vagus indigestion

Rumination diminished

Regurgitation and cud-chewing are part reflex, part voluntary acts. Causes of absence include:

+ Low fiber diets
+ Distraction, harassment
+ Reduced ruminoreticular motility

Splashing sounds ballottement right abdomen

Occurs in:
+ Intestinal obstruction
+ Enteritis
+ Right abomasal dilation/torsion

Splashing sound ballottement over rumen

Occurs in:
+ Carbohydrate engorgement
+ Pyloric obstruction

Stomach tube passage

+ Passage of a properly placed tube by a foreign body in esophagus
+ Reflux of alkaline fluid in vagus indigestion and abomasal reflux due to high intestinal or pyloric obstruction
+ Frothy or porridge-like contents which will not flow through the tube may be evacuated by lavage

Teeth grinding

See Pain, abdominal spontaneous

Viscus (firm) palpable in right flank

+ Omasal impaction
+ Abomasal impaction
+ Grossly enlarged ventral ruminal sac extending across abdominal floor, in vagus indigestion
+ Liver enlargement, rarely

DISEASES OF THE RUMEN, RETICULUM AND OMASUM

SIMPLE INDIGESTION [VM8 p. 259]

Etiology

+ Too much of a highly digestible feed, e.g. grain, palatable, e.g. ensilage
+ Indigestible feed, e.g. chopped straw, tree loppings
+ Mouldy feed
+ Frozen feed
+ Insufficient drinking water
+ Depraved appetite
+ Prolonged, heavy feeding antibiotics, sulfonamides
+ Improperly formulated formalin or caustic-treated feeds
+ Industrial junk feeds, e.g. coffee grounds, shredded paper

Clinical findings

+ Anorexia
+ Sharp, moderate fall in milk yield
+ Ruminal movements reduced or absent
+ Rumination ceases
+ Rumen moderate distension when gorged on palatable feed

+ Rumen firm, doughy, may be slight tympany
+ Feces dry, firm; voluminous, smelly, soft in convalescence
+ Spontaneous recovery or good response to treatment in 48 hours

Clinical pathology

Ruminal contents pH 5.5–6.0 in cattle on grain diets.

Diagnosis

Resembles:
+ Acetonemia
+ Traumatic reticuloperitonitis
+ Carbohydrate engorgement
+ Left abomasal displacement
+ Right abomasal displacement
+ Abomasal volvulus
+ Vagus indigestion
+ Phytobezoar

Treatment

+ Magnesium sulfate 0.5–1 kg in water as a drench
+ 15–20 liters water by stomach tube when rumen contents inspissated

• Cud transfer in patients with history of more than a week anorexia, especially cases caused by prolonged oral antibacterials
• Rumenotomy in obstinate cases of impaction with dry fiber

INDIGESTION IN CALVES FED MILK REPLACERS (RUMINAL DRINKERS) [VM8 p. 261]

Etiology

Imperfect esophageal reflex in veal calves 5–6 weeks after beginning bucket feeding on milk replacer.

Clinical findings

• Recurrent ruminal tympany
• Anorexia
• Unthriftiness
• Clay-like feces
• Spontaneous recovery in a few days after change to normal feeding
• Distended ventral abdomen , especially left side
• Splashing sounds on ballottement left flank
• Splashing sounds left flank during drinking
• Siphoning ruminal contents produces foul, acid-smelling, gray–white fluid

Clinical pathology

Milk entering rumen–reticulum visible radiologically

Necropsy findings

• Rumen distended
• Marked ruminal hyperkeratosis
• Villous atrophy in proximal jejunum
• Casein clot in rumen

Treatment

• Weaning onto dry feed, recovery in 1–2 weeks

ACUTE CARBOHYDRATE ENGORGEMENT (RUMEN OVERLOAD) [VM8 p. 262]

Etiology

Large intake carbohydrate-rich feed, e.g. grain, apples, standing sweet corn, bread, dough, sugar beet, concentrated sugar solutions, incompletely fermented brewers grains.

Epidemiology

• Cattle, sheep, goats, farmed deer
• Sudden, often accidental, change to carbohydrate-rich diet
• Common in feedlots, especially when starting cattle on feed
• Grazing on stubble fields with much spilt grain
• Wheat, barley, corn most toxic; oats, sorghum least
• Ground grain more toxic than whole
• Toxic dose very variable depending on type and digestibility of feed and prior adaptation of animals to feed
• Morbidity 10–50%; case fatality rate in untreated up to 90%; in treated 30–40%

Clinical findings

• Sudden onset complete anorexia
• Profound depression, reluctant to move
• Complete ruminal stasis
• Fluid splashing sounds in rumen
• Severe dehydration up to 12% body weight
• Very rapid heart rate, small amplitude pulse
• Soft to watery, light-colored, smelly feces; may contain undigested evidence of toxic feed
• Actions indicate blindness
• Stumbling gait, muscle tremor, recumbency, coma
• Death in 24–72 hours
• Some mild cases in affected group may recover spontaneously after 2–3 days; others respond to treatment for simple indigestion

Sequels include:
• Chemical rumenitis leading to fatal peritonitis
• Laminitis
• Abortion

Clinical pathology

• Ruminal fluid pH <5 in clinical cases
• No protozoa in ruminal fluid
• Hematocrit 50–60%
• Blood lactate, inorganic phosphate elevated
• Blood pH, bicarbonate fall markedly
• Mild hypocalcemia

Necropsy findings

Ruminal contents thin, porridge-like, fermented smell

Rumenitis – ruminal epithelium in patches peels off, revealing hemorrhagic surface, mostly in ventral sac

Abomasitis, enteritis

Gangrenous patches of ruminal wall at 3–4 days

Diagnosis

Standing cases resemble lead poisoning

Recumbent cases resemble:
- Many profound toxemias especially
  - Coliform mastitis
  - Acute diffuse peritonitis
- Milk fever

Treatment

Animals known to have been exposed

- Remove from feed, shut off water supply
- Feed small ration of hay only
- Vigorous exercise every hour for 12 hours
- Segregate cows showing anorexia, staggery gait, depression
- Treat mild cases for simple indigestion and return to water
- Salvage by slaughter or treat for ruminal acidosis the rest

Mild cases

- 500 g magnesium hydroxide/450 kg body weight, in 10 liters warm water by stomach tube, external ruminal kneading
- Treat dehydration and acidosis by intravenous isotonic sodium bicarbonate (1.3%) or balanced electrolyte solution

Moderate clinical cases, those still standing

- Warm water rumen lavage with large bore tube, repeated 10–15 times
- Treat systemic acidosis: I/V 5% sodium bicarbonate solution, 5 liters during 30 minutes/450 kg body weight, followed by isotonic bicarbonate (1.3%), 150 ml/kg during 6–12 hours

Severe clinical cases – recumbent, rumen pH 5 or less, heart rate 110+/minute

- Rumenotomy plus rumen lavage
- Cud transfer plus handful of hay in rumen
- Treat systemic acidosis as above

Miscellaneous, ancillary treatments

Antihistamines, corticosteroids, thiamin, parasympathomimetics, oral antibiotics used but usefulness doubtful.

Follow-up

Sudden deterioration in apparently recovering animals may be due to mycotic rumenitis if cases treated too late or acidosis not adequately treated.

Prevention

- Adaptation to grain by 50% grain ration for 10 days, then decrease roughage by 10% every 2–4 days down to 10–15%. Roughage and grain should be mixed, not fed separately
- Feeding alkalis, e.g. sodium bicarbonate, of doubtful value and some disadvantages
- Feeding regimens offering some value include:
  - Thiopeptin antibiotic, alone or with sodium bicarbonate
  - Salinomycin, monensin, lasolocid
  - Ruminal inoculation with cud transfer from grain adapted to non-adapted cattle

RUMINAL PARAKERATOSIS [VM8 p. 269]

Etiology

Heat-treated feed pellets containing alfalfa.

Clinical findings

Nil but weight gain may be reduced.

Necropsy findings

Large, dark, leathery ruminal papillae, some fused together into clumps, mostly in dorsal half of rumen, and at level of fluid surface.

RUMINAL TYMPANY (BLOAT) [VM8 p. 270]

Etiology

Primary ruminal tympany (frothy bloat)

- Grazing legume pasture
- Feedlot cattle on high grain diets
- Some cases of vagus indigestion, diaphragmatic hernia

Secondary ruminal tympany (free gas bloat)

+ Esophageal obstruction
+ Tetanus
+ *Rhizoctonia leguminicola* poisoning
+ *Actinomyces bovis* lesions, papilloma or carcinoma, in reticular wall, near esophageal groove
+ Anaphylaxis
+ Hypocalcemia, as in milk fever
+ Some cases of feedlot bloat due possibly to esophagitis, rumenitis, failure of eructation due to all-grain diets
+ Persistent enlarged thymus
+ Chronic idiopathic tympany in calves up to 6 months old
+ Some cases of vagus indigestion, diaphragmatic hernia

Epidemiology

Pasture bloat commonest in:

+ Lush, immature (pre-bloom) legume pasture
+ Some legumes, e.g. subterranean, crimson clovers not tympanogenic
+ Cases also in highly fertilized young grass pasture, cereal crops, vegetables
+ Spring and autumn

Feedlot bloat commonest in:

+ Cattle on heavy grain, little roughage (<20%) diets
+ Finely ground or pelleted feeds

All bloat:

+ Losses due to deaths plus
+ Loss of production in subclinical cases due to constant fullness of rumen with foam
+ Predominantly a disease of cattle. Does occur in sheep

Clinical findings

+ Sudden onset of bloat
+ Often not till second day on tympanogenic pasture
+ As soon as 15 minutes, usually 1 hour, after going onto pasture
+ Deaths usually commence 3–4 hours later
+ Often patients found dead
+ Obvious distension entire abdomen, mostly on left
+ Lying down and getting up frequently, kicking at belly
+ Frequent defecation of a stream of sloppy feces, urination
+ Severe dyspnea, mouth breathing, head extended, tongue protruded, profuse salivation
+ Tachycardia and systolic murmur, disappears when bloat relieved
+ Projectile vomiting in some
+ Ruminal movements continuous earl later atony
+ **Trocarization** yields rush of gas and defla tion in free gas bloat; dribble of froth onl in frothy bloat
+ **Stomach tube** relieves free gas bloat (tub may need clearing), no effect in frothy bloat
+ No feed taken, no eructation, no rumina tion
+ Sudden collapse and death without strug gle
+ Many animals may be affected at same time
+ In affected herd many cattle will have mil bloat without other clinical signs

Chronic bloat

+ Rumen distended, usually hypermotile, fo weeks; usually free gas bloat, may be frothy
+ Little feed taken
+ Weight loss, emaciation
+ Scant pasty feces

Clinical pathology

Insufficient time available for in-depth contemplation.

Necropsy findings

+ Tongue protrusion
+ Vascular congestion more obvious in front quarters
+ Lungs compressed
+ Rumen distended but froth disappears soon after death
+ Liver pale
+ Diaphragm or rumen may be ruptured
+ Subcutaneous emphysema

Diagnosis

Primary bloat resembles secondary bloat caused by:

+ Esophageal obstruction,
+ Ruminal drinkers – esophageal groove dysfunction
+ Vagus indigestion
+ Tetanus
+ Idiopathic bloat in young cattle – cattle not under close supervision may be found dead and need to be differentiated as set out under sudden death.

Treatment

+ Remove animals from feed supply
+ Extreme cases trocarize or perform emergency rumenotomy and clean up later

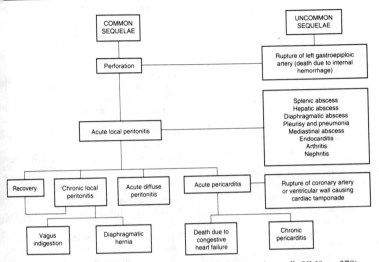

Figure 6.2 Sequelae of traumatic perforation of the reticular wall (VM8 p. 279).

♦ Less urgent cases attempt relief with wide bore stomach tube; administer 250–500 ml of non-toxic oil, usually mineral oil, or 150–200 g sodium bicarbonate in water
♦ Other effective oral medications include:
  • Oil containing detergent, e.g. dioctyl sodium sulfosuccinate
  • Poloxalene 25–50 g
  • Alcohol ethoxylates (e.g. Rx Teric)
♦ Mild cases drench with one of the above treatments
♦ Forcibly walk all cattle on treatment or in affected group and likely to develop bloat
♦ Kneading of the rumen through the left flank recommended

Prevention

Pasture bloat
♦ Daily administration during the danger period of one of the following:
  • Non-biodegradable, non-toxic oil or fat 60–120 ml
  • Poloxalene 10–20 g
  • Alcohol ethoxylate 17–19 g
as a drench, spray on the pasture to be eaten, in a special ration of hay or grain before the cattle are turned into the pasture, in the drinking water, by lick, roller drum lick, or spray or paint on each cow's flank
♦ Ruminal installation of a slow-release device delivering 300 mg/day monensin

Feedlot bloat
♦ Procedures used in pasture bloat less effective

♦ Ensure ration contains >15% roughage, preferably mature cereal or grass hay
♦ Use only rolled or cracked grain, not finely ground, nor pelleted
♦ Avoid sudden fluctuations in amounts of grain fed

TRAUMATIC RETICULOPERITONITIS [VM8 p. 278]

Etiology

Perforation of reticular wall by swallowed sharp foreign bodies e.g. nails, short pieces of fencing wire, cause acute local peritonitis, or other sequelae (Fig. 6.2).

Epidemiology

♦ Mostly dairy cows because of exposure to hand-feeding
♦ Rare cases in dairy bulls and yearlings, beef cattle, sheep, goats
♦ Lesion morbidity may be as high as 70% in a herd; clinical morbidity much less
♦ With treatment 75% recover, 25% develop sequelae with poor recovery rate or die
♦ Mortality rate greater in late pregnancy

Clinical findings

Acute local peritonitis
♦ Sudden onset, during a 12 hour period
♦ Complete anorexia

- Drop in milk yield to <33%
- Reluctant to move, walks slowly, often with grunting
- Standing preferred; some recumbent
- Arching and rigidity of back
- Abdominal wall tense; gives tucked-up or gaunt appearance
- Infrequent urination, defecation
- Some grunt with each respiration
- Mild fever
- Pulse, respiratory rates marginally elevated
- Respirations shallow
- No ruminal movements, no rumination, no eructation
- Left paralumbar fossa full, rumen pack firm, doughy with small gas cap
- Constipation or scant feces
- Grunt elicited by firm pressure behind xiphoid on left, best heard by tracheal auscultation or by pressure by fist, knee or rail lifted by two persons, one on each side
- Short course 48–72 hours but may recur with exercise

Chronic local peritonitis
- Continuation of acute stage
- Incomplete return of appetite
- Incomplete return of milk yield
- Depression
- Mild or intermittent fever
- Slow, careful walk
- Some grunt during rumination, defecation, urination
- Chronic, mild bloat; ruminal movements present
- Rumination depressed
- Feces dry, firm
- Abdomen may be distended with fluid or
- Abdomen gaunt with no fluid and many adhesions on rectal

Acute diffuse peritonitis
- Mostly in puerperal cows
- Profound depression
- Complete anorexia
- Cessation milk flow
- Complete ruminal stasis
- Pain on percussion over ventral abdomen soon disappears
- May be fever, usually severe hypothermia
- Tachycardia >100/minute
- Recumbency, coma terminally

Clinical pathology
- Metal detectors effective in diagnosing presence of ferrous foreign bodies in reticulum, but most cows react positively

- Radiological examination is used in large hospitals
- Fiberoptoscopic examination through a laparotomy also used

Acute peritonitis
- Neutrophilia and regenerative left shift
- Total leukocyte count varies with degree of segregation of leukocytes in peritoneal cavity
- Elevated mean plasma protein concentrations
- Abdominocentesis may reveal inflammatory fluid

Chronic peritonitis
- Moderate leukocytosis, neutrophilia, monocytosis
- Large volume clear serous inflammatory fluid may be found on abdominocentesis. When adhesions extensive no fluid may be collectable

Acute diffuse peritonitis
- Leukopenia, degenerative left shift, lymphopenia
- Elevated plasma fibrinogen levels
- Abdominocentesis may confirm clinical diagnosis

Necropsy findings
- In acute diffuse peritonitis fibrinous or suppurative peritonitis over entire serous surface
- Foreign body in fibrous tissue track to diaphragm or fallen back into reticulum
- Chronic peritonitis – massive adhesions walling off pus-filled cavities; extensive inflammatory fluid accumulation in a few
- Associated lesion in other organs in some cases (see Fig. 6.2)

Diagnosis
Acute local peritonitis resembles:
- Peritonitis due to other causes
- Indigestion
- Acetonemia
- Ephemeral fever usually involves a number of animals
- Acute intestinal obstruction
- Abomasal displacement, abomasal torsion
- Carbohydrate engorgement
- Postpartum metritis
- Pleurisy

Chronic peritonitis resembles:
♦ Pyelonephritis
♦ Liver abscess
♦ Splenic abscess
♦ Diaphragmatic abscess
♦ Mediastinal abscess

Acute diffuse peritonitis resembles:
♦ Milk fever
♦ Coliform mastitis
♦ Septic metritis

Treatment

Acute diffuse or chronic peritonitis
Not susceptible to any form of treatment.

Acute local peritonitis
Three programs used: conservative medical, rumenotomy, and medical rumenotomy if response poor.
♦ **Medical treatment:**
  • Immobilization of patient with fore limbs elevated
  • Systemic antibacterial treatment for 3–5 days
  • Contraindicated for cows pregnant more than 6 months
♦ **Rumenotomy:**
  • Has the advantage of being diagnostic
  • Recovery rate good if performed early
♦ **Combined treatment:**
  • If response to medical treatment by 72 hours is not good perform laparotomy

Prevention

♦ Use only string-baled hay
♦ Neutralize foreign bodies by:
  • Passing all feed over electromagnets
  • Fit all cows in the milking herd with reticular magnets

VAGUS INDIGESTION [VM8 p. 284]

Etiology

In many cases the cause is obscure but some appear to be the result of:
♦ Traumatic reticuloperitonitis causing injury to vagus nerve branches over the anterior wall of the reticulorumen
♦ Perireticular abscess near the reticulo-omasal orifice
♦ Induration of medial reticular wall without vagus nerve involvement
♦ Reticulum–diaphragm adhesions impairing reticulum mobility

♦ Liver abscess
♦ Actinobacillosis of rumen and reticulum
♦ Fibropapillomas of the cardia
♦ After surgery for right abomasal displacement or volvulus
♦ Pyloric achalasia secondary to septicemia, toxemia
♦ Thoracic involvement of vagus nerve by mediastinal involvement in tuberculosis, viral leukosis, diaphragmatic hernia

Clinical findings

Three well-defined syndromes, all with a basic syndrome:
♦ A slow onset over several weeks of:
  • Anorexia
  • Weight loss
  • Scant feces
  • Abdominal distension, with or without bloat
  • Abdominal contour is pear-shaped on right, apple-shaped on left (**papple-shaped**)
  • Enlarged, impacted abomasum palpable through flank or rectally
  • Enlarged rumen palpable rectally
  • Vital signs normal
  • No response to treatment of any sort
♦ Additional signs in each of the characteristic syndromes:
  Ruminal distension with hypermotility
  • Ruminal hypermotility with continuous, forceful contractions
  • Ruminal sounds soft because of frothy contents
  • May be fluid sounds on left flank ballottement
  • Feces normal or scant and pasty
  • Bradycardia in some
  • Systolic murmur in some
  • Rumen dorsal sac pushed into pelvis, ventral sac protrudes into and fills lower right segment. Not detectable in late pregnancy
  Ruminal distension with atony
  • Occurs mostly in late pregnancy
  • Anorexia
  • Emaciation
  • Scant, pasty feces
  • Distended abdomen
  • Ruminal movements diminished to absent
  • Persistent mild bloat in some
  • Fluid splashing sounds on ballottement left and right flanks
  • Rumen distension almost fills pelvic inlet
  • Terminal recumbency, coma, quiet death

Pyloric obstruction and abomasal impaction:

- In late pregnancy
- Anorexia, emaciation, scant, pasty feces as above
- Abdomen normal size
- No ruminal movements
- Tachycardia terminally
- Enlarged, doughy abomasum palpable by ballottement through right flank and rectally in lower right abdomen
- Commonly combined with ruminal distension with atony
- Terminal recumbency, coma, quiet death

Clinical pathology

♦ Hematology usually normal; may be mild neutrophilia with left shift and monocytosis
♦ Hemoconcentration if fluid accumulates in rumen
♦ Hypochloremia with hypokalemic alkalosis in abomasal distension
♦ May be high chloride levels in rumen from abomasal reflux

Necropsy findings

♦ Abomasal impaction with fine fiber and sand and rumen-type undigested fiber contents
♦ Abomasal ulcer common
♦ Ruminal contents in distended cases are finely digested; if no distension contents are clear, watery
♦ Intestines almost empty; ingesta scant, pasty
♦ Adhesions, fibrous fistulae, some with foreign body embedded, abscesses, residual scar tissue, on anterior reticular wall in some

Diagnosis

Ruminal distension–atony syndrome resembles:
♦ Chronic traumatic reticuloperitonitis
♦ Dietary abomasal impaction
♦ Omasal impaction
♦ Pyloric obstruction by phytobezoar
♦ Non-hemorrhaging abomasal ulcer
♦ Reticulo-omasal orifice obstruction by foreign body

Ruminal hypermotility syndrome resembles diaphragmatic hernia.

Treatment

Ruminal distension with hypermotility cases respond reasonably well over a period of 8–10 days to rumenotomy and emptying of the rumen. A temporary fistula is necessary because of the continued formation of foam.

Abomasal impaction cases:

♦ Abomasotomy is unsuccessful because the condition recurs immediately
♦ Temporary, rarely permanent, recovery may be achieved by draining and lavaging the forestomachs via a large-bore stomach tube, followed by oral administration of a lubricant, e.g.:
  - mineral oil (6–10 liters daily for 3 days), or
  - dioctyl sodium sulfosuccinate (120–180 ml of 25% solution for 450 kg body weight daily for 3 days)
♦ Late pregnant cows may be induced with dexamethazone (20 mg I/M) and may recover permanently
♦ These cases suffer dehydration and need supportive treatment with fluids and electrolytes to survive

DIAPHRAGMATIC HERNIA
(RETICULAR) [VM8 p. 288]

Etiology

♦ Most cases due to weakening of diaphragm by foreign body penetration from the reticulum and protrusion of small (20 cm diameter) sac of reticulum into thorax
♦ Sporadic congenital cases
♦ A spectacular incidence in buffalo in India

Clinical findings

♦ Gradual development over several weeks
♦ Capricious appetite
♦ Loss of weight
♦ Ruminal, abdominal distension
♦ Persistent ruminal tympany
♦ Continuous ruminal contractions
♦ No ruminal sounds because of frothy ruminal contents
♦ Grinding of teeth
♦ Feces scant, pasty
♦ Rumination absent
♦ Vomiting in some, especially at passage of stomach tube
♦ Temperature normal
♦ Bradycardia
♦ Systolic cardiac murmur
♦ Heart sounds displaced anteriorly and to left

♦ Rare cases with peristaltic sounds in thorax, interference with respiration, and pain with each reticular contraction
♦ Death from starvation after some weeks

Clinical pathology

♦ Radiological examination with barium meal contrast can identify the lesion
♦ Lesion palpable on exploratory rumenotomy

Necropsy findings

♦ Fistulous tract, sometimes with foreign body
♦ Reticulum adhered to diaphragm and protruding into thorax through a 15–20 cm dia. hernial ring
♦ Omasum, abomasum empty, rumen overfilled with frothy ingesta

Diagnosis

Resembles:
♦ Chronic esophageal obstruction
♦ Vagus indigestion

Treatment

No response to medical or surgical treatment and animals should be salvaged.

TRAUMATIC PERICARDITIS [VM8 p. 289]

Etiology

Penetration of pericardial sac by foreign body through reticulum wall and diaphragm.

Epidemiology

♦ Most common in late pregnant (6–9 months) cows or at parturition
♦ All affected animals die or are euthanized because of ill-health

Clinical findings

Acute pericarditis
♦ Profound depression
♦ Complete anorexia
♦ Rapid weight loss
♦ Scant feces early, severe diarrhea late
♦ Teeth grinding, salivation, nasal discharge in some
♦ Posture is back arched, elbows abducted
♦ Respiration shallow, fast rate, grunting

♦ Jugular veins engorged and prominent pulse
♦ Submandibular, brisket and ventral abdominal wall edema
♦ Conjunctival edema protruding over eyelids in bad cases
♦ Tachycardia (>100/minute)
♦ Fever
♦ Ruminal movements decreased, weak
♦ Grunt on percussion over xiphoid or cardiac area
♦ Pericardial friction sound early, washing-machine sounds obscuring heart sounds later. In chronic cases these sounds restricted to small areas of heart
♦ Most cases die in 1–2 weeks. Some persist in chronic state

Chronic pericarditis
♦ Variable appetite
♦ Thin to emaciated
♦ Milk yield negligible
♦ Bright, no toxemia
♦ Jugular engorgement without local edema
♦ Heart sounds muffled, fluid splashing or squeaking sounds over small areas
♦ Heart rate fast, sometimes irregular, pulse small amplitude

Clinical pathology

♦ Pronounced leukocytosis with neutrophilia
♦ Pericardial paracentesis in acute cases yields inflammatory fluid

Necropsy findings

♦ Distension pericardial sac with foul-smelling, grayish fluid containing flecks of fibrin
♦ Fibrous track containing foreign body adhered to sac
♦ Pleurisy, pneumonia common accompaniments
♦ **Chronic cases** show thickened sac adherent to myocardium over much of its surface. Some loculi filled with pus or serous fluid

Diagnosis

Resembles congestive heart failure caused by:
♦ Endocarditis
♦ Cardiomyopathy
♦ Cor pulmonale
♦ Bovine viral leukosis
♦ Congenital (inherited) cardiomyopathy
♦ Miscellaneous congenital cardiac defects

Resembles also space-occupying lesions of the anterior thorax, e.g. thymic tumor.

Treatment

♦ Complete recovery not possible. Life prolongation achievable in some early cases with:
  • Prolonged treatment with broad spectrum antibacterials
  • Pericardiotomy

TRAUMATIC SPLENITIS AND HEPATITIS [VM8 p. 290]

Etiology

♦ Penetration of liver or spleen by foreign body protrusion from reticulum
♦ May be continuation of an initial reticuloperitonitis or relapse after apparent recovery from an attack

Clinical findings and clinical pathology

♦ Fever
♦ Tachycardia
♦ Decline in feed intake, milk yield
♦ Ruminal movements near enough to normal
♦ Grunt on percussion over spleen or liver
♦ Marked leukocytosis, with regenerative left shift

Diagnosis

Resembles:
♦ Traumatic reticuloperitonitis
♦ Hepatic abscess
♦ Other, unspecified local infection

DISEASES OF THE ABOMASUM

ABOMASAL REFLUX [VM8 p. 292]

Etiology

♦ An outcome in cases where abomasal fluid does not pass the pylorus and refluxes into the rumen
♦ Occurs in cases of:
  • Pyloric obstruction by phytobezoar
  • Abomasal displacement, left, right
  • Vagus indigestion

Treatment

Broad-spectrum antibacterial cover for 1 week.

IMPACTION OF THE OMASUM [VM8 p. 291]

Etiology

♦ Diet of tree loppings, alfalfa stalks
♦ Fed on ground with large sand intake

Clinical findings

♦ Recurrent bouts of indigestion
♦ Ruminal hypomotility
♦ Scanty feces
♦ Anorexia
♦ Disinclination to move or lie down
♦ Pain on percussion behind right costal arch
♦ Rarely palpable as hard, round, firm mass in midline behind right costal arch or per rectum
♦ Rectum empty

Necropsy findings

♦ Gross distension of omasum
♦ Necrotic patches in wall and leaves
♦ Necrosis ruminal mucosa in some

Diagnosis

Resembles:
♦ Chronic reticuloperitonitis
♦ Abomasal ulcer

Treatment

Repeated doses of mineral oil.

• Peritonitis
• Intussusception
• Abomasal compression in late pregnancy
• Abomasal emptying defects in sheep

Clinical findings

♦ Abdominal, ruminal distension
♦ Ruminal stasis
♦ Regurgitation overflow via mouth, nostrils of ruminal fluid
♦ Plus other signs of primary disease

TRAUMATIC
ABOMASOPERITONITIS [VM8
p. 291]

Etiology

♦ Perforation abomasal wall by metallic foreign body causes local peritonitis

Clinical findings and clinical pathology

♦ Anorexia
♦ Fall in milk yield
♦ Depression
♦ Humped back, disinclined to move
♦ Fever
♦ Ruminal stasis
♦ Grunt on percussion behind xiphoid, right side
♦ Peritoneal fluid on paracentesis inflammatory
♦ Leukocytosis, left shift
♦ Positive result on metal detector over abomasum

Treatment

♦ Immobilization of patient
♦ Broad-spectrum antibacterial systemically for 5 days

LEFT-SIDED DISPLACEMENT OF
THE ABOMASUM (LDA) [VM8
p. 292]

Etiology

♦ High level concentrate feeding to dairy cows
♦ Unidentified factor, possibly low fiber content of diet, in cows on lush pasture

Epidemiology

♦ Commonest in large, adult, high-producing cows; rare cases in calves and yearlings
♦ Immediately after calving (90% cases seen during 6 weeks after calving)
♦ Feeding diet containing 17% crude fiber reduces incidence
♦ Few cases in late pregnancy
♦ Commonest in housed or closely confined cattle; lack of exercise may be a factor
♦ Losses due to lost production; mortality rate is negligible unless severe diarrhea

Clinical findings

♦ Cows in early lactation eat less and produce less milk than normal
♦ Ketosis, ketonuria, relapse after treatment for acetonemia
♦ Vital signs normal; paroxysmal tachycardia in some
♦ Left abdominal contour slab-sided; small rumen
♦ Scant feces; episodes of diarrhea
♦ Ruminal movements reduced, sounds inaudible
♦ Infrequent, tinkling, splashing, peristaltic sounds auscultatable ventrally behind left costal arch
♦ Ping on finger flick over area between left ribs 9 and 12 in upper third abdominal wall; may disappear transiently after exercise or transport
♦ Rumen small on rectal examination; feeling of emptiness in upper right flank
♦ Syndrome persists for lactation; cow thin, milk yield poor

Exertional LDA

♦ Rare cases in other than puerperal cows, including males, after unusual activity, e.g. mounting other cows
♦ Sudden onset moderate abdominal pain
♦ Tachycardia initially
♦ Visible gaseous, tympanitic distension in anterior half upper left paralumbar fossa
♦ Acute signs subside but standard LDA syndrome persists

Clinical pathology

♦ Ketonuria; normal blood glucose level
♦ Leukocytosis in cases with leaking abomasal ulcer

Necropsy findings

♦ Not a fatal disease
♦ Normal abomasal wall trapped under rumen
♦ Fixed by adhesions in cases with abomasal ulcer
♦ Abomasal rupture through ulcer rarely

Diagnosis

Resembles:
♦ Acetonemia
♦ Chronic reticuloperitonitis
♦ Vagus indigestion
♦ Diaphragmatic hernia
♦ Anterior abomasal displacement (displace-

ment between reticulum and diaphragm) signs similar to LDA except normal ruminal sounds in left flank; abomasal sounds audible above and behind heart on both sides

Treatment and prevention

♦ Recommended surgical procedures include:
  • Right paramedian abomasopexy
  • Right paralumbar fossa abomasopexy, favored because surgery performed on standing patient
♦ Rolling and manipulating previously starved cow reduces some displacements but relapses common
Restriction of heavy grain feeding in late pregnancy and ensuring cows take exercise recommended as preventive.

RIGHT-SIDED DISPLACEMENT OF THE ABOMASUM (RDA) AND ABOMASAL VOLVULUS [VM8 p. 296]

Etiology

♦ **Dilation—volvulus type.** Cause unclear but, as in LDA, due probably to heavy feeding on high grain diet in heavy producing dairy cows
♦ **Acute abomasal volvulus** Can occur spontaneously, without prior dilation, usually after violent exercise or transport
♦ Idiopathic pylorus obstruction in calves

Epidemiology

♦ Adult dairy cows
♦ Recognized during weeks 3–6 after calving
♦ Heavy grain diets during late pregnancy/ early lactation
♦ Inactive cows, usually housed or closely confined
♦ In similar circumstances to LDA but incidence ratio LDA:RDA is 7.4:1
♦ Also in calves up to 6 months old; thought to be accidental
♦ Rarely in pregnant cows and bulls

Clinical findings

Dilation–volvulus type
♦ Calved during past few weeks
♦ Depression
♦ Anorexia, sham drinking
♦ Milk yield reduced
♦ Feces scant, soft, dark
♦ Heart rate increased to 100/minute
♦ Pale dry mucosae
♦ Dehydrated
♦ No ruminal movements
♦ Rumen pack doughy
♦ Deep palpation behind right costal arch may detect distended abomasum
♦ Ballottement right flank detects fluid, splashing sounds, percussion elicits ping
♦ **Dilation** occurs after 3–4 days; abdomen distended on right
♦ Tense, fluid-distended abomasum palpable per rectum in lower right quadrant
♦ **Volvulus** occurs at 10–14 days
♦ Gross distension, grunting respiration
♦ Abomasum now fills right half of abdomen
♦ Feces scant, soft, dark
♦ Recumbent within 24 hours
♦ Death at 48–96 hours due to shock and dehydration
♦ Unexpected, early deaths usually due to abomasal rupture

Spontaneous acute abomasal volvulus – adult and calf
♦ Sudden onset acute abdominal pain, bouts of kicking at belly, depression of back, straining, bellowing
♦ Abdomen distended, tense
♦ High-pitched tympanitic sounds heard over right flank
♦ Splashing, fluid sounds heard on ballottement
♦ Tense, distended viscus palpable behind right costal arch
♦ Tachycardia
♦ Distended viscus may be palpable rectally
♦ Feces become diarrheic, blood-stained or melenic terminally

Clinical pathology

♦ Dehydration, hemoconcentration
♦ Hypochloremia, hypokalemia, metabolic alkalosis, possibly paradoxic aciduria
♦ Abomasal paracentesis yields fluid with acid pH; serosanguineous in torsion
♦ Great prognostic store set on degree of dehydration and other biochemical indicators such as serum alkaline phosphatase, serum anion gap

Necropsy findings

♦ Gross distension abomasum with fluid and gas
♦ Rumen may also be full of fluid due to abomasal reflux

+ May be pyloric obstruction with sand or fibre, or ulcer
+ In **volvulus** twisted abomasum, distended with sanguineous fluid. Wall may be hemorrhagic, gangrenous, ruptured

Diagnosis

Resembles other causes of right-side, tympanitic resonance (ping):
+ Abomasum dilation–volvulus
+ Spontaneous abomasal volvulus
+ Cecal dilation/torsion
+ Cranial duodenal obstruction
+ Ascending colon dilation
+ Intussusception
+ Small intestine volvulus
+ Pneumoperitoneum

Other causes of distended viscus in the right caudal abdomen include:
+ Fetal hydrops
+ Subacute abomasal ulcer with abomasal dilation

Acute diffuse peritonitis resembles acute abomasal volvulus.

Treatment

Dilation/torsion
+ Early cases before abomasal dilation large, salvage slaughter of commercial cattle
+ **Early, mild cases** – calcium borogluconate (500 ml 25% solution I/V), feed no grain, just quality hay for 3–5 days
+ Intravenous fluids and electrolytes in mild cases with moderate distension and dehydration
+ Additional therapy is oral mineral oil (5–10 liters daily) plus magnesium hydroxide (500 g daily for adults every second day)
+ **Alternative therapy** – hyoscine-*n*-butyl bromide plus dipyrone, and complete fasting
+ **Advanced cases** – right flank laparotomy to drain abomasum, plus intensive fluid–electrolyte therapy before and after surgery, plus cud transplant to restore forestomach motility

DIETARY ABOMASAL IMPACTION IN CATTLE [VM8 p. 301]

Etiology

+ Diet of excessive quantities of poor roughage, low in digestible protein, energy
+ Ingestion of excessive sand or soil contaminating feed, or when fed on the ground

Epidemiology

+ Commonest in young, pregnant, beef cows kept outdoors in cold climate winters and fed poor feed containing inadequate nutrients, especially when roughage is chopped
+ Feedlot cattle fed on low grain, high roughage diets
+ Cattle fed industrial residues, e.g. almond shells
+ Occurs as outbreaks

Clinical findings

+ Slow onset
+ Complete anorexia
+ Moderate abdominal distension
+ Scant feces
+ Emaciation, recumbency
+ Temperature may be subnormal
+ Heart rate up to 120/minute
+ Dehydration
+ Dyspnea, sometimes grunting
+ Mucoid nasal discharge
+ Cracked muzzle
+ No ruminal movements
+ Rumen packed with dry fiber, possibly fluid-filled
+ Impacted abomasum may be palpable behind right costal arch
+ May elicit grunt by percussion over abomasum
+ Impacted abomasum may be palpable on abdomen floor by rectal examination
+ Weakness, recumbency
+ Severe cases die in 4–6 days.
+ Sudden death if abomasum ruptures
+ Most average cases go down and die in 2–3 weeks

Clinical pathology

+ Hemoconcentration
+ Hypochloremia, hypokalemia, metabolic alkalosis

Necropsy findings

+ Abomasum, usually omasum also, twice normal size, filled with impacted, dry, rumen-like contents
+ Rumen grossly distended and filled with –
  • Dry, impacted contents **or**
  • Clear fluid
+ Intestines dry, empty
+ Carcase dehydrated, emaciated
+ Some case have abomasal ulcer, abomasal rupture, patchy necrosis of walls of rumen, omasum, abomasum

Diagnosis

Resembles:
♦ Vagus indigestion
♦ Omasal impaction
♦ Chronic traumatic reticuloperitonitis
♦ Intestinal obstruction

Treatment

♦ Severe cases with badly distended aboma-sum, high heart rate and recumbency best slaughtered
♦ Treatment includes:
  • Electrolyte–fluid therapy to relieve dehy-dration
  • Dioctyl sodium sulfosuccinate (120–180 ml of 25% solution by stomach tube per 450 kg daily for 3–5 days) mixed with warm water and 10 liters mineral oil
  • Abomasotomy or rumenotomy, empty-ing of rumen and addition of dioctyl sodium sulfosuccinate and oil as above
♦ Induction of parturition (20 mg dexameth-azone) in late pregnant cows
♦ Readjust diet of remainder to ensure ade-quate energy intake for cold weather plus late pregnancy

ABOMASAL IMPACTION IN SHEEP
[VM8 p. 304]

Etiology

Abomasal emptying defect of ewes
♦ Cause unknown
♦ In 2–6 years old Suffolk ewes, rarely rams
♦ Ewes in late gestation or puerperium
♦ Diet of grain and good quality hay

Dietary impaction of lambs
Probably insufficient milk from ewe leads to too early roughage intake.

Clinical findings and clinical pathology

♦ Duration of illness – days to weeks
♦ Progressive weight loss to emaciation
♦ Anorexia
♦ Distension lower right abdomen
♦ Palpable masses in lower right abdomen
♦ Metabolic alkalosis, hypochloremia, hypo-kalemia present but only in some patients

Necropsy findings

♦ Grossly distended abomasum contains impacted material like ruminal contents
♦ Rumen may be filled with clear fluid
♦ Some lambs have phytobezoars, rubbery milk clots in abomasum

Treatment

Ineffective; case fatality rate may exceed 90%.

ABOMASAL ULCERS OF CATTLE
[VM8 p. 304]

Etiology

♦ Causes unknown except for those associ-ated with:
  • Bovine leukosis
  • Viral erosive diseases
  • Vagus indigestion
  • Abomasal impaction/torsion
  • Abomasal displacement
♦ Speculative causes include:
  • Stress of parturition
  • Heavy grain feeding
  • Stress of lactation
  • Stress of prolonged transport, painful conditions, extensive surgery, prolonged illness
♦ Subclinical ulcers are very frequent in calves changing from milk diet to roughage
♦ Case fatality rate high with perforating ulcer

Non-perforating ulcer
♦ In calves intractable indigestion with anor-exia, weight loss, intermittent diarrhea
♦ Thought to cause no illness in adults unless chronic, then chronic indigestion, reduced feed intake, milk yield

Bleeding ulcer
♦ Acute onset mild abdominal pain
♦ Anorexia, drop in milk yield
♦ Melena after 24 hours
♦ Scant pasty feces, occasional bouts of diarr-hea
♦ Rumen stasis
♦ Tachycardia
♦ Mucosal pallor
♦ Spontaneous recovery in most
♦ Course 4–6 days
♦ Death in as little as 24 hours

Perforating ulcer

- Rarely sudden death due to abomasal rupture
- Most cases have subacute illness
- Fluctuating fever
- Anorexia
- Rumen stasis
- Intermittent diarrhea
- Pain on deep palpation lower right abdomen behind costal arch
- Some cases distended abomasum with splashing sounds on ballottement lower right abdomen
- Teeth grinding
- Sham drinking
- Dehydration
- Apparent recovery with relapse common
- Periabomasal abscess causes chronic peritonitis in some

Clinical pathology

- Blood in feces indicated by melena or positive test for occult blood
- Hemorrhagic anemia
- Leukocytosis with left shift in perforating ulcer
- Abdominal paracentesis may collect inflammatory fluid

Necropsy findings

- Deep well-defined ulcers usually on ventral part of fundic region
- Blood in ingesta
- Adhesions to omentum
- Periabomasal abscess

Diagnosis

Bleeding ulcer resembles:
- Duodenal ulcer
- Bovine leukosis

Perforating ulcer resembles traumatic reticuloperitonitis. In **calves** resembles chronic abomasitis.

Treatment

- Oral protectants, e.g. kaolin, pectin
- Oral antacids, e.g. magnesium oxide (500–800 g/450 kg daily for 2–4 days) or magnesium silicate (100 g/day)
- Blood transfusion (4–8 liters) in anemic patients
- Abomasotomy and surgical excision hazardous; may be multiple ulcers. Usually attempted only in recurrent or chronic cases

OMENTAL BURSITIS [VM8 p. 307]

Etiology

A complication of:
- Perforating abomasal ulcer
- Perforation of ventral wall of blind sac of rumen
- Traumatic reticuloperitonitis
- Spread from umbilical infection
- Extension of abdominal abscess
- Extension from postparturient parametritis

Clinical findings

- Course several days
- Anorexia
- Dehydration
- Fluid splashing sounds in right lower abdomen
- Large, soft, poorly defined mass palpable in right upper abdomen

Clinical pathology

- Peritoneal fluid indicates chronic inflammation
- Neutrophilia, serum fibrinogen elevated

Necropsy findings

- Diffuse fibrinous, necrotizing peritonitis
- Omental bursa distended with purulent exudate

Diagnosis

Resembles:
- Chronic reticuloperitonitis
- Retroperitoneal abscess

Treatment

- Long-term, broad-spectrum antibiotics
- Surgical drainage if possible

ABOMASAL BLOAT IN LAMBS
AND CALVES [VM8 p. 307]

Etiology

- Lambs and calves fed milk replacer
- Feeding of large quantities of warm milk at infrequent intervals
- Lambs on deep litter on silage feed predisposed

Clinical findings

♦ Gross abdominal distension within an hour after feeding
♦ Death in a few minutes

Necropsy findings

♦ Grossly distended abomasum
♦ Filled with gas and unclotted milk replacer

Diagnosis

Resembles rumen bloat in ruminal drinkers.

Prevention

♦ *Ad lib* feeding of cold milk containing no insoluble ingredients prevents
♦ 0.1% formalin (37% formaldehyde) added to milk replacer containing 20% solids

DISEASES OF THE INTESTINES OF RUMINANTS

CECAL DILATION AND VOLVULUS
[VM8 p. 308]

Etiology

♦ Unknown
♦ Sheep, and well-fed dairy cows
♦ Few weeks after parturition
♦ Heavy carbohydrate feeding

Clinical findings

Cecal dilation without volvulus
♦ Gradual onset, several days
♦ Mild abdominal pain
♦ Anorexia
♦ Drop in milk yield
♦ Scant feces
♦ Upper right flank may be distended
♦ Ping on percussion right paralumbar fossa
♦ Splashing sounds on ballottement of right flank
♦ Long (<90 cm), cylindrical (20 cm diameter) movable organ with blind end palpable rectally

Cecal dilation with volvulus
♦ Sudden onset
♦ Mild abdominal pain, treading, kicking at belly
♦ Anorexia
♦ Ruminal stasis
♦ Scant or no feces
♦ Dehydration
♦ Tachycardia
♦ Right paralumbar fossa distended, tympanitic; ping on percussion, splashing sounds on ballottement
♦ Cecum tightly distended, blunt end displaced
♦ May be distension of colon and ileum
♦ Cecal rupture followed by sudden death

Clinical pathology

♦ Mild dehydration
♦ Compensated hypochloremia, hypokalemia

Necropsy findings

Cases with torsion show compromised vasculature and ischemic necrosis of cecal wall, possibly rupture.

Diagnosis

Resembles right abomasal dilation and volvulus.

Treatment

Cecal dilation
♦ Saline purgative and feed hay for a few days
♦ Neostigmine hourly for 2–3 days is used

Cecal volvulus
♦ Surgical correction
♦ Relapsing cases partial resection advisable

INTESTINAL OBSTRUCTION IN
CATTLE [VM8 p. 309]

Etiology

Intestinal accidents
♦ Volvulus – distal jejuno-ileum
♦ Mesenteric torsion
♦ Intussusception (enteric, ileo-colic, ceco-colic, colonic); may be related to intestinal polyposis
♦ Strangulation by mesenteric tear, persistent vitello-umbilical band, ventral or lateral bladder ligament, adhesion, persistent urachus, inverted bladder, ductus deferens segment

➧ Compression stenosis, e.g. by ovarian clot, duodenitis
➧ Cecal dilation/torsion

Luminal blockage
✦ Fat necrosis, lipoma
✦ Phytobezoars, e.g. due to Romulea bulbocodium
✦ Trichobezoar
✦ Rectal paralysis in late pregnant cows

Clinical findings

✦ Sudden onset brief bouts of abdominal pain for 8–12 hours – treading with hind feet, kicking at belly, depression of back, groaning or bellowing, lying down, occasionally rolling
✦ Complete anorexia
✦ No feces passed; in rectum are hard turds covered with mucus in some, may be blood as thick red slurry dries as flakes around anus, or mucoid, even a plug of mucus. In phytobezoar obstruction feces in rectum pasty, smelly, yellow–gray
✦ Heart rate elevated to 100 if gut blood supply compromised or in late stages of others

After pain subsides
✦ Complete anorexia
✦ No feces passed
✦ Depression
✦ No rumination
✦ Ruminal stasis in most cases
✦ Feces as above
✦ Distended loops of intestine on rectal examination rarely except in colon or cecum obstruction
✦ Bowel section affected by intussusception or volvulus mobile and difficult to locate; often not palpable
✦ Marginal abdominal distension except in ileus or other intestinal dilation, then right side distension
✦ Splashing sounds left and right flanks in upper small intestine obstruction
✦ Splashing sounds only on right in pylorus obstruction
✦ Fluid regurgitation from nose in some
✦ Death due to dehydration, shock, endotoxemia on day 3–8, depending on severity of lesion

Special signs in coiled colon torsion (mesenteric root torsion)
✦ Short course; may die by 24 hours
✦ Right flank distended, coils may be visible

Special signs in cecal dilation/torsion
Single, transverse distended segment on rectal, usually mobile blind end palpable.

Special signs in fat necrosis
Hard, irregular shaped masses on rectal examination; mobile in mesentery, fixed retroperitoneally, encircling rectum.

Special signs in phytobezoar
May be palpable as 10 cm dia. smooth roundish mass in lower right abdomen.

Clinical pathology

✦ Dehydration, hemoconcentration; not marked until late stages or cases with marked distension and compromised blood supply to gut
✦ Hypochloremia, hypokalemia, metabolic alkalosis

Necropsy findings

✦ Distended loops of intestine oral to obstruction; or independent of lesion, as in idiopathic ileus
✦ Physical lesion of intussusception, strangulation, volvulus, phytobezoar
✦ Dehydration

Diagnosis

Resembles:
✦ Abomasal displacement
✦ Abomasal torsion
✦ Pyloric obstruction
✦ Abomasal impaction
✦ Abomasal ulcer
✦ Renal, ureteric calculus
✦ Photosensitive dermatitis

Treatment

✦ Spontaneous recovery recorded; usually after truck ride
✦ In cecal dilation prior to torsion –
  • Withhold feed
  • Saline purgative
✦ Surgical correction

INTESTINAL OBSTRUCTION IN SHEEP [VM8 p. 312]

✦ Heavy Oesophagostomum columbianum infestation

- High intussusception incidence in travelling sheep
- Cecal torsion (red gut) in up to 20% of sheep flock on lush legume pasture. Die in 24 hours. Signs include abdominal pain, distension, fluid sounds in right abdomen
- Phytobezoars

TERMINAL ILEITIS [VM8 p. 312]

- No cause identified
- Lambs 4–6 months old show ill-thrift
- Necropsy lesion is thickening, ulceration o terminal ileum, mesenteric lymph node en largement

7 DISEASES OF THE LIVER AND PANCREAS

DISEASES OF THE LIVER

CLINICAL INDICANTS

The principal clinical signs and clinicopathological findings on which clinical diagnoses of liver diseases are based include the following.

Abdominal pain

Clinical findings Subacute pain caused by:
♦ Distension of capsule
♦ Inflammatory lesions of capsule

Occurs in:
♦ Liver abscess
♦ Neoplasia
♦ Cholangiohepatitis

Biopsy specimen abnormal

♦ Transabdominal needle biopsy – using special animal-size equipment and well-defined location guides and techniques; specimens collected for histopathology, nutrient and toxin assay
♦ Disadvantages are small sample, uncertainty as to representative character, possible laceration of hilar vessels and fatal internal hemorrhage, or bile ducts and biliary peritonitis, or attack of focal necrotic hepatitis
♦ Alternative is peritoneoscopy, visualization of liver edge, incisional biopsy

Black livers in sheep

♦ Lipofuscin deposits probably due to *Acacia aneura* in diet
♦ Melanin deposits in livers of mutant Corriedale sheep

Bleeding tendency

Clinical findings Clotting time prolonged.

Occurs in Hepatitis.

Defecation – feces abnormality

Clinical findings:
♦ Anorexia, vomiting (pigs), constipation alternating with bouts of diarrhea, due to bile salt deficiency in gut contents, and portal hypertension
♦ Pale feces (steatorrhea) due to bile pigment deficiency

Occurs in Hepatitis.

Edema

Occurs in:
♦ Moderate anasarca, e.g. submandibular edema due to hypoproteinemia
♦ Ascites due to portal hypertension, e.g. in hepatic fibrosis

Encephalopathy, hepatic

Clinical findings:
♦ Hyperexcitability, mania, convulsions, or
♦ Dullness, somnolence, failure to respond to signals
♦ Muscle tremor, weakness
♦ Aimless wandering, compulsive walking, head-pressing

Occurs in:
♦ Hepatitis
♦ Porto-caval shunts

Jaundice

Clinical findings:
♦ Staining of mucosae, sclera by accumulation of bilirubin
♦ Severity of jaundice greatest in cases in

117

which bilirubin has been conjugated in the liver; thus more obvious in obstructive than in hemolytic jaundice
♦ Bilirubin accumulates preferentially in elastic tissue, thus jaundice most obvious in sclera and peritoneum

Occurs in:
♦ Hemolytic anemia
♦ Biliary system obstruction due to intra- or extraluminal obstructions or aplasia of bile ducts
♦ Hepatitis, hepatic fibrosis due to interference with the passage of bilirubin from the liver to the biliary system
♦ Blood levels of bilirubin (thus severity of jaundice) greater in obstructive than hemolytic jaundice; levels intermediate in hepatic disease

Laboratory tests, liver

♦ Need to be integrated with clinical signs, history
♦ Combinations of tests to suit individual disease best
♦ Serum enzyme tests, liver clearance tests, blood ammonia, albumin, globulin, and glucose measurements, serological tests
♦ Serum bile acids elevation is a sensitive measure of hepatic disease
♦ Icteric index as measure of blood level of bilirubin
♦ Hemogram; e.g leukocytosis, neutrophilia and left shift in hepatic abscess

Liver, displacement

Occurs in:
♦ Acquired diaphragmatic hernia
♦ Torsion of a liver lobe in a pig

LIVER DISEASES

HEPATITIS [VM8 p. 321]

Etiology

Toxic hepatitis
♦ Poisonous plants:
  • Weeds – *Amsinckia, Astragalus, Crotalaria, Echium, Encephalartos, Heliotropum, Myoporum, Pimelea, Senecio, Trachyandra, Tribulus* spp.
  • Commercial plants – *Lupinus* spp.,

Liver enlarged

Clinical findings Alteration in size only detectable clinically if grossly enlarged in ruminants. Liver protrudes beyond right ribs, e.g. in:
♦ Advanced congestive heart failure
♦ Multiple liver abscesses, tumors

Liver painful

Clinical findings Pain elicited by percussion over caudal right ribs.

Occurs in:
♦ Hepatitis
♦ Liver abscess
♦ Cholangiohepatitis
♦ Liver neoplasm

Photosensitization

Clinical findings Phylloerythrin, chlorophyll metabolite, accumulates in blood stream causing photosensitive dermatitis.

Occurs in:
♦ Hepatitis
♦ Cholangiohepatitis

Ultrasonography, liver

Size, location and parenchymal pattern identifiable.

Weight loss

Due to anorexia and failure of protein anabolism.

Medicago sativa (lucerne, alfalfa) hay water-damaged, *Panicum effusum, Trifolium hybridum* (alsike clover)
  • Trees and shrubs – *Lantana camara, Myoporum* spp. (ngaio), *Terminalia oblongata* (yellow-wood), *Zamia* spp. (seeds)
  • Fungi – *Aspergillus, Fusarium, Myrothecium, Penicillium, Periconia, Phomopsis, Pithomyces* spp.
  • Algae–cyanobacteria e.g. *Anacystis* spp. (slow death factor)

- Insects – *Lophyrotoma* spp. (sawfly) lar-
  vae
♦ Miscellaneous farm chemicals:
  - Dried poultry wastes
  - Cottonseed cake (*Gossypolium* spp.)
  - Herring meal

Infectious hepatitis
♦ Rift Valley fever
♦ Tyzzer's disease (*Bacillus piliformis*)
♦ Equid herpesvirus-1 infection in aborted
  foals
♦ *Chlamydia* spp. infection in aborted calves
  (epizootic abortion)
♦ Idiopathic postvaccinal hepatitis
♦ Severe cases of equine viral arteritis
♦ Histoplasmosis
♦ **Toxic perfusion hepatitis,** e.g. in salmonel-
  losis, septicemic listeriosis, leptospirosis, or
  endotoxins from mixed bacterial infection
  such as mastitis, metritis

Parasitic hepatitis
Migrating larvae of:
♦ Fascioliasis
♦ Ascariasis

Nutritional hepatitis
♦ **Dietary hepatic necrosis** of pigs prevent-
  able by selenium–vitamin E
♦ White liver disease in cobalt-deficient sheep

Congestive hepatopathy
Congestive heart failure.

Functional hepatopathy
inherited photosensitization, an hepatic
insufficiency in sheep.

Congenital defects
Portosystemic shunt.

Clinical findings

Acute hepatitis
♦ Anorexia
♦ Dullness, somnolence, yawning, lack of re-
  sponse to stimuli **or**
♦ Excitement, mania, convulsions
♦ Weakness, tremor, terminal recumbency,
  coma
♦ Jaundice
♦ Photosensitization
♦ Constipation, bouts of diarrhea
♦ Vomiting, pale feces in pigs
♦ Arched back, pain on palpation over liver

Hepatic fibrosis
♦ Alopecia
♦ Photosensitization
♦ Dummy syndrome
  - Apparent blindness
  - Head-pressing, aggression
  - Aimless wandering
  - Compulsive walking
♦ Anasarca
♦ Weight loss, susceptibility to nutritional
  stress

Portosystemic shunt
♦ Growth retardation (stature and weight)
♦ Dummy syndrome, as above
♦ Ascites

Clinical pathology

♦ Serum bilirubin levels, ratio of conjugated
  and unconjugated
♦ Serum bile acids
♦ Serum liver enzymes in acute hepatitis
♦ Bromsulfalein clearance test, serum biliru-
  bin in chronic cases
♦ Blood sugar, ammonia, protein levels
♦ Leukocytosis, neutrophilia, left shift in
  bacterial infections

Necropsy findings

Acute
♦ Liver enlarged, edges swollen
♦ Pale, red
♦ Cut surface varies

Toxic
♦ Lobular pattern accentuated due to engor-
  gement of centrilobular vessels
♦ Jaundice
♦ Edema
♦ Photosensitization

Infectious
♦ Patchy or focal lesion

Parasitic
♦ Focal hemorrhages under capsule
♦ Trauma and necrosis definable as tracks

Congestive
♦ Marked enlargement of liver
♦ Marked accentuation of lobular pattern

Hepatic fibrosis
Liver either:
♦ Grossly enlarged, or
♦ Much shrunken

Diagnosis

Hepatic encephalopathy resembles:
♦ Encephalitis
♦ Encephalomalacia
♦ Carbohydrate engorgement
Liver fibrosis resembles congestive heart failure

Treatment

Acute

♦ No specific treatment of any value
♦ Attempt to keep the patient alive to allow spontaneous regeneration of hepatic tissue
♦ Maintain on parenteral normal glucose saline injections

Chronic, diffuse hepatic disease

No treatment of any sort attempted.
♦ Ensure calcium intake maintained
♦ Diet high in carbohydrate and calcium, low in protein and fat, if patient will eat
♦ Periodic injections of water-soluble vitamins
♦ Oral broad-spectrum antibiotic used to control protein digestion and ammonia poisoning

HEPATIC ABSCESS [VM8 p. 323]

Etiology

♦ Mixed infections with *Actinomyces pyogenes, Streptococcus, Staphylococcus* spp., *Fusobacterium necrophorum* secondary to:
  • Rumenitis caused by heavy grain feeding
  • Omphalophlebitis
  • Ruminal parakeratosis
♦ Traumatic hepatitis associated with reticuloperitonitis
♦ Infectious necrotic hepatitis (black disease) caused by *Clostridium novyi*, and necrotic abscesses by *Clostridium sordelli*
♦ In bacillary hemoglobinuria caused by *Clostridium hemolyticum*
♦ Tyzzer's disease caused by *Bacillus piliformis*
♦ Yersiniosis caused by *Yersinia pseudotuberculosis*
♦ In strangles in horses
♦ In lamb septicemia caused by *Haemophilus agni*

Clinical findings

Most liver abscesses are asymptomatic but at high incidence cause significant losses at abattoirs because of condemnation of livers. In rare cases of clinical illness, signs include:
♦ Anorexia
♦ Depression
♦ Fever
♦ Pain on percussion over liver area, behind caudal right ribs

Sequel

♦ May develop caudal vena caval syndrome

Clinical pathology

♦ Leukocytosis, neutrophilia, left shift
♦ Elevation blood levels mucoprotein, sialic acid

Necropsy findings

♦ Single or multiple abscesses in parenchyma
♦ Single necrotic abscess specifically located under capsule on diaphragmatic curvature of liver in infections due to *Clostridium* spp.
♦ Contiguous local peritonitis over subcapsular abscesses

Diagnosis

Resembles other localized infections, especially:
♦ Endocarditis
♦ Traumatic splenitis
♦ Subperitoneal abscess
♦ Pyelonephritis
♦ Caudal vena caval syndrome

Treatment

♦ Long-term (>2 weeks) broad-spectrum antibiotics with high probability of relapse
♦ Intensive antibacterial therapy in clostridial infections

LIVER NEOPLASMS [VM8 p. 324]

♦ Rare; still rarer as causes of clinical illness
♦ Can be anticipated to cause:
  • Local enlargement of liver, possibly palpable behind right rib cage if very extensive
  • Subacute abdominal pain due to stretching of capsule
  • Weight loss

- Tumors of biliary tissue or compressing it cause obstructive jaundice

LIVER TORSION [VM8 p. 317]

Etiology Adult sows after farrowing.

Clinical findings

- Anorexia
- Restless, refuses to suckle young
- Prolonged vomiting
- Severe abdominal pain
- Dyspnea
- Sudden death due to internal hemorrhage if capsule ruptures

LIVER RUPTURE [VM8 p. 317]

Etiology
- Acute abdominal trauma
- Severe liver or lobe distension
- Amyloidosis in horses, with extreme distension
- Inherited short sternum in North Country Cheviot lambs, permitting compression-rupture of exposed liver during birth

Clinical findings

Sudden death due to internal hemorrhage.

DISEASES OF THE BILIARY SYSTEM

CHOLANGITIS [VM8 p. 324]

Etiology
- Extension from parasitic duodenitis
- Parasite invasion of bile duct by *Fasciola* spp., *Dicrocelium dendriticum*
- More severe cases occur as **gall bladder empyema**

Clinical findings

- Fever
- Anorexia, depression
- Pain on percussion over liver
- Jaundice
- Photosensitization
- Secondary multiple hepatic abscess

Clinical pathology

- Leukocytosis, neutrophilia, left shift

Treatment

Potentiated sulfonamide or broad-spectrum antibiotic course for 7 days.

OBSTRUCTIVE CHOLELITHIASIS [VM8 p. 324]

Clinical findings

Horses

- Intermittent or continuous colic
- Jaundice
- Weight loss
- Fever

Clinical pathology

- Leukocytosis
- Delayed bromsulfalein clearance

Cattle
Concretions usually associated with fascioliasis:
- Anorexia
- Pain on percussion over liver
- Recurrent bouts severe abdominal pain
- Ruminal stasis
- Jaundice in some late cases

BILE DUCT ATRESIA [VM8 p. 324]

Clinical findings

Foals
- Illness commencing at 2–3 weeks of age
- Anorexia, depression
- Severe jaundice
- Gray pasty feces
- Death in 1 week

DISEASES OF THE PANCREAS

DIABETES MELLITUS [VM8 p. 325]

Rare, sporadic occurrences in cows, horses, donkeys.

Clinical findings

♦ Weight loss
♦ Polydipsia, polyuria

Clinical pathology

♦ Intense hyperlipemia
♦ High blood levels glucose, cholesterol, triglycerides

♦ Glycosuria
♦ Ketonuria

HYPERINSULINISM [VM8 p. 325]

♦ Recorded, possibly, in one pony with pancreatic beta-cell adenoma
♦ Signs included convulsions, hypoglycemia

PANCREATIC ADENOCARCINOMA
[VM8 p. 325]

♦ Caused biliary duct obstruction in a horse
♦ Signs included emaciation, abdominal pain, variable fecal texture and intermittent jaundice

8 DISEASES OF THE CARDIOVASCULAR SYSTEM

The principal clinical signs, clinicopathological findings and basic syndromes on which clinical diagnoses of cardiovascular disease are based include the following.

BASIC SYNDROMES

There are four syndromes that are part of the clinical manifestations of most diseases of the cardiovascular system.
♦ Congestive heart failure
♦ Acute heart failure
♦ Peripheral circulatory failure
♦ Cardiac arrhythmia

CONGESTIVE HEART FAILURE
[VM8 p. 329]

Etiology

Valvular disease
♦ Endocarditis
♦ Congenital valvular defects
♦ Valve or chordae tendinae rupture

Myocardial disease
♦ Myocarditis
♦ Myocardial degeneration
♦ Cardiomyopathy, congenital, hereditary

Pericardial disease
♦ Pericarditis
♦ Cardiac tamponade

Blood pressure increase
♦ Pulmonary hypertension, e.g. high altitude disease, cor pulmonale

Congenital shunts, constrictions
♦ Septal defects
♦ Fibro-elastosis
♦ Aorta coarctation
♦ Patent ductus arteriosus

Clinical findings

Left side failure
♦ Resting respiratory rate, depth increased
♦ Cough
♦ Moist crackles at lung base
♦ Dull percussion note over ventral lungs
♦ Dyspnea, cyanosis at rest
♦ Tachycardia
♦ Possibly murmur referable to left AV or aortic valves

Right side failure
♦ Listlessness, depression
♦ Reluctant to walk
♦ Shuffling, staggery gait, eventual recumbency
♦ Anasarca ventrally under the jaw, down the neck and under the abdomen
♦ Ascites
♦ Hydrothorax
♦ Possibly palpable enlargement of liver beyond right costal arch
♦ Urine volume small, concentrated, minor albuminuria
♦ Profuse diarrhea terminally
♦ Anorexia

♦ Condition lost, weight may increase due to edema
♦ Jugular vein distension (other veins also)
♦ Abnormally high and visible jugular pulse
♦ Epistaxis in some horses
♦ Hydropericardium

Prognosis

♦ Horses with rhythm defects capable of surviving
♦ Rarely survive; survival is with permanently reduced cardiac reserve

Clinical pathology

♦ Increased venous pressure
♦ Paracentesis from all body cavities; fluid is edema transudate but has high protein content due to anoxic damage to capillary walls
♦ Proteinuria

Necropsy findings

♦ Left side – pulmonary congestion and edema
♦ Right side – anasarca, ascites, hydrothorax, hydropericardium, liver enlargement, engorgement

Diagnosis

Resembles:
♦ Peritonitis
♦ Bladder rupture
♦ Liver fibrosis
♦ Hypoproteinemia
♦ Urine accumulation in ventral abdominal wall due to urethral perforation
♦ Edema of late pregnancy in mares and cows involving perineum udder edema, ventral abdominal wall
♦ Pulmonary edema occurs also in:
  • Acute bovine pulmonary emphysema and edema
  • Organophosphorus compound poisoning
♦ Jugular engorgement also caused by space-occupying thoracic lesions, e.g. thymus lymphosarcoma

Treatment

Limited value in cattle because lesions not reparable. Impractical in all species because rest-of-life treatment not eminently practicable.
♦ Digoxin orally or intravenously in horses;

intravenously only in cattle. *Not* intramuscular in any species.
Horse: I/V loading dose 1.0–1.5 mg/100 kg then maintenance dose every 24 hours at half the dose. Oral loading dose: 7 mg/100 kg, plus daily maintenance oral doses at half the rate.
Cattle and sheep: I/V loading dose 2.2 mg. 100 kg, then maintenance doses 0.34 mg. 100 kg every 4 hours. Any animals under treatment require daily potassium chloride (100 g cattle, 30 g horses) if not eating, with blood potassium levels being monitored
♦ Furosemide (0.25–1.0 mg/kg for horses. 2.5–5.0 mg/kg for cattle) when edema a problem; also reduce salt intake
♦ Stall rest

ACUTE HEART FAILURE [VM8 p. 332]

Etiology

♦ Cardiac tamponade
♦ Aortic or pulmonary arterial rupture
♦ Myocarditis
♦ Nutritional deficiency myopathy
♦ Plant poisoning myopathy
♦ Electrocution, lightning strike
♦ Iatrogenic intravenous injection calcium, potassium solutions, xylazine
♦ Aortic valve rupture
♦ Anaphylaxis
♦ Induction stage of halothane or barbiturate anesthesia

Clinical findings

Acute syndrome

♦ Commonest during exercise or excitement; a significant cause of death in horses during training or racing
♦ Dyspnea
♦ Staggering, falling, recumbency
♦ Marked mucosal pallor
♦ Sporadic, incoordinated limb movements; short of actual convulsions
♦ Bradycardia, tachycardia or heart sounds absent
♦ No pulse
♦ Death within minutes, with deep, asphyxial gasps

Subacute syndrome

♦ Course 12–24 hours
♦ Tachycardia, often tachyarrhythmia
♦ Severe dyspnea
♦ Lung base crackles

♦ Hydrothorax, ascites in those with longer course

Clinical pathology

♦ Not applicable in most cases
♦ Elevated serum levels of creatine kinase, aspartase aminotransferase, lactate dehydrogenase

Necropsy findings

♦ Acute cases may show:
  • Visceral vein engorgement
  • Only microscopic lesions of pulmonary vessels dilation, pulmonary edema
♦ Less acute cases – lesions of congestive heart failure
♦ Myocardial inflammatory or degenerative lesions

Diagnosis

Acute cases resemble other causes of sudden death. Less acute cases resemble:
♦ Congestive heart failure
♦ Pulmonary edema
♦ Pneumonia

Treatment

Usually impractical because of short course.

PERIPHERAL CIRCULATORY
FAILURE [VM8 p. 333]

Etiology

Hypovolemic failure
♦ Hemorrhagic anemia
♦ Dehydration

Distributive failure (including vasogenic shock)
♦ Severe burns injury
♦ Surgical shock after extensive surgery or trauma
♦ At uterine prolapse
♦ Too sudden reduction of pressure in body cavity
♦ Severe pain as in equine colic

Non-toxic general vasogenic shock
♦ Hypocalcemia as in milk fever

Toxic and septic shock
♦ Endotoxemia
♦ Exotoxins, e.g. gangrenous mastitis, acute diffuse peritonitis

Clinical findings

♦ Depression, dullness, coma terminally
♦ Muscle weakness,
♦ Subnormal temperature
♦ Tachycardia
♦ Small amplitude, low pressure pulse
♦ Skin cool
♦ Mucosal pallor, prolonged capillary refill time
♦ Muzzle dry
♦ Shallow respirations, rapid rate
♦ Anorexia, thirst in some
♦ Clonic convulsions in a few
♦ Reversal relatively easy provided no toxic component

Clinical pathology

♦ Arterial blood pressure reduced from 120 to 60 mmHg
♦ Disseminated intravascular coagulation
♦ Other parameters indicative of primary condition, e.g. leukocytosis, hemoconcentration, anemia, hypocalcemia
♦ Metabolic acidosis in untreated peripheral circulatory failure

Necropsy findings

♦ The only lesions are those of the primary condition
♦ There are no lesions characteristic of peripheral circulatory failure

Diagnosis

Resembles:
♦ Shock
♦ Dehydration
♦ Hemorrhagic anemia

Treatment

Restoration of the circulating blood volume by:
♦ Plasma in cases of shock when plasma protein concentration <3.5 g/dl
♦ Isotonic fluids required in cases of dehydration where PCV >50%; may be desirable when PCV >40%
♦ Fluid replacement continued until urine flow rate restored to normal or PCV reduced to <40% or central venous pressure <5 cm H_2O
♦ Specific bicarbonate therapy when blood pH <7.1
♦ Blood transfusion in cases of hemorrhagic anemia where PCV <12%
♦ Large doses of corticosteroids (dexametha-

zone 5–10 mg/kg or methylprednisolone 30 mg/kg) may be beneficial

♦ In cases of endotoxic shock flunixin meglumine valuable

ARRHYTHMIAS

PRINCIPLES

♦ Diagnosis at slow heart rates can be by auscultation but electrocardiography more accurate and the only valid method at high heart rates
♦ Those which occur commonly are:
  • **Horses:** first degree heart block, second degree heart block, sinoatrial block, ventricular extrasystoles, atrial extrasystoles, atrial fibrillation
  • **Cattle:** ventricular extrasystoles, atrial fibrillation, atrial extrasystoles
♦ Many are of no known clinical significance e.g. sinus arrhythmia, wandering pacemaker, sinoatrial block, first and second-degree atrioventricular block
♦ Arrhythmia in horses at rest which disappears with exercise thought to be of no significance
♦ Transient arrhythmia common in newborn foals
♦ Cardiac arrhythmia may be associated with gastrointestinal disease in cows and horses; resolves spontaneously when primary disease corrected
♦ Most cases of arrhythmia dealt with by treating the primary condition

Sinus tachycardia [VM8 p. 344]

Significance Physiologically normal fast rate.

Occurs in Painful states, excitement, exercise, etc.; disappears when stimulus removed.

Signs include Rate per minute >48 in horses, >80 in cows.

Sinus bradycardia [VM8 p. 344]

Significance A normal, decreased rate.

Occurs in:
♦ Highly trained horses
♦ High blood pressure

♦ Space-occupying cranial lesions
♦ Pituitary abscess
♦ Hypothermia
♦ Hypoglycemia
♦ Following xylazine administration
♦ Cases of vagus indigestion, diaphragmatic hernia in cows, disappears with exercise or atropine administration

Signs include Heart rates down to 26/minute in horses, 48 beats/minute in cows.

Sinus arrhythmia [VM8 p. 344]

Significance A physiologically normal arrhythmia.

Occurs in:
♦ Uncommon in large animals compared with dogs
♦ Commonest in young, and tame sheep, goats
♦ Occurs during hypercalcemia of early milk fever treatment in cows

Clinical signs include:
♦ Occurs at slow heart rate
♦ Rate increases in inspiration, decreases in expiration; also unassociated with respiration in horses
♦ Abolished by exercise or atropine

ECG Variations in P–P intervals, sometimes in P–R intervals; often associated with a **wandering pacemaker**.

Sinoatrial block [VM8 p. 344]

Significance Considered physiologically normal unless it persists during and immediately after exercise.

Occurs in Fit horses at rest.

Clinical signs include:
♦ Dropped heart beats, pulse waves with regular underlying rhythm
♦ For one heart beat period complete absence

heart sounds, jugular atrial wave, arterial pulse

ECG Complete absence PQRST complexes for one beat

Atrioventricular block [VM8 p. 344]

First-degree atrioventricular block

Significance None.

Occurs in Transient episodes.

Clinical signs include Detectable only by electrocardiograph.

ECG P–R interval prolonged.

Second-degree atrioventricular block (partial heart block)

Significance:
◆ Can be a physiological variation when abolished by exercise or atropine
◆ Considered abnormal in horses when it persists during exercise; in other species always indicates myocardial disease
◆ May progress to complete to third-degree block

Occurs in:
◆ Up to 20% light horses at rest, in quiet surroundings
◆ In some horses accompanies myocarditis and reduced performance
◆ At fast heart rates occurs in horses with alkalosis in cases of duodenitis/proximal jejunitis
◆ In electrolyte disturbances in all species
◆ Overdosing with calcium salts
◆ Digitalis poisoning
◆ Cardiomyopathy, myocarditis in infectious or nutritional deficiency disease

Clinical signs include:
◆ Random or regular occurrence of absence of first and second heart sounds, arterial pulse
◆ In horses fourth heart sound audible in block period
◆ Jugular pulse detectable
◆ Intensified first heart sound in first cardiac cycle after block

ECG P wave present but QRS and T waves absent in blocked beat

Treatment:
◆ Not usually necessary, but treat primary disease
◆ Short-term relief with atropine injection

Third-degree atrioventricular block (complete heart block)

Significance:
◆ Almost always fatal
◆ Not well defined clinically

Occurs:
◆ During anesthesia; possibly associated with arrhythmogenic drugs
◆ During hypoxia, hypercarbia, acid–base imbalances

Clinical signs include:
◆ Bradycardia unresponsive to exercise or atropine
◆ Rarely audible atrial tachycardia
◆ Periodical atrial cannon waves shoot up jugular
◆ Variable intensity of first heart sound
◆ Very poor exercise tolerance
◆ General signs of heart failure
◆ History of syncopal attacks

ECG QRS complexes completely dissociated from faster P waves

Treatment:
◆ Prognosis very poor
◆ Correct acid–base balance
◆ Corticosteroid and dextrose intravenously
◆ Atropine (0.02 mg/kg) used but may not alleviate; dopamine hydrochloride (3–5 μg/kg/minute) effective

Premature beats (extrasystoles) [VM8 p. 345]

◆ These may be atrial, junctional (arising in the atrioventricular node or conducting tissue), or ventricular
◆ Careful exercise usually increases severity and occurrence
◆ All indicate myocardial disease except atrial premature beats which occur commonly in gastrointestinal disease in cattle

Atrial premature beats [VM8 p. 346]

◆ Normal rhythm to gross, variable arrhythmia; usually periodic interruption of a nor-

mal rhythm by a dropped pulse or one markedly decreased in amplitude
♦ Can progress to atrial fibrillation

ECG P wave early and abnormal configuration.

Junctional premature beats
[VM8 p. 346]

♦ Irregularity usually consisting of a premature heart beat followed by a longer than normal interval, a compensatory pause, then a regular rhythm

ECG P wave vector opposite to normal but P and QRS configurations normal.

Ventricular premature beats
[VM8 p. 346]

♦ Arrhythmia similar to that in junctional premature beats

ECG Bizarre configurations of QRS complexes, T waves have greater duration and magnitude. Vector orientation, opposite of normal.

Arrhythmias with tachycardia
[VM8 p. 346]

Includes paroxysmal and ventricular tachycardias and atrial and ventricular fibrillation.

Paroxysmal tachycardia [VM8 p. 346]

Occurs in Spontaneously or following excitement.

Clinical signs include:
♦ Bouts of tachycardia with abrupt commencements and endings
♦ Rate during bout excessively high

Ventricular tachycardia [VM8 p. 347]

Significance:
♦ Indicates severe cardiac disease
♦ May progress to fatal ventricular fibrillation

Clinical signs include:
♦ Either a regular or irregular rhythm with a very rapid rate
♦ The defect with regular rhythm is easily missed clinically

♦ The irregular rhythm is grossly abnormal and marked by pulse deficits and cannon waves in the jugular veins
♦ Signs of acute heart failure

ECG Multiple, irregular extrasystoles with abnormal amplitude and duration of the QRS and T complexes. P waves may be missing or have no relationship to QRS and T complexes.

Treatment of horses:
♦ Standard remedy in horses is quinidine sulfate 20 mg/kg orally, then 10 mg/kg every hours
♦ Lignocaine intravenously used also but has disadvantages
♦ No recommended treatment for cows; quinidine has been used but therapeutic index narrow
♦ Excitement exacerbates the condition

Ventricular fibrillation [VM8 p. 347]

Occurs in:
♦ Lightning stroke
♦ Anesthetic overdose
♦ Plant poisonings, e.g dimethyl tryptamines cardiac glycosides
♦ Terminal stages of most acquired cardiac disease

Clinical findings:
♦ Complete absence heart sounds, pulse
♦ Not usually observed clinically because sudden death the usual outcome

Treatment Impractical.

Atrial fibrillation in horses
[VM8 p. 348]

Occurrence:
♦ One of the common arrythmias in large animals
♦ Common cause of poor racing performance

Significance:
♦ **Benign fibrillators** – horses with heart rates of 26–48 beats/minute. Can elevate rate with exercise to perform modestly but not effective as racehorse
♦ May persist for life of horse if not defibrillated
♦ **Heart disease fibrillators** – complication of heart disease, usually valvular disease

Clinical findings include:
- Exercise intolerance
- Examination must be just after exercise; may be normal at rest
- Gross irregularity of heart and pulse with a very variable rate
- At fast rates pulse deficit common
- No atrial fourth sound or atrial wave at jugular inlet
- Third heart sound grossly accentuated
- Variable degree of heart failure
- **Benign fibrillator** horses have gross irregularity
- At rest 3–6 second episodes of no ventricular activity
- Periodic syncope
- **Heart disease fibrillator** horses have tachycardiac arrhythmia with resting heart rates of 80–100/minute, and rapidly develop heart failure

ECG:
- No P waves but 300–600 f waves/minute
- QRS complexes normal but wide variations in Q–Q intervals

Treatment Benign fibrillators:
- Used in horses required to work, e.g. may race again
- Quinidine sulfate orally 20 mg/kg every 2 hours until conversion (total dose usually <40 g) or toxicity (total dose >60 g)
- Signs of toxicity include depression, anorexia, urticaria, mucosal congestion, colic, death
- Conversion more likely in young horses and when condition present for less than 4 months
- Rest for 3 months after treatment
- May recur; reconversions possible

Heart disease fibrillators: treatment not undertaken.

Atrial fibrillation in cattle
[VM8 p. 348]

- Commonly functional related to gastrointestinal disease, abdominal pain, metabolic disease, enteritis, left abomasal displacement, uterine torsion.
- Treatment not undertaken; revert spontaneously when lesion corrected

Atrial fibrillation in goats
[VM8 p. 349]

- Sequel to interstitial pneumonia with cor pulmonale
- Signs include dyspnea, ascites, jugular distension, irregular jugular pulse,

- Response to treatment poor
- May be result of atrial hypertrophy in cardiac disease

CLINICAL INDICANTS

Apex beat displacement

Clinical findings Area of maximum palpability of heart action displaced caudally or to right.

Occurs in:
- Mass in chest, e.g.:
  - Thymoma
  - Mediastinal abscess
  - Mediastinal lymph node enlargement
- Mediastinum displacement by pleural:
  - Fluid in hydrothorax
  - Air in pneumothorax
- Gross heart enlargement

Arrhythmias

Irregularities of cardiac rate and rhythm may be detected by auscultation of heart sounds or palpation of the pulse but some will be missed without electrocardiographic examination.

Arteriolar–capillary circulation

- Capillary engorgement indicated by mucosal reddening
- Capillary emptiness indicated by mucosal pallor
- Skin coldness suggests poor capillary flow
- Skin warmth suggests good capillary flow
- Mucosal petechiae usually indicates capillary fragility
- Retinal hemorrhages suggests increased vascular fragility

Blood pressure

Arterial blood pressure
- Indirect measurement practicable only in the horse by application of sphygmomanometer to the tail and measurement of pressure in ventral coccygeal artery
- Mean systolic/diastolic pressures in the coccygeal artery in normal horses are 112–77 mm Hg
- Raising or lowering head significantly alters pressure
- Hypertension in horses occurs in:
  - Epistaxis

- Laminitis
- Painful lower limb fractures
- Intestinal obstruction

Intracardiac blood pressure
Cardiac catheterization can provide evidence of blood pressure in each of the heart chambers and in the larger vessels. Abnormalities can provide conclusive diagnostic information about such diseases as congenital cardiac, atrial or large vessel defects. Largely supplanted by the less hazardous echocardiography.

Blood volume

A research tool, based on measurement of degree of dilution of Evans blue dye injected intravenously.

Cardiac output

Circulating blood volume estimated by the dilution of an intravenously injected dye over time. Output per kg body weight per minute is estimated by dividing the circulating blood volume by the time taken for one complete circulation. Not a test suitable for everyday clinical use.

Cardiac reserve depletion

Compensation for an additional load on the heart is to call on the cardiac reserve. Its depletion represents less reserve for countering additional loads, and a step further towards eventual cardiac and hence circulatory failure. Signs indicating depletion include:

- **Increased resting heart rate** to compensate for the decrease in stroke volume resulting from reduced myocardial contractility
- **Increased heart sound intensity** suggesting cardiac dilation or possibly hypertrophy
- **Wide pulse amplitude** suggesting an increase in stroke volume
- **Cardiac enlargement** indicated by:
  - Increased area of audibility or **palpability of apex beat**
  - Backward **displacement of apex beat**
  - Increased **visibility of cardiac impulse** at the base of the neck and behind the elbow
- Decrease in **exercise tolerance** as measured by heart rate, and time taken to return to normal, after standard exercise
- **Echocardiographic** evidence of changes in cardiac chamber size, wall thickness, valve structure and function, and determination

of the existence of cardiac hypertrophy or dilation

Cardiac thrill

Clinical:
- Thrill (fremitus) palpated over cardiac area
- Synchronous with cardiac cycles
- Turbulent blood flow sufficient to cause murmur may cause a thrill; the bigger the aperture, the stronger the thrill

Occurs in:
- Valvular disease
- Congenital heart defects
- Hemic thrill

Echocardiographic changes

- Ultrasonic recordings of heart movements combined with an electrocardiograph, can measure ventricle wall thickness, chamber dimensions, observe valve motion, and rate of blood flow
- Valuable in diagnosis of valve defects, endocarditis, congenital cardiac defects especially shunts, abnormalities of contractility, presence of tumor masses, presence of pleural or pericardial effusions, and in the vascular part of the system, the diagnosis of iliac thrombosis
- The procedure has the enormous advantage for the clinician of being non-invasive

Edema

See also Chapter 9.

Clinical:
- Aggregations of serous fluid especially at:
  - Intermandibular space
  - Brisket
  - Ventral underline
- Swellings cold, pit on pressure

Occurs in:
- Congestive heart failure
- Blood loss anemia
- Low protein intake
- Renal failure

Electrocardiographic abnormality

- In ruminants and horses the electrocardiogram's usefulness is limited to detection and differentiation of conduction abnormalities and arrhythmic heart disease
- The recommended lead system is the traditional:

- Bipolar limb leads I, II, III plus
- Augmented, unipolar limb leads aVR, aVL, aVF
- With an exploring unipolar chest lead
- Recordings must be taken with the patient standing square or with the left fore foot slightly in advance of the right
- Electrolyte imbalances, e.g. hypocalcemia and hyperkalemia, can cause abnormalities in the electrocardiogram
- Electrocardiographic parameter for horses and cattle are in Table 8.1

Exercise tolerance reduced

- Determined as a subjective estimate by a clinician during a standard clinical examination
- Standardized tests, useful for general clinical use, with normal parameters defined, are not available but tests using telemetry in horses running on the track or on treadmills are used in special horse medicine institutes. There is also much data about the effects of equine endurance rides
- Fitness is determined by the top rate achieved and the time lapse before the rate returns to normal

Heart sounds irregular

Irregular heart sounds occur in:
- Gallop rhythms (variable audibility of third and fourth heart sounds in horses; in cattle similar variable audibility of these additional sounds or true splitting of the first heart sound) occur in normal animals

- Conduction disturbances
- Errors in the pacemaker of the heart

Heart murmurs

Occur in:
- Endocarditis
- Distortion of atrioventricular orifice by external compression, e.g. in ruminal tympany,
- Atrial deformity by tumor, e.g. viral leukosis
- Abnormal orifices, e.g. aneurysm, patent ductus arteriosus
- Pericardial or pleural friction sounds synchronous with cardiac cycles

Heart sounds, loud

Occur in:
- Hemorrhagic anemia
- Hypomagnesemic tetany
- Excitement

Heart sounds, muffled

Occur in:
- In soft sounds the heart action is weak; in muffled sounds the heart action is often very vigorous
- Myocardial asthenia
- Hydropericardium, pericarditis
- Fluid of hydropericardium or pericarditis in pericardial sac
- Fluid of hydrothorax or pleuritis in pleural cavity
- Interposition of other tissue e.g. emphyse-

Table 8.1 Electrocardiographic parameters in cattle and horses [VM8 p. 337]

	Holstein	Jersey	Thoroughbred
Duration (sec)			
Lead II			
P	0.1 ± 0.011	0.08 ± 0.022	0.132 ± 0.012
P–R	0.208 ± 0.022	0.16 ± 0.006	0.325 ± 0.065
QRS	0.088 ± 0.008	0.070 ± 0.003	0.110–0.009
Q–T	0.398 ± 0.034	0.38 ± 0.010	0.524 ± 0.034
T	0.114 ± 0.081	0.10 ± 0.011	—
Mean electrical axis – frontal plane			
P	+23.5 ± 12	—	Majority +50–+90
QRS	+196 ± 70	—	Majority +30–+90
T	+129 ± 76	—	Majority +60–+160

matous lung, intestine in diaphragmatic hernia

Jugular inlet abnormalities

♦ Atrial contraction waves, visible in the jugular inlet, may be unaccompanied by a heart sound in second-degree heart block when the atrium contracts but the ventricle does not
♦ **Cannon atrial waves** occur in complete heart block when the atrium contracts against a closed atrioventricular valve

Jugular pulse excessive

See jugular vein engorgement, this section.

Jugular vein engorgement

Clinical:
♦ Obvious distension of vein when animal standing at attention
♦ Tip of distension may reach as high as the jaw angle
♦ A jugular pulse usually accompanies, not in space occupying lesion of anterior thorax

Occurs in:
♦ Congestive heart failure
♦ Thymoma
♦ Valvular disease
♦ Endocarditis
♦ Pericarditis

Pericardial friction sounds

Clinical:
♦ Loud, rasping sounds with each cardiac cycle
♦ For few days only; replaced by muffled heart sounds
♦ Accompanying signs of pericarditis

Occurs in:
♦ Traumatic pericarditis
♦ Pericarditis

Phonocardiographic abnormalities

♦ Better definition and dissection of heart sounds and murmurs is possible with a phonocardiogram
♦ Recorded simultaneously with an electrocardiogram the timing of the sounds and intervals can be more accurate
♦ An advantage in examining hearts with very fast rates

Pulse, arterial, changes

Changes in the arterial pulse are reflections of the changes more readily found by examination of the heart, including arrhythmias, except for:
♦ Pulse deficit when the stroke volume of the heart is insufficient to create a pulse wave, detected by simultaneous pulse palpation and cardiac auscultation
♦ Pulse amplitude, the digital pressure required to obliterate the pule; an indicator of stroke volume
Special artery examinations include:
♦ External iliac and volar digital arteries in iliac thrombosis
♦ Middle uterine arteries in pregnancy diagnosis for cows in late pregnancy
♦ Cranial mesenteric artery in verminous arteritis and thromboembolic colic

Radiographic changes

Limited to use in neonates because of the patient's size. Combined with angiography can be diagnostic in congenital cardiac defects.

DISEASES OF THE HEART

MYOCARDIAL DISEASE AND CARDIOMYOPATHY
[VM8 p. 350]

Etiology

Bacterial myocarditis
♦ Strangles, navel-ill, other bacteremia
♦ Tuberculosis especially horses
♦ Tick pyemia in lambs
♦ Extension from endocarditis, pericarditis

♦ Emboli, e.g. from *Pteridium aquilinum* poisoning
♦ *Clostridium chauvoei*
♦ *Hemophilus somnus*

Viral myocarditis
♦ Bovine viral leukosis
♦ Foot and mouth disease, especially young animals
♦ African horse sickness
♦ Equine viral arteritis

♦ Equine infectious anemia
♦ Swine vesicular disease
♦ Encephalomyocarditis of pigs
♦ Bluetongue of sheep

Parasitic myocarditis
♦ *Strongylus* spp., migrating larvae
♦ Cysticercoses
♦ Sarcocystosis
♦ *Neosporum caninum* in neonatal calves

Nutritional deficiency
♦ Vitamin E/selenium deficiency in all species
♦ Copper deficiency (falling disease) of cattle
♦ Iron deficiency in calves and piglets
♦ Copper – cobalt deficiency in lambs

Poisonings
♦ Selenium, arsenic, mercury, phosphorus, thallium
♦ Gossypol
♦ Fluoracetate
♦ Cardiac glycoside in plants
♦ Dimethyl tryptamine in plants
♦ Tunicamycin and corynetoxins in algae, fungi, cyanobacteria
♦ Cantharidin
♦ Succinylcholine, catecholamines, xylazine, ionophores especially monensin, salinomycin, lasolocid
♦ Vitamin D and plants containing analogues, e.g. *Cestrum* spp., *Solanum malacoxylon*

Inherited
♦ Malignant hyperthermia, swine
♦ Congenital cardiomyopathy, cattle
♦ Glycogen storage disease (α-1,4-glucosidase deficiency), cattle, sheep

Unknown causes
♦ Secondary to acute central nervous system disease
♦ Exertional rhabdomyolysis, capture myopathy, restraint stress
♦ Young calves, precipitated by intense excitement, e.g. at feeding time
♦ Myocardial lipofuscinosis, in aged, cachectic cattle; also in normal cattle
♦ In horses exercised when affected by mild upper respiratory disease

Clinical findings

♦ Decreased exercise tolerance
♦ Increased heart rate
♦ Tachyarrhythmias associated with ventricular extrasystoles

♦ Patients with suspected heart disease but no clinical signs may need to be exercised gently and observed in the period immediately afterwards
♦ Attacks of cardiac syncope, falling unconscious
♦ Sudden death due to acute heart failure
♦ Dyspnea due to left congestive heart failure
♦ Generalized edema due to right congestive heart failure
♦ Hemic heart murmur with first heart sound and peaking at peak of inspiration

Clinical pathology

♦ Electrocardiography defines abnormalities of conduction, but not myocardial lesions nor the state of the myocardium
♦ Echocardiography can define wall thickness and volume of cavities
♦ Because of importance of systemic states in development of heart disease, full hematological, biochemical profiles recommended
♦ Serum levels of creatine kinase, lactate dehydrogenase elevated in cases with significant lesions

Necropsy findings

♦ Discrete abscesses, areas of inflammation in bacterial infections
♦ Areas or streaks of pallor, sometimes restricted to inner wall layers, in viral infections, poisonings or nutritional deficiency
♦ Petechial or linear hemorrhages in acute cases
♦ Infarction of an area of wall in coronary thrombosis
♦ Calcification in enzootic calcinosis
♦ Fibrous tissue replacement of damaged tissue; may lead to rupture and fatal cardiac tamponade
♦ Large masses of lymphoid tissue in atrium in bovine viral leukosis

Diagnosis

Resembles other causes of:
♦ Sudden death
♦ Congestive heart failure
♦ Increased audibility of lung sounds, e.g. retraction of lung
♦ Decreased audibility of lung sounds, e.g. that caused by lung emphysema
♦ Space-occupying lesions of chest including:
  • Diaphragmatic hernia
  • Mediastinal abscess
  • Mediastinal tumor

Treatment

Treatment is directed at:
♦ Specific causes, e.g bacterial myocarditis
♦ Individual arrhythmia
♦ Acute or congestive heart failure

RUPTURE OF HEART OR MAJOR VESSELS [VM8 p. 353]

Etiology

Cattle
♦ Penetration of ventricular wall by foreign body from reticulum
♦ Coronary vessel laceration by reticular foreign body
♦ Aorta rupture subsequent to damage by *Onchocerca* spp. larvae
♦ **Marfan syndrome** in calves; an inherited collagen defect causing aorta dilation, which may rupture, loud systolic murmur, long, thin limbs, joint and tendon laxity, and lenticular opacity, displacement

Horse
♦ Left atrium rupture following chronic fibrotic myocarditis
♦ Base of aorta rupture, subsequent to damage by migration of strongyle larvae, and during exercise, e.g. in stallions at mating
♦ Laceration of epicardium in foal during difficult parturition
♦ **Aorta to pulmonary artery fistula** causing sudden onset cardiac failure; possibly familial in origin

Pigs
♦ Nutritional deficiency of copper; rupture of heart wall or major blood vessel

Clinical findings

♦ Sudden death due to acute heart failure following cardiac tamponade
♦ Rapidly developing congestive heart failure due to dissecting aneurysm into myocardium or vessel wall

HEART VALVE RUPTURE [VM8 p. 353]

Etiology

♦ Rupture of mitral valve chordae tendineae in foals and adult horses, either independently or sequel to endocarditis
♦ Rupture of medial cusp of aortic valve in horse

Clinical findings

♦ Acute heart failure in healthy horse, or
♦ Complication of existing endocarditis syndrome
♦ Heart failure may be right or left sided depending on valve affected

COR PULMONALE [VM8 p. 353]

Etiology

♦ Genetic predisposition
♦ Cattle residing at altitudes above 1500 m predisposed
♦ Ingestion *Oxytropis sericea* (locoweed), possibly also *Crotalaria* spp., intensifies effects of high altitude
♦ *Pimelea* spp. poisoning causing pulmonary venule constriction
♦ Fat cattle with fat deposits reducing pulmonary ventilation
♦ Chronic obstructive pneumonia
♦ Pulmonary thromboembolic disease

Clinical findings

Generalized edema and venous distension due to right-sided congestive heart failure

VALVULAR DISEASE [VM8 p. 354]

Etiology

Congenital
♦ Fenestration of aortic, pulmonary semilunar valves in horses
♦ Hematocysts in atrioventricular valves

Acquired
♦ Bacterial endocarditis
♦ Endocardiosis in pigs
♦ Valve laceration
♦ Valve detachment
♦ Chordae tendineae rupture
♦ Functional insufficiency due to atrioventricular annulus dilation, e.g. in brisket disease

Clinical findings

Include signs of acute or congestive heart failure. Additional signs specific to valvular disease include heart murmurs, cardiac thrills and abnormalities of the arterial pulse.

Heart murmurs

Heart murmurs characterised by their **timing**, e.g.:

- **Systolic** (due to stenosis of arterial valves or insufficiency of atrioventricular valves
- **Diastolic** (due to insufficiency of arterial valves, or stenosis of atrioventricular valves)
- **Continuous** (due to stenosis and insufficiency of the same valve, involvement of multiple valves or flow from high to low pressure system, e.g. patent ductus arteriosus) as indicated by simultaneous palpation of arterial pulse, e.g. posteromedial carpal artery

Heart murmurs characterized by their **duration**, e.g. **pansystolic** or **pandiastolic** compared with early or late systole, etc.

Heart murmurs characterized by their **loudness** (intensity) and the presence or absence of a thrill, graded by a score of *I* to *V*

Heart murmurs characterized by their **location** relative to the anatomical location of the valves

Cardiac thrills

Vibrations palpated over the cardiac area and matching murmurs but more indicative of severity of lesion than murmurs.

Arterial pulse abnormalities

These include:

- Very wide amplitude (**water-hammer**) pulse of aortic semilunar valve incompetence
- Narrow amplitude, slow-rising pulse of aortic valve stenosis

These clinical signs can be used to determine location and severity of the valve lesion but not its nature or cause. The syndromes caused by individual valvular lesions include:

Aortic valve stenosis

- Harsh murmur replacing or modifying first sound
- Most audible over left heart base, posteriorly
- Systolic thrill over base
- Cardiac impulse increased
- Pulse small amplitude, slow rising, delayed peak
- May be syncope
- May be left-sided failure (dyspnea, pulmonary edema)

Aortic valve insufficiency

- Commonest valve defect in horses
- Loud murmur modifying second sound or immediately after it
- Audible over entire left cardiac area
- Frequently thrill during diastole
- Pulse in significant defect has very wide amplitude (water-hammer)

Pulmonary arterial valve stenosis–insufficiency

- Acquired lesions rare in large animals
- Harsh murmur replacing or modifying first or second sound or both
- Most audible right side
- Pulse unaffected
- Heart failure right-sided if it occurs

Left atrioventricular valve insufficiency

- Caused by endocarditis or rupture of valve chordae
- Second most common valvular lesion in large animals
- Loud, pansystolic murmur most intense mitral area (lower third, anterior to mid left thorax)
- Modification first and second sounds, accentuation of third sound
- Pulse unchanged
- Heart failure initially left-sided but followed by right-sided failure
- May predispose to atrial fibrillation in horse
- Acute heart failure with rupture of chordae

Right atrioventricular valve insufficiency

- Commonest acquired valvular lesion in ruminants, pigs
- Cause may be dilation of valve annulus in altitude sickness, cor pulmonale, anemia
- Harsh, pansystolic murmur modifying first sound
- Most audible tricuspid area (right lower third mid thorax but audible both sides)
- Exaggerated systolic part of jugular pulse
- Heart failure will be right sided, if it occurs

Right or left atrioventricular valve stenosis

- Either is uncommon
- Diastolic murmur over heart base either side, depending on lesion location
- Accentuation of atrial part of jugular pulse if stenosis is of right atrioventricular valve

Clinical pathology

No findings specific to valvular disease.

Necropsy findings

- Lesions of valves relevant to specific disease
- Congestive heart failure in some

Diagnosis

Valvular murmurs resemble:
- Friction rub of early pericarditis
- Friction rub of early pleuritis
- Murmurs associated with shunts
- Aneurysm of aorta in horses causing aortic valve insufficiency

Valvular murmurs may occur without structural lesions of valves, e.g. in:
- Anemia
- Hypoproteinemic states
- In debilitated, emaciated animals
- Dilation of valvular annulus
- Dilation of nearby vessel
- Distortion of annulus in recumbency, ruminal tympany, diaphragmatic hernia
- When critical velocity of blood flow exceeded, e.g. ejection murmur in horses after exercise
- Newborn calves, foals and piglets due possibly to patent atrial septum or temporary patency of closing ductus arteriosus

Treatment

Is of congestive heart failure and endocarditis.

ENDOCARDITIS [VM8 p. 357]

Etiology

Cattle
- Alpha-hemolytic streptococci
- *Actinomyces pyogenes*
- *Clostridium chauvoei* (blackleg)
- *Mycoplasma mycoides*
- *Erysipelothrix insidiosa* (rare)

Horses
- *Actinobacillus equuli*
- *Streptococcus equi, S. zooepidemicus*
- Migrating *Strongylus* spp. larvae

Pigs and sheep
- *Erysipelothrix insidiosa*
- *Streptococcus equisimilis, S. dysgalactiae, S. suis*
- *Escherichia coli*
- *Actinomyces pyogenes*

Clinical findings

- Low body condition; history of ill-thrift
- Periodic, dramatic, transient drops in milk yield
- Often history of intermittent lameness
- Mild cases have poor exercise tolerance
- Bad cases show congestive heart failure
- Moderate, fluctuating fever
- Mucosal pallor
- Tachycardia
- Heart murmur and/or cardiac thrill in most cases
- Pulse mostly normal; rarely water-hammer in aortic valve insufficiency, slow-rising small amplitude in aortic valve stenosis
- Jugular pulse exaggerated in right atrioventricular valve disease (see under valvular disease)
- Course in all species may be sudden death without premonitory signs, often during exercise or excitement, or illness for several months

Sequels
- Signs of peripheral lymphadenitis, embolic pneumonia, nephritis, arthritis, tenosynovitis, myocarditis in a few cases
- Atrial fibrillation in horses with left atrioventricular valve endocarditis
- Valve rupture in foals or adult horses, causing acute heart failure

Clinical pathology

- Non-regenerative anemia
- Leukocytosis, neutrophilia, left shift, monocytosis, elevation of plasma fibrinogen levels in cases with active lesions. Normal levels in healed lesions on scarred valves
- Hypergammaglobulinemia common
- Blood culture essential; often negative unless repeated
- Antibacterial sensitivity of cultured organisms
- Echocardiography a major aid in diagnosis

Necropsy findings

- Vegetative or verrucose valve lesions
- Rarely healed lesions with shrunken, distorted valves with thickened edges

◆ Embolic lesions in other organs; smear and culture often negative

Diagnosis

Resembles:
◆ Pericarditis with friction rub
◆ Altitude disease with right atrioventricular valve insufficiency
◆ Bovine viral leukosis involving right atrium

Principal sources of error in diagnosis are:
◆ Cases without valvular murmur
◆ Cases without leukocytosis

Treatment

◆ Success rate poor without identification of bacteria
◆ Where bacteria not identified a broad-spectrum antibacterial. Penicillin, possibly combined with gentamicin or potentiated sulfonamide
◆ Course of treatment needs to be long, often repeated, and of dubious financial benefit except in very valuable animals
◆ Not recommended in cases with congestive heart failure

PERICARDITIS [VM8 p. 360]

Etiology

◆ Traumatic perforation
◆ Blood-borne infection in some specific diseases
◆ Extension from pleurisy, myocarditis

Specific causes include:

Cattle
◆ Traumatic pericarditis
◆ Pasteurellosis
◆ Black disease
◆ Tuberculosis
◆ Sporadic bovine encephalomyelitis
◆ *Haemophilus somnus* infection
◆ *Pseudomonas aeruginosa* infection
◆ *Mycoplasma* spp. infection

Horses
◆ Many cases sterile, after respiratory tract infection
◆ Idiopathic effusive pericarditis
◆ *Streptococcus equi, S. zooepidemicus, S. fecalis*
◆ Tuberculosis
◆ *Actinobacillus equuli*

Sheep
◆ Pasteurellosis
◆ *Staphylococcus aureus*
◆ *Mycoplasma* spp.

Pigs
◆ Pasteurellosis
◆ *Mycoplasma* spp., especially *M. hyorhinis*
◆ *Haemophilus* spp.
◆ *Streptococcus* spp.
◆ Salmonellosis

Clinical findings

Description refers to cows but horse cases very similar.

Acute pericarditis
◆ Reluctance to move, lies down carefully
◆ Elbows abducted
◆ Arched back
◆ Rapid, shallow, abdominal respiration
◆ Pain on percussion over cardiac area
◆ Fever
◆ Pericardial friction sound first 24–48 hours then muffled heart sounds
◆ Splashing sounds over cardiac area in most cases
◆ Pulse amplitude reduced
◆ Tachycardia
◆ Toxemia
◆ Signs of congestive heart failure
◆ Additional signs of pleurisy, pneumonia, peritonitis in a few cases
◆ Death in 1–3 weeks due to combined effects of toxemia and congestive heart failure

Chronic pericarditis
◆ Congestive heart failure and toxemia subside gradually
◆ Chronic stage persists more or less indefinitely
◆ Heart rate continues fast
◆ Venous engorgement, anasarca subside
◆ Feed intake limited
◆ Emaciation
◆ Heart sounds audible, gassy sounds may persist over limited areas

Clinical pathology

Acute cases
◆ Marked leukocytosis, neutrophilia, left shift
◆ Paracentesis of pericardial fluid may be culturally positive, inflammatory
◆ Electrocardiographic changes include dim-

inished amplitude of QRS complex and electrical alternans
♦ Echocardiography allows differentiation of fibrinous and effusive pericarditis

Chronic cases

♦ Leukon approximates normality
♦ Paracentesis not feasible

Necropsy findings

Acute cases

♦ Early cases have hyperemia of and fibrin deposits on endothelial lining of pericardial sac
♦ Later effusion of turbid fluid containing tags of fibrin
♦ Epicardium and pericardium thick and edematous
♦ Putrid odor and gas present if infecting bacteria include *Actinomyces pyogenes, Fusobacterium necrophorum*

Chronic cases

♦ Pericardium, epicardium adherent; some serous fluid-filled loculi

Diagnosis

Pericardial friction sounds resemble:
♦ Pleurisy friction sounds
♦ Endocarditis murmurs
♦ Congenital cardiac defect murmurs
Muffled heart sounds also caused by:
♦ Pleurisy effusion
♦ Pulmonary emphysema
♦ Hydropericardium
♦ Congestive heart failure due to other causes.

Treatment

♦ Broad-spectrum antibiotic, preferably chosen on basis of pericardial fluid culture; penicillin and gentamicin combination preferred
♦ Non-steroidal anti-inflammatories in non-bacterial, idiopathic pericarditis
♦ Needle or indwelling catheter drainage of sac in horses
♦ Thoracotomy and marsupialization of sac in septic pericarditis of cattle

CONGENITAL DEFECTS OF THE HEART AND MAJOR VESSELS

Etiology

♦ Causes of most defects are unknown. Inherited defects include interventricular septal defect in cattle and miniature swine

Clinical findings

♦ Most defects cause clinical illness in the newborn and death during the first few weeks of life
♦ Compensation for the defect may enable the patient to survive for up to a year
♦ Congenital murmurs, especially in piglets and foals, are often caused by defects which correct themselves quickly, e.g. partly closed ductus arteriosus; prognosis should always be guarded
♦ Common signs are:
  • Dyspnea
  • Cyanosis
  • Cardiac enlargement
  • Cardiac murmur
  • Signs of acute heart failure or congestive heart failure
♦ Echocardiography very helpful in differentiating between individual defects

ECTOPIC HEART [VM8 p. 363]

In cattle, mostly in lower cervical region, accompanying divergence of first ribs, ventrodorsal compression of sternum. These survive only a few days. May survive for long periods when heart located in abdomen.

PATENT FORAMEN OVALE [VM8 p. 363]

Sporadic cases in cattle, but asymptomatic unless with other defects.

VENTRICULAR SEPTAL DEFECTS [VM8 p. 363]

♦ Common defect in sheep, cattle, horses
♦ Causes shunt of blood from left to right
♦ Loud, blowing, pansystolic murmur both sides of chest
♦ Normal heart sounds audible also
♦ Thrill both sides of chest
♦ Confirmable by cardiac catheterization and comparison of pressures in the ventricles

♦ Sudden death at birth usually accompanied by signs of left-sided failure; deaths later accompanied by right-sided congestive failure syndrome; at 1–3 years old in cattle may be **Eisenmenger complex** with marked cyanosis
♦ When defect large:
  • Dead at birth or in first few months
  • Poor exercise tolerance
  • Severe dyspnea
  • Growth retarded
  • Lassitude
♦ When defect small: clinically normal or signs delayed till late in life

Sequels

♦ Endocarditis of right atrioventricular valve in calves
♦ Endocarditis of aortic valve in foals
♦ Valve prolapse into defect causing aortic insufficiency
♦ Valve rupture causing sudden death
♦ Commonly concurrent with microphthalmia in calves, lambs

Treatment

♦ None practicable
♦ Cases with murmur but no cardiac insufficiency can survive and breed but not race; genetic implications suggest breeding may not be wise

TETRALOGY OF FALLOT [VM8 p. 364]

Commonly fatal defect in foals and calves. Includes:
♦ Ventricular septal defect
♦ Pulmonary stenosis
♦ Dextraposition of aorta
♦ Secondary right ventricular hypertrophy
Clinical signs at birth or very early with quick death. Signs include:
♦ Lassitude
♦ Dyspnea
♦ Cyanosis in most cases, especially after exercise
♦ Murmur, sometimes thrill, over left third intercostal space
  Diagnosis confirmed by cardiac catheterization, echocardiography.

PATENT DUCTUS ARTERIOSUS [VM8 p. 364]

♦ Commonest in foals; the murmur may be transiently audible in survivors for up to 5 days

♦ Loud, continuous murmur over heart base, waxing and waning, the so-called **machinery murmur**
♦ Diagnosis confirmed by angiography or oxygen saturation differences above and below shunt
♦ Surgical correction feasible

COARCTATION OF THE AORTA [VM8 p. 364]

Signs include systolic murmur, slow-rising, small amplitude pulse.

PERSISTENCE OF THE RIGHT AORTIC ARCH [VM8 p. 364]

Causes esophageal constriction at birth with signs of:
♦ Dysphagia
♦ Regurgitation
♦ Resistance to stomach tube at first rib
♦ Confirmable radiologically
♦ Surgical repair feasible

PERSISTENT TRUNCUS ARTERIOSUS [VM8 p. 364]

♦ Common trunk to pulmonary and somatic circuits persists into fetal life
♦ Incompatible with life

FIBROELASTOSIS [VM8 p. 364]

♦ Occurs in calves and pigs; cause unknown
♦ Signs of congestive heart failure without localizing signs such as murmurs
♦ Illness may not be apparent till late in life
♦ Endocardium is a thick fibroelastic coat; ventricular capacity reduced

SUBVALVULAR AORTIC STENOSIS [VM8 p. 364]

♦ Common in pigs; possibly inherited
♦ Aortic stenosis at or below point of attachment of semilunar valves
♦ Sudden death after dyspnea, frothing at mouth, nostrils **or**
♦ Recurrent dyspnea attacks over long period

ANOMALOUS ORIGIN OF CORONARY ARTERIES [VM8 p. 364]

♦ Recorded calves, piglets
♦ One or both coronary arteries affected

♦ Arteries originate from pulmonary artery instead of aorta
♦ Congestive heart failure syndrome

CARDIAC NEOPLASIA [VM8 p. 365]

♦ Primary neoplasms extremely rare; recorded cases include:
  • Aortic body adenoma
  • Pericardial mesothelioma

♦ Metastases uncommon; recorded cases include:
  • Lymphosarcoma commonest; cattle, horses
  • Melanoma
  • Hemangiosarcoma
  • Testicular embryonal carcinoma
  • Squamous cell carcinoma
♦ Benign adenomas recorded as cause of heart failure in young calf

DISEASES OF THE BLOOD VESSELS

ARTERIAL THROMBOSIS AND EMBOLISM [VM8 p. 365]

Etiology

Parasitic arteritis
♦ *Strongylus vulgaris* – horses
♦ Onchocerciasis, elaeophoriasis in cattle, sheep, goats, horses

Viral arteritis
♦ Bovine malignant catarrh
♦ Equine viral arteritis
♦ African horse sickness
♦ African swine fever
♦ Hog cholera
♦ Bluetongue

Bacterial arteritis
♦ Septicemic salmonellosis
♦ Erysipelas
♦ *Haemophilus pleuropneumoniae*
♦ *Haemophilus somnus*

Embolic arteritis and thromboembolism
♦ From endocarditis or arterial thrombus
♦ Hyperlipemia, hyperlipidemia in horses
♦ Fat emboli following surgery
♦ In subclinical *Salmonella dublin* infection in calves
♦ Pulmonary embolism from jugular or caudal vena caval thrombosis
♦ From intravenous, indwelling catheters

Microangiopathy
♦ Vitamin E/selenium deficiency
♦ Cerebrospinal angiopathy
♦ Terminally in most septicemias

Calcification
♦ Enzootic calcinosis
♦ Vitamin D poisoning

♦ Chronic hypomagnesemia in calves
♦ Lymphosarcoma in some horses

Vasoconstrictive agents
♦ *Claviceps purpurea* poisoning
♦ *Acremonium coenophialum* poisoning

Clinical findings

Signs at specific anatomic locations listed under those headings.

AORTIC-ILIAC THROMBOSIS [VM8 p. 366]

Etiology and epidemiology

♦ Unknown, possibly verminous arteritis, or idiopathic degenerative vascular disease
♦ Horses older than 3 years

Clinical signs – limb form

One or both hind limbs.

Chronic onset – most common
♦ Poor performance due to lameness at maximum exertion
♦ Lameness disappears after rest
♦ Lameness due to weakness, limb gives way on the turn
♦ Frequent lifting or kicking out in some cases
♦ Refusal to work in severe cases

Acute onset – rarely
♦ Sudden onset of severe pain and anxiety
♦ Marked dyspnea, tachycardia
♦ Profuse sweating; affected limb dry
♦ May be recumbent
♦ Limb cool from gaskin down
♦ Pulse amplitude small in common digital artery of affected limb

- Slow filling of saphenous vein in affected limb
- Enlargement, firmness at aortic quadrification; irregularity, asymmetry internal, external iliac arteries, absence of pulse

Testicular form – rare in stallions

- Testicular atrophy
- Ejaculatory failure but libido and coupling good

Clinical pathology

- Leukocytosis, left shift, serum fibrinogen level elevated
- In acute cases serum creatine kinase, lactate dehydrogenase levels elevated
- Secondary hyperkalemia, uremia in some
- Ultrasonography a more sensitive method of detection than rectal examination

Necropsy findings

- Thrombus in terminal aorta or one iliac artery
- Thrombus adherent to intima, often laminated
- Local ischemia, infarction and abscessation

Diagnosis

Resembles:
- Azoturia
- Tying-up
- Non-specific lamenesses
- Enzootic incoordination

Treatment

- The prognosis is for chronically progressive disease so treatment not highly effective
- Parenteral anticoagulants, fibrinolytic enzymes, sodium gluconate have been used, including by retrograde catheterization up coccygeal artery
- Stallion impotence responds to phenylbutazone plus gonadotrophin releasing hormone
- Broad-spectrum antibiotic regimen needed if infection still active

PULMONARY EMBOLISM [VM8 p. 367]

Etiology

- Embolus from jugular vein phlebitis, thrombosis, tricuspid valve endocarditis

- Caudal vena caval syndrome
- Vascular surgery

Clinical findings

- Severe acute dyspnea
- Anxiety
- Profuse sweating
- Temperature, pulse rate elevated
- No toxemia
- Lungs clear on auscultation
- Usually spontaneous recovery in 24–48 hours

Sequels

- Possibly blindness, imbecility
- Pulmonary abscess
- Pulmonary hypertension leading to cor pulmonale
- Pulmonary arterial aneurysm leading to rupture and pulmonary hemorrhage

Clinical pathology

Leukocytosis, left shift, serum fibrinogen level elevated.

Necropsy findings

Large thrombus, often lamellated, in pulmonary artery.

Diagnosis

Resembles:
- Pneumonia
- Pneumothorax
- Hemothorax

Treatment

As for iliac thrombosis, see above.

VENOUS THROMBOSIS [VM8 p. 368]

Etiology

- Irritant injections, e.g. phenylbutazone, chloral hydrate
- Long-term venous catheterization
- Extension from surrounding infection
- Infection umbilical veins in neonates
- Localization from blood-borne infection, e.g. in strangles, many septicemias in pigs

Clinical findings

* Marked local swelling, pain, local edema especially if periphlebitis present
* Local sloughing
* Rarely rupture
* Subsequent cicatricial contraction
* Purple discoloration, later sloughing of ears in pigs

Clinical pathology

* Leukocytosis, neutrophilia, left shift, hyperfibrinogenemia
* Culture of affected tissue desirable

Necropsy findings

* Vessel obstructed by thrombus
* Local edema, hemorrhage

Diagnosis

Resembles other local edemas:
* Local pressure by tumor, lymphadenopathy, hematoma, fibrous tissue contraction
* Perineal–udder edema in late pregnancy
* Sporadic lymphangitis

Treatment

* Parenteral broad-spectrum antibacterial treatment
* Hot fomentations to external lesions
* Anti-inflammatory drugs, including topicals, e.g. bi-methyl sulfoxide
* Anticoagulant therapy not recommended in horses because of risk of bleeding while racing

VASCULAR NEOPLASMS

HEMANGIOMA
[VM8 p. 369]

Occurrence

* Mostly in young
* May be congenital
* Mostly cutaneous, rarely ovarian in sows, generalized

Clinical findings

* Continuous growth
* Skin lesions ulcerate and bleed
* May necessitate euthanasia
* Similar outcome with mouth lesions

Treatment

* Surgical excision, thermocautery or radiation therapy used

HEMANGIOSARCOMA
[VM8 p. 369]

Occurrence

* Middle-aged and older animals
* Usually widely disseminated

Clinical findings

* Hemorrhagic anemia; bleeding into tumor or body cavity, especially thorax
* Space-occupying lesion in thoracic cavity causing dyspnea, resembling pleurisy
* Spleen the usual site of primary; causes peritoneal bleeding
* Metastases can be in any organ
* Secondaries in muscle cause pain and difficult movement
* Appetite good but serious weight loss, weakness

Treatment

Not applicable; profuse bleeding if tumor incised.

9 DISEASES OF THE BLOOD-FORMING ORGANS

CLINICAL INDICANTS

The principal clinicopathological findings on which clinical diagnoses of hemopoietic system diseases are based are mostly hematological and biochemical and are included in Appendix tables (pp. 684–687). Additional indicants are listed below.

Capillary refill slow

Clinical findings The time required for the mucosa, previously blanched by digital pressure, to return to normal pink color is prolonged beyond the usual several seconds.

Occurs in:
♦ Peripheral circulatory failure
♦ Shock

Edema, intermandibular

Occurs as part of general edema.

Eye, anterior chamber, blood in (hyphema)

Occurs in:
♦ Hemorrhagic disease
♦ Trauma

Lymph node enlargement (lymphadenectasis)

♦ Local lymph node enlargement, without inflammation in neoplasia primary or metastases
♦ Generalized lymph node enlargements without inflammation in lymphosarcoma, bovine viral leukosis
♦ Single or multiple lymph node enlargements with pain, heat in acute forms, cold,

containing pus on needle biopsy in chronic infections

Occurs in Lymphadenitis.

Lymphatic vessels thickened (lymphangiectasis)

Clinical findings:
♦ Thickened, corded subcutaneous lymph vessels, visible
♦ Acute lesions painful, hot with spread to surrounding tissue
♦ Most are chronic, cold, hard, tortuous cords
♦ Many connected to enlarged lymph nodes

Occurs in Sporadic lymphangitis, epizootic lymphangitis, skin tuberculosis, cutaneous farcy.

Methemoglobinemia

Clinical findings:
♦ Dyspnea
♦ Mucosal brown discoloration

Occurs in:
♦ Nitrate–nitrite poisoning
♦ Inherited methemoglobinemia of horses

Mucosal hemorrhages

Clinical findings:
♦ Mucosal, conjunctival petechiation
♦ Cutaneous, internal involvement also, but not usually visible
♦ Prolonged bleeding time in some

Occurs in:
♦ Hemorrhagic disease

143

Mucosal/corneal pallor

Clinical findings Paleness, most visible in mucosae.

Occurs in:
♦ Anemia
♦ Shock

Spleen enlarged/displaced

Clinical findings Detectable only in horses.

Occurs in Dorsal displacement of left colon.

Spleen painful

Clinical findings:
♦ Pain elicited over upper, last ribs on left side of ruminants
♦ Pain elicited on rectal in horses by palpation spleen against left, ventral abdominal wall

Occurs in Splenic abscess.

HEMOPOIETIC DISEASES [VM8 p. 370]

HEMORRHAGIC DISEASE [VM8 p. 370]

Etiology

Vasculitis
♦ Septicemia, viremia
♦ Purpura hemorrhagica
♦ Idiopathic necrotizing vasculitis
♦ Fungal toxins, e.g. citrinin, trichothecenes

Coagulation defects
♦ Thrombocytopenia, thrombasthenia, thrombopathy
♦ Coumarol poisoning from:
  • Warfarin poisoning and other rodenticides
  • Plants including moldy *Melilotus, Anthoxanthum, Apium, Ferula* spp.
♦ Some snake venoms
♦ Anticoagulants secreted by *Parafilaria* spp. in subcutaneous sites
♦ Inherited defects:
  • Hemophilia A
  • Von Willebrand disease
  • Factor XI deficiency
  • Prekallikrein deficiency
♦ Idiopathic, vitamin K responsive, bleeding disease in young, grower pigs with prolonged prothrombin, activated partial thromboplastin times; related to feeding of antibacterials and interference with vitamin K intake from feces, bedding
♦ Idiopathic, vitamin C-responsive, navel bleeding, newborn pigs. Possibly due to collagen immaturity preventing proper clot formation. Navel cords thick, fleshy, do not shrink, ooze, drip blood; mortality can be high. Prevented by feeding vitamin C for >6 days before farrowing
♦ Disseminated intravascular coagulopathy (consumption coagulopathy, DIC)

Clinical findings

Generally:
♦ Mucosal and cutaneous petechiation
♦ Spontaneous bleeding into cavities, tissues
♦ Excessive bleeding from injuries, after surgery
♦ Signs of anemia, hemorrhagic blood loss
♦ External blood losses via hematemesis, melena, hematochezia, dysentery, epistaxis, hemoptysis, hematuria
♦ Other specific organ involvement, e.g. renal cortical necrosis, acute renal failure in horses

Clinical signs associated with bleeding from specific sites dealt with under hemorrhagic blood loss.

Clinical pathology

♦ Thrombocytopenia, or
♦ Deficit of one or more coagulation factors, or
♦ Prolonged prothrombin or partial thromboplastin times
♦ The clinical pathology of hemorrhagic anemia
♦ Blood in paracentesis samples or excretions, secretions

DIC
♦ Subclinical cases can only be detected by these examinations; early detection re-

quires frequent monitoring in hazardous situations

♦ Diagnostic clinicopathological pattern includes:
  • Erythrocyte distortion, fragmentation
  • Hypofibrinogenemia (not always in horses)
  • Abnormal prothrombin (or activated partial thromboplastin time)
  • Fibrin degradation products present
  • Thrombocytopenia

Necropsy findings

♦ Blood in body cavities or tissue extravasations
♦ Subserosal, submucosal petechiae, ecchymoses or splashes
♦ Pallor of tissues, thin blood in cases of blood loss

Diagnosis

Differentiation between causes of hemorrhagic anemia or excessive bleeding, as listed under etiology, dependent on clinical pathology, detection of poisons in environment, history of repeated attacks, cases in related animals.

Treatment

♦ Principal objective is treatment of primary disease
♦ Response in terms of existing extravasations poor
♦ Empirical supportive treatment includes:
  • Antihistamines in allergies
  • Corticosteroids in auto-immune disease
  • Epinephrine on a pad applied locally, including nasal mucosa
  • Parenteral coagulants used extensively, often without effect if endothelial damage already present

DIC
♦ Active therapy of primary disease, especially toxemia
♦ Intravenous fluid and electrolyte therapy to ensure proper tissue perfusion
♦ Blood transfusion

HEMORRHAGIC BLOOD LOSS
[VM8 p. 374]

Etiology

Primary excessive bleeding:

Cattle
♦ Pulmonary hemorrhage in caudal vena caval syndrome
♦ Abomasal ulcer; some related to bovine viral leukosis
♦ Enzootic hematuria
♦ Pyelonephritis
♦ Ruptured middle uterine artery during uterine prolapse
♦ Cardiac perforation, aorta, atrium rupture
♦ Intraluminal bleeding due to intestinal ulcer, hematoma
♦ Juvenile angiomata

Horse
♦ Nasal bleeding at rest from guttural pouch mycosis
♦ Ethmoidal hematoma
♦ Exercise-induced pulmonary hemorrhage
♦ Uterine artery rupture during foaling
♦ Mesenteric artery rupture secondary to verminous arteritis
♦ Splenic hematoma, hemangioma, hemangiosarcoma
♦ Ulceration varicose veins in dorsal vaginal wall
♦ Congenital venous aneurysm

Pig
♦ Esophagogastric ulcer
♦ Proliferative hemorrhagic enteropathy
♦ Congenital umbilical bleeding
Secondary excessive bleeding:
♦ Hemorrhagic disease

Clinical findings

♦ Visible blood loss in many cases
♦ Blood in secretions or excretions may be visible only if complete clinical examination carried out
♦ Mucosal pallor
♦ Weak, staggery gait, recumbency
♦ Tachycardia
♦ Cold extremities
♦ Hypothermia
♦ Respirations deep, not seriously dyspneic
♦ Dull, depressed
♦ Coma, death in lateral recumbency
♦ **Localizing signs** in hemothorax, hemopericardium, umbilical bleeding, pulmonary hemorrhage, abomasal ulcer

Clinical pathology

♦ Erythrocyte count, hematocrit, hemoglobin count, serum protein level depressed;

degree dependent on efficiency of compensatory back up; after 4 days evidence of regeneration
- Paracentesis for identification of intracavity hemorrhage
- Special tests in cases of suspected hemorrhagic disease

Necropsy findings

- Tissue pallor
- Thin, watery blood
- Blood extravasations in cases of internal hemorrhage
- Anemia and/or edema in chronic cases

Diagnosis

Resembles:
- Other causes of peripheral circulatory failure
- Other causes of anemia

Treatment

- Correction of cause of blood loss
- If PCV less than 12% give blood transfusion (using 10 ml 0.85 sodium citrate solution per 100 ml of blood as anticoagulant); 10–15 ml/kg is adequate for survival; chances of an incompatibility reaction are very small unless transfusions repeated
- If PCV >12 and less than 20% represents hypovolemia and fluid therapy (40–80 ml/kg of isotonic saline) advisable. Small volumes 3–5 ml/kg hypertonic (7.2% sodium chloride) solutions also used
- Frequent monitoring of blood parameters when PCV <20%

SHOCK [VM8 p. 377]

Etiology

Hypovolemic shock
- Severe hemorrhage with loss of >35% total blood volume
- Dehydration due to severe diarrhea, intestinal obstruction

Cardiogenic shock
Acute heart failure due to myocardopathy or arrhythmia.

Distributive shock
Includes vasogenic shock:
- Severe trauma or burn
- Extensive surgery
- Uterine prolapse

- Too rapid withdrawal fluid or gas from body cavity
- Severe pain, e.g. colic in horse

Toxic shock
Toxins, including endotoxin, microorganisms gain access to circulation via:
- Septicemia
- Absorption of toxins from gut, e.g. infarction of segment of gut wall
- Absorption of toxins from a local infection, e.g. coliform mastitis

Clinical findings

Early stages
- Mucosae congested, vessels injected
- Normal capillary refill time
- Tachycardia
- Normal blood pressure

Late stages
- Weak, dull,
- Skin cold
- Hypothermia
- Rapid, shallow breathing
- Tachycardia
- Small amplitude, low pressure pulse
- Veins difficult to raise, venous pressure low
- Mucosae pale, gray, muddy
- Capillary refill time more than 3–4 seconds
- Terminally coma, recumbency, death

Clinical pathology

- In severe shock systolic blood pressure falls from 120 to terminal 60 mmHg
- See toxemia, septicemia, dehydration, hemorrhagic blood loss for specific variations in total and differential leukocyte counts, packed cell volume, total serum protein levels, blood gas analysis, arterial blood lactic acid level, serum enzyme levels indicative of tissue and myocardial damage, and indicators of renal function

Necropsy findings

- Widespread petechial and ecchymotic hemorrhages
- In toxic shock splanchnic vessel congestion, pulmonary edema in some
- Lesions of the primary disease

Diagnosis

- Shock is a secondary diagnosis in cases of severe trauma, intestinal obstruction, septicemia, toxemia, peripheral circulatory failure, and necessary to the proper treatment of the patient

Treatment

♦ Elimination of the precipitating cause, often a surgical procedure
♦ Aggressive fluid therapy, before irreversible stage, to maintain tissue perfusion
♦ See other sections for details of treatment of hemorrhagic blood loss, dehydration, heart failure, peripheral circulatory failure
♦ Treatment for toxic shock includes:
  • **Antibiotics** – broad-spectrum, bactericidal antibiotic until specific infection identified, especially in cases where systemic infection present
  • **Fluid therapy** – crystalloid solutions (containing electrolytes), e.g. isotonic saline, preferably Ringer's solution, other sodium-containing solutions **but not** glucose solutions used; 50–100 ml/kg initially and repeated to effect. Beneficial effect short-lived; ceases soon after administration ceases
  • **Corticosteroids** – large doses of dexamethasone (5–10 mg/kg I/V) commonly used but little evidence of benefit
  • Cyclooxygenase inhibitors, e.g. **flunixin meglumine**, inhibit formation prostaglandins, thromboxane A_2, maintain blood pressure, tissue perfusion better in horses with toxemia

WATER INTOXICATION [VM8 p. 381]

Etiology

♦ Excessive drinking by thirsty animals, or dosing with water compensated very quickly by increased urine flow
♦ Intoxication more likely if:
  • Environmental temperature high
  • Patient salt deprived beforehand
  • Antidiuretic hormone administered
  • Young animals

Clinical findings

♦ Intravascular hemolysis, hemoglobinuria, *or*
♦ Cerebral edema, muscle weakness, tremor, restlessness, staggering gait, convulsions, coma in some

Diagnosis

Resembles:
♦ Polioencephalomalacia
♦ Salt poisoning

Treatment

♦ Diuretics
♦ Sedation
♦ Intravenous hypertonic saline

EDEMA [VM8 p. 382]

Etiology

Increased hydrostatic pressure as in:
♦ Congestive heart failure
♦ Portal hypertension causing ascites
♦ Local pressure, e.g. large fetus causing mammary edema in late pregnancy
Decreased plasma osmotic pressure, due principally to hypoproteinemia as in:
♦ Blood-sucking parasites, e.g. *Haemonchus, Strongylus, Bunostomum* spp.
♦ Urinary protein loss in nephrosis caused by *Quercus, Terminalia* spp. poisoning
♦ Protein-losing enteropathy in Johne's disease, *Ostertagia* spp. infestations
♦ Liver damage, e.g. fascioliasis
♦ Malnutrition, e.g. drought time in ruminants, piglets when dams on low-protein diet
♦ **Lymphatic obstruction**
♦ Local tumors, inflammatory lesions, granulomas on serous surfaces
♦ Congenital inherited lymphatic aplasia in calves and pigs
♦ Sporadic lymphangitis in horses
♦ Enzootic calcinosis
♦ Horses immobilized for long periods by injury
♦ **Vascular damage**
♦ Allergic, e.g. angioedema, urticaria, purpura hemorrhagica
♦ Damage by infection, e.g. anthrax, gas gangrene, equine viral arteritis, equine infectious anemia
♦ Damage by toxin, e.g. gut edema, mulberry heart disease, plant toxins in *Verbesina, Galega, Wedelia* spp.

Clinical findings

Fluid accumulates in:
♦ Subcutaneous tissue in dependent parts with loose skin, e.g. ventral abdomen, brisket, intermandibular space, eyelids – **anasarca**
♦ Peritoneal cavity – **ascites**
♦ Thoracic cavity – **hydrothorax**
♦ Pericardial sac – **hydropericardium**
♦ Local sites, e.g. head in African horse sickness, purpura hemorrhagica; udder in puerperal cows, mares; lower limbs in

horses; intermandibular space in grazing animals
- Edematous swellings soft, cool, pit on pressure
- Ascites causes abdominal distension, fluid thrill on percussion, fluid flow on paracentesis
- Hydrothorax causes dyspnea, muffling of breath sounds with level top line, fluid flow on paracentesis
- Hydropericardium causes muffling of heart sounds, jugular engorgement, fluid flow on paracentesis
- Local swellings cause obstructive dyspnea, pulmonary edema causes dyspnea, frothing from the nostrils; idiopathic, self-limiting, local plaque around umbilicus in yearling horses

Clinical pathology

- Clear serous fluid on aspiration; inflammatory cells absent, protein content varies depending on cause and severity
- Changes due to primary disease

Necropsy findings

- General or local aggregations of sterile, clear fluid
- Lesions of primary lesion, e.g. cardiac, liver disease, local tissue mass

Diagnosis

Resembles:
- Subcutaneous accumulation of urine at ventral abdomen in urethral rupture
- Peritonitis, pericarditis, pleurisy
- Renal amyloidosis
- Local trauma, e.g. damage to brisket of cattle feeding from troughs with sharp front edges

Treatment

- Correction of hypoproteinemia, parasite infestation, or other cause
- Drainage of fluid accumulations by aspiration, administration of diuretics

ABNORMALITIES OF THE CELLULAR ELEMENTS OF THE BLOOD

ANEMIA [VM8 p. 384]

Etiology

Hemorrhagic anemia
As for hemorrhagic blood loss.

Hemolytic anemia

Cattle
- Babesiosis, anaplasmosis, eperythrozoonosis, trypanosomiasis, theileriosis
- Bacillary hemoglobinuria
- Leptospirosis in calves (*Leptospira interrogans* serovar *pomona*)
- Postparturient hemoglobinuria
- Plant poisons in *Brassica* spp., *Mercurialis*, *Pimelea*, *Allium* spp.
- Feeding cannery offal of onions, tomatoes
- Poisoning by phenothiazine, guaifenesin, chronic copper, especially in calves
- Rarely in treatment with long-acting tetracycline
- Calves drinking large volumes of very cold water
- In a transfusion reaction

- Congenital isoerythrolysis due to vaccination of dam with blood-derived vaccination, e.g. anaplasmosis
- Autoimmune hemolytic anemia in young calves
- Inherited dyserythropoiesis in Polled Herefords
- Congenital anemia in Murray Grey cattle due to cell membrane defect

Sheep
- Chronic copper poisoning, primary due to excessive intake, secondary due to ingestion pyrrolizidine alkaloids
- Eperythrozoonosis, babesiosis
- Plant toxins in *Brassica*, *Allium* spp.
- *Fasciola*, *Haemonchus* spp infestations
- Lambs fed cow colostrum from rare individual cows

Pigs
- Eperythrozoonosis recorded, hemolytic anemia rare
- Neonatal isoerythrolysis rarely
- Thrombocytopenic purpura
- Generalized cytomegalovirus infection

Horses

- Equine infectious anemia
- Babesiosis
- Phenothiazine poisoning
- Alloimmune hemolytic anemia
- Autoimmune hemolytic anemia
- Penicillin-induced hemolytic anemia

Nutritional deficiency anemia

- Copper – ruminants
- Cobalt – ruminants
- Iron – piglets and calves
- Potassium, possibly in calves
- Pyridoxine, experimentally
- Folic acid. Some response to supplementation in horses

Anemia secondary to chronic disease

- Chronic suppurative processes
- Radiation injury
- Poisoning by:
  - Ptaquiloside
  - Trichlorethylene-extracted soybean meal
  - Arsenic
  - Furazolidone
  - Phenylbutazone
- Sequel to inclusion body rhinitis of pigs
- Ostertagiasis, trichostrongylosis in calves and lambs
- Temporarily after moving to high altitude

Myelophthisic anemia

- Lymphosarcoma in calves
- Plasma cell myelomatosis in calves, pigs and horses
- Myelofibrosis in horses

Miscellaneous anemias

- Equine unspecified anemia

Clinical findings

All signs

- Except reduced physical performance, as in racing – limited to occurrence when anemia already severe
- Mucosal pallor
- Depression
- Anorexia
- Weakness, shuffling gait, tremor, terminal recumbency
- Tachycardia
- Large amplitude (bounding) pulse
- Marked increase in heart beat intensity; loud sounds, exaggerated apex beat
- Heart dilation
- Hemic systolic murmur, maximum at inspiration peak
- Deep sighing respiration short of dyspnea until late stages

Associated signs include edema, hemoglobinuria, jaundice.

Clinical pathology

- Hemoglobin level reduced; clinical signs at 50% reduction, below 20% incompatible with life
- Erythrocyte count, packed cell volume reduced
- Immature erythrocyte numbers increased in hemorrhagic, hemolytic anemia **except in horses**
- No evidence of erythrocyte regeneration in chronic disease anemia
- Hypoproteinemia in hemorrhagic anemia
- Serum and plasma discolored due to hemoglobin, and hemoglobinuria in hemolytic anemia
- Hypochromasia in nutritional deficiency of iron
- Bone marrow biopsy essential for diagnosis of myelophthisic anemia

Necropsy findings

- Tissue pallor
- Thin, watery blood
- Spleen contracted
- Additional lesions of a primary chronic or tissue-invasive disease in some cases

Diagnosis

Resembles:
- Hemorrhagic blood loss
- Hemorrhagic disease
- Shock
- Shortfall
- Performance
- Ill-thrift
- Poor racing performance

Treatment

- Blood transfusion in critical cases
- Treatment of specific cause, possibly verified by response trial
- Hematinic preparations, especially iron administered orally, supportively; organic iron parenterally for more prolonged effect
- Corticosteroids in autoimmune anemia

POLYCYTHEMIA [VM8 p. 370]

Etiology

♦ Familial polycythemia vera
♦ Inappropriate secondary polycythemia
♦ Inherited methemoglobinemia

Clinical findings

♦ Stunted growth
♦ Congested mucosae
♦ Dyspnea

Clinical pathology

Erythrocyte count, packed cell volume elevated.

LEUKEMIA [VM8 p. 387]

Etiology

♦ Enzootic bovine leukosis
♦ Myelogenous leukemia, rarely, in all species
♦ Erythroblastic, plasma cell, monocytic leukemias rarer still
♦ Chronic lymphocytic leukemia in horses
♦ Monomyelocytic leukemia in horses
♦ Eosinophilic myeloproliferative disease in horses
♦ Bovine leukocyte adhesion deficiency an example of a leukemia but the pathogenesis is of a leukopenia because of the defect in neutrophil function

Clinical findings

♦ Lymph node enlargement
♦ Splenomegaly
♦ Poor performance
♦ Dullness
♦ Weight loss

Additional signs of related lesions include:
♦ Ventral edema
♦ Predisposition to infection
♦ Mucosal pallor
♦ Hemic murmur
♦ Mucosal petechiation

Clinical pathology

♦ Leukocytosis, many immature cells
♦ Proliferative lesions in bone marrow biopsy

LEUKOPENIA [VM8 p. 387]

Etiology

♦ Virus diseases, e.g. hog cholera
♦ Some bacterial infections, e.g. early leptospirosis
♦ Acute local bacterial infections; leukocytes sequestered to site, e.g. peracute diffuse peritonitis
♦ In pancytopenias when all marrow functions depressed:
  • Ptaqiloside poisoning
  • Radiation injury
  • Furazolidone poisoning
  • Granulocytopenic disease
  • Mycotoxins e.g. *Stachybotrys* spp.
  • Chediak–Higashi syndrome
  • Toluene poisoning
  • Trichlorethylene extracted soybean meal poisoning

Clinical findings

♦ No specific signs
♦ Susceptible to infection

Clinical pathology

♦ Pancytopenia

THROMBOCYTE DISEASES [VM8 p. 372]

Includes:
♦ **Thrombocytopenia**, a quantitative deficiency in the number of platelets
♦ **Thrombopathy**, any qualitative or functional disorder of platelets, **including**
♦ **Thrombasthenia**, impaired ADP-induced platelet aggregation and defective clot retraction
Examples are:

Thrombocytopenia
♦ Deficient production caused by –
  • Toxemia
  • Megakaryocyte infections, e.g. by viruses of hog cholera, African swine fever, bovine virus diarrhea
  • Specific poisonings with ptaqiloside, the toxin of *Stachybotrys* spp., furazolidone, trichlorethylene extracted soybean meal, radiation injury
♦ Excessive withdrawal from circulation – consumption coagulopathy, e.g. as part

of disseminated intravascular coagulopathy

♦ Excessive destruction in:

• Maternal isoimmunization causing **thrombocytopenic purpura**, a rare, fatal disease of neonatal piglets, normal at birth but developing generalised hemorrhages, after sucking colostrum containing antiplatelet antibody. Affected sows should be culled

• Idiopathic **thrombocytopenia**, an immune-mediated thrombocytopenia in horses and cattle. Hemorrhages may be confined to a single system, e.g. respiratory or reproductive systems, or be generalized. Treatment includes blood transfusion, corticosteroids

• Other **immune-mediated thrombocytopenias** occur, e.g. in drug intoxications, infectious or neoplastic diseases. Prothrombin and partial thromboplastin times are normal and there is no disseminated intravascular coagulopathy

Thrombopathy and thrombasthenia
Non-thrombocytopenic purpuras, e.g.:
♦ Chediak–Higashi syndrome
♦ Inherited Simmental thrombopathia

DISEASES OF THE SPLEEN, LYMPHADENOPATHY AND THYMIC DISEASE

SPLENOMEGALY [VM8 p. 388]

Etiology

♦ Acute, fatal infectious diseases, e.g. anthrax, salmonellosis
♦ Acute hemolytic diseases, e.g. babesiosis, equine infectious anemia
♦ Sudden deaths, e.g. electrocution, barbiturate euthanasia
♦ Congestive heart failure
♦ Portal obstruction
♦ Tumor, e.g. hemangiosarcoma, lymphosarcoma, myelocytic leukemia, malignant melanoma in horses

Clinical findings

♦ Virtually symptomless
♦ Palpated accidentally on rectal examination in horses
♦ Displaced spleen, e.g. in left dorsal displacement of colon, may give impression of splenomegaly
♦ Bleeding from hemangiosarcoma may cause signs of anemia and hemoperitoneum
♦ Rupture of enlarged spleen may cause death due to hemorrhagic anemia

SPLENIC ABSCESS [VM8 p. 388]

Etiology

♦ Extension of infection from perforated stomach, reticulum
♦ Hematogenous spread by bacteremia or embolus, e.g. in strangles

Clinical findings

♦ Anorexia
♦ Fever
♦ Tachycardia
♦ Pain on palpation over spleen
♦ Inflammatory fluid on paracentesis
♦ Anemia, mucosal pallor
♦ Ventral edema as a late sign
♦ Enlarged spleen rarely palpable rectally
♦ If peritonitis concurrent additional signs of:
• Arched back
• Disinclination to move
• Mild, recurrent colic in horses

Clinical pathology

Marked leukocytosis, neutrophilia, left shift.

Treatment

♦ Broad-spectrum antibacterial treatment for at least 7 days, preferably longer; response good but relapse frequent; dubious value in severe cases in low-value animals
♦ Splenectomy an option if adhesions and peritonitis absent

LYMPHADENECTASIS (LYMPHADENOPATHY) [VM8 p. 388]

Etiology

♦ Lymphadenitis
♦ Neoplasms, primary of lymphoid tissue or secondary of many tumors

Clinical findings

- Visible, palpable enlargement
- Lymphatic obstruction, local edema
- Obstruction of surrounding tissues, e.g. mediastinal nodes compressing esophagus

LYMPHADENITIS [VM8 p. 389]

Etiology

- Caseous lymphadenitis
- Tuberculosis
- Actinobacillosis in cattle and sheep
- Ulcerative lymphangitis (*Corynebacterium pseudotuberculosis*) in horses and cattle
- Anthrax in pigs and horses
- Strangles
- Cervical adenitis (jowl abscess) in pigs
- Granulomatous cervical adenitis of pigs caused by *Rhodococcus equi*, atypical mycobacteria, *Mycobacterium bovis, M. tuberculosis, M. avium.* No illness but lesions resemble tuberculous adenitis at meat inspection
- Tularemia
- Melioidosis
- Tick pyemia
- Bovine malignant catarrh
- Bright green algal (*Prototheca* spp.) retropharyngeal adenitis in cattle
- *Pasteurella multocida* lymphadenitis in lambs
- Bovine farcy
- Atypical skin tuberculosis

Clinical findings

- Node enlarged
- May be painful, mostly not
- Obstruction to surrounding organs, e.g. pharyngeal choke
- Node biopsy allows identification of infection

ABSCENCE OF LYMPHOID TISSUE [VM8 p. 389]

Etiology

- Combined immunodeficiency of Arabian foals, calves; combined with lymphopenia
- Inherited lymph node aplasia of calves

LYMPHOPROLIFERATIVE AND THYMIC DISEASE [VM8 p. 389]

Etiology

Cattle

- Juvenile multicentric lymphosarcoma involving lymph nodes and bone marrow, at birth or early weeks of life
- Thymic lymphosarcoma, 3 months to 2 years, mostly thymus only, some lymph nodes in some cases
- Cutaneous lymphosarcoma; nodules at multiple skin sites; at 1–3 years old
- Adult multicentric lymphosarcoma (bovine viral leukosis)

Sheep

- Lymphosarcoma rare
- Lymphocytic leukemia recorded

Pigs

- Thymic lymphoma reported
- Lymphosarcoma seen at slaughter

Horses

- Any age
- Multicentric
- Common relative to other neoplasms

Clinical findings

- Chronic wasting
- Multiple lymphadenectasis, palpable, visible
- Dyspnea in some
- Anasarca
- Anemia
- Masses palpable per rectum in abdomen
- Signs of space-occupying lesion in chest:
  • Pectoral edema
  • Jugular engorgement
  • Absent jugular pulse
  • Heart murmur
  • Dysphagia
  • Dyspnea
- Signs of intestinal lymphosarcoma in horses:
- Weight loss
- Diarrhea in some
- Colic initially in some

Clinical pathology

- Leukemia infrequent
- Anemia common
- Thrombocytopenia in some
- Hypergammaglobulinemia in some
- Hypoalbuminemia in some
- Immunodeficiency in some
- Cytology of biopsy or needle aspirate often diagnostic

10 DISEASES OF THE RESPIRATORY SYSTEM

The principal clinical signs and clinicopathological findings on which clinical diagnoses of respiratory diseases are based include basic syndromes and individual clinical indicants. (Special examination techniques listed include bronchoalveolar lavage, endoscopic examination, nasal swabs, pharyngeal swabs, pleuroscopy, pulmonary function tests, radiographic examination, sputum cup, thoracocentesis, transtracheal (tracheobronchial) aspiration, ultrasonography.)

BASIC SYNDROMES

Anoxia–hypoxia [VM8 p. 391]

Clinical findings:
⧫ Hyperpnea, increased depth of respiratory movement
⧫ Increased heart rate
⧫ Increased pulse amplitude
⧫ Signs of cerebral anoxia
⧫ Signs of dysfunction in other body systems
⧫ Splenic contraction
⧫ Increased erythropoiesis in long-standing cases

Occurs in:
Any failure of tissues to receive adequate (hypoxia) or any (anoxia) oxygen as in:
⧫ Defective oxygenation of blood in the pulmonary circuit – **anoxic anoxia**, e.g. pulmonary edema, pneumonia, pulmonary emphysema
⧫ Deficiency of hemoglobin per unit volume of blood – **anemic anoxia**, e.g. anemia, methemoglobinemia
⧫ Deficient blood flow through capillaries – **stagnant anoxia**, e.g. congestive heart failure
⧫ Defective tissue oxidation systems cause failure of tissues to take up oxygen even though the blood is fully oxygenated – **histotoxic anoxia**, e.g. cyanide poisoning

Respiratory failure [VM8 p. 392]

The terminal stage of respiratory insufficiency; compensatory responses fail to maintain oxygen and carbon dioxide tensions in the blood at sustainable levels and the respiratory centre fails to function, respiration ceases. Failure may be:
⧫ **Asphyxial** – dyspnea, gasping, terminal apnea; occurs in:
  • Pneumonia
  • Pulmonary edema
  • Upper respiratory obstruction
⧫ **Paralytic** – respirations become shallower, then cease; occurs in:
  • Respiratory center depressant poisoning
  • Nervous shock
⧫ **Tachypneic** – rapid shallow respirations due to hypocapnia. Occurs in:
  • Hyperthermia
  • Mechanical overventilation

CLINICAL INDICANTS

Abdominal respiration

Clinical findings:
Inspiration and expiration accomplished mainly by movements of abdominal muscles, diaphragm.

Occurs in:
♦ Pleurisy
♦ Intercostal muscle paralysis, e.g. tick paralysis

Breath sounds abnormal

See also respiratory sounds.
♦ Auscultation necessary over larynx, trachea, tracheal bifurcation, bronchi, upper and lower lungs both sides
♦ Characteristics of absent sounds, abnormal sounds and their significance in Table 10.1

Bronchoalveolar lavage

♦ Gives best evaluation of pathogens and cytology in lung tissue of part of lung examined, e.g. pneumonia, pulmonary neoplasm
♦ But no information provided about other lobes of lung; false negatives common; best examination of entire lungs is tracheobronchial aspiration
♦ No information provided about interstitial tissue, fluid

Coughing

♦ Indicates inflammation of respiratory mucosa due to laryngitis, tracheitis, bronchitis, bronchopneumonia, lung abscess
♦ **Simple, short cough** indicates mild inflammation
♦ **Paroxysmal cough** indicates chronic, persistent inflammation and irritation
♦ **Suppressed cough** indicates pain of acute laryngitis, bronchitis or pleurisy
♦ **Loud, explosive cough** indicates painlessness but extensive inflammation
♦ **Productive cough** (expulsion of mucus, debris from nostrils, mouth) indicates exudative lesion
♦ **Dry cough** indicates non-exudative lesion

Cyanosis

Clinical findings:
♦ Blue discoloration mucosa, skin, conjunctivae caused by increase in reduced hemoglobin in blood
♦ Can occur only if blood concentration of hemoglobin normal

Occurs in:
♦ Only in anoxic, stagnant anoxia, not histotoxic or anemic anoxia
♦ Polycythemia predisposes
♦ Most marked in congenital cardiac defects, severe laryngeal obstruction not in pulmonary disease

Dyspnea

Clinical findings:
Laboured, distressing respiration at rest. Signs include:
♦ Head extended
♦ Deep, labored breaths
♦ Breathing rate increased
♦ Nostrils flared
♦ Mouth-breathing in some

Occurs in:
♦ **Respiratory disease**
  • Pneumonia, pulmonary edema; due to filled alveoli
  • Pleural effusion, hydrothorax, hemothorax, pneumothorax, emphysema, diaphragmatic hernia; due to compressed alveoli
  • Nasal, pharyngeal, laryngeal, tracheal, bronchial obstruction by foreign body, collapse, exudate – due to blocked air passages
♦ **Cardiovascular disease**
  • Congestive or acute heart failure
  • Shock, dehydration causing peripheral circulatory failure
  • Polycythemia vera, disseminated intravascular coagulopathy, causing increased circulating blood viscosity
♦ **Hemopoietic disease**
  • Anemia (hyperpnea only)
  • Methemoglobinemia
  • Carboxyhemoglobinemia
♦ **Systemic states**
  • Pain
  • Hyperthermia
  • Acidosis
♦ **Environmental circumstances**

- Oxygen lack in altitude disease, exposure to fire and smoke, toxic gas
- Poisons
  - Metaldehyde, dinitrophenols
  - Organophosphatic compounds, carbamates
  - Urea
  - Poisonous plants – *Albizia*, *Erythrophleum*, *Eupatorium*, *Helenium*, *Ipomoea*, *Laburnum*, *Taxus* spp.

Elbows abducted

Occurs in Pleurisy.

Endoscopic examination

Flexible fiberoptic endoscope gives best view of lesions in pharynx, larynx, trachea in horses and cattle.

Epistaxis

Clinical findings:
Bleeding from the nose; does not include:
- Serosanguineous exudate, e.g. in equine infectious anemia
- Blood-stained froth, as in pulmonary edema

Occurs in:
- Equine exercise-induced pulmonary hemorrhage
- Caudal vena caval thrombosis
- Lung abscess
- Any hemorrhagic disease

Exercise tolerance reduced

Subjective estimates made on basis of severity of dyspnea, rapidity of return to normal after exercise. No objective tests documented. Some data available on effects of endurance rides in horses.

Head extended

See dyspnea, this section.

Hypercapnia and hypocapnia

- Hypercapnia, excessive retention of CO_2, due to respiratory insufficiency stimulates respiratory effort and contributes to respiratory acidosis
- Hypocapnia, due to hyperventilation with a mechanical ventilator, or as a response to hypoxia in lower respiratory tract disease, can contribute to **respiratory acidosis**

Hyperpnea

Increased respiratory depth, a principal response to hypoxia, preliminary to dyspnea, and not clinically differentiated from it.

Nasal breath foul (ozena)

Occurs in:
- Necrotic tissue in tract, e.g. guttural pouch infection
- Gangrenous pneumonia
- Aspiration pneumonia

Nasal breath reduced

Clinical findings:
- Volume reduced from one nostril compared with other
- Tested by palm of hand or suspended thread
- Usually nasal stridor

Occurs in Nasal obstruction.

Nasal discharge

Clinical findings:
- Cattle often lick most of it away
- **Copious, bilateral, serous** – early rhinitis
- **Copious, bilateral, mucoid** – rhinitis several days old
- **Copious, bilateral, purulent** – severe inflammation upper (rhinitis) or lower respiratory tract (bronchitis)
- **Copious, bilateral, caseous** – allergic or bacterial rhinitis
- **Bilateral discharge containing feed particles** – cleft palate, aspiration pneumonia, dysphagia or other cause of regurgitation, vomiting
- **Unilateral, necrotic discharge** – involvement of one nasal cavity
- **Bilateral** discharge indicates both nasal cavities involved or lesion caudal to nasal system

Nasal foreign body

Clinical findings:
- Respiratory stertor
- Dyspnea
- Purulent nasal discharge
- Reduced nasal air flow
- Related often to nasal irritation, muzzle rubbing

Table 10.1 Identification and clinical significance of respiratory sounds [VM8 p. 396]

Sounds	Identifying characteristics	Significance
Increased loudness of breath sounds	Mild to moderate increase in loudness of breath sounds audible on inspiration and expiration	Occurs in fevers, after exercise, high environmental temperatures, early pneumonia
Decreased loudness of breath sounds	Decreased loudness of breath sounds	Obese animal, cold ambient temperature
Loud breath sounds	Marked increase in loudness of breath sounds, begin and end abruptly, on inspiration and expiration	Any disease resulting in collapse or filling of alveoli and leaving bronchial lumen open; consolidation and atelectasis; heard commonly in cattle with severe pneumonia and calves with enzootic pneumonia where there is consolidation of the cranial lobes of the lungs
Crackles	Discontinuous, bubbling, sizzling, moist sounds primarily on inspiration; may be characterized as coarse or fine crackles	Suggests the presence of secretions and exudate in airways and edematous bronchial mucosa as in exudative bronchopneumonia, exudative tracheobronchitis, aspiration pneumonia
Loud crackling sounds	Harsh crackling sounds on inspiration and expiration	Interstitial pulmonary emphysema in cattle
Wheezes	Continuous musical-type squeaking and whistling, occur primarily on expiration although they are frequently heard during both inspiration and expiration	Indicates narrowing of airways; expiratory polyphonic wheezing common in animals with chronic obstructive pulmonary disease, chronic bronchopneumonia, any species; inspiratory monophonic wheezing occurs when upper extrathoracic airways are constricted, such as in laryngeal disease

Pleuritic friction rubs	'Sandpapery' sound; dry, grating sounds close to the surface, on inspiration and expiration, tend to be jerky and not influenced by coughing	Pleuritis, diffuse pulmonary emphysema in cattle with dry pleural surfaces; diminish or disappear with pleural effusion
Absence of lung sounds (silent lung)	Lung sounds not audible	Bronchial lumen filled with exudate, space-occupying mass, pleural effusion, diaphragmatic hernia, pneumothorax (dorsal aspects of thorax)
Peristaltic sounds	Intermittent intestinal sounds	Normal in cattle thoraces after eating. Does not indicate diaphragmatic hernia unless other signs present
Expiratory grunting and/or groaning	Loud grunting on expiration which is usually forced against a closed glottis with sudden release, audible on auscultation of the thorax, over the trachea and often audible without the aid of a stethoscope	Severe diffuse pulmonary emphysema, extensive consolidation; in acute pleurisy and peritonitis a groan is more characteristic
Laryngeal stertor (stridor)	Loud stenotic sounds on incpiration audible with or without stethoscope over the trachea	Obstruction of larynx (due to edema, laryngitis, paralysis of vocal cord); prime example is calf diphtheria

157

Occurs in:
♦ Nasal obstruction
♦ Enzootic nasal granuloma
♦ Rhinosporidiosis

Nasal mucosal congestion

Clinical findings Reactive hyperemia, an essential part of respiratory mucosal inflammation.

Occurs in:
♦ Rhinitis
♦ Rhinotracheitis
♦ Upper respiratory tract infections generally

Nasal mucosal erosions, ulcers, necrosis

Clinical findings:
♦ Nasal discharge, purulent, blood-stained
♦ Respiratory stertor

Occurs in:
♦ Bovine malignant catarrh
♦ Bovine virus diarrhea
♦ Rinderpest
♦ Peste des petits ruminantes
♦ Bluetongue
♦ Infectious bovine rhinotracheitis

Nasal polyp

Clinical findings:
♦ Intermittent nasal obstruction
♦ Usually unilateral
♦ Respiratory stertor
♦ Reduced nasal air flow
♦ Dyspnea
♦ Bilaterally causes asphyxia

Occurs in Nasal obstruction.

Nasal swabs

♦ Culture of limited value because of mixed flora in normal animals
♦ Best indicator of nasal cavity pathogen, e.g. infectious bovine rhinotracheitis
♦ Cytological examination may indicate neoplasm or allergic state
♦ Best results with nasal wash to ensure adequate volume of liquid and avoid loss of viruses due to drying

Nostril dilation

Occurs in:
♦ Part of **dyspnea** syndrome (above)
♦ Tetanus

Peristaltic sounds in chest

See Table 10.1.

Pharyngeal swabs

♦ Culture represents microbial population upper respiratory tract
♦ Swab is sheathed for passage through nasal cavity, exposed and resheathed in pharynx
♦ Unless used immediately swab immersed in transport fluid
♦ Vacuum-aspirated fluids provide more volume
♦ More accurate results with transtracheal aspirates, tracheal lavage, bronchoalveolar lavage

Pleuroscopy

Pleural lesions viewable via rigid endoscope.

Pulmonary function tests

♦ Aim to detect early pulmonary inefficiency
♦ Tests include:
  • Arterial pO_2 before and after hard exercise
  • Respiratory exchanges during exercise on treadmill
  • A forced oscillation technique used in cattle

Radiographic and ultrasonographic abnormality

♦ X-rays give excellent results in imaging pulmonary lesions in foals and calves
♦ Ultrasonography valuable in identification pleural fluid, bullous emphysema, lung consolidation, abscess, neoplasm

Respiratory movements, double

Occurs in Pulmonary emphysema.

Respiratory noises, laryngopharyngeal

Snoring (stertor) Indicates chronic inflammation of pharyngeal mucosa causing vibration with each breath.

Stridor Inspiratory stenotic sound caused by reduction in laryngeal lumen.

Expiratory grunt Common in diffuse pulmonary disease.

Painful grunt In painful disease of chest, e.g. pleurisy; unassociated with inspiration, expiration.

Roaring Air passing through narrowed larynx, e.g. laryngeal hemiplegia.

Snuffling, bubbling sounds Most audible on inspiration indicate exudate accumulation.

Respiratory noises, nasal

Sneezing Indicates rhinitis, nasal obstruction.

Wheezing (high-pitched sound of air coming through a narrowed orifice) indicates stenosis or chronic rhinitis.

Sputum cup

♦ Old-fashioned small spoon on long handle passed orally, via mouth gag to pharyngeal area exposed to view by pulling tongue. Fluid, mucus scraped up with spoon

Thoracocentesis

♦ Pleural fluid may be inflammatory, have neoplastic cytology
♦ Introduction of needle low down in 6–7 interspace risks penetration pericardial sac

Thoracic pain

Spontaneous pain causes expiratory grunt occurs in:
♦ Fractured rib
♦ Torn intercostal muscle
♦ Subpleural hematoma
♦ Pleurisy
♦ Pain on chest percussion occurs in the same conditions, but of less severe degree, as for expiratory grunt

Tracheal sounds

See breath sounds, this section.

Transtracheal (tracheobronchial) aspirates

♦ Polyethylene tube passed through tracheal incision to tracheal bifurcation and into bronchus; normal saline introduced and aspirated
♦ Also obtained via fibreoptic endoscope
♦ Gives best result for examination of entire lung field
♦ Culture gives most representative result of upper tract
♦ Cytological examination may indicate neoplasm or allergic state:
  • Many neutrophils, much mucus in suppurative pneumonia, bronchiolitis
  • Eosinophils suggest allergy , parasitic invasion
  • Hemosiderin-packed macrophages suggest hemorrhage
♦ Pathogenic microorganisms in many clinically normal animals
♦ Poor correlation between findings and necropsy lesions

DISEASES OF THE LUNGS

PULMONARY CONGESTION AND EDEMA [VM8 p. 404]

Etiology

Primary congestion
♦ Early pneumonia
♦ Smoke, fumes inhalation
♦ Anaphylaxis
♦ Hypostasis in recumbent patients

Secondary congestion
♦ Congestive heart failure
♦ Severe overexertion, horses

Pulmonary edema
♦ Sequel to congestion in:
  • Acute anaphylaxis
  • Acute interstitial pneumonia
  • Congestive heart failure
  • Acute heart failure
  • Smoke, fumes inhalation
♦ Specific diseases including:
  • Mulberry heart disease
  • African horse sickness
  • Organophosphatic compound poisoning
  • alpha-naphthyl   thiourea   (ANTU) poisoning

- Plants, *Hymenoxis, Sphenosciadium* spp.
- Barker–wanderer syndrome foals
- Barker syndrome in pigs
- In **acute lung injury** where increased pulmonary microvascular permeability results from non-pulmonary sepsis (in humans is adult respiratory distress syndrome). In farm animals occurs mostly in systemic sepsis as in peracute coliform mastitis in cows, experimental septic peritonitis in sheep

Clinical findings

- Dyspnea, often extreme with head extended, mouth breathing, heaving respiratory movements
- Posture of fore limbs spread, elbows abducted, head lowered
- Respiratory rate fast
- Hyperthermia in most
- Tachycardia
- Mucosa congested early, cyanotic later
- Abnormal breath sounds:
  - In congestion hard sounds, no crackles
  - Early edema, increased sounds, crackles
  - Long-standing edema crackles, wheezes in dorsal lungs
- Percussion sounds dull in edema
- Cough softer, moist, painless
- Nasal discharge moderate serous early, in severe edema voluminous, frothy, sometimes blood-stained

Clinical pathology

- Used to differentiate causes
- Complete hematological examination, bacterial culture of exudate are standard, eosinophilia an important criterion

Necropsy findings

- **Acute congestion** – lungs dark red, excessive blood exudes from cut surface; microscopically visible engorged capillaries
- **Edema** – lungs pale, swollen, inelastic, pit on pressure, excess serous fluid from cut surface; microscopically fluid in alveoli, parenchyma

Diagnosis

Resembles:
- Pneumonia
- Pulmonary hemorrhage
- Acute bovine pulmonary emphysema and edema

Treatment

- Correct primary cause
- **Anaphylaxis** – ephedrine, followed by corticosteroids. Antihistamines much used but usefulness debated. Sodium meclofenamate probably beneficial
- **Edema, congestion** – oxygen therapy; aminophylline by slow intravenous injection to dilate bronchioles; furosemide to extract tissue fluid; corticosteroids in large doses to reduce capillary permeability; inhalation nebulized 20% ethanol to reduce foaming

PULMONARY HYPERTENSION
[VM8 p. 406]

Etiology

Excessive pulmonary arterial blood pressure, due usually to structural changes in pulmonary vasculature in:
- Altitude disease
- Phytotoxins in *Crotalaria* spp.
- Alveolar hypoxia, eliciting potent pulmonary constrictive response

Clinical findings

Right-side congestive heart failure syndrome.

ATELECTASIS [VM8 p. 407]

Etiology

Extensive alveolar collapse due to:
- Failure of lung to inflate in neonates
- Compression of lung
- Acute airway construction, e.g. horses in flotation tanks unable to lower heads, fluid accumulates

Clinical findings

- Dyspnea
- Cyanosis
- Lung sounds over atelectatic area decreased or absent, loud over rest of lung
- Reversible if obstruction, compression relieved
- Weakness, staggery gait, tremor, recumbency

PULMONARY HEMORRHAGE
[VM8 p. 407]

Etiology

Hemorrhage into parenchyma and airways due to:

- **Horses** – following exercise; due to rupture of vessels adjacent to diseased parts of lung
- **Cattle** – spontaneous rupture vessels adjacent to embolic pneumonia lesions in cases of caudal vena caval syndrome

Clinical findings

Horse

Exercise-induced hemorrhage very common but clinical epistaxis in few:
- Blood from nostrils, especially if head lowered
- Many swallow blood, make frequent swallowing movements but no blood evident
- Rarely profuse epistaxis, sudden death during race
- Epistaxis causes disqualification from racing because of risk to other participants
- Fiberoptoscopic examination of trachea after hard exercise best test for pulmonary hemorrhage

Cattle

Cow at rest, usually bleed profusely from the nostrils and dies within the hour:
- Dyspnea
- Continuous swallowing
- Mucosal pallor
- Tremor, staggering gait, recumbency
- May be repeated minor attacks

Treatment

- Not very effective
- Furosemide alleviates severity in horses

PULMONARY EMPHYSEMA [VM8 p. 408]

Etiology

Lung distension due to alveolar overdistension, wall rupture, with interstitial emphysema resulting. Always secondary to other pulmonary disease. Occurs in:

Cattle

- Acute bovine pulmonary emphysema and edema
- Parasitic pneumonia
- Anaphylaxis
- Traumatic reticuloperitonitis with lung laceration
- Lung abscess
- Poisoning by *Senecio* spp., *Zieria arborescens*, *Perilla frutescens*, *Periconia* spp., rape

Horses

- Bronchiolitis in mature horses due to inhalation moldy, dusty feed
- Bronchiolitis in young horses due to respiratory viral infection

All species

- Secondary to bronchopneumonia
- Fumes inhalation, e.g. chlorine gas, welding fumes
- Local around pneumonic lesions, e.g. aspiration pneumonia pigs; mostly nonpathogenic

Clinical findings

- Severe expiratory dyspnea with grunting
- Loud crackling sounds on auscultation
- In cattle subcutaneous emphysema
- In horse chronic obstructive pulmonary syndrome

Clinical pathology

- Compensatory polycythemia
- Increased alkali reserve
- With associated bronchopneumonia leukocytosis with left shift
- Check for lungworm larvae in feces
- Eosinophils in nasal swabs or washings, eosinophilia in allergic disease
- Precipitins against *Micropolyspora faeni* in some horses

Necropsy findings

- Lungs pale, distended, show rib imprints
- Interstitial emphysema marked by air in interalveolar septa, under pleura to mediastinum, subcutaneous tissues
- Bronchiolitis in most cases; some with associated bronchopneumonia

Diagnosis

Resembles:
- Pulmonary congestion and edema; all three commonly occur together
- Pneumonia, especially parasitic in young animals
- pneumothorax
- Spontaneous acute transient pulmonary emphysema in horses at pasture probably an allergy. Responds to antihistamines followed by corticosteroids

Treatment

- Most cases recover spontaneously provided the primary lesion relieved
- Oxygen necessary for life-threatening phase in valuable animals
- Antihistamines, atropine, corticosteroids all used enthusiastically and empirically

PNEUMONIA [VM8 p. 410]

Etiology

Cattle

- Pneumonic pasteurellosis (*Pasteurella* spp. with or without parainfluenza-3 virus)
- *Haemophilus somnus*
- Calf enzootic pneumonia
- Bovine respiratory syncytial virus
- Contagious bovine pleuropneumonia
- Bovine interstitial pneumonia
- *Ascaris suum* larvae massive infestation
- *Dictyocaulus viviparus*
- *Klebsiella* spp.
- *Mycobacterium bovis*
- *Fusobacterium necrophorum* in calf diphtheria

Pigs

- Enzootic pneumonia
- Pneumonic pasteurellosis
- Pleuropneumonia
- Septicemic salmonellosis
- *Bordetella bronchiseptica*
- Lungworm pneumonia
- Pulmonary anthrax

Horses

- Pleuropneumonia due to β-streptococci, *Pasteurella* spp., *Escherichia coli*, *Enterobacter*, *Bacteroides*, *Clostridium* spp.
- Foal septicemia due to *Streptococcus* spp., *Escherichia coli*, *Actinobacillus equuli*
- Combined immunodeficiency with adenovirus, *Pneumocystis carinii*
- *Rhodococcus equi*
- Equine herpesvirus-1
- Equine influenza virus 1A/E2
- Idiopathic bronchointerstitial pneumonia of foals
- *Dictyocaulus arnfieldi*, *Parascaris equorum*, rarely
- Strangles
- Glanders
- Epizootic lymphangitis

Sheep

- Pneumonic pasteurellosis
- *Streptococcus zooepidemicus*, *Salmonella abortus-ovis* in neonatal lambs

- Kageda due to *Mycoplasma* spp.
- *Corynebacterium pseudotuberculosis* rarely
- Melioidosis
- *Dictyocaulus filaria*
- Maedi
- Jaagsiekte
- Post-dipping aspiration pneumonia

Goats

- *Mycoplasma* spp. pleuropneumonia
- Chronic interstitial pneumonia *Mycoplasma mycoides* var. *mycoides*
- Retrovirus

All species

- Toxoplasmosis
- Systemic mycoses
- Aspiration pneumonia
- Sporadic secondary pneumonia due to *Streptococcus, Corynebacterium, Dermatophilus* spp.
- Interstitial pneumonia, pulmonary consolidation, fibrosis due to phytotoxins in *Eupatorium glandulosum, Zieria arborescens, Astragalus* spp.

Clinical findings

Basic syndrome

- Rapid shallow respiration early
- Dyspneic later
- Fever
- Cough
- Gurgles or moist crackles of exudate in air passages, cleared by coughing
- May be pleuritic friction rub, muffled breath sounds later if pleurisy develops
- Cyanosis rarely
- Nasal discharge in some
- Nasal breath rotten with much discharge, putrid with anaerobic infection

Additional signs with acute bacterial pneumonia

- Toxemia syndrome of:
  - Anorexia
  - Depression
  - Tachycardia
- Reluctance to lie down
- Severe dyspnea with expiratory grunt
- Moist cough
- Good response to standard systemic antibacterial treatment, but relapse due to reinfection or recurrence from abscess

Additional signs with chronic bacterial pneumonia

- Weight loss
- Rough hair coat

- Moderate fever
- Moderate tachycardia
- Moderately rapid respiration
- Respiration deeper than normal
- Expiratory grunt and open-mouthed breathing in advanced cases
- Copious bilateral mucopurulent nasal discharge
- Moist productive cough
- Loud breath sounds over ventral lungs, crackles and wheezes over entire lungs

Additional signs with viral pneumonias

- *Not* toxemic *but* are anorexic, febrile
- No response to antibacterial therapy
- Dry, harsh cough
- Loud, dry breath sounds
- Dyspnea can be severe
- Some deaths within a few days

Acute interstitial pneumonia of cattle

- Acute bovine emphysema and edema syndrome

Pleuropneumonia of horses

- Commonly a history of long distance travel
- Dyspnea, fever
- Inappetence
- Lethargy
- Cough
- Purulent nasal discharge
- Thoracic pain on percussion
- Malodorous breath in some
- Tachycardia
- Jugular vein engorgement
- Caudal displacement of heart sounds
- Pointing of fore limb

Clinical pathology

- Tracheobronchial lavage most reliable source for microbiological, cytological examination
- Culture and cytology of thoracocentesis aspirate recommended if pleurisy suspected
- Acute and convalescent sera for immunological examination in suspected viral pneumonia
- Herd serological sampling advised for accurate serotype identification
- Fresh fecal samples when lungworm suspected
- Hematology may be normal in viral pneumonia, leukocytosis with left shift in bacterial infection

- Thoracocentesis, ultrasonography, radiography, pleuroscopy all relevant diagnostic procedures especially in equine pleuropneumonia

Necropsy findings

- Lesions concentrated in anterior and ventral lobes
- **Bronchopneumonia** has serofibrinous or purulent exudate in bronchioles, congestion or hepatization of parenchyma
- Fibrinous pleurisy between lobe in some
- Chronic cases consolidation, fibrosis, emphysema, bronchi filled with purulent exudate, bronchiectasis, abscessation
- **Interstitial pneumonia** bronchioles clear of exudate, affected lung sunken, dark red,

Diagnosis

Resembles:
- Congestive heart failure
- Histotoxic anoxia due to cyanide poisoning
- Anemic anoxia due to nitrate–nitrite poisoning
- Hyperthermia
- Acidosis
- Pulmonary congestion and edema
- Caudal vena caval syndrome
- Pulmonary emphysema
- Pleurisy
- Pneumothorax
- Pulmonary consolidation, fibrosis caused by *Eupatorium glandulosum*, *Zieria arborescens*, *Astragalus* spp., plant poisonings tracheitis

Common errors are:
- Failure to detect abnormal lung sounds
- Failure to consider other causes of dyspnea

Treatment

Bacterial pneumonia

- Rapid recovery (24 hours) in early cases with broad-spectrum antibacterial or combination
- Late or severe cases take 3–5 days; adequate doses of long-acting preparations eliminate daily treatments
- Chronic cases likely to relapse
- In anaerobic bacterial pneumonia in horses antibacterial regimen may be supplemented with metronidazole (15 mg/kg orally every 6 hours, *or* 20 mg/kg of a 40% solution I/M daily for several days)

Viral and mycoplasmal pneumonias

No effective treatment but broad-spectrum antibacterial regimen usual because of risk of secondary bacterial infection.

Supplementary treatments

♦ Corticosteroids, bronchodilators, respiratory stimulants widely used but efficacy debated
♦ Oxygen therapy valuable in critical phase especially in foals
♦ Fluid therapy used with caution to avoid overloading compromised vascular system and precipitate pulmonary edema or acute heart failure

Herd outbreaks

Alternative procedures include:

♦ Treat clinical cases, maintain close surveillance, treat new cases
♦ Treat clinical cases, single injection of long-acting antibacterial to remainder
♦ Mass medication in drinking water or feed

ASPIRATION PNEUMONIA [VM8 p. 416]

Etiology

♦ Careless drenching, drenching of recumbent or lethargic patient
♦ Passage of stomach tube into trachea
♦ Feeding, especially pigs and calves, in inadequate troughing; animals struggle to get some feed
♦ Rough handling during plunge dipping, animals too crowded, head held under for too long
♦ Vomiting, regurgitation in horses and ruminants, especially in milk fever cows, during passage of stomach tube:
  • Rupture of pharyngeal abscess during manipulation
  • During swallowing attempts in patients with esophageal paralysis or obstruction
  • In crude oil poisoning

Clinical findings

♦ Profound toxemia
♦ Dyspnea
♦ Cough
♦ Gurgles, crackles, friction rub on auscultation anterior and ventral lung lobes, often over very small area

♦ Friction rub
♦ Respiration painful
♦ Breath putrid in most
♦ Most patients die; survivors have chronic lung abscess

Clinical pathology

♦ May be marked leukocytosis, left shift but severe cases may be leukopenic
♦ Infection likely to be mixed but culture of aspirate or lavage sample may be advantageous

Necropsy findings

Necrotic or gangrenous pneumonia of anteroventral parts of lung, sometimes on only one side; acute fibrinous pleurisy.

Diagnosis

Resembles:

♦ Pneumonia
♦ Caudal vena caval thrombosis
♦ Pulmonary emphysema
♦ Pulmonary congestion, edema
♦ Pulmonary hypertension
♦ Pulmonary hemorrhage
♦ Pleurisy
♦ Hydrothorax
♦ Pneumothorax

Treatment

♦ Intensive broad-spectrum antibiotic regimen but prognosis very poor
♦ Animals known to have aspirated material should receive immediate intensive treatment with broad-spectrum antibiotic for 5–7 days

CAUDAL VENA CAVAL THROMBOSIS [VM8 p. 416]

Includes embolic pneumonia, cranial vena caval thrombosis.

Etiology

Occurs in heavily grain-fed cattle in the UK and Europe.

Clinical findings

♦ May be found dead with blood from nostrils
♦ Usually history of respiratory disease for some weeks

- Dyspnea, grunting with each breath
- Cough
- Bouts of epistaxis, hemoptysis
- Mucosal pallor
- Hemic murmur
- Pain on thoracic percussion
- Lung sounds normal at first, then wide-spread crackles, wheezes
- Anorexia
- Ruminal stasis
- Liver enlargement, ascites, melena in some
- Scant feces
- Course 2–18 days
- Death due to hemorrhagic anemia, acute or subacute

Clinical pathology

- Radiographic evidence of increased lung density, markings
- Ultrasonographic evidence of changes in vena cava
- Neutrophilia with left shift
- Hypergammaglobulinemia

Necropsy findings

- Large, pale thrombus in vena cava between liver and right atrium
- Liver enlarged, ascites
- Liver abscesses especially close to vena cava
- Multiple lung abscesses; streptococci, staphylococci, *Escherichia coli*, *Fusobacterium necrophorum*
- Suppurative pneumonia
- Erosion of wall of pulmonary artery
- Intrapulmonary hemorrhage
- Lung emphysema, edema
- Sudden death patients have clotted blood in bronchi and trachea

Diagnosis

Resembles:
- Verminous pneumonia
- Chronic aspiration pneumonia
- Pulmonary endoarteritis due to endocarditis
- Chronic atypical interstitial pneumonia

Treatment

- No effective treatment
- Early recognition may enable patient to be salvaged

CRANIAL VENA CAVAL THROMBOSIS [VM8 p. 417]

Etiology

- Occurs in cattle, possibly originating from umbilical infection
- Thrombus in vena cava, multiple lung abscesses but no pulmonary hypertension

Clinical findings

- Cough
- Hyperpnea
- Poor exercise tolerance
- Jugular vein dilation
- Intermandibular, brisket edema

PULMONARY ABSCESS [VM8 p. 418]

Etiology

Primary
- Tuberculosis
- Actinomycosis
- Coccidioidomycosis, aspergillosis, histoplasmosis, cryptococcosis, moniliasis
- Strangles
- Caseous lymphadenitis
- *Rhodococcus equi*

Secondary
- Sequestration of a pneumonia focus, e.g. contagious bovine pleuropneumonia
- Emboli from endocarditis, metritis, mastitis, omphalophlebitis, caudal vena caval thrombosis
- Residual abscess after aspiration pneumonia
- Penetration by foreign body in traumatic reticuloperitonitis

Clinical findings

Single, large abscess
- Dullness, decline in appetite, weight, milk yield
- Fluctuating, mild fever
- Severe, short, harsh cough
- Bouts of bilateral epistaxis, hemoptysis
- May terminate with fatal pulmonary hemorrhage
- Breath sounds often normal; crackles around a local area of dullness in a few

Miliary abscesses

♦ Severe dyspnea
♦ Putrid, purulent nasal discharge if concurrent bronchopneumonia

Termination

♦ Euthanasia because of chronic ill-health
♦ Some deaths due to bronchopneumonia or emphysema
♦ Rarely hypertrophic pulmonary osteoarthropathy

Clinical pathology

♦ Leukocytosis and left shift in some but leukon often normal because lesion encapsulated
♦ Culture of swab, aspirate, lavage material from various levels may indicate nature of infection
♦ Radiographic or ultrasonographic examination may indicate location and size of abscess

Necropsy findings

♦ Large abscesses mostly in anterior, ventral lobes
♦ Pus at varying levels of inspissation, surrounded by:
  • Thick-walled fibrous capsule
  • Zone of bronchopneumonia
  • Pressure atelectasis or emphysema
  • Local emphysema
  • May obliterate the lung
  • Miliary abscesses through lungs

Diagnosis

Resembles:
♦ Other internal abscess, e.g. liver, spleen
♦ Focal parasitic lesions, e.g. hydatid cyst
♦ Pulmonary neoplasm

Treatment

Long-term broad-spectrum antibacterial treatment best but rarely effective.

PULMONARY NEOPLASMS [VM8 p. 419]

Etiology

♦ Pulmonary carcinoma, adenocarcinoma rare in cattle
♦ Squamous cell type papillomas recorded in goats
♦ Granular-cell myoblastomas in horses
♦ Malignant melanomas in young cattle and old horses may metastasize to lungs
♦ Thymomas, as part of lymphosarcoma in cattle, resembles pulmonary tumor
♦ Many single specimens of tumors recorded; most are asymptomatic

Clinical findings

Signs in basic syndrome include:
♦ Weight loss, appetite declines
♦ Increasing dyspnea
♦ Dry, harsh cough
♦ Areas of dullness on percussion, absence of sounds on auscultation

Additional signs include:
♦ Tachycardia
♦ Hemic systolic murmur
♦ Pleural effusion with muffling of heart and lung sounds
♦ Backward displacement of heart
♦ Hydropericardium
♦ Jugular vein engorgement
♦ Ventral edema
♦ Edema of limbs
♦ Dysphagia
♦ Chronic bloat in cattle
♦ Radiographic or ultrasonic demonstration of tumors

Necropsy findings

Tumor masses in parenchyma, lymph nodes, mediastinum, pleura

DISEASES OF THE PLEURA AND DIAPHRAGM

HYDROTHORAX AND HEMOTHORAX [VM8 p. 419]

Etiology

Hydrothorax occurs in:
♦ Congestive heart failure
♦ Hypoproteinemia
♦ African horse sickness
♦ Bovine viral leukosis

Chylothorax occurs in:
♦ Rupture of thoracic duct (very rare)

Hemothorax occurs in:
♦ Trauma to chest wall

- Pleural hemangiosarcoma
- Dicoumarol derivative poisoning

Clinical findings

- Dyspnea
- Absence of breath sounds, dullness over ventral lungs; bilateral in horses, may be unilateral in other species
- Intercostal spaces bulge in thin patients
- Jugular vein engorgement, increased jugular pulse in some

Clinical pathology

- Sterile blood or clear serous fluid on thoracocentesis
- Low hematocrit and hemoglobin level in hemothorax

Necropsy findings

- Thorax contains unclotted blood or serous transudate
- Other hemorrhages in anticoagulant poisoning
- Injury to thorax wall in some
- In hydrothorax other edema accumulations, congestive heart failure lesions in some

Diagnosis

Resembles:
- Pleurisy
- Pleural implants of neoplasms
- Space-occupying lesions of thorax, e.g. bovine viral leukosis

Treatment

- Treat primary condition
- Drain fluid from chest
- Blood transfusion, parenteral coagulants in severe hemothorax

PNEUMOTHORAX [VM8 p. 420]

Etiology

- Spontaneous lung rupture, e.g. during coughing in an emphysematous lung
- Injury to chest wall, rib fracture
- Surgical opening of chest

Clinical findings

- Acute onset of dyspnea
- Death within a few minutes in horses
- One side of rib cage immobilized in unilateral pneumothorax
- Also compensatory extra movement in unaffected side
- Breath sounds absent on affected side
- Displacement heart sounds, apex beat
- Hyperresonance on percussion affected side

Clinical pathology

Radiographic or ultrasound examination may be practicable.

Necropsy findings

- Collapsed lung on affected side(s)
- Pre-existing bullous emphysema in spontaneous cases
- Hemothorax, pleurisy present also in some trauma cases

Diagnosis

Resembles:
- Diaphragmatic hernia
- Hydrothorax, hemothorax

Treatment

- Patient must be kept still and quiet
- Surgically close chest wound
- Prophylactic antibiotic therapy in trauma cases
- Simple pneumothorax recovers spontaneously
- Tension pneumothorax should be relieved by thoracocentesis

DIAPHRAGMATIC HERNIA [VM8 p. 421]

All forms rare in large animals.

Congenital diaphragmatic hernia
- Diaphragm rudimentary or large defect in dorsal part with liver, stomach and intestine in thoracic cavity
- In some pericardial sac also incomplete
- Severe dyspnea at birth
- Survive usually only few hours, some several weeks
- Surgical repair has been effected

Acquired diaphragmatic hernia
- Very small hernias associated with traumatic reticuloperitonis; no respiratory signs
- Cases deriving from trauma mostly in

horses; signs vary with size of defect and organs displaced:

- No signs or moderate dyspnea with chance of conversion to acute colic with exercise, transport
- Acute colic, negative rectal findings, hyperresonance over chest, gut sounds in chest, severe dyspnea, signs of shock, negative abdominal paracentesis, stomach distension with nasal tube reflux or vomiting. Radiography or ultrasonography may identify lesion

SYNCHRONOUS DIAPHRAGMATIC FLUTTER IN HORSES (THUMPS)
[VM8 p. 422]

Etiology

- Idiopathic in adult ponies used for pleasure riding
- Horses in endurance contests

Clinical findings

- Violent hiccough synchronous with each heart beat
- Accentuated apex beat felt more strongly on one side
- Eating impeded
- Respiratory difficulty
- Recovers spontaneously within 24 hours
- In endurance horses
  - Additional signs of muscle rigidity and fasciculation, high-stepping gait

Clinical pathology

- Hypocalcemia, hypochloremia and hypokalemia
- Hemoconcentration
- Alkalosis
- Elevated creatine kinase levels

Treatment

Recover with slow intravenous injection of calcium solution.

PLEURISY [VM8 p. 422]

Etiology

- Traumatic or surgical penetration of chest wall
- Penetration of diaphragm by reticular foreign body
- Spread via lymphatics from peritonitis, from pneumonia or lung abscess, e.g. equine strangles
- As part of specific infectious diseases:
  - **All species** – pasteurellosis
  - **Pigs** – Glasser's disease, *Actinobacillus pleuropneumoniae*, swine influenza
  - **Cattle** – tuberculosis, sporadic bovine encephalomyelitis, contagious bovine pleuropneumonia, *Haemophilus somnus*
  - **Sheep, goats** – *Mycoplasma, Haemophilus* spp. pleuropneumonia
  - **Horses** – rupture or extension from a lung abscess. Pleuropneumonia caused by *Bacteroides* spp., *Klebsiella pneumoniae*, *Streptococcus zooepidemicus*

Clinical findings

Early stage
- Anxious facial expression
- Respiration rapid, shallow, mostly abdominal, fixed thorax
- Short, dry cough
- Elbows abducted
- Disinclined to move or lie down; stand quietly
- To-and-fro, dry, abrasive pleuritic friction sound; not cleared by coughing
- Pain on deep palpation, percussion over affected pleura
- Fever
- Tachycardia
- Anorexia
- Depression

Later (2–3 days)
- Friction rub disappears
- Local pain on palpation reduced
- Breath and heart sounds absent ventrally, up to a well defined horizontal top line; percussion dull below line
- Dyspnea; pleuritic ridge at costal arch
- Little rib movement on affected side
- Toxemia more severe
- Anorexia

Sequels
- Pericarditis
- Chronic adhesive pleurisy
- Never complete recovery to racing standard in horse
- Chronic emaciation
- Fatal, acute hemothorax with adhesion rupture

Additional signs in horses
- Mild, intermittent colic
- Ventral edema
- Weight loss

Clinical pathology

Leukocytosis and left shift in acute stage
Inflammatory fluid on thoracocentesis;
positive on aerobic, anaerobic culture
Radiography, ultrasonography reveal:
• Heart, mediastinum displacement to one
  side
• Fluid with level top line
• Atelectasis
Pleuroscopy gives direct view of pleura

Necropsy findings

Acute phase
→ Marked pleural edema, hyperemia, thick-
  ening
→ Fibrin tags, shreds between lung lobes

Exudative phase
→ Large quantity turbid fluid; fibrin flakes,
  clots
→ Thick pleura
→ Ventral lung collapsed, dark red
→ Concurrent pneumonia, possibly pericar-
  ditis

Healing phase
→ Adhesions between parietal, visceral
  pleurae

Diagnosis

Resembles:
♦ Pneumonia
♦ Pulmonary congestion/edema
♦ Pericarditis
♦ Pulmonary emphysema
♦ Hemothorax, hydrothorax

Treatment

♦ Commonly in an advanced stage when
  recognized
♦ Prognosis usually bad; negative for com-
  plete racing-ready recovery; may survive as
  pet or for breeding
♦ Specific therapy difficult because bacteria
  not identified
♦ Aggressive, specific or broad-spectrum
  antibacterial treatment long term up to 3
  weeks
♦ May require metronidazole or chloram-
  phenicol in combination in horses
♦ Pleural fluid drainage by:
  • Cannulation; difficult because of fibrin
    blockage, possible laceration of lung;
    permits antibiotic perfusion
  • Thoracotomy with chronic drainage
  • Diuresis ineffective

DISEASES OF THE UPPER RESPIRATORY TRACT

RHINITIS [VM8 p. 425]

Etiology

♦ Minor lesion in most pneumonias
♦ Significant part of syndrome in:
  Cattle
  • Bovine malignant catarrh
  • Bovine virus diarrhea
  • Rinderpest
  • Infectious bovine rhinotracheitis
  • Adenoviruses 1, 2, 3 infection
  • Respiratory syncytial virus infection
  • Rhinosporidiosis
  • *Schistosoma nasalis* infection
  • atopic rhinitis (summer snuffles)
  • familial allergic rhinitis

  Horses
  • Glanders
  • Epizootic lymphangitis
  • Strangles
  • Equine viral rhinopneumonitis
  • Equine viral arteritis

  • Influenza virus infection
  • Equine rhinovirus, reovirus, adenovirus
    infection
  • Dust, smoke inhalation
  • Nasal granuloma due to *Pseudoalles-
    cheria boydii* infection

  Sheep
  • Melioidosis
  • Bluetongue
  • Ecthyma rarely
  • Sheep pox rarely
  • *Oestrus ovis* infestation
  • *Elaeophora schneideri* infestation
  • Allergic rhinitis

  Pigs
  • Atrophic rhinitis
  • Inclusion body rhinitis
  • Swine influenza
  • Aujeszky's disease (some outbreaks)

Clinical findings

♦ Nasal discharge, serous → mucoid → purulent

♦ Unilateral originates in nasal cavity
♦ Bilateral may be nasal origin or pharyngeal, pulmonary
♦ Persistent, weeks or months, purulent discharge suggests sinus lesion or allergic or mycotic infection
♦ **Sneezing** early → **snorting** gobs of mucopurulent material
♦ Head shaking
♦ Erythema, or erosive, granular, necrotic, vesicular viewable with difficulty

Clinical pathology

♦ Examination of swabs, scrapings may help identify bacterial, viral, fungal, protozoal, parasitic, neoplastic, allergic causes
♦ Endoscopic examination may identify location of lesion

Diagnosis

Resembles:
♦ Facial sinusitis
♦ Guttural pouch infection in horses

Treatment

♦ Treat primary disease
♦ Nasal irrigation with normal saline
♦ Nasal decongestant spray may allow neonates to suck
♦ Allergic rhinitis cases confined indoors

OBSTRUCTION OF THE NASAL
CAVITIES [VM8 p. 426]

Etiology

Cattle
♦ Enzootic nasal granuloma
♦ Allergic rhinitis, including impacted twigs in cavity
♦ Cystic enlargement ventral nasal conchae
♦ Mucus-filled nasal mucosal polyps in posterior nares
♦ *Rhinosporidium* spp., granuloma
♦ *Schistosoma nasalis* infestation

Sheep
♦ *Estrus ovis* infestation
♦ Neoplasm; enzootic nasal adenocarcinoma, sometimes in outbreak form

Horse
♦ Ethmoidal hematoma
♦ *Coccidioides immitis* pyogranuloma
♦ Nasal amyloidosis

Clinical findings

Basic syndrome
♦ Sneezing, snorting, head shaking
♦ Loud, wheezing inspiration if obstruction incomplete
♦ Variable nasal discharge depending on cause, serous, hemorrhagic, purulent
♦ Unilateral detected by breath stream absence from one nostril or inability to pass nasal tube
♦ Bilateral – severe dyspnea, terminal gasping
♦ Intermittent with pedunculated polyps

Other signs in cases with specific causes
♦ **Nasal amyloidosis** – painless nodules on rostral nasal septum, floor
♦ **Nasal adenocarcinoma** – unilateral occasionally bilateral; on ethmoid turbinates; locally invasive, not metastatic retrovirus suspected; in sheep and goats
♦ **Ethmoidal hematoma** – in horses; unilateral, chronic nasal discharge, then obstruction; recognized by endoscopy; surgical resection advised
♦ **Enzootic ethmoidal tumor** – Sweden Brazil. Invades paranasal sinuses

Clinical pathology

♦ Endoscopy the only satisfactory examination
♦ Lesional biopsy may reveal swelling's composition

Diagnosis

Resembles:
♦ Laryngitis, tracheitis, bronchitis
♦ Guttural pouch disease

Treatment

♦ Treat specific disease
♦ Remove foreign body by forceps traction
♦ Oral organic iodine preparations, I/V iodide solutions widely used

EPISTAXIS AND HEMOPTYSIS
[VM8 p. 427]

Etiology

Horses
♦ Guttural pouch mycosis
♦ Exercise-induced pulmonary hemorrhage
♦ Hemorrhagic polyps in nasal cavity, paranasal sinus

Ethmoidal hematoma
Nasal mucosal erosions, e.g. glanders
Nasal granulomas
Trauma from inept nasal intubation
Purpura hemorrhagica
Congestive heart failure

Cattle
- Pulmonary abscess
- Caudal vena caval thrombosis
- Ptaquiloside poisoning
- Dicoumarol poisoning
- Enzootic ethmoidal tumor

Clinical findings

Basic syndrome
- Bouts, often recurrent, of bleeding from nostrils (epistaxis) or mouth (hemoptysis)
- May be as little as blood flecks or pink staining in clear serous fluid to profuse whole blood
- Blood not in clots where clotting defect present
- Melena or occult blood in feces
- Reduced racing performance in horses
- Regenerative anemia
- Lung auscultation normal even with pulmonary hemorrhage

Epistaxis
- May be visible nasal lesions
- Whole blood from nostrils varies from blood stained serous fluid, to few clots to profuse stream
- Bleeding at rest or after mild exercise, usually from guttural pouch lesion,
- During a race profuse bleeding precedes sudden death during the race, or sudden slowing and baulking horses behind
- Repeated bouts occur in cattle and horses

Hemoptysis
Whole blood pouring from mouth, usually accompanied by coughing, continuous licking and swallowing movements, or just continuous swallowing movements, followed by melena.

Other signs in specific diseases
- **Ethmoidal hematoma** (horse)
  - Dyspnea
  - Cough
  - Choking while swallowing
  - Persistent unilateral epistaxis
- **Guttural pouch arteritis** – acute unilateral epistaxis at rest or after mild exercise

Clinical pathology

- Check clotting mechanisms in case of defect
- Packed cell volume, hemoglobin content of blood may be low with chronic blood loss
- Radiographic examination may identify guttural pouch lesion; endoscopic examination essential

Necropsy findings

- Cadaver anemic
- Lungs and or airways filled with blood

Diagnosis

Resembles sudden death due to any cause, especially acute heart failure

Treatment

- Surgical correction necessary for most upper respiratory tract lesions characterized by epistaxis
- Epistaxis in a racehorse during a race disqualifies the horse from racing for a specified period; resumption of racing is usually dependent on horse completing a test performance without bleeding. Most horses that bleed once are predisposed to do so again and leave the racing industry
- Treatment for exercise-induced pulmonary hemorrhage is of the resting horse after disqualification; many drugs used, e.g. coagulants, estrogens, furosemide, Clenbuterol, atropine, but without demonstrable advantage

LARYNGITIS, TRACHEITIS,
BRONCHITIS [VM8 p. 430]

Etiology

Diseases in which inflammation of the larynx, trachea or bronchioles is a significant feature include:

Cattle
- Infectious bovine rhinotracheitis
- Calf diphtheria
- *Haemophilus somnus* infection
- Congenital arytenoid cavitation

Sheep
- Chronic *Actinomyces pyogenes* infection

Horses
+ Equine viral rhinopneumonitis
+ Equine viral arteritis
+ Equine influenza
+ Strangles

Pigs
+ Swine influenza

Clinical findings

+ Cough, dry, easily induced by tracheal compression initially
+ Moist, painful cough if secondary bacterial infection; may cough up blood-flecked mucus
+ In acute laryngitis tissues around larynx may be swollen, painful
+ Fever
+ Toxemia
+ Anorexia
+ Inspiratory dyspnea
+ Loud stridor
+ Loud breath sounds over trachea, lung base; loudest in inspiration
+ Cyanosis, anxiety, death from asphyxia in worst cases
+ Excitement of transport, examination, may precipitate asphyxia

Sequels
+ Chronic laryngeal chondritis
+ Local abscess
+ Pneumonia

Clinical pathology

+ Examination via endoscope in horse, or illuminated cylindrical speculum in cow, permits visualization of larynx and first part of trachea; lesions, collections of mucus may be visible; specimens for bacteriological, cytological examination collected
+ Microbiological examination of nasal, tracheal or bronchoalveolar lavage or aspirate samples for evidence of specific infection

Necropsy findings

+ Lesions vary from acute catarrhal to chronic granulomatous
+ Diphtheritic pseudomembrane in secondary bacterial infection
+ Exudate accumulation at trachea bifurcation, dependent bronchi

Diagnosis

Resembles:
+ Pneumonia, especially viral pneumonia often concurrent
+ Obstruction of upper respiratory tract
+ Rhinitis

Treatment

+ Most cases recover spontaneously in a few days
+ Avoid exertion, inclement environment dust
+ Broad-spectrum antibiotic a common prophylaxis against, treatment for, secondary bacterial infection; 3–5 days usually up to 3 weeks for chondritis
+ Corticosteroids may be used to reduce swelling provided infection under control by antibacterial treatment
+ Surgical repair of resulting chronic lesions or distortions is attempted

TRAUMATIC
LARYNGOTRACHEITIS, TRACHEAL
COMPRESSION AND TRACHEAL
COLLAPSE [VM8 p. 431]

Etiology

+ Pressure of tube or inflatable cuff in endotracheal intubation, endoscopy cause traumatic injury to nasal meatus, arytenoid cartilages, trachea, dorsal pharyngeal recess, vocal cords, entrance to guttural pouch
+ Tracheal injury, including fractured first ribs, in calves during dystokia
+ Idiopathic congenital defect of cartilages
+ Sequel to tracheitis in horses
+ Trauma causing rupture
+ Compression by swollen cranial mediastinal lymph nodes

Clinical findings

+ Stridor, including **honking** spontaneously or when trachea squeezed
+ Cough
+ Reduced exercise tolerance
+ Short-term tracheotomy when asphyxial death threatens
+ Loud, referred breath sounds auscultated over trachea
+ Subcutaneous emphysema, pneumomediastinum in tracheal rupture

Necropsy findings

- Restriction of lumen, injury to cartilage, dorsal tracheal ligament lax
- Local emphysema in rupture

Diagnosis

Resembles:
- Nasal, pharyngeal, laryngeal obstruction, paralysis
- Laryngitis, tracheitis, bronchitis

Treatment

- Conservative treatment usually successful because of spontaneous recovery or adaptation to lesion
- Tracheotomy for an emergency
- Long-term tracheal prostheses have been used

OBSTRUCTION OF THE LARYNX
[VM8 p. 432]

Air flow impaired at rest.

Etiology

Acute obstruction

- Laryngeal edema in allergic reaction
- Laryngeal edema due to smoke, fumes inhalation
- Gut edema, swine; not usually so severe
- Pharyngeal phlegmon
- Anthrax (horses, pigs)
- Solid food lodgement after vomiting, regurgitation
- Sharp foreign body lodgement locally
- Chronic laryngitis in sheep due to *Actinomyces pyogenes* in sheep
- Acute, bilateral vocal cord paralysis due to organophosphatic compound poisoning

Chronic obstruction

Cattle Retropharyngeal abscess obstruction in:
- Tuberculosis
- Actinobacillosis
- *Actinomyces pyogenes* infection

Horse:
- Pharyngeal lymphoid hyperplasia
- Laryngeal chondroma
- Laryngeal papilloma
- Foreign body

Clinical findings

- Dyspnea, worst when stressed
- Prolonged inspiration
- Inspiratory stridor
- Loud breath sounds over larynx
- Fremitus over larynx

Diagnosis

Resembles:
- Exercise-induced upper respiratory obstruction
- Laryngitis, tracheitis, bronchitis
- Tracheal compression, collapse

Treatment

- Prognosis not good because of nature of obstruction
- Surgical removal of foreign body
- Emergency tracheotomy in acute cases

EXERCISE-INDUCED UPPER
RESPIRATORY OBSTRUCTION
[VM8 p. 432]

Horses only; solely for differential diagnosis. List of conditions in which dyspnea occurs only during exercise includes:
- Pharyngeal lymphoid hyperplasia, a variant of pharyngitis
- Left laryngeal hemiplegia due in some to guttural pouch mycosis; the cause of classical roarers
- Soft palate paresis
- Soft palate dorsal displacement; some accompanied by foreshortened epiglottis
- Epiglottis entrapment
- Subepiglottic cysts; besides respiratory difficulty, foals also show:
  - Dysphagia
  - Chronic cough
  - Bilateral nasal discharge
  - Aspiration pneumonia
- Other minor defects

DISEASES OF THE GUTTURAL
POUCH [VM8 p. 433]

For purposes of differential diagnostic completeness a list is included.

Guttural pouch mycosis

- Thrombus formation in internal carotid artery shedding emboli unilaterally in

brain, causes mycotic encephalitis, blindness and ataxia
♦ Profuse epistaxis at rest due to erosion of internal carotid or maxillary artery
♦ Inflammation of nearby cranial nerves causes:
  • Dysphagia
  • Laryngeal hemiplegia
  • Facial paralysis
  • Horner's syndrome

Guttural pouch empyema
Signs include:
♦ Toxemia
♦ Pain on swallowing, palpation
♦ Cough
♦ Purulent nasal discharge in some, especially if patient fed on ground

Guttural pouch tympany
In neonatal foals:
♦ Pouches distend to enormous size
♦ After several weeks, swallowing and respiration may be impaired

Guttural pouch laceration and penetration
Causes epistaxis.

CONGENITAL DEFECTS [VM8 p. 434]

♦ Tracheal collapse
♦ Accessory lungs; when bronchi vestigia accessory lungs resemble tumor masses occupy most of thoracic cavity
♦ Defects of face, oral cavity and crania vault may affect respiratory function

11 DISEASES OF THE URINARY SYSTEM

The principal clinical signs, clinicopathological findings and special examination techniques on which clinical diagnoses of urinary system diseases are based include the following lists of basic syndromes and clinical indicants.

BASIC SYNDROMES

RENAL INSUFFICIENCY [VM8 p. 435]

Etiology

Specific causes of renal insufficiency are as for renal failure (see below).

Reduction in the kidney's functional activity in producing glomerular filtrate and actively and selectively reabsorbing substances from it through its renal tubules occurs for three reasons:

♦ Abnormal rate of renal blood flow, e.g. in shock, dehydration, hemorrhage, congestive heart failure causing reduction in glomerular filtration rate and renal ischemia
♦ Damage to the glomerular epithelium causing loss of plasma protein into the filtrate, e.g. in glomerulonephritis; even cessation of filtration (or complete back diffusion of all filtrate through damaged tubules)
♦ Reduced tubular reabsorption efficiency, e.g. in hemoglobinuric nephrosis

After renal damage occurs some nephrons cease to function and renal reserve is lost but surviving nephrons can maintain metabolic equilibrium by increasing their filtration rate often beyond the tubules' capacity to reabsorb the filtrate; a state of **renal insufficiency** exists. Loss of sufficient nephrons can be so severe that compensation does not occur; **renal failure** prevails. In many diseases both glomerular and tubular efficiencies are affected.

Clinical findings

Increased urine volume (polyuria).

Clinical pathology

♦ Reduced urine specific gravity
♦ Retention of metabolites causing elevation of blood levels of:
  • Urea
  • Phosphate
  • Sulphate
  and excessive loss of metabolites causing depression of blood levels of:
  • Sodium
  • Calcium (hypercalcemia may also occur in horses)
♦ Possible development of renal metabolic acidosis
♦ Susceptibility to dehydration, possibly clinical dehydration
♦ Susceptibility to circulatory emergencies; renal failure may supervene

RENAL FAILURE (UREMIA) [VM8 p. 436]

Etiology

♦ Renal ischemia due to acute cardiac or peripheral circulatory failure
♦ Glomerulonephritis
♦ Interstitial nephritis
♦ Nephrosis (including hemoglobinuric, myoglobinuric, and toxic)
♦ Pyelonephritis
♦ Embolic nephritis

♦ Amyloidosis

The pathological physiology of renal **insufficiency** is so severe that the patient's continued existence is impossible; the clinical syndrome is **uremia**.

Clinical findings

♦ Reduced or complete absence of urine flow (oliguria, anuria); often a history of polyuria
♦ Dehydration
♦ Anorexia
♦ Often a history of polydipsia
♦ Weight loss, emaciation due to continued proteinuria
♦ Depression, terminating as coma
♦ Muscle weakness, tremor, staggering gait, terminating as recumbency
♦ Myocardial asthenia due to hyponatremia, hypokalemia, hypocalcemia
♦ Diarrhea (horses)
♦ Temperature normal or depressed
♦ Heart rate increased
♦ Respiratory rate, depth slightly increased; periodic terminally
♦ Breath smell reputed to be ammoniacal
♦ Inexorably fatal
♦ Some horses have history of renal colic
♦ Ventral edema in cattle with nephrosis

Clinical pathology

Elevated blood levels of:
♦ Urea
♦ Creatinine

Diagnosis

Differentiation of cause of uremia from renal causes need to be made between:
♦ Complete urinary tract obstruction as in obstructive urolithiasis, and
♦ Bladder rupture, urethral rupture

RENAL COLIC [VM8 p. 439]

Etiology

♦ Pyelonephritis (renal pelvis distension)
♦ Obstructive urolithiasis (renal pelvis, ureter, urethra, bladder)
♦ Kidney infarction

Clinical findings

♦ Intermittent bouts of abdominal pain:
  • Downward arching of back
  • Paddling with hind feet; kicking at belly
  • Grunting or bellowing
  • Rolling
♦ Urethral peristaltic movement on palpation
♦ Distended bladder in urethral obstruction
♦ Repeated vigorous urination attempts with grunting
♦ Tail switching, rubbing of tail head

Diagnosis

Resembles:
♦ Alimentary tract colic
♦ Obstructive bililithiasis
♦ Acute photosensitive dermatitis

INDIVIDUAL CLINICAL INDICANTS

Anuria

Clinical findings:
♦ Cessation of urine flow
♦ Empty bladder

Occurs in:
♦ Water deprivation
♦ Dehydration
♦ Congestive heart failure
♦ Peripheral circulatory failure
♦ Acute tubular nephrosis
♦ Urethral obstructive urolithiasis
♦ Terminal stages of all forms of nephritis

Bladder distended, painful

Occurs in:
♦ Obstructive urolithiasis
♦ Bladder paralysis – cauda equina neuritis syndrome

Bladder wall thickened

Occurs in:
♦ Cystitis
♦ Pyelonephritis

Casts, cells in urine

♦ Individual epithelial cells, and agglomer

ations of cells and protein, occur in some cases of active inflammatory or degenerative renal disease; they are worthy of note but are of no differential diagnostic significance (See also hematuria, pyuria.)

Casts dissolve in alkaline, including stale, urine

Crystalluria

* Calcium carbonate, triple phosphate crystals common in normal herbivore urine
* Large numbers indicate urine concentrated, possible potential urolithiasis

Discoloration

Red–brown urine discoloration, with negative protein, guaic, specific hemoglobin or myoglobin, tests.

Occurs in:
* Inherited congenital porphyria
* Poisoning by *Xanthorrhea* spp., phenolphthalein

Dysuria

Clinical findings:
* Frequent urination
* Small amounts of urine per urination, dribbling
* Straining to urinate
* Lengthy retention of urination posture after completion
* Often associated urine signs of inflammation, pyuria, hematuria

Occurs in:
* Cystitis
* Cystic urolithiasis, without obstruction
* Cystic neoplasm; enzootic hematuria
* Pyelonephritis

Glycosuria

Clinical findings Positive strip or tube test for glucose in urine.

Occurs in:
* Diabetes mellitus, rarely in domestic animals
* In *Clostridium perfringens* type D intoxication
* After therapy with:
  * Parenteral glucose
  * Glucocorticoids or analogs
* Acute tubular nephrosis
* Often concurrent with ketonuria

Hematuria

Clinical findings:
* Clots or deep red to brown color, or
* Cloudiness forming red deposit (deposit also with hemoglobinuria), or
* Red cells on microscopic examination
* In bad cases, signs of blood loss anemia
* Positive tests for hemoglobin, myoglobin, and protein
* Sample may be contaminated by blood from vagina, prepuce; catheter sample most accurate, midstream sample the practical solution

Occurs in:
* Trauma to kidney
* Septicemia
* Purpura hemorrhagica
* Hemorrhagic diseases
* Acute glomerulonephritis
* Renal infarction
* Renal artery embolism
* Toxic nephrosis
* Pyelonephritis
* Urolithiasis
* Cystitis
* Enzootic hematuria
* Proximal urethral ulceration in horses causing hematuria at end of urination

Hemoglobinuria

Clinical findings:
* Deep red to almost black color of urine
* Other signs of hemolytic anemia
* Positive urinalysis for hemoglobin, protein
* No red cells in urine sediment
* Haemoglobinaemia
* Signs of hemoglobinuric nephrosis rarely

Occurs in Cases of hemolytic anemia when hemoglobin blood levels exceed reticuloendothelial system capacity to metabolize it and exceeds renal threshold.

Hypoproteinemia

Clinical findings Low blood protein level.

Occurs in:
* Chronic glomerulonephritis
* Acute tubular nephrosis
* Amyloidosis
* Protein starvation
* Liver insufficiency
* Blood loss
* Protein-losing enteropathy

Ketonuria

Clinical findings Positive strip or tablet test.

Occurs in:
♦ Starvation in ruminants
♦ Acetonemia, pregnancy toxemia
♦ Fat cow syndrome
♦ Parturition syndrome
♦ Left abomasal displacement
♦ Marginal ketone levels in normal lactating dairy cows; test needs to be selective for high levels

Kidney enlarged

Clinical findings:
♦ Usually only one palpable
♦ Painful also in most cases

Occurs in:
♦ Hydronephrosis
♦ Pyelonephritis, some cases
♦ Neoplasm
♦ Renal amyloidosis
♦ Obstructive urolithiasis

Myoglobinuria

Clinical findings:
♦ Red–brown urine
♦ Proteinuria
♦ Laboratory test for myoglobin

Occurs in Severe muscle damage especially equine azoturia, not in enzootic muscular dystrophy.

Oliguria

Clinical findings Reduced daily urine output.

Occurs in:
♦ Water deprivation
♦ Dehydration
♦ Congestive heart failure
♦ Peripheral circulatory failure
♦ Acute tubular nephrosis
♦ Terminal stages of all forms of nephritis

Polyuria

Clinical findings:
♦ Urine output impossible to assess accurately
♦ If urine isosthenuric with specific gravity constant at 1.008–1.012 renal problem exists

♦ Blood urea, creatinine levels usually elevated
♦ Water deprivation test fails to concentrate urine; serious dehydration, uremia in some patients with renal insufficiency

Occurs in:
♦ Central diabetes insipidus; very rare except in horses with pituitary tumor; responsive to antidiuretic hormone
♦ Peripheral diabetes insipidus; tubules unresponsive to antidiuretic hormone
♦ Voluntary increased water intake
♦ After therapy with:
  • Diuretics
  • Parenteral fluids
♦ Normal neonates on fluid diets
♦ Nephrosis

Proteinuria

Clinical findings Positive reaction to tests for protein in urine.

Occurs in:
♦ False positives with dipsticks in highly alkaline urine of herbivores; protein precipitation tests free from this error
♦ Normal neonates for 40 hours after receiving colostrum
♦ Hemoglobinuria
♦ Myoglobinuria
♦ Hematuria
♦ Urinary tract infections
♦ Glomerulonephritis
♦ Renal infarction
♦ Tubular nephrosis
♦ Amyloidosis

Pyuria

Clinical findings: Usually cloudy
♦ Leukocytes, casts or pus in urine
♦ Often microbiology culture positive
♦ Signs of urinary tract infection (frequency dysuria, and retention of urination posture)

Occurs in:
♦ Pyelonephritis
♦ Embolic nephritis
♦ Cystitis

Renal function tests

♦ Test that urine being voided; dry pen or cloth under patient for 12 hours
♦ Urine specific gravity abnormal; normal is 1.028–1.032; in chronic renal disease is about 1.010

Urine osmolality has same use as specific gravity; more direct

Elevated blood urea, creatinine levels when 75% nephrons lost; levels subject also to other factors including protein catabolism

Tests of rate of elimination of injected substance e.g. sodium sulfanilate and phenolsulfonthalein

Tests of kidney concentrating function (see in **polyuria**, above)

- Contrast radiography useful in neonates
- Ultrasound used to evaluate equine urinary system
- Percutaneous kidney biopsy used in cattle and horses

Uremia

See renal failure, this section.

Urination small amounts, dribbling

See dysuria, this section.

Urination straining

See dysuria, this section.

Urine cloudy

See pyuria, this section.

Urine red

See **discoloration**, this section.

DISEASES OF THE KIDNEY

NEPHROSIS [VM8 p. 442]

- The most important cause of acute kidney failure in farm animals
- Nephrotic uremia may be acute or chronically terminal
- Caused by:
  • Renal ischemia
  • Poisons (toxic nephrosis)

RENAL ISCHEMIA [VM8 p. 442]

Etiology

Acute ischemia
- Dehydration
- Shock
- Acute blood loss
- Acute heart failure
- Renal artery embolism (horse)
- Extreme ruminal distension (cattle)

Chronic ischemia
- Congestive heart failure

Clinical findings

See renal failure above.

Clinical pathology

See renal function tests above.

Necropsy findings

- Kidney cortex pale and swollen
- Line of necrosis at corticomedullary junction visible in some
- Tubular, glomerular possibly, epithelium necrotic
- Hyaline tubular casts in hemoglobinuric, myoglobinuric nephrosis

Diagnosis

Antemortem differentiation from other primary renal disease not possible.

Treatment

Correct circulatory problem as early as possible.

TOXIC NEPHROSIS [VM8 p. 443]

Etiology

- **Metals** – mercury, arsenic, cadmium, selenium, copper (organic compounds), potassium dichromate
- **Antibacterials** – aminoglycoside antibiotics, sulfonamides, excessive treatment with long-acting tetracyclines
- Parenteral menadione sodium bisulfite (vitamin K_3) to horses
- Cholecalciferol, ergocalciferol to horses
- Non-steroidal anti-inflammatories to horses; cause also interstitial nephritis, renal crest necrosis

♦ Some benzimidazole anthelmintics, e.g. thiabendazole
♦ Aldrin (low dosage) to goats
♦ Highly chlorinated naphthalenes
♦ Monensin to ruminants
♦ Ethylene glycol
♦ Oxalates in plants, fungi
♦ Tannins in plants
♦ Ingested *Lophyrotoma* spp. larvae
♦ Cantharidin
♦ Most endogenous or exogenous toxemias

Clinical findings

The basic uremic syndrome of renal failure (see above).

Clinical pathology

♦ **Urinalysis** – proteinuria, glycosuria, hematuria
♦ Gamma-glutamyl transferase present in urine (experimental cases)
♦ In chronic cases urine isosthenuric and may contain no protein
♦ **Blood chemistry** – hypoproteinemia in some
♦ Blood urea nitrogen and creatinine levels elevated in late stages

Necropsy findings

♦ **Acute** – kidney swollen and wet
♦ Edema, especially renal tissues
♦ Tubular epithelium necrotic desquamated; hyaline casts in tubules
♦ Ulcers in any part of alimentary tract – mouth to colon

Diagnosis

Resembles:
♦ Acute glomerulonephritis
♦ Diabetes mellitus
♦ Cushing's syndrome (chronic hyperadrenocorticism); characterized in horses by polyuria, glycosuria, debilitation, hirsutism, polyphagia, hyperglycemia
♦ Equine undifferentiated diarrhea

Treatment

♦ Remove patient from toxin source
♦ Isotonic fluids parenterally until dehydration corrected
♦ Avoid overhydration by ensuring urine flows
♦ If dehydration corrected but urine flow inadequate administer furosemide

GLOMERULONEPHRITIS [VM8 p. 445]

Uncommon in farm animals. Proliferative glomerulonephritis considered an important cause of chronic renal failure in horses.

Etiology

Primary glomerulonephritis – only kidney involved
♦ Immune response in which antibodies are directed against intrinsic or deposited antigens in the glomerulus
♦ Circulating antigen–antibody complexes (e.g. streptococci, equine infectious anemia virus antigens) deposited in and damage glomerulus, and surrounding interstitial tissue and blood vessels
♦ In Finnish Landrace sheep mesangiocapillary glomerulitis antigen absorbed from colostrum initiates immune reaction and deposition of complexes in glomerulus

Secondary glomerulonephritis
Occurs in:
♦ Equine infectious anemia
♦ Chronic hog cholera

Clinical findings

Glomerular damage leads to proteinuria, renal failure (see above).

INTERSTITIAL NEPHRITIS [VM8 p. 445]

A rare cause of clinical illness, but a common necropsy finding, in farm animals.
♦ **Focal interstitial nephritis** (white spotted kidney) in bacteremic calves
♦ **Diffuse interstitial nephritis** in pigs with leptospirosis; the lesion is an important source of the infection; clinical illness does nor occur because of it
♦ **Chronic interstitial fibrosis** a common necropsy finding in horses with chronic renal failure terminating in uremia

EMBOLIC NEPHRITIS [VM8 p. 446]

Uncommon cause of clinical illness; an incidental finding at necropsy.

Etiology

A sequel to bacteremia, septicemia, e.g.:
♦ Valvular endocarditis
♦ Suppurative metritis, mastitis, omphalo-phlebitis, peritonitis
♦ Shigellosis in foals
♦ Coliform septicemia in neonates
♦ Porcine erysipelas
♦ Strangles

Clinical findings

♦ Toxemia in a few
♦ Transient abdominal pain rarely
♦ Enlarged, lumpy, painful kidney rarely
♦ Uremia rarely

Clinical pathology

♦ Transient proteinuria, hematuria, pyuria
♦ Leukocytosis, left shift
♦ Transient, intermittent bacteriuria

Necropsy findings

♦ In acute cases microabscesses, infarcts evident grossly
♦ In chronic cases large abscesses, fibrous capsules, scarring; kidney may be mis-shapen

Diagnosis

Resembles:
♦ Pyelonephritis
♦ Ischemic tubular nephrosis in neonates
♦ Acute intestinal obstruction

Treatment

♦ Broad-spectrum antibacterial treatment if identity of infection unknown; potentially nephrotoxic drugs should be avoided
♦ Treatment needs to be 7–14 days; checked by negative urine culture

PYELONEPHRITIS [VM8 p. 447]

Etiology

♦ *Corynebacterium renale*, cattle
♦ *Eubacterium suis*, pigs
♦ Secondary to lower urinary tract infection
♦ Spread from embolic nephritis

Clinical findings

♦ Blood-stained urine, or blood clots
♦ Fluctuating fever
♦ Anorexia
♦ Weight loss
♦ Reduced milk yield
♦ Frequent urination
♦ Dysuria
♦ Bladder wall thickened; bladder shrunken, ureters thickened, kidney enlarged, painful, in late stages
♦ Urine contains blood, pus, tissue debris; may be intermittently
♦ Terminal anemia, toxemia and uremia

Clinical pathology

♦ Erythrocytes, leukocytes, cell debris in urine, grossly or microscopically
♦ Urine culture to identify organism

Necropsy findings

♦ Necrosis, ulceration of renal pelvis, papillae
♦ Pelvis dilated, contains blood clots, pus
♦ Streaks of gray, necrotic material radiate from pelvis through renal medulla, into cortex, between normal tissue, contracted scar tissue
♦ Necrosis, suppuration in ureters, bladder

Diagnosis

Resembles:
♦ Cystitis
♦ Embolic nephritis
♦ Enzootic hematuria
♦ Bladder neoplasm

Treatment

♦ Emphasis on early detection and instant treatment
♦ Prolonged antibacterial treatment for 2–3 weeks in established cases; prognosis fair, relapse common
♦ Penicillin in infection with *Corynebacterium renale*; broad spectrum, renal toxicity free if infection not identified

HYDRONEPHROSIS [VM8 p. 447]

Etiology

♦ Congenital obstruction to urine flow
♦ Acquired, especially unilateral, chronic, incomplete, obstruction, e.g.:
  • Bladder papilloma

- Irregular shaped uroliths
- External compression by tumor material in bovine viral leukosis

Clinical findings

♦ Grossly enlarged kidney
♦ Chronic renal failure in bilateral lesion
♦ Ultrasonography helps to identify

RENAL NEOPLASM [VM8 p. 448]

♦ Carcinomas recorded in cattle and horses; cause renal enlargement

♦ Adenocarcinomas in horses cause:
  - Weight loss
  - Anorexia
  - Intermittent colic
  - Ascites in some
  - Hemoperitoneum
  - Hematuria
  - Masses in abdomen on rectal examination
  - Metastases in liver, lungs
♦ Nephroblastomas recorded in pigs; may cause palpable, visible enlargement
♦ Metastases appear as palpable local or diffuse enlargement of kidney

DISEASES OF THE BLADDER, URETERS AND URETHRA

CYSTITIS [VM8 p. 448]

Etiology

Trauma, introduction of infection, stagnation of urine initiate most cases of cystitis caused principally by *Escherichia coli*, e.g. in:
♦ Bladder urolithiasis
♦ Bladder paralysis
♦ Horses eating cyanogenetic plant causing cystitis/ataxia
♦ Dystokia
♦ Late pregnancy
♦ Contaminated catheterization

Secondary cystitis
Escherichia coli, Streptococcus, Pseudomonas spp. infections in cases of:
♦ Bovine pyelonephritis (*Corynebacterium renale*)
♦ Porcine pyelonephritis (*Eubacterium suis*)

Clinical findings

♦ Frequent urination, small amounts
♦ Urination painful; tail swishing, treading with hind feet, sometimes kicking at belly, grunting
♦ Patient retains urinating posture for prolonged time, makes additional expulsive efforts
♦ Mild fever in some
♦ Rarely urethral blockage, acute retention, bladder distension
♦ **Acute cases** – bladder not palpable but pain response on palpation
♦ **Chronic cases** – thick wall, contracted bladder on rectal palpation
♦ Bladder calculus palpable in some horses

Clinical pathology

♦ **Acute cases** – blood, pus in urine
♦ **Chronic cases** – urine turbid or normal grossly
♦ Urine contains erythrocytes, leukocytes, epithelial cells
♦ Quantitative bacteriology needed for prognosis and treatment guide

Necropsy findings

♦ **Acute** – mucosa edematous, hemorrhagic, hyperemic; urine cloudy, contains mucus
♦ **Chronic** – wall thick, mucosa roughened, granular, vascular papillary projections with eroded tips; urine contains blood
♦ **Equine cystitis/ataxia** – soft masses of calcium carbonate in bladder, on vaginal wall

Diagnosis

Resembles:
♦ Pyelonephritis
♦ Bladder urolithiasis
♦ Enzootic hematuria
♦ Bladder neoplasm
♦ *Terminalia oblongata* poisoning

Treatment

♦ **Acute** – broad-spectrum antibacterial, or specific medication directed by culture identification of bacteria; continued 7–14 days; relapse common
♦ **Chronic** – prognosis very poor if bladder wall thickened

PARALYSIS OF THE BLADDER
[VM8 p. 449]

Etiology

Cauda equina lesion, as in mounting injury by heavy bull on young males, females
Equine herpesvirus myelitis
After prolonged bladder distension, e.g. obstructive urolithiasis
Equine cystitis/ataxia
Idiopathic distension with overflow in horses

Clinical findings

Incontinence with dribbling or intermittent overflow
Urine may be expelled jerkily during exercise
Bladder enlarged, full on rectal; urine easily expelled
Heavy calcium carbonate sludge in horses
Ataxia, tail paralysis in cases due to spinal cord disease
Cystitis a common sequel

Clinical pathology

Urine may contain cells, bacteria, erythrocytes, and leukocytes if cystitis or uroliths present.

Diagnosis

Resembles:
♦ Obstructive urolithiasis
♦ Cystitis

Treatment

♦ Relieve bladder distension by catheter; lavage
♦ Continuous antibacterial cover
♦ Prognosis fair for return of function if traumatically neurogenic; poor in most others

RUPTURE OF THE BLADDER [VM8 p. 449]

Etiology

♦ Obstructive urolithiasis; commonest in castrated males
♦ Sequel to dystokia
♦ After normal parturition in mares
♦ Congenital bladder rupture in foals

Clinical findings

♦ Anuria
♦ Anorexia
♦ Depression and coma
♦ Abdominal distension
♦ Fluid thrill in abdomen
♦ Ruminal stasis
♦ Constipation
♦ Bladder not palpable when distension expected
♦ Paracentesis delivers urine
♦ Death due to uremia

Clinical pathology

♦ Blood levels urea, potassium, phosphorus elevated
♦ Blood levels of phosphorus best indicator of survival in cattle (>9 mg/dl indicates fatal outcome)

Diagnosis

Resembles:
♦ Ascites
♦ Chronic peritonitis

Treatment

♦ Surgical repair via laparotomy
♦ Installation of indwelling catheter or urethrostomy, encouraging spontaneous repair has good recovery rate, reduces costs

UROLITHIASIS IN RUMINANTS
[VM8 p. 450]

Etiology

Urolith formation
♦ Management system includes:
  • Water deprivation
  • High salt intake in high salinity water
  • Hot arid climates
  • High phosphorus intake on heavy grain diets
  • High magnesium content milk replacers to calves
  • Rapid growth of livestock
  • Heavy grain–low roughage rations
  • Pelleted rations
  • Diethylstilbestrol implants
♦ Enzootic areas where feeds contain high levels of:
  • Silicon
  • Estrogen, e.g. *Trifolium subterraneum* in pasture
  • Oxalate

Obstructive urolithiasis

♦ High estrogen intake
♦ Early castration (females and entire males usually pass mobile calculi through their wider caliber urethras)
♦ Urine stasis encourages urolithiasis by encouragement of infection, providing niduses

Obstruction by calculus

♦ Obstruction can be by single stone or unformed sediment
♦ Obstruction favored by:
  • Small bore urethra, e.g. early castrates,
  • Enlarged accessory sex glands, e.g. high estrogen intakes in pasture, implants
  • Optimum conditions for rapid calculus formation

Clinical findings

Non-obstructive calculi

♦ Asymptomatic; not diagnosed antemortem
♦ Associated cystitis, pyelonephritis

Renal pelvis/ureter obstruction

♦ Acute abdominal pain
♦ Stiff gait
♦ Pain on pressure over loins
♦ Sequel of enlarged hydronephrosis in some

Urethra obstruction

♦ The common obstruction syndrome
♦ Kicking at belly
♦ Swishing tail
♦ Repeated penis twitching, shakes prepuce
♦ Vigorous, grunting straining to urinate
♦ May pass few drops of, sometimes blood-stained urine
♦ On rectal urethra, bladder distended, urethra pulsates on palpation
♦ Crystalline precipitate on preputial hairs, inside thighs in some
♦ Tranquilizer or epidural then passage of catheter or lead wire may identify site of obstruction
♦ Incomplete obstructions due to irregularly shaped calculi cause dribbles of small amounts frequently

Sequels

♦ Bladder rupture after 48 hours
♦ Urethral perforation, leakage into ventral abdominal connective tissue; signs include:
  • Pitting, fluid-filled swelling reaches from prepuce to brisket

  • Swelling becomes inflamed and painful skin may slough
  • Uremia syndrome

Variation

Top-shaped calculi in prepuce, act as valve block urine flow, may cause urine leakage into belly wall.

Clinical pathology

♦ Erythrocytes, epithelial cells, crystals in urine in early, asymptomatic stage
♦ Secondary cystitis accompanied by leukocytes and bacteria in urine
♦ Identification of fluid from paracentesis subcutaneous aggregation, as urine
♦ Elevated blood urea, creatinine levels in obstructed animals and in bladder rupture or urethral perforation

Calculus composition

♦ Semi-arid great plains North America, Australia, silica content of pasture high siliceous calculi common
♦ On clover or oxalate-containing pasture calcium carbonate calculi common
♦ Pastured animals generally – ammonium, calcium, magnesium carbonate calculi common
♦ In feedlot animals calculi usually struvite (magnesium–ammonium phosphate) especially on high magnesium feeds
♦ Oxalate calculi rare
♦ Xanthine calculi on some poor pastures
♦ High estrogen content subterranean clover pasture can produce soft, moist, yellow calculi or unformed sediments containing benzocoumarins and other related compounds

Necropsy findings

♦ Calculi in renal pelvis, ureter, bladder, and urethra
♦ Hydronephrosis, cystitis, pyelonephritis, and cystitis in some
♦ Ventral abdominal, subcutaneous urine accumulation, urethra perforation at obstruction site with local cellulitis
♦ Identification of calculus composition assists in planning prevention

Diagnosis

Non-obstructive urolithiasis resembles:
♦ Cystitis
♦ Pyelonephritis
Obstructive urolithiasis resembles:

Embolic nephritis
Acute intestinal obstruction
Urethral perforation resembles:
  Edema due to congestive heart failure, hepatic fibrosis
Bladder rupture resembles:
» Ascites
» Chronic peritonitis

Treatment of obstructive urolithiasis

» Slaughter for salvage an important option in feeder steers or lambs
» Treatment is necessarily surgical; outcome good if bladder not yet ruptured; prognosis is for recurrence in same animals, probability of occurrence in others
» Urethrostomy, with passage of long catheter if necessary, to relieve bladder pressure; salvage as soon as possible (see also bladder rupture)

Prevention

Delay castration; limited benefit.

Feedlots
♦ Avoid excess phosphorus in ration (Ca:P ratio should be close to 1.2:1)
♦ Ensure high water intake; ample trough space; 4% salt in total ration increases water intake in steers and lambs. High concentrations cause anorexia

Pasture
♦ Increase water intake, e.g. feeding lucerne hay
♦ Avoid saline drinking water in high-risk areas
♦ Feed imported hay, legumes when silica calculus outbreak threatens
♦ Creep feed high salt (up to 12%) concentrate ration to calves; calves to get 200 mg/kg salt per day; commence 2 months before weaning, prevents all calculi
♦ Alternative to salt is ammonium chloride (435 g/day to steers, 10 g/day to lambs); not effective for siliceous calculi
♦ Use females to graze dangerous pasture

UROLITHIASIS IN HORSES [VM8 p. 455]

♦ Most occur in bladder
♦ Most are single, calcium carbonate stones
♦ Occasional cases bilateral nephrolithiasis

Clinical findings

Cystitis syndrome
♦ Frequent urination
♦ Dysuria
♦ Hematuria in most
♦ Thick bladder wall, calculus palpable rectally
♦ Calculus detectable with ultrasonography and cystoscopy

Obstructive urolithiasis syndrome
♦ Acute abdominal pain, kicking at belly, crouching, flank watching
♦ Penis protruded, grunting efforts to urinate, may pass small amounts of blood-tinged urine
♦ Bladder distended on rectal
♦ Calculus palpable from exterior or by catheter

Bladder rupture
♦ Pain, straining cease
♦ Bladder no longer distended
♦ Urine accumulates in peritoneal cavity
♦ Urine identifiable in paracentesis aspirate
♦ If rupture at bladder neck, urine leakage is retroperitoneal producing a large, soft, diffuse swelling
♦ Uremia syndrome in 48 hours; depression to recumbency to coma, hypothermia, tachycardia

Nephrolithiasis
♦ Bilaterally affected patients develop chronic renal failure
♦ Weight loss

Clinical pathology

♦ Identification of bacteria if cystitis present
♦ Assessment of uremia development via estimation of blood urea, nitrogen, plasma creatinine levels

Diagnosis

Resembles:
♦ Acute intestinal obstruction
♦ Cystitis

Treatment

♦ Surgical removal with bladder repair if necessary
♦ Prophylaxis for cystitis

URINARY BLADDER NEOPLASMS
[VM8 p. 455]

Etiology

♦ Sporadic cases, mostly at abattoirs, in cattle and horses

♦ Multiple cases associated with ptaquilosid poisoning

Clinical findings

♦ Hematuria
♦ Straining to urinate
♦ Weight loss
♦ Secondary cystitis

CONGENITAL DEFECTS OF THE URINARY TRACT

PATENT OR PERVIOUS URACHUS
[VM8 p. 455]

♦ Urine drips/leaks from umbilicus; variable amount from moist umbilicus to continuous stream
♦ Cystitis, omphalitis, urachal abscess common sequels
♦ Chemical cauterization or surgical correction

BLADDER RUPTURE IN NEWBORN
FOAL [VM8 p. 456]

Etiology

♦ Traumatic due to rupture of full bladder during birth
♦ Defective closure of bladder wall during organogenesis

Clinical findings

♦ Almost all cases in colts
♦ Signs commence at 24–36 hours old
♦ Subacute colic
♦ Early vigorous sucking ceases
♦ Frequent straining to urinate
♦ Amount of urine passed varies from nil to 50% normal; mostly small amount
♦ Catheter passes easily
♦ No retained meconium
♦ Fluid in abdomen on succussion
♦ Uremia syndrome develops (depressed, hypothermia, recumbency, coma)

Clinical pathology

♦ Elevated blood urea, plasma creatinine
♦ Urine on abdominal paracentesis
♦ If doubt about paracentesis fluid being urine
  • Sterile dye solution introduced into bladder collectable from peritoneal cavity
  • Contrast radiography

• Creatinine content in paracentesis sample double the serum value

Necropsy findings

♦ Urine in peritoneal cavity
♦ Dorsal bladder wall defective with thin, undamaged edges **or**
♦ Ragged-edged tear in wall
♦ Defect in urachus, or ureter with retroperitoneal accumulation of urine

Diagnosis

Resembles:
♦ Intestinal obstruction
♦ Meconium retention
♦ Congenital defect of ureter

Treatment

♦ Surgical repair
♦ Intravenous fluids to correct dehydration, urea accumulation

URETHRAL ATRESIA [VM8 p. 456]

♦ Recorded in calves
♦ No urine passed
♦ Distension of bladder, patent part of urethra

URETERAL DEFECT [VM8 p. 456]

♦ Uni- or bilateral in foals, may be more common in fillies
♦ Syndrome not clinically distinguishable from bladder rupture

POLYCYSTIC KIDNEYS [VM8 p. 456]

Etiology

♦ Most species, relatively commonly; considered to be inherited

- Most cases congenital; acquired cases recorded
- Sporadic cases; multiple cases, with other defects, in offspring of sows vaccinated against swine fever with attenuated virus

Clinical findings

- Most cases asymptomatic because normal renal tissue compensates
- Patients with one cystic kidney may be encountered because of a very large other kidney
- Residual tissue may be lost late in life; uremia develops and cystic lesion discovered
- Gross abdominal distension, gross cystic distension kidneys and tract in some pigs

HYPOSPADIAS [VM8 p. 456]

Incomplete closure of external male urethra, with other defects, including atresia ani, diaphragmatic hernia, recorded in lambs.

RENAL HYPOPLASIA AND
DYSPLASIA [VM8 p. 456]

- Partial or complete absence of kidney tissue recorded as a probable inherited defect in piglets; piglets stillborn or die soon afterwards
- Cases recorded in horse; most die at birth, some survive for years; die after gradual onset of uremia syndrome; kidneys small and nodular

ECTOPIC URETER [VM8 p. 457]

- Recorded cattle, horses
- Uni- or bilateral
- Urinary incontinence since birth; urine dribbles intermittently, especially with movement
- Secondary ascending infection, hydronephrosis, ureter dilation frequent sequels
- Definitive diagnosis requires contrast radiography

12 DISEASES OF THE NERVOUS SYSTEM

Disease of the nervous system should be suspected when there are one or more of the following:
♦ Mental disturbance
♦ Involuntary movements
♦ Posture or gait abnormalities
♦ Paralysis
♦ Sensory, including visual, disturbances
♦ Autonomic nervous system defects

The principal clinical signs, clinicopathological findings and special examination techniques on which clinical diagnoses of nervous system disease are based are included in the following list.

CLINICAL INDICANTS

Aggression

Clinical findings:
♦ Charging
♦ Head-butting
♦ Biting
♦ Trampling

Occurs in:
♦ Encephalitis
♦ Chronic cerebral anoxia
♦ Neuroses, e.g. sow farrowing hysteria, granulosa-cell tumors of ovary
♦ Normally aggressive animals
♦ Trapped or physically handicapped animals

Aimless wandering

See wandering aimlessly, this section.

Anesthesia/Hypoesthesia, cutaneous

Clinical findings Loss of sensation indicated by failure to respond to needle prick or forceps pinch.

Occurs in:
♦ Local sensory innervation interrupted
♦ May be generalized, due to:
• Trauma
• Meningitis
• Toxemia, shock

Anal paralysis

Clinical findings:
♦ Anus open
♦ No anal or perineal reflex
♦ Straining in some

Occurs in:
♦ Spinal cord injury at S1–S3 due to:
• Trauma
• Local myelitis, meningitis
♦ Rabies
♦ Flaccid paralysis, generalized

Anal reflex absent

See anal paralysis, this section.

Ataxia

See cerebellar ataxia, this section.

Bellowing continuously

See mania, this section.

Blindness

See also night blindness.

Clinical findings:
♦ Patient bumps into objects
♦ Fails obstacle test
♦ Menace reflex absent
♦ Pupillary light reflex absent in patients with lesion in:

- Eye
- Optic nerve
pupillary light reflex present in patients with lesion in optic cortex

Occurs in:
  Cerebral hypoxia
  Brain edema
  Increased intracranial pressure
♦ Hydrocephalus
♦ Encephalitis
♦ Encephalomalacia, especially polio-encephalomalacia
♦ Brain trauma
♦ Cerebral nematodiasis
♦ Meningitis
♦ Toxic, metabolic encephalopathies, e.g.:
  • Lead poisoning
  • Plant poisonings, e.g. *Stypandra* spp.
♦ Pregnancy toxemia
♦ Hepatic encephalopathy
♦ Carbohydrate engorgement
♦ Nutritional deficiency vitamin A
♦ Congenital retina dysplasia, goats
♦ Brain, especially pituitary *rete mirabile* abscess
♦ Coenurosis
♦ Hyphaema
♦ Congenital defects
  • Microcephaly
  • Miscellaneous eye defects

Catalepsy

See narcolepsy, this section.

Cerebellar ataxia

See also incoordination, sensorimotor ataxia, sensory ataxia.

Clinical findings:
♦ Errors of exaggerated strength (hypermetria), distance, wrong direction (dysmetria) cause gross incoordination of limb movements
♦ Frequent falling due to poor foot placement
♦ Head-bobbing
♦ Intention tremor

Occurs in:
♦ Cerebellum disease, e.g.:
  • Inherited cerebellar defects
  • Congenital fetal viral infection, e.g. bovine virus diarrhea, hog cholera virus
♦ Inherited familial ataxia, Angus cattle

♦ bovine, caprine mannosidosis
♦ neonatal maladjustment syndrome, foals, some cases
♦ *Claviceps paspali* poisoning
♦ Hematoma in 4th ventricle
♦ Idiopathic cerebellar degeneration adult cattle

Cerebrospinal fluid contains cells

Clinical findings:
♦ Normal fluid is perfectly clear, contains <5 cells/μml
♦ Inflammatory fluid is turbid and contains large numbers of cells

Occurs in:
♦ meningitis in, e.g.:
  • Listeriosis
  • Pasteurellosis
  • Streptococcal infection
♦ Brain abscess
♦ Spinal cord abscess
♦ Cerebrospinal nematodiasis (erythrocytes only)

Chewing, licking objects

See mania, this section.

Chewing movements

See mania, this section.

Circling

See head rotation, head deviation.

Coma

See depression, this section.

Compulsive rolling

Clinical findings:
♦ Cannot stand
♦ Rolls to one side when placed on the other
♦ Nystagmus

Occurs in:
♦ Vestibular lesions
♦ Brain abscess
♦ Otitis media

Compulsive walking

See head-pressing, this section.

Convulsions (fit, seizure)

Clinical findings:
♦ Recumbent
♦ Paddling movements with limbs
♦ Opisthotonus
♦ Eyelid-snapping
♦ Jaw-champing
♦ Frothy salivation

Occur Because of lesions or other abnormalities within the brain (intracranial convulsions) or because of abnormalities external to the brain (extracranial convulsions).

Intracranial fits occur in:
♦ Encephalitis
♦ Encephalomalacia
♦ Meningitis
♦ Encephalomalacia
♦ Acute brain edema
♦ Brain ischemia
♦ Increased intracranial pressure
♦ Hydrocephalus
♦ Trauma, e.g. concussion, contusion
♦ Brain abscess
♦ Brain tumor
♦ Cerebrospinal nematodiasis
♦ Coenurosis
♦ Brain hemorrhage
♦ Epilepsy, inherited, traumatic, idiopathic
♦ Doddler calves
♦ Inherited familial convulsions/ataxia, Angus cattle

Extracranial fits occur in:
♦ Hypoxia
♦ Neonatal maladjustment syndrome
♦ Toxic, metabolic encephalopathies
♦ Acute heart failure
♦ Hepatic encephalopathy
♦ Hypoglycemia
♦ Pancreas tumor
♦ Hypomagnesemia
♦ Poisons including
  • Chlorinated hydrocarbons
  • Pluronics
  • *Clostridium* spp.

Corneal reflex absent

Clinical findings Light touch to cornea fails to elicit eyelid closure.

Occurs in:
♦ Facial paralysis
♦ Unconsciousness
♦ Death

Crossed limb stance

See paresis, this section.

Deafness

Clinical findings Lack of response to auditory stimuli.

Occurs in:
♦ Injury to cochlear portion of vestibulocochlear nerve, cortical hearing center
♦ Congenital defect
♦ Aminoglycoside antibiotic poisoning

Depression/coma

See hyporesponsive, this section.

Drifting sideways gait

See paresis, this section.

Dumb

See larynx paralysis, this section.

Dysmetria

See also cerebellar ataxia, this section)

Clinical findings:
♦ Incoordinated direction, force of limb movements
♦ Includes hypermetria (exaggerated movements), hypometria (subdued movements)

Occurs in:
♦ Inherited cerebellar disease
♦ Cerebellar defect due to fetal virus infection, e.g. hog cholera, bovine virus diarrhea
♦ *Claviceps paspali* poisoning

Dysphagia

See swallowing ineffectual, this section.

Ear paralysis or ear droop

See facial paralysis, this section.

Eyeball deviation, squint or strabismus

Clinical findings:
♦ Abnormal orientation one or both eyeballs
♦ Dorsomedial orientation – trochlear nerve

Ventrolateral orientation – oculomotor nerve
Medial orientation – abducens nerve

Occurs in:
♦ Polioencephalomalacia (trochlear nerve compression)
♦ Local compressive lesion, e.g. abscess, tumor
♦ Inherited strabismus, cattle

Eyeball protrusion, exophthalmos

Clinical findings One or both (rarely) eyeballs protrude beyond normal position.

Occurs in:
♦ Abducens nerve compression by abscess or tumor
♦ Periorbital space-occupying lesion, e.g. bovine viral leucosis
♦ Inherited combined with strabismus, cattle
♦ Part of inherited cardiomyopathy syndrome, Hereford cattle

Eyelid paralysis (ptosis)

Clinical findings:
♦ Eyelid droops
♦ No palpebral reflex

Occurs in:
♦ Facial nerve paralysis
♦ Listeriosis
♦ Petrous temporal bone fracture

Eyelid snapping

See convulsions, this section.

Facial nerve paralysis

Clinical findings:
♦ Paralysis with drooping of ear, eyelid, and lip
♦ Absence of menace reflex
♦ Ear droops or fails to prick

Occurs in:
♦ Injury to facial nerve
♦ Otitis media
♦ Petrous temporal bone fracture
♦ Guttural pouch mycosis

Falling to one side

Clinical findings:
♦ Forms part of circling syndrome
♦ Associated with tail deviation

Occurs in:
♦ Vestibular system lesion
♦ Caudal spinal cord injury
♦ Otitis media
♦ *Xanthorrhea* spp. poisoning

Falls easily

Occurs in:
♦ General weakness
♦ Myaesthenia
♦ Myopathy
♦ Peripheral (e.g. femoral, perineal, radial, tibial, sciatic) nerve injury; weak limb syndrome
♦ Paresis, hemiparesis
♦ Circling due to vestibular system lesions

Fetlock knuckled

Clinical findings Sole flat to the ground, fetlock flexed and held in a forward position.

Occurs in:
♦ Peripheral (e.g. femoral, peroneal, radial, tibial, sciatic, obturator) nerve paralysis, paresis
♦ Gastrocnemius muscle rupture
♦ Ischemic muscle necrosis
♦ Myopathy
♦ Maternal obstetric paralysis
♦ Weak limb syndrome

Frenzy/restless

Clinical findings:
♦ Violent, uncontrolled, dangerous activity
♦ Sometimes aggression

Occurs in:
♦ Encephalitis, especially rabies, Aujeszky's disease
♦ Toxic, metabolic encephalopathies
♦ Brain abscess
♦ Brain tumor
♦ Coenurosis
♦ Meningitis
♦ Severe skin irritation, e.g. early photosensitization
♦ Equine colic

♦ Panic, e.g. stampeding cattle, bolting horses

Head-pressing/compulsive walking

Clinical findings:
♦ Pushing against fixed objects
♦ Compulsive walking, straight ahead, will not be restrained, looks aggressive
♦ Blind
♦ Nystagmus

Occurs in:
♦ Toxic, metabolic encephalopathies, e.g. hepatic encephalopathy
♦ Increased intracranial pressure
♦ Encephalitis
♦ Encephalomalacia, e.g. polioencephalomalacia
♦ Brain neoplasm
♦ Brain abscess
♦ Brain injury
♦ Coenurosis

Head deviation

Clinical findings:
♦ Head turned to one side
♦ Circles most times, some can walk straight

Occurs in:
Focal lesion in cerebral cortex or medulla, e.g.
♦ brain abscess
♦ Listeriosis
♦ Brain tumor
♦ Coenurosis

Head rotation

Clinical findings:
♦ Always walks in circles in the one direction
♦ Falls easily

Occurs in:
♦ Encephalitis
♦ Lesion in vestibular nerve, nucleus or canals
♦ Brain abscess
♦ Listeriosis
♦ Brain trauma
♦ Otitis media
♦ Coenurosis
♦ Fracture equine petrous temporal bone

Head-shaking

Clinical findings Frequent bouts of violent head-shaking

Occurs in:
♦ Pruritus, e.g. otitis externa, ear mites
♦ Mucosal irritation, e.g. rhinitis, conjunctivitis
♦ Idiopathic cranial sensory nerve paresthesia
♦ Guttural pouch mycosis
♦ Dental periapical osteitis

Head tilt

See head rotation, this section.

Hoof dragged along ground

As in:
♦ Myaesthenia
♦ Peripheral (e.g. femoral, perineal, radial, tibial, sciatic) nerve paralysis, paresis, weak limb syndrome
♦ Gastrocnemius muscle rupture
♦ Patellar luxation or subluxation

Hoof dorsum, walks on

Extreme case of hoof-dragging (see above).

Horner's syndrome

Clinical findings:
Hemilateral:
♦ Drooping upper eyelid
♦ Pupil constriction
♦ Eyeball sunken
♦ Sweating on face and upper neck

Occurs in Lesions causing damage to cervical, cranial thoracic sympathetic trunks, e.g.:
♦ Anterior mediastinal mass, e.g. thymoma
♦ Guttural pouch mycosis
♦ Periphlebitis of jugular vein
♦ Xylazine injection normal horses
♦ Periorbital tumor

Hyperesthesia (hypersensitivity)

Clinical findings:
♦ Excessive response to normal touch stimuli
♦ Usually refers to cutaneous sensitivity but includes paresthesia (a subjective heightening of sensitivity) in animals
♦ Nibbling reaction in scrapie

Occurs in:
♦ Nervous acetonemia
♦ Rabies (some species)
♦ Aujeszky's disease (cattle)
♦ Scrapie
  See also pruritus

Hypermetria

See cerebellar ataxia, this section.

Hyperresponsive (= frenzy/ restless, excitable)

See frenzy/restless, this section.

Hyphaema

Clinical findings Hemorrhage into the anterior chamber of the eye.

Occurs in:
♦ Hemorrhagic disease
♦ Trauma

Hyporesponsive (= depression/coma, somnolent, lethargy)

Clinical findings:
♦ Anorexia
♦ Isolation from group
♦ Disinterest in surroundings, unresponsive to stimuli

Occurs in:
♦ Encephalitis
♦ Encephalomalacia
♦ Meningitis
♦ Hydrocephalus
♦ Toxic, metabolic encephalopathies, e.g.
  • Hypoglycemia
  • Hepatic encephalopathy
  • Uremia
  • Toxemia
♦ Cerebral hypoxia/anoxia
♦ Brain edema
♦ Trauma (concussion, contusion)
♦ Brain abscess
♦ Starvation

Imbecility

Clinical findings:
♦ Standing, will suck, drink, or feed
♦ Blind
♦ No response to external stimuli

Occurs in:
♦ Hydranencephaly
♦ Encephalomalacia
♦ Hepatic encephalopathy
♦ Survivors of polioencephalomalacia

Incoordination

See also cerebellar ataxia, this section.

Clinical findings:
♦ Abnormality of movements, usually referring to gait, so that they do not achieve objectives smoothly and accurately
♦ In common usage includes **limb weakness, proprioceptive defects, cerebellar ataxia, weaving gait**, leaning gait

Occurs in:
♦ Impaired functions of spinal nerve tracts, cerebellum in some cases, nerve impulse transmission including:
♦ Poisoning by *Claviceps paspali*, *Acremonium*, *Phalaris* spp, many other poisonous plants
♦ Encephalitis
♦ Brain abscess
♦ Petrous temporal bone fracture
♦ Coenurosis
♦ Cerebellar disease
♦ Ovine enzootic ataxia
♦ Equine enzootic incoordination
♦ Minor spinal cord trauma
♦ Spinal cord compression due to developing mass in vertebral canal
♦ Many congenital spinal cord defects, e.g. atlanto-occipital dysplasia, spinal cord hypoplasia
♦ Progressive ataxia, Charolais cattle
♦ Myelomalacia
♦ Myaesthenia

Jaw champing

See convulsions, this section.

Jaw paralysis

See prehension/mastication ineffectual, Chapter 5.

Knuckling

See fetlock knuckled, this section.

Larynx paralysis

Clinical findings:
♦ Respiratory stertor at exercise
♦ Poor racing performance
♦ Loss of voice

Occurs in:
- Unilateral vocal cord paralysis (idiopathic laryngeal hemiplegia)
- Bilateral in delayed organophosphate poisoning
- Loss of voice in vocal cord paralysis of rabies

Leaning gait

See paresis, this section.

Licking, chewing, rubbing of self

See mania, below.

Mania

Clinical findings:
- Bizarre behavior including:
  - Intensive licking, chewing foreign objects or themselves
  - Constant bellowing, neighing
  - Aggression
  - Blindness
  - Disregards normal commands
  - Often precedes paralysis

Occurs in:
- Encephalitis, e.g. rabies
- Brain hypoxia, e.g. terminal pneumonia
- Meningitis
- Brain tumor
- Coenurosis
- Nervous acetonemia
- Hypomagnesemia
- Chlorinated hydrocarbon poisoning
- Farrowing hysteria

Menace reflex absent

Clinical findings Patient does not blink, recoil when finger stabbed at eye.

Occurs in:
- Blindness
- Facial nerve paralysis

Muscle atrophy (neurogenic)

Clinical findings:
- Visible atrophy skeletal muscle masses related to distribution of a specific nerve
- Other parts of body usually normal

Occurs in:
- Injury to or compression of a specific nerve, e.g.:

- Sweeney (suprascapular nerve paralysis)
- Facial nerve paralysis

Myoclonus

Clinical findings:
- Brief, intermittent contraction all skeletal muscles
- Causes whole of body rigidity

Occurs in Inherited congenital myoclonus, Hereford calves.

Narcolepsy/catalepsy

Clinical findings:
- Uncontrollable sleep episodes
- Recumbency during episodes

Occurs in Inherited narcolepsy/catalepsy in Shetland ponies, Suffolk horses, possibly cattle.

Neck rigid

See tetany, this section: osteomyelitis Chapter 13.

Nibbling reaction

See hyperesthesia, this section.

Night blindness

Clinical findings:
- Blindness in dim light
- Fails nocturnal obstacle test

Occurs in:
- Nutritional deficiency vitamin A
- Inherited defect, Appaloosas

Nystagmus

Clinical findings:
- Involuntary periodic slow movements both eyeballs in unison
- Pendular nystagmus – both movements equal velocity

Occurs in Lesions of vestibular apparatus, *or* midbrain and cerebellopontine area, *or* diseases with no lesion:
- Encephalitis
- Encephalomalacia, e.g. polioencephalomalacia

- Brain edema
- Hydrocephalus
- Brain trauma
- Brain abscess
- Meningitis
- Brain tumor
- Coenurosis
- Otitis media
- Otitis interna
- Fracture petrous temporal bone
- Listeriosis
- Inherited pendular nystagmus

Opisthotonus

Clinical findings:
- Rigid fixation of head, neck, and trunk
- Head dorsiflexed
- Back arched down

Occurs in:
- Spastic paralysis syndrome
- Brain edema
- Encephalitis
- Encephalomalacia, e.g. polioencephalomalacia
- Hydrocephalus
- Brain abscess
- Brain tumor
- Meningitis
- Epilepsy
- Tetany
- Tetanus

Orthotonus

Clinical findings:
- Rigid fixation of head, neck, and trunk in a straight line
- Limbs extended caudally

Occurs in:
- Extreme tetany state
- Severe tetanus in young ruminants and horses

Palpebral reflex absent

Clinical findings No eyelid closure when eyelid touched.

Occurs in:
- Lesion of sensory branch of trigeminal nerve
- Facial trauma

Panniculus reflex absent

Clinical findings Absence of the quick twitch of the superficial cutaneous muscle along the entire back when patient pricked with a pin beside the spine in the thoracolumbar area.

Occurs in Trauma, compression of spinal cord at C8–T2.

Paralysis, flaccid, generalized

Clinical findings:
- Recumbency
- Flaccid paralysis of limbs, neck, and tail
- Jaw, tongue, and eye movements may be normal
- Tendon reflexes weak or absent
- Consciousness may be unaffected

Occurs in:
- Terminal encephalitis
- Cervical spinal cord injury
- Myelitis
- Myelomalacia
- Spinal cord congenital defects
- Enzootic ataxia
- Tick paralysis
- Carbon tetrachloride poisoning
- Botulism
- Milk fever

Paralysis, flaccid, pelvic limb only

Clinical findings:
- Flaccid hind limbs
- No anal reflex

Occurs in:
- Injury, compression of cord at L4–L8
- Early paralytic rabies
- Vertebral osteomyelitis
- Vertebral fracture
- Lymphosarcoma

Paralysis, flaccid, thoracic and pelvic limbs

Clinical findings:
- Flaccid paralysis all four limbs and neck
- Unable lift head off ground

Occurs in:
- Damage to cord at C1–C5
- Injury, lymphosarcoma

Paresis

Clinical findings:
- Staggery gait
- Leaning, drifting sideways gaits
- Easy falling
- Difficulty rising
- Cross-legged stance in a few
- Unilateral paresis causes **weak limb syndrome** (see below)

Occurs in:
- Spinal cord compression
- Early milk fever
- Peripheral nerve injury

Paresthesia

See hyperesthesia, this section.

Patellar reflex absent

Clinical findings Tap on the patellar tendon fails to elicit standard extension response.

Occurs in:
- Lesion of spinal cord at L5–S3
- Peripheral nerve injury

Perineal reflex absent

Clinical findings Light pin prick of perineal skin fails to cause normal contraction of anal sphincter, clamping down of tail.

Occurs in Lesion in spinal cord segments S1–CQ.

Pharynx paralysis

Clinical findings:
- Attempts to swallow followed by coughing up feed, and nasal regurgitation
- Drools saliva
- In some horses combined with laryngeal paralysis
- Aspiration pneumonia common sequel

Occurs in:
- Traumatic injury to glossopharyngeal, recurrent laryngeal nerves or nuclei
- Rabies
- Botulism
- *Centaurea* spp. poisoning

Prehension/mastication ineffectual

Clinical findings:
- Attempts to prehend and chew food are ineffectual
- Patient drops food from mouth
- Drops cuds

Occurs in:
- Cranial nerve lesions:
  - Sensory branch of trigeminal (prehension)
  - Hypoglossal (tongue movements)
  - Facial (lip movements)
  - Motor branch of trigeminal (chewing)
- Focal medullary lesion affecting cranial nerve nuclei due to trauma, listeriosis
- *Phalaris* spp. poisoning
- Guttural pouch lesion (facial nerve)
- Petrous temporal bone fracture (facial nerve)

Proprioceptive deficit

See sensorimotor ataxia, this section.

Pupil constriction

Clinical findings:
- Pupil constricted, unresponsive to light
- May be combined with blindness, coma, or spastic paralysis

Occurs in:
- Transient cholinesterase inactivation, e.g. organophosphate, carbamate poisoning
- Lead poisoning
- Horner's syndrome
- Diffuse optical cortical lesion, e.g. polio-encephalomalacia

Pupil dilation

Clinical findings:
- Pupil dilated; does not constrict with increased light intensity
- Pupillary light reflex absent
- Transient dilation is without blindness
- Permanent dilation accompanies blindness, with or without retinal lesion

Occurs in:
- Part of general paresis
- Retina lesion
- nervous shock
- Optic nerve lesion, e.g. constriction in avitaminosis A

Transient in milk fever, snakebite, atropine poisoning
Retinal lesion in ophthalmitis, trauma, toxoplasmosis

Pupillary light reflex absent

Clinical findings Pupil does not contract or dilate in response to changes in incident light intensity.

Occurs in:
* Lesion in eye, retina or optic nerve, e.g. pituitary gland abscess
* Traumatic or compressive lesion of oculomotor nerve

Recumbency

Clinical findings:
* Patient is unable to rise
* Lateral recumbency
* Unable to lift neck from ground – indicates severe upper cervical lesion; *or* head and neck can be lifted but patient not able to maintain sternal recumbency – indicates lower cervical lesion; *or* sternal recumbency unable to rise indicates thoracolumbar cord lesion; *or* musculoskeletal lesion, e.g. 'downer cow' syndrome

Occurs in:
* General paresis
* Skeletal muscle asthenia
* Cerebral hypoxia
* Increased intracranial pressure
* Encephalitis
* Brain tumor
* Coenurosis
* Meningitis
* Cord injury, compression
* Spondylosis
* Congenital spinal cord defects
* Myelitis

Restlessness

See frenzy/restless, this section.

Rigid stance

See tetany, this section.

Rising difficult

See paresis, this section.

Sensorimotor ataxia

Clinical findings:
* Paresis plus incoordination
* Fetlock knuckling (= knuckling)

* Toe scuffing
* Incomplete flexion, extension
* Wobbly, wandering gait
* Easy falling
* Difficulty rising

Occurs in:
* Compression causes moderate damage to spinal cord motor and sensory tracts, e.g. cervical vertebral compression spinal cord (Wobblers)
* Degenerative myelopathy
* Myelitis
* Myelomalacia
* Congenital spinal cord defects
* *Sorghum, Phalaris, Zamia* spp. poisoning

Sensory ataxia

Clinical findings:
* Timing of limb movements wrong; no paresis
* Limbs incoordinated when pivoting; limbs cross

Occurs in:
* Spinal cord injury damaging spinocerebellar tracts
* Cervical cord damage affects thoracic limbs
* Thoracolumbar cord injury affects pelvic limbs

Slap test (laryngeal adductor reflex) negative

Clinical findings Slap on saddle region causes endoscopically visible adduction of contralateral arytenoid cartilage.

Occurs in:
* Absence of reflex indicates laryngeal hemiplegia, *or*
* A tense or frightened horse

Spastic pareses, intermittent

Clinical findings Intermittent contractions of large muscle masses cause limb movements.

Occurs in:
* stringhalt
* Bovine spastic paresis (Elso heel)
* Bovine periodic spasticity
* Neuraxial edema
* Inherited myotonia

Stiff gait

Occurs in:
♦ peritonitis
♦ Arthritis
♦ Meningitis
♦ Myositis
♦ tetany

Strabismus, squint

See eyeball deviation, this section.

Stumbling gait

♦ General weakness
♦ myaesthenia
♦ myopathy
♦ Peripheral (e.g. femoral, perineal, radial, tibial, sciatic) nerve injury, weak limb syndrome
♦ paresis

Sway response

Clinical findings:
♦ Affected animals stumble, may fall because of wide hindquarter sway when tail pulled laterally or hindquarters pushed while on the move
♦ Incoordination in most cases

Occurs in Patients with weakness of limb or poor proprioception fail to maintain erect stance because of compromised spinal cord tracts due to spinal cord compression, or myelitis.

Syncope (fainting)

Clinical findings:
♦ Suddenly falling unconscious
♦ May be other signs, e.g. of cardiac failure

Occurs in:
♦ Acute heart failure
♦ Nervous shock
♦ Cerebral hemorrhage
♦ Contusion, concussion
♦ Lightning strike, electrocution

Tail paralysis

Clinical findings Anesthesia, flaccidity of tail.

Occurs in:
♦ spinal cord injury, caudal segments, e.g. mounting
♦ Local meningitis, cauda equina abscess
♦ Early rabies

Tenesmus

Clinical findings:
♦ Straining as if to defecate
♦ Often associated with anus paralysis
♦ Limb weakness also in some

Occurs in Irritation to peripheral nerves a or near cauda equina, e.g.:
♦ caudal equina neuritis, e.g sexual mounting injury
♦ Early rabies

Tetany

Clinical findings:
♦ Continuous muscle contraction without tremor
♦ Entire body or part maintained in state of continuous, rigid extension
♦ Stiff gait, reduced joint flexion
♦ Rigid stance
♦ Stiff neck
♦ Third eyelid prolapse
♦ Tetanic convulsions

Occurs in:
♦ Tetanus
♦ Hypomagnesemia
♦ Spinal cord injury resulting in upper motor neurone lesion

Third eyelid prolapse

See tetany, above.

Tongue paralysis

Clinical findings:
♦ Prehension difficult
♦ Tongue tip hangs or protrudes from mouth
♦ Tongue easily pulled out, cannot be withdrawn
♦ May be fibrillation of tongue muscles
♦ Drooling saliva in some

Occurs in:
♦ Injury to hypoglossal nerve or nerve nucleus
♦ Medullary abscess

Tremor

Clinical findings Palpable, visible, continuous, repetitive skeletal muscle contractions sufficient to move parts of body.

Occurs in:
♦ Most diffuse diseases of brain including:
  • Hypoxia

- Increased intracranial pressure
- Encephalitis
- Encephalomalacia
- Meningitis
- Toxic, metabolic encephalopathies, e.g. shaker foals, hyperkalemic periodic paralysis, border disease (lambs), poisonings by *Swainsona* spp. *Phalaris* spp., *Acremonium* spp.
- Congenital defects nervous system, e.g.- congenital tremor piglets, calves; hypomyelinogenesis, neuraxial edema

Tremor, intention

Clinical findings Tremor of head, neck when patient fixes gaze on something.

Occurs in:
- Cerebellar dysfunction, e.g. cerebellar hypoplasia
- *Claviceps paspali* poisoning

Trismus (lockjaw)

Clinical findings:
- Spasm of masseter muscles; mouth cannot be opened passively
- Mild cases in cattle can eat with difficulty
- Muscle fibrillation in masseter muscles

Occurs in Tetanus.

Voice absent

See laryngeal paralysis, this section.

Wandering aimlessly

Clinical findings:
- Aimless walking, head-pressing
- Continuous, chewing movements

- Tongue protrusion
- Unable to drink or eat

Occurs in:
- Toxic, metabolic encephalopathies
- Encephalomalacia, e.g. hepatic encephalopathy, equine nigropallidal encephalomalacia
- Ovine ceroid lipofuscinosis

Weak limb

See also paresis, this section.

Clinical findings:
- Stumbling or sideways drifting or leaning gait
- Falls easily
- Foot misplacement on pivoting
- Knuckling at fetlock
- Toe worn
- Positive sway test
- Difficulty rising on affected limb

Occurs in:
- Single limb paresis
- Peripheral nerve trauma
- Musculoskeletal defect

Withdrawal reflex absent

Clinical findings Pricking, pinching skin at coronet does not elicit withdrawal of limb.

Occurs in:
- Severe peripheral nerve trauma
- Bovine viral leukosis lesion at nerve root
- Vertebral abscess
- Deficit in pelvic limb indicates lesion in cord segments L5–S3
- Absence in thoracic limb indicates lesion in segments C6–T2

DISEASES OF THE BRAIN

CEREBRAL HYPOXIA/ANOXIA
[VM8 p. 481]

Etiology

Systemic hypoxia/anoxia
- Cyanide poisoning
- Nitrate-nitrite poisoning
- Acute heart failure, e.g. falling disease, cattle

- Anesthetic accidents
- Terminal congestive heart failure
- Terminal pneumonia
- During prolonged parturition in all species
- Neonatal adjustment syndrome of foals

Local cerebral anoxia
- Increased intracranial pressure
- Brain edema

Clinical findings:

Acute

- Sudden onset of
  - Unconsciousness
  - Tetraparesis, *or*
- Tremor
- Recumbency
- Convulsions
- Death or temporary or complete recovery depending on cause

Chronic

- Lethargy
- Dullness
- Stumbling gait
- Falls easily
- Disinclined to rise
- Blindness in some
- Tremor/convulsions in some

Fetal hypoxia:

- Chronic syndrome present at birth
- Too weak to suck, dies of starvation

Clinical pathology and necropsy findings

- Principally lesions and chemical, cytological changes of primary disease
- Cerebrocortical necrosis in long-term hypoxia

Diagnosis

Resembles:
- Hypoglycemia
- Polioencephalomalacia
- Lead poisoning
- Arsenic poisoning
- Many plant poisonings, e.g. cardiac glycosides
- Encephalitis
- Encephalomalacia

Treatment

- Remove primary cause
- Supply oxygen
- Artificial respiration
- Respiratory stimulant

INCREASED INTRACRANIAL PRESSURE, CEREBRAL SWELLING AND BRAIN EDEMA [VM8 p. 481]

Etiology

Secondary to:
- Hypoxia
- Polioencephalomalacia in ruminants
- Salt poisoning, swine
- Hydrocephalus
- Brain abscess
- Brain hemorrhage
- Purulent meningitis
- Lead encephalopathy
- Trauma
- Encephalitis
- Propylene glycol poisoning in horses
- Intracarotid injection promazine
- Neonatal septicemia in foals

Clinical findings

- Develops over 12–24 hours
- Blindness, isolation from group, unwilling to move
- Dullness
- Bouts of:
  - Opisthotonus
  - Tremor
  - Convulsions
  - Nystagmus
- Staggery then recumbency
- Permanent opisthotonus, tremor, convulsions, nystagmus
- Death after 1–6 days, *or*
- Survival with residual signs of:
  - Blindness
  - Imbecility, usually have to be hand fed

Clinical pathology

None other than those of primary disease.

Necropsy findings

- Brain gyrae flattened
- Brain soft, sags over cranium edges
- Cerebellum herniated into foramen magnum
- Caudal parts of occipital lobes herniate under tentorium cerebelli

Diagnosis

Resembles:
- Encephalitis
- Encephalomalacia
- Hypovitaminosis A
- Carbohydrate engorgement of ruminants
- Pregnancy toxemia
- Hypomagnesemic tetany of ruminants
- *Clostridium perfringens* type D enterotoxemia
- Gut edema in swine

Treatment

- Treat primary disease
- Decompression by intravenous injection of hypertonic solutions (e.g. 20% solution mannitol 2 g/kg), followed 3 hours later by corticosteroids (e.g. dexamethazone 1 mg/kg)
- Diuretics mostly valuable only as supportive to decompression

HYDROCEPHALUS [VM8 p. 483]

Etiology

Congenital
- Sporadic cases with lateral mesencephalon narrowing
- Inherited in Hereford, Holstein, Ayrshire, Jersey cattle
- Inherited combined with chondrodysplasia
- Inherited combined with retinal dysplasia, microphthalmia in white Shorthorn cattle
- Idiopathic, high prevalence occurrences

Acquired
- Hypovitaminosis A in young calves and piglets
- Cholesteatoma of lateral ventricle choroid plexuses in aged horses
- Tumor, chronic inflammatory swelling obstructing lateral ventricle

Clinical findings

Chronic onset cases (the commonest)
- Depression, somnolence
- Vacant expression
- Leans on or against object for support
- Blind, disinclined to move; pupillary light reflex present
- Stumbling gait, incoordination, imprecise movements
- Circling in some
- Slow, incomplete, intermittent; feed hangs from mouth
- Bradycardia, arrhythmia in some
- Optic papilledema

Terminally
- Recumbency
- Opisthotonus
- Paddling convulsions

Acute cases
- Episodes up to several weeks apart
- Wild expression
- Head-pressing, charging
- Tremor
- Convulsions

Congenital
- Recumbent
- Nystagmus
- Exophthalmos in some
- Cranium domed in some
- Meningocele rarely

Clinical pathology

- Cerebrospinal fluid pressure high
- Serum creatine kinase elevated in congenital hydrocephalus in calves

Necropsy findings

- Congenital cases – cranium enlarged, soft
- Ventricles distended, cerebrospinal fluid under pressure
- Cerebral tissue thin

Diagnosis

Resembles:

Congenital
- Hydranencephaly
- Hypovitaminosis A in piglets
- Toxoplasmosis

Acquired
- Encephalitis
- Encephalomalacia
- Hepatic encephalopathy

ENCEPHALITIS [VM8 p. 484]

Includes **encephalomyelitis**

Etiology

Most are caused by viruses

All species
- Toxoplasmosis
- Sarcocystosis
- Viruses of:
  - Rabies
  - Pseudorabies
  - Japanese B encephalitis
- Bacterial infections in neonates

Cattle
♦ Bacteria:
  • *Listeria* spp.
  • *Haemophilus* spp.
  • *Cowdria ruminantium* – heartwater
  • Mixed infections or *Clostridium* spp. after calf dehorning
♦ Viruses of:
  • Bovine malignant catarrh
  • Sporadic bovine encephalomyelitis
  • Bovine spongiform encephalopathy due to scrapie virus
  • Bovine herpes virus

Sheep
♦ Viruses of:
  • Louping-ill
  • Scrapie
  • Visna
♦ Idiopathic meningoencephalitis

Goats
♦ Caprine arthritis/encephalitis

Pigs
♦ Bacterial systemic infections with:
  • *Salmonella* spp.
  • *Erysipelas* spp.
  • *Listeria monocytogenes* rarely
♦ Viruses of:
  • Hog cholera
  • African swine fever
  • Swine vesicular disease
  • Encephalomyocarditis
  • Hemagglutinating encephalomyelitis virus
  • Porcine encephalomyelitis virus

Horses
♦ Viruses of:
  • Infectious equine encephalomyelitis
  • Borna disease
  • Near eastern equine encephalomyelitis
  • West Nile equine encephalomyelitis
  • Equine herpesvirus
  • Equine infectious anemia
  • Louping-ill, rarely
♦ Protozoal encephalomyelitis
♦ *Strongylus* spp. larval migration

Clinical findings

Most encephalitides have an acute course. Chronic diseases, e.g. scrapie and bovine spongiform encephalopathy, have a much longer course but may show the same symptomatology but over a greatly extended period (months).

Initial signs of excitation occur in some cases, some diseases:
♦ Sudden onset, short course
♦ Maniacal bouts in some
♦ Easily startled
♦ Hypersensitive to stimuli, hyperesthesia, paresthesia
♦ Aggression
♦ Bellowing, neighing
♦ Self-mutilation, nibbling, fleece-pulling
♦ Convulsions with tremor, nystagmus, jaw champing, frothy salivation
♦ Blindness
♦ Aimless wandering, compulsive walking, head-pressing
♦ Leaning or propping head on object
♦ Circling
♦ Ataxia
♦ Fever
♦ Anorexia
♦ Depression
♦ Tachycardia

Later signs of function loss:
♦ Drooling saliva (pharyngeal paralysis)
♦ Feed hangs from mouth
♦ Limb knuckling
♦ Ataxia, recumbency
♦ Circling
♦ Ascending paralysis, commencing in hind limbs

Residual signs, usually only in bacterial infections:
♦ Head rotation
♦ Facial paralysis

Diseases not truly neurotropic show other signs pathognomonic of the disease, e.g.:
♦ Mucosal erosions in bovine malignant catarrh
♦ Respiratory signs in equine herpesvirus-1 infection

Clinical pathology

♦ Used extensively but mostly specific to the individual disease, including:
♦ Complete hemogram, total biochemical profile in horses
♦ Acute-convalescent sera if specific infectious disease suspected
♦ Microbiological, cytological, chemical examination of cerebrospinal fluid recommended to aid differentiation

Necropsy findings

♦ In many encephalitides no macroscopic lesions, other than those in other systems, characteristic of the specific disease
♦ Hemorrhagic necrosis visible in some bacterial meningoencephalitides
♦ Most viral diseases have no gross lesions; necropsy activity limited to collecting specimens for histopathology, transmission experiments

Diagnosis

Resembles:
♦ Encephalomalacia
♦ Meningitis
♦ Brain edema
♦ Increased intracranial pressure
♦ Focal space-occupying lesions of brain
♦ Salt poisoning
♦ Lead poisoning
♦ Rotenone poisoning
♦ Chlorinated hydrocarbon poisoning
♦ Hypoglycemia

Treatment

♦ Supportive treatment, intravenous fluid, electrolytes or alimentary feeding during acute phase
♦ Sedation to avoid self-injury

ENCEPHALOMALACIA [VM8 p. 486]

Etiology

All species
♦ hepatic encephalopathy
♦ Organic mercurial poisoning
♦ Lead poisoning, some cases
♦ Selenium poisoning, possibly
♦ Prolonged parturition, principally in calves

Cattle
♦ Plant poisoning – Astragalus, Oxytropis, Swainsona, Vicia spp., Kochia scoparia
♦ Polioencephalomalacia
♦ Lysosomal storage diseases:
  • Mannosidosis
  • Gangliosidosis
  • Progressive ataxia, Charolais
♦ Hypomyelinogenesis congenita due to in utero infection with bovine virus diarrhea virus
♦ Weavers in Brown Swiss
♦ Ammoniated forage poisoning

Sheep
♦ Plant poisoning – Astragalus, Oxytropis, Swainsona, Vicia spp., Kochia scoparia
♦ Polioencephalomalacia
♦ Focal symmetrical encephalomalacia
♦ Nutritional deficiency copper:
  • Enzootic ataxia
  • Swayback
♦ Globoid cell leukodystrophy
♦ Idiopathic bilateral multifocal cerebrospinal poliomalacia [VM8 p. 486]
♦ Congenital hypomyelinogenesis, dysmyelinogenesis in lambs (hairy shakers) due to in utero infection with border disease virus

Horses
♦ Fumonisin poisoning (Fusarium moniliforme on moldy corn)
♦ Sesquiterpene lactone poisoning (Centaurea solstitialis)
♦ Thiamin deficiency induced by ptaquiloside (Pteridium, Equisetum spp.) poisoning
♦ Neonatal maladjustment syndrome
♦ Equine degenerative myeloencephalopathy

Pigs
♦ Mulberry heart disease
♦ Subclinical enterotoxemia similar to gut edema
♦ Organic arsenical poisoning
♦ Salt poisoning
♦ Cerebrovascular disorders comparable with those in man; minor importance
♦ Congenital hypomyelinogenesis (myoclonia congenita) due in some cases to in utero infection with hog cholera virus

Clinical findings

♦ Initial excitation phase in some diseases, e.g. polioencephalomalacia:
  • Tremor
  • Opisthotonus
  • Nystagmus
  • Convulsions
♦ Then prolonged function loss phase:
  • Dullness, somnolence
  • Blindness
  • Stumbling gait
  • Head pressing
  • Circling
  • Coma terminally, or
  • Long period of imbecility with no change

Clinical pathology

The only findings are those of the specific disease.

Necropsy findings

Softening, cavitation, laminar necrosis varying between specific diseases.

Diagnosis

Resembles:
- Encephalitis
- Hypovitaminosis A
- Carbohydrate engorgement of ruminants
- pregnancy toxemia

Treatment

Prognosis is negative in most cases. Early treatment in polioencephalomalacia may result in complete recovery.

TRAUMATIC INJURY TO THE
BRAIN [VM8 p. 487]

Etiology

- Direct trauma to head in:
  - Accidental collisions, e.g. gate posts
  - Rearing forwards
  - Rearing and falling backwards
  - Hot iron debudding in young ruminants
- Violent extension or flexion of head—neck articulation in fall, excessive pull on halter shank:
  - Pulling back when tethered
  - Extricated from bog, river, or sump by tractor pulling on halter
- Parasitic larval migration (cerebral or cerebrospinal nematodiasis)
  - *Micronema deletrix*
  - *Setaria* spp.
  - *Parelaphostrongylus tenuis*
  - *Draschia megastoma*
  - *Strongylus vulgaris*
  - *Angiostrongylus cantonensis*
- Parasitic insect larval migration
  - *Hypoderma bovis*
  - *Oestrus ovis*
- Brain injury during parturition
- Spontaneous hemorrhage rare; recorded as multiple small hemorrhages in medulla and brainstem in cows at parturition
- Electrical current in lightning strike, electrocution

Clinical findings

- Initial nervous shock including:
  - Falling unconscious
  - Transient clonic convulsion in some
- Fails to recover or does so in minutes to hours
- Pupil dilation
- Pupillary light reflex absent
- Menace reflex absent
- Slow, irregular respiration
- May be bleeding from nose, ears
- Bone fracture, e.g. periorbital, forehead visible

Residual defects include:
- Blindness
- Nystagmus
- Hemiplegia
- Quadriplegia
- Traumatic epilepsy
- Head rotation, circling
- Falling backwards
- Bleeding into guttural pouches, retropharyngeal tissues causing asphyxia

Special traumatic cases
Petrous temporal bone fracture:
- From rearing, falling backwards, rarely stress fracture with no fall
- Facial, vestibular nerves damaged
- May be unable to stand due to lack of balance
- Head rotated, damaged side down
- Nystagmus early
- Ear, eyelid, lip on affected side paralyzed, sag
- Ataxia, falls easily
- Permanent recovery unusual; patient improves by adaptation to defect

Basisphenoid and/or basioccipital, midline facial bone fracture Bone fragments damage large vessels in area causing fatal hemorrhage

Cerebral nematodiasis Acute or chronic onset of:
- Incoordination
- Dysmetria
- Leaning
- Head-pressing
- Intermittent clonic convulsions
- Blindness, uni- or bilateral
- Cranial nerves, uni- or bilateral paralysis

Clinical pathology

- Cerebrospinal fluid may contain erythrocytes, heme pigments
- Eosinophils or hypersegmented neutrophils suggests parasitic invasion

Necropsy findings

Gross hemorrhagic lesion, *or* only histological lesion.

Diagnosis

Resembles:
* Encephalitis
* Encephalomalacia
* Meningitis
* Brain edema
* Increased intracranial pressure
* Focal space-occupying lesions of brain
* Salt poisoning
* Lead poisoning
* Rotenone poisoning
* Chlorinated hydrocarbon poisoning
* Hypoglycemia

Treatment

* Patients recovering within a few hours need no treatment
* Coma persisting more than 6 hours prognosis unfavorable
* Brain decompression with intravenous hypertonic fluid followed by corticosteroids (p. 201) may be used

BRAIN ABSCESS [VM8 p. 489]

Etiology

* Hematogenous spread from lesions in other organs in:
  * Glanders
  * Strangles
  * Tuberculosis
  * Actinomycosis
  * *Fusobacterium necrophorum*
  * Melioidosis
  * Tick pyemia
  * Cryptococcosis
* Local spread from:
  * Oropharynx, e.g. listeriosis
  * Abscesses of pituitary gland or *rete mirabile* from local lesion, e.g. nasal septal nose-ringing abscess
  * Dehorning abscess
  * Otitis media

Clinical findings

* Depression
* Clumsy movements
* Head-pressing
* Blindness, uni- or bilateral, in some
* Unequal pupil size
* Nystagmus in some
* Transient attacks of:
  * Restlessness, excitement
  * Frenzy

* Convulsions
* Temperature normal or mild fever
* Localizing signs in some include:
  * Cerebellar ataxia
  * Head deviation
  * Circling, falling
  * Hemiplegia
  * Paralysis of individual or groups of cranial nerves, some unilaterally

Special lesions include:
* Acute necrotizing, hemorrhagic encephalitis of cerebral cortex caused by *Clostridium* spp. with death in 48 hours, after dehorning
* Pituitary gland abscess in 2–5 year old cattle. Signs include:
* Depression
* Bradycardia in 50% of cases
* Wide-based stance
* Head and neck extended
* Ataxia
* Unable to chew or swallow, dropped jaw, drools saliva
* Blindness
* Pupillary light reflex absent
* Strabismus
* Head tilt in some
* Facial paralysis in some
* Tongue paralysis in some
* Terminally nystagmus, balance deficit, recumbency, opisthotonus

Clinical pathology

* Cerebrospinal fluid may contain leukocytes, protein, bacteria
* Drug sensitivity of causative bacteria detectable
* Leukocytosis with left shift in some cases

Necropsy findings

* Peripheral abscesses accompanied by meningitis
* Deep abscesses may extend to lateral ventricles causing diffuse ependymitis
* Microabscesses visible only microscopically
* Primary lesion may be located in other organ

Diagnosis

Resembles:
* encephalitis
* Tumor
* Parasitic larval migration

- Otitis media
- Polioencephalomalacia

Treatment

Prolonged parenteral treatment with broad-spectrum antibiotic used but prognosis poor.

NEOPLASMS OF THE BRAIN [VM8 p. 491]

Etiology

- Equine cholesteatoma, an aggregation of cholesterol causing granuloma in choroid plexus of lateral ventricles
- Bovine viral leukosis
- Pituitary carcinoma, neuroblastoma in cattle
- Meningeal tumors in cattle

Clinical findings

- Dullness
- Head-pressing
- Ataxia
- Bouts of restlessness, frenzy, sometimes precipitated by rapid movement of head; patient may be normal between bouts
- Localizing signs in some cases including
  - Head deviation, circling
  - Loss of balance, fall easily
  - Diabetes insipidus
  - Cushings syndrome
- Terminal recumbency, opisthotonus, nystagmus, convulsions

Clinical pathology

No positive indicators available.

Necropsy findings

Deep-seated lesions may be found only after fixation and careful sectioning.

Diagnosis

Resembles:
- Brain abscess
- Brain trauma
- Any other space-occupying lesion

Treatment

Surgical excision unlikely to be attempted.

COENUROSIS (GID, STURDY) [VM8 p. 492]

Etiology

Taenia multiceps, the tapeworm of canidae, passes eggs in its feces; embryos from the eggs ingested by sheep, invade the brain, spinal cord, via the bloodstream, developing into the coenurid stage (*Coenurus cerebralis*).

Clinical findings

Larval migration stage
- Blindness
- Nystagmus
- Frenzy
- Ataxia
- Muscle tremor
- Collapse

Acute stage of coenurus irritation
- Wild expression
- Salivation
- Frenzy
- Convulsions
- Deviation head, eyes

Chronic stage of coenurus irritation
- Blindness, partial or complete, usually in one eye
- Dullness
- Clumsiness
- Ataxia
- Head-pressing
- Incomplete mastication
- Periodic convulsions
- Papilledema in some
- Localizing signs include
  - Head deviation with circling
  - Head rotation
  - Local skull softening in young; may rupture
- Death after several months

Spinal cord lesions
Gradual onset of paresis, recumbency.

Clinical pathology

- Serological tests to identify *C. cerebralis* not yet commercially available
- Radiological examination may identify exact location of cyst

Necropsy findings

♦ Thin-walled cysts mostly on external surface of cerebrum; in cord at cervical or lumbar sites
♦ Local pressure atrophy of nervous tissue, softening of overlying bone

Diagnosis

Resembles:
♦ Brain abscess
♦ Brain tumor
♦ Brain trauma, hemorrhage
♦ Encephalitis, in early stages

Treatment and control

♦ Surgical drainage allows salvage
♦ Excision can achieve recovery

OTITIS MEDIA/INTERNA [VM8 p. 493]

Etiology and pathogenesis

♦ Mostly young (1–4 weeks old) animals, all species
♦ Infection usually hematogenous, may be from otitis externa

Clinical findings

♦ Head rotation
♦ Facial paralysis on down side
♦ Falls easily; falls to affected side

Necropsy findings

Tympanic bullae contain pus

Diagnosis

Resembles:
♦ Otitis externa with head-shaking and transient rotating of head, pawing at ear, exudate, offensive smell in ear cavity
♦ Brain abscess
♦ Brain injury
♦ Spinal cord, cervical, injury

Treatment

Prolonged parenteral treatment with broad-spectrum antibacterial; poor prognosis for complete recovery; progress of disease may be halted.

MENINGITIS [VM8 p. 493]

Etiology

All species
Deriving from omphalophlebitis or septicemia in very young. Often accompanied by arthritis, endocarditis, panophthalmitis. Common infections are:
♦ Calves – *Escherichia coli*
♦ Lambs – *Streptococcus zooepidemicus*
♦ Piglets – *Streptococcus zooepidemicus, S. suis* type 2

Cattle
♦ Bovine malignant catarrh
♦ Sporadic bovine encephalomyelitis
♦ Listeriosis
♦ Haemophilus somnus infection
♦ Leptospirosis
♦ Tuberculosis, rarely

Sheep
♦ Melioidosis
♦ Tick pyemia, in neonate lambs
♦ *Pasteurella multocida, P. hemolytica,* lambs

Pigs
♦ Glasser's disease
♦ Erysipelas
♦ Salmonellosis
♦ *Streptococcus suis* type 2, weaned, feeder pigs

Horses
♦ Strangles
♦ *Pasteurella haemolytica* infection

Clinical findings

♦ Anorexia
♦ Sudden onset
♦ Fever
♦ Respiration slow, deep, sometimes phasic
♦ Toxemia, vomiting in pig
♦ Mania, frenzy early in some
♦ Cutaneous hyperesthesia, light touch causes pain in some
♦ Blindness in some
♦ Trismus
♦ Opisthotonus
♦ Rigidity of neck and back
♦ Tonic neck spasms causing head retraction
♦ Tremor
♦ Convulsions
♦ Most die

Terminally
♦ Recumbency
♦ Depression, coma

Neonates
♦ Accompanying omphalitis
♦ Ophthalmitis with hypopyon

Clinical pathology

♦ Cerebrospinal fluid (csf) has:
  • Elevated protein level
  • High cell count
  • Bacteria; sensitivity determination critical because of low antibacterial levels in csf
♦ Severe leukocytosis, left shift in hemogram

Diagnosis

Resembles:
♦ Encephalitis
♦ Brain edema
♦ Spinal cord compression

Treatment

♦ High doses parenterally of broad-spectrum antibacterial
♦ Penicillin–streptomycin combination, potentiated sulfonamides (with or without gentamicin) widely used
♦ Third-generation cephalosporins likely to be highly effective

TOXIC AND METABOLIC ENCEPHALOMYELOPATHIES AND NEUROPATHIES [VM8 p. 495]

♦ Poisons and metabolic diseases which cause:
  • Nervous dysfunction
  • Without detectable lesions
♦ Those causing lesions listed in encephalomalacia

  • Chlorinated hydrocarbons, organophosphates, carbamates insecticides
  • Propylene glycol
  • Metaldehyde
  • Strychnine

Abnormalities of consciousness and behavior
♦ Hypoglycemia and ketosis (some degenerative lesions in hypoglycemia)
♦ Metabolic acidosis, causing depression
♦ Hypomagnesemia – tetany
♦ Hyperammonemia of hepatic insufficiency – hepatic encephalopathy
♦ Uremia – depression, coma
♦ Chlorinated hydrocarbons – unconsciousness·
♦ Plants containing cyanide, nitrate – histotoxic hypoxia
♦ Poisonous plants (*Helichrysum, Pennisetum, Descurainia, Dryopteris, Stypandra* spp.) – range of signs including drowsiness, blindness

Tremor, ataxia, paralysis
♦ Plants – *Conium, Eupatorium, Sarcostemma, Euphorbia, Karwinskia* spp.
♦ bacterial toxins – *Clostridium botulinum,* shaker foal syndrome
♦ Fungal toxins, e.g. *Acremonium* spp.
♦ Agricultural chemicals:
  • Piperazine, levamisole, toluene, carbon tetrachloride, nicotine sulfate – anthelmintics
  • 2,4-D, 2,4,5-T herbicides

Ataxia/paralysis due to proprioceptive defect
♦ *Phalaris* spp.
♦ *Lolium rigidum*
♦ *Echinopogon ovatus*
♦ *Romulea bulbocodium*
♦ *Erythrophloeum* spp.
♦ *Eupatorium* spp.
♦ *Indigophera* spp.
♦ *Xanthorrhea* spp.
♦ *Zamia* spp.

Gait abnormality due to spastic contraction muscle masses
Australian stringhalt – due to the plant *Arctotheca calendula.*

Convulsions
♦ Hypoglycemia
♦ Hypomagnesemia
♦ Nutritional deficiencies:
  • Vitamin A
  • Pyridoxine (experimentally)
♦ Inorganic poisons
  • Lead
  • Mercury
  • Organic arsenicals
  • Organophosphates
  • Chlorinated hydrocarbons

- Strychnine
- Urea
- Metaldehyde
♦ Bacterial toxins:
  - *Clostridium tetani*
  - *Clostridium perfringens* type D
♦ Fungal toxins:
  - *Claviceps* spp.

- *Acremonium* spp.
♦ Plant toxins in:
  - *Echinopogon ovatus*
  - *Pennisetum* spp. (or fungal or caterpillar toxin)
  - *Lupinus* spp.
  - *Oenanthe* spp.
  - *Cicuta* spp. and many others

PSYCHOSES OR NEUROSES

CRIB-BITING [VM8 p. 496]

Signs include:

♦ Horse grasps feed box rim or other solid object with teeth, arches neck, pulls up and back, gulps air with loud grunt
♦ Variant is the same routine but resting teeth or chin on the object without grasping it
♦ Habitual crib biting causes:
  - Incisor teeth wear
  - Flatulence, colic
♦ Resembles:
  - Wood chewing due to boredom
  - Pica due to nutritional deficiency, possibly of fiber

WIND-SUCKING [VM8 p. 496]

Horse repeatedly flexes, arches neck, swallows air with grunting, but does not grasp object.

GRASPING [VM8 p. 496]

Similar vice of perpetually grasping the solid object without swallowing air.

MISCELLANEOUS NEUROTIC VICES [VM8 p. 496]

In horses include:

Kicking – persistent wall-kicking
Pawing – persistent floor-pounding
Circling – walking ceaselessly around the pen in either direction
Weaving – rocking from side to side on the fore feet, swinging head and neck with the movement
Self-mutilation – skin injuries due to repeated biting of itself

FARROWING HYSTERIA IN SOWS [VM8 p. 496]

♦ Commonest in gilts; likely to repeat at subsequent farrowings

♦ Hyperactive, restless
♦ Savage piglets if they come near her head
♦ Piglets killed, not eaten
♦ Control program includes:
  - Sedating sow, removing suckers temporarily
  - Put sow in farrowing place 4–6 days before farrowing to permit settling in
  - Minimize disturbances in farrowing environment
♦ Cull sow

CANNIBALISM IN PIGS [VM8 p. 497]

♦ A problem in intensive pig-rearing units
♦ *Tail-biting* – begins as sucking; spreads as epidemic of biting, eating down to stump; serious sequelae of abscessation
♦ *Ear-biting* – begins as sucking, symmetrical loss of ventral part of ear
♦ *Flank-sucking* – progresses to bite wounds; some outbreaks associated with mange occurrence
♦ *Snout-rubbing* – causes erosions on flanks
♦ Cannibalism due to inadequate total environment including:
  - Large group size
  - Active, restless pigs
  - High pen population density
  - Limited feed supply; strong competition for feed
  - Low protein content in ration
  - Boredom
  - Inadequate ventilation
  - Inadequate temperature
♦ Preventive measures include:
  - Improving environment
  - Docking tails
  - Clipping incisor teeth was used at one time but is no longer favored

EPILEPSY [VM8 p. 497]

Very rare in farm animals. Occurs in:

♦ Inherited in Brown Swiss cattle
♦ Due to residual lesion after encephalitis

Clinical signs include:

♦ Recurrent, infrequent convulsive episodes
♦ Some preceded by local sign, e.g. tremor of one limb
♦ Initial period of alertness followed by general tetany, patient falls, loses consciousness, clonic convulsion, with paddling, jaw champing, opisthotonus
♦ Relaxation period, patient regains consciousness

DISEASES OF THE SPINAL CORD

TRAUMATIC INJURY [VM8 p. 498]

Etiology

External injury
♦ Falling through barn floor
♦ Falling off vehicle
♦ Spontaneous in osteoporotic patients
♦ Spontaneous fracture of spondylotic thoracolumbar vertebra in aged bull during mating
♦ Excessive mobility upper cervical vertebrae in wobbles in horses
♦ Dislocation atlanto-occipital joint
♦ Cervical vertebral canal stenosis in young rams; due possibly to head butting
♦ Fracture T1 vertebra, calves turning violently in narrow alley
♦ Neonates due to forced traction during difficult birth
♦ Lightning stroke causing tissue damage in vertebral canal
♦ Spontaneous vertebral body fracture in presence of pre-existing necrotic condition, e.g vertebral body abscess

Parasite invasion
♦ Cerebrospinal nematodiasis in sheep and goats, due to:
  • *Parelaphostrongylus tenuis*
  • *Setaria* spp.
♦ *Toxocara canis* in pigs
♦ *Strongylus vulgaris* in horses and donkeys
♦ *Hypoderma bovis* larvae in cattle

Local ischemia
♦ Embolism in cord, including fibrocartilaginous embolism in pigs
♦ Caudal vena caval compression reducing drainage, e.g. in horses during prolonged dorsal recumbency for surgery

Clinical findings

Severe trauma
♦ Immediate spinal shock includes:
  • Flaccid paralysis caudally
  • Local sweating
  • Stretch, flexor reflexes, cutaneous sensitivity disappear
♦ Return of reflexes but not muscle tone in 1–2 hours but:
  • Unable to rise; sternal (thoracolumbar injury) or lateral (cervical injury) recumbency
  • Eventual flaccid paralysis, absence of reflexes, wasting in areas supplied from damaged cord segments
♦ Skeletal abnormalities include:
  • Excessive mobility of vertebrae
  • Pain on pressure
  • Spinous process malalignment
  • Radiographically visible displacements, fractures
♦ Sequels include:
  • Stumbling gait, toe scuffing, knuckling, inability to mount
  • Torticollis, humped back, neck deformity

Acute compression without transection
Return to normal and able to stand in 3 weeks

Parasite larvae invasion
♦ As for acute trauma above, but
♦ No spinal shock
♦ Further increments of function loss may occur

Gradual compression
♦ Gradual onset of staggering gait, difficulty rising, recumbency
♦ Radiographically visible vertebral exostoses

Cervical fracture/dislocation horse
♦ Lateral recumbency
♦ Unable to lift head from ground in cranial lesions, can lift head but not shoulders in caudal cervical lesions
♦ Conscious, able to drink and eat
♦ Tendon, withdrawal reflexes strong

Spondylosis in bulls
After vigorous ejaculation by aged bull, often in artificial insemination center, fracture of ossified ventral vertebral ligament, associ-

ated vertebral body with subsequent minor displacement and compression of cord causes:

♦ Immediate recumbency for some days then standing in some
♦ Arched back
♦ Slow, stiff gait with trunk rigid
♦ Unilateral hind limb lameness in some

Clinical pathology

Radiological examination may indicate site, nature of injury, and compression.

Necropsy findings

♦ Lesion visible macroscopically but may require longitudinal section for clear observation
♦ Acute cases, especially calves with traction injury, hemorrhages around kidneys, in perivertebral muscles, rib fractures

Diagnosis

Resembles:
♦ Myelitis
♦ Meningitis
♦ Azoturia in horses
♦ Enzootic muscular dystrophy
♦ Peripheral nerve injury, e.g. in cows at parturition

Treatment

Where prognosis reasonable good nursing including avoidance of compression sores and ischemic myopathy includes:
♦ Slinging in horses and to a lesser extent, in cows
♦ Periodic slinging, in a hip sling, for brief periods (30 minutes) combined with recumbency nursing is a practicable procedure for periods up to 3 weeks in cows
♦ Problem animals are uncooperative, overweight, flighty
♦ Deep bedding with good footing
♦ Frequent turning from side to side

SPINAL CORD COMPRESSION
[VM8 p. 500]

Etiology

Tumors
♦ Lymphomatosis is the common neoplasm
♦ Rare tumors, e.g. fibrosarcomas, plasma cell myelomas

Abscesses
♦ Vertebral body abscess associated with chronic suppurative lesion elsewhere in body
♦ Hematogenous spread of *Corynebacterium pseudotuberculosis, Actinomyces pyogenes*
♦ Epidural abscesses

Bony lesions
♦ Exostosis over non-displaced vertebral body fracture
♦ Vertebral body exostoses in lambs grazing near old lead mines
♦ Hypovitaminosis A in young pigs causing compression of peripheral nerves passing through vertebral foraminae
♦ Congenital deformity atlanto-occipito-axial joints
♦ Congenital spinal stenosis in calves
♦ Intervertebral disk protrusion, diskospondylitis of horses
♦ Intervertebral disk degeneration with vertebral osteophytes in pigs cause lameness rather than paralysis

Equine ataxia
(See also equine enzootic ataxia.) Compressive lesions in equine ataxia include:
♦ Non-fatal skull fractures; basisphenoid, basioccipital, petrous temporal bones
♦ Non-fatal cervical vertebral fractures
♦ Atlanto-occipital instability
♦ Stenosis of cranial vertebral orifice C3–C7
♦ Abnormal growth interarticular surfaces
♦ Dorsal enlargement of caudal vertebral epiphyses, bulging of intervertebral disks
♦ Formation, protrusion false joint capsules, extrasynovial bursae
♦ Spinal abscess, usually intervertebral body
♦ Meningeal tumors

Clinical findings

♦ Congenital defects manifested by stumbling gait or recumbency at birth
♦ With acquired lesions signs develop during a course as short as 4 days
♦ Local pain may be first sign, pain on passive movement or palpation
♦ Difficulty rising first motor sign
♦ Stumbling gait
♦ Toes drag while walking
♦ Fetlock knuckles at rest
♦ Recumbency
  • With thoracolumbar cord lesions sternal recumbency, with assumption of dog-sitting position in a few cases

- With caudal cervical lesions lateral recumbency able to lift head
- With cranial cervical lesions lateral recumbency unable to lift head
♦ In recumbent animal, paralysis of affected limbs may be spastic or flaccid depending on exact location of lesion and tracts involved; degree of paralysis also variable; the cow which is unable to rise usually has sufficient limb muscle tone to move limbs vigorously

Wobbler horse (see p. 672)

Clinical pathology

♦ Myelography will help locate lesion, identify its nature and magnitude
♦ Cerebrospinal fluid may contain inflammatory or neoplastic cells

Necropsy findings

♦ Gross abnormalities of vertebrae or cord easily seen
♦ Degenerative lesions of spinal cord often not obvious

Diagnosis

Resembles:
♦ Myelitis
♦ Myelomalacia
♦ Spinal meningitis
♦ Congenital spinal cord defects
♦ Polyradiculoneuritis
♦ Generalized peripheral nerve degeneration
♦ Back muscle sprain, dorsal spinous process injury, spondylosis
♦ tying-up

Treatment

♦ Surgical relief of many equine problems in this area is now possible
♦ Treatment is not usually undertaken in farm animals

MYELITIS [VM8 p. 502]

Etiology

♦ Usually part of an encephalomyelitis dominated by the encephalitis

♦ Diseases in which the signs of myelitis may dominate those of encephalitis are:
♦ Listeriosis in sheep
♦ Equine protozoal myeloencephalitis
♦ Cauda equina neuritis

Clinical findings

♦ Hyperesthesia, paresthesia, and paralysis
♦ Most cases recumbent
♦ Bright, alert, and able to eat

MYELOMALACIA [VM8 p. 503]

Etiology

♦ Rarely a separate entity from encephalomalacia
♦ Diseases in which myelitis dominates or is a separate entity include:
  - Focal spinal poliomalacia in sheep
  - Enzootic ataxia; lesions often restricted to spinal cord
  - Caprine arthritis/encephalitis in young goats
  - Sorghum cystitis/ataxia in horses
  - 3-nitro-4-hydroxyphenylarsonic acid poisoning in pigs
  - Selenium poisoning in ruminants
  - Zamia spp. poisoning
  - Inherited ovine degenerative axonopathy (Murrurrundi disease)
  - Equine degenerative myeloencephalopathy

Clinical findings

Syndrome includes paralysis without cerebral signs.

Diagnosis

Resembles:
♦ myelitis
♦ Spinal cord compression by space-occupying lesions of vertebral canal, cervical vertebral malformations and articulations

CONGENITAL DEFECTS OF THE CENTRAL NERVOUS SYSTEM

DEFECTS WITH OBVIOUS
STRUCTURAL ERRORS [VM8 p. 504]

◆ Hydrocephalus with cranial enlargement, some inherited
◆ Meningocele, inherited in some pigs
◆ Hydrocephalus with spina bifida – the **Arnold—Chiari syndrome** in cattle
◆ Hydrocephalus with achondroplasia – Bulldog calves
◆ Cranium bifidum in pigs, some with meningocele
◆ Microphthalmia
◆ Exophthalmos, with or without strabismus in Jersey, Shorthorn cattle
◆ Neurofibroma in cattle; enlargements on peripheral nerves
◆ Hydranencephaly – in ruminants, intra-uterine infection with Akabane virus
◆ Porencephaly – in ruminants with intra-uterine infection bluetongue, Wesselbrons viruses
◆ Spina bifida with skin defect – calves born alive, flexion, contracture, muscle atrophy hind limbs
◆ Congenital spinal stenosis, calves

DISEASES CHARACTERIZED BY
CONGENITAL PARESIS/PARALYSIS

◆ Enzootic ataxia
◆ Inherited congenital posterior paralysis
◆ Spinal dysraphism – Charolais, Angus
◆ Syringomyelia
◆ Hydromyelia
◆ Atlanto-occipital dysplasia – foals, tetra-paresis, tetraplegia, head deviation, ataxia, clicking sound on passive movement. Also Angora goats, Devon calves

DISEASES CHARACTERIZED BY
CEREBELLAR ATAXIA

◆ Inherited cerebellar hypoplasia, all species
◆ Cerebellar hypoplasia and hypomyelinogenesis of calves due to bovine virus disease virus
◆ Cerebellar hypoplasia of piglets due to hog cholera virus
◆ Familial convulsions, ataxia in Angus cattle
◆ Mannosidosis in cattle, goats
◆ Intracranial hemorrhage in foals – in neonatal adjustment syndrome
◆ Spinal cord hypoplasia in ruminants, in Akabane virus infection

DISEASES CHARACTERIZED BY
TREMOR

◆ Congenital paresis/tremor piglets
◆ Inherited congenital spasms in cattle
◆ Inherited neonatal spasticity in Jersey and Hereford calves
◆ Border disease in lambs
◆ Inherited myoclonus in Hereford calves
◆ Myoclonia congenita in piglets due to hog cholera and Aujeszkys disease viruses
◆ Hydranencephaly, porencephaly, calves infected in utero with bovine virus diarrhea virus – tremor with rigidity
◆ Shaker calves

NEUROGENIC ARTHROGRYPOSIS,
MUSCLE ATROPHY

Akabane virus in utero infection in all ruminants

MUSCLE MASSES SPASMS

◆ Inherited spastic paresis (Elso-heel)
◆ Inherited periodic spasticity (stall cramp)

CONVULSIONS

◆ Brain injury during birth
◆ Brain compression due to hypovitaminosis A in pigs and calves
◆ Neonatal adjustment syndrome in foals
◆ Congenital toxoplasmosis
◆ Inherited idiopathic epilepsy in Brown Swiss
◆ Familial convulsions/ataxia in Angus calves
◆ Doddler calves

IMBECILITY

◆ Microcephaly, possibly inherited, calves; cranium normal size, cerebrum, cerebellum, brainstem small, corpus callosum, fornix absent
◆ Microcephaly, lambs; many dead at birth, survivors incoordinate, recumbent, blind, tremor
◆ Anencephaly, calves; cerebrum and midbrain absent
◆ Hydranencephaly, ruminants; in utero Akabane virus infection
◆ Porencephaly, lambs; in utero infection bluetongue virus

EYE DEFECTS

- Sporadic cases microphthalmia, anophthalmia in calves
- Congenital lenticular cataracts in calves and lambs
- Blindness after birth in gangliosidosis in cattle; ceroid lipofuscinosis in sheep
- Optic nerve constriction due to hypovitaminosis A
- Optic nerve constriction in calves; in utero infection bovine virus diarrhea virus
- Inherited exophthalmos and strabismus
- Familial undulatory nystagmus

13 DISEASES OF THE MUSCULOSKELETAL SYSTEM

Diseases of the organs of support and loco-motion, the muscles, bones and joints, should be suspected when there are one or more of the following:

♦ Lameness
♦ Failure of bodily support
♦ Insufficiency of movement, reduced or excessive
♦ Deformity
♦ Posture abnormality

Many clinical signs referable to the musculoskeletal system are also characteristic of the nervous system and are described in Chapter 12, e.g. falling easily, fetlock knuckled, hoof dragged, walking on hoof, incoordination, stiff gait, stumbling gait, rising with difficulty, recumbency.

CLINICAL INDICANTS

The principal clinical signs, clinicopathological findings and special examination techniques on which clinical diagnoses of musculoskeletal disease are based include the following.

Abdomen ventral wall swollen

Clinical findings Thickening, pits on pressure, of ventral abdominal wall reaching from sternum to udder; bad cases reach from brisket to vulva.

Occurs in:
♦ Urethral perforation
♦ Congestive heart failure
♦ Udder edema
♦ Other causes of anasarca
♦ Late pregnancy

Abdomen ventral wall sunken

Clinical findings Wall dropped to well below normal level; may be unilateral; some local edema, hemorrhage.

Occurs in Ventral abdominal hernia.

Arthrocentesis

Fluid from joint cavity obtained by needle aspiration can provide information about synovial fluid content of cells, infectious agents, chemical constituents.

Arthroscopic abnormality

Endoscopic examination of joint cavities, articular surfaces reveals actual site, nature of lesion. Biopsy specimens from synovial membrane can be retrieved.

Back arched

Clinical findings:
♦ Back arched upward, head held low
♦ Other signs of subacute abdominal pain

Occurs in:
♦ Subacute abdominal pain, e.g. traumatic reticuloperitonitis cattle
♦ Moderate pain in all four limbs, e.g. osteodystrophia fibrosa, horse
♦ Back pain in bovine spondylosis

Back pain elicited

Clinical findings:
♦ Horse lame when ridden, especially heavy rider
♦ Pain on manual pressure on back

Occurs in:
♦ Spondylosis
♦ Dorsal spinous process injury
♦ Muscle sprain

Blood biochemistry

♦ Serum levels of muscle enzymes
  • Creatine kinase
  • Glutamic oxaloacetic transaminase (SGOT)
elevated where recent muscle breakdown has occurred
♦ Serum levels of calcium, phosphorus, alkaline phosphatase can give some information about state of bone metabolism

Body weight low

Clinical findings:
♦ Condition score 2.5–3.5 out of a possible of 8 = **poor condition**
♦ Condition score less than 2.5 out of a possible of 8 = **emaciated**

Occurs in:
♦ Starvation
♦ Inanition
♦ All diseases in which food intake is reduced in the presence of an adequate supply

Bone deformity, limb

Clinical findings:
♦ Any deformity from normal size, shape of bones
♦ Mostly limb bones, includes pelvic collapse

Occurs in:
♦ Congenital skeletal deformity, absence
♦ Rickets
♦ Bent-leg
♦ Marie's disease

Bone, discharging sinus

Occurs in:
♦ Osteomyelitis
♦ Bone sequestrum

Bone pain

Clinical findings:
Pain on palpation, manipulation in:

Occurs in:
♦ Osteomyelitis
♦ Neoplasm
♦ Traumatic injury

Bones soft

Clinical findings:
♦ Frontal bone bends on digital pressure
♦ Easy fracture

Occurs in:
♦ Osteomalacia
♦ Rickets

Brisket swollen

Occurs in:
♦ Anasarca
♦ Hematoma due to injury by feeder edge

Bursa inflamed

Clinical findings:
Fluid-filled, some painful, sac-like swelling.

Occurs in:
♦ Carpal hygroma, cattle, *Brucella abortus*
♦ Fistulous wither, horse, *Brucella abortus*

Condition poor

See body weight low, this section.

Conformation – asymmetrical

♦ Front-to-back – hyena disease
♦ Side-to-side – asymmetric hindquarters

Conformation – dwarf

♦ Congenital skeletal deformity:
  • Inherited miniature calves
  • Inherited achondroplastic dwarfs
  • Inherited osteopetrosis
♦ Nutritional deficiency of manganese
♦ Acorn calves

Conformation – giant

Not recorded. Fetal giants occur in prolonged gestation are stillborn and not likely to maintain their giant status after birth.

Coronet skin lesion (coronitis)

Clinical findings:
♦ Lameness
♦ Lesions mostly at rear, extending up to back of pastern
♦ Some with horizontal fissures

- Knuckling of fetlock because of pain on extension
- Lesion varies from erosions through vesicles to seborrheic dermatitis
- May resemble oozing of pus from badly under-run wall

Occurs in:
- greasy heel, horses, cattle
- Vesicular diseases, foot and mouth disease, vesicular stomatitis, vesicular swine disease, vesicular exanthema swine, fungal toxin (furocoumarins) poisoning
- Gangrene in *Claviceps purpurea* poisoning
- Erosive lesions in bovine malignant catarrh, bovine virus diarrhea, ovine bluetongue, caprine pemphigus foliaceous, porcine dermatosis vegetans
- Granulomatous lesions in contagious ecthyma, strawberry footrot
- Ulcerative lesions, ovine ulcerative dermatitis
- Erythema, ovine strongyloidosis
- Congenital skin absence, in epitheliogenesis imperfecta (calves, lambs, piglets), familial acanthosis (cattle), epidermolysis bullosa (cattle, sheep), hereditary junctional mechanobullous disease (calves, lambs, foals), redfoot disease (lambs)

Cranium domed

See skull deformity, this section.

Cyclopian defect

See skull deformity, this section.

Dwarf

See stature.

Elbows abducted

Occurs in:
- Severe dyspnea
- Pleurisy, pericarditis pain
- Winged shoulder in Jersey cows

Emaciation

See body weight low, this section.

Fracture susceptibility increased

Occurs in:
- Osteodystrophia fibrosa in horse and pig
- Rickets
- Osteomalacia
- Nutritional deficiency, copper
- Chronic fluorine poisoning

Hoof deformity

Clinical findings:
- Wall overgrown
- Horizontal ridges
- Concave anterior wall
- Dropped sole
- Vertical cracks

Occurs in:
- Shelly hoof
- Laminitis
- Selenium poisoning
- Hypovitaminosis A

Hoof pain

Clinical findings:
- Hoof lameness
- Pain on squeezing

Occurs in:
- Sole penetration or crack
- Sole under-run with pus or debris
- Wall crack
- Oozing at coronet in some
- Pododermatitis
- Sole abrasion
- Third phalanx (pedal bone) fracture, injury
- Pedal ostitis
- Navicular bone fracture
- Navicular disease
- Tenosynovitis flexor tendons

Hoof (dew claws), sloughing

Clinical findings:
- Separation from sensitive laminae causes severe lameness
- Finally sloughing of hoof wall

Occurs in:
- Limb edema or lymphangitis
- Burn injury from grass fires
- Coronitis as in pemphigus
- Mushroom poisoning
- Terminally in laminitis
- Due to peripheral gangrene of ergotamine poisoning

♦ Selenium poisoning
♦ Familial acantholysis
♦ Bluetongue

Hoof sole under-run

See hoof pain, this section.

Inguinal region swollen

Occurs in:
♦ Inguinal hernia, strangulated hernia
♦ Scirrhous spermatic cord

Interdigital skin lesion

Clinical findings:
♦ Lameness
♦ Necrotic fissure, dermatitis
♦ Papilloma
♦ Fibrous granuloma
♦ Lifting of horn-skin junction without extensive under-running

Occurs in:
♦ Pododermatitis
♦ Ovine footrot
♦ Ovine foot abscess
♦ Ovine interdigital dermatitis
♦ Bovine footrot
♦ Bovine interdigital fibroma
♦ Bovine interdigital papilloma

Joint enlargement

Occurs in:
♦ Arthritis
♦ Rickets
♦ Peripheral osteophytes

Joint creaking, crepitus

Clinical findings:
♦ Lame
♦ Joint creaks while walking, crepitus on passive movement

Occurs in:
♦ Arthritis
♦ Osteoarthritis
♦ Osteodystrophia fibrosa
♦ Round ligament rupture

Joint fixation

Clinical findings:
♦ Joint in permanent fixation; cannot be moved passively
♦ Severe lameness

Occurs in:
♦ Traumatic, infectious ankylosis
♦ Congenital fixation (congenital articular rigidity)
  • Inherited ankylosis
  • Inherited arthrogryposis

Joint hot, painful

Occurs in Arthritis.

Joint hypermobility

Occurs in:
♦ Luxation, subluxation
♦ Congenital joint hypermobility cattle Occurs in:
  • Hyperelastosis cutis
  • Ehlers–Danlos syndrome
  • Osteogenesis imperfecta

Joint pain

Clinical findings Pain on palpation, passive movement in –

Occurs in:
♦ Arthritis
♦ Neoplasm
♦ Traumatic injury

Lameness

Clinical findings:
The following material is based largely on the diseases of farm animals, including horses only coincidentally. It does not include a detailed description of lameness in racing horses.
♦ Abnormal gait due to pain or deformity, including contracture, shortness of limb
♦ Disinclined to move
♦ Resting of limb
♦ Pain during support phase indicated by:
  • Short step
  • Body rises on the lame limb; head rises on the lame forelimb, falls on the lame hind
  • Grunting or groaning
♦ Pain during forward advancement of limb causes wider, or narrower, swing of the limb, plus a lifting of the hind quarter
♦ Pain on pressure, passive movement of limb, hoof
♦ Muscle atrophy in chronic cases
♦ Clinical signs in lameness due to **deformity** include:
  • Shortness of step
  • Reduced movement, extension, flexion of limb or part

Occurs in:
♦ Myositis
♦ Osteodystrophy
♦ Osteomyelitis
♦ Arthropathy (osteoarthritis)
♦ Arthritis
♦ Arthrogryposis
♦ tenosynovitis
♦ Cellulitis
♦ Lymphangitis
♦ Bursitis
♦ Pododermatitis
♦ Laminitis
♦ Hoof horn damage, including:
  • Sole abrasion
  • Cracks, penetrations
  • Under-horn bruising
  • Under-horn infection
♦ Coronet dermatitis

Lameness, shifting

Clinical findings:
♦ Lameness shifts between limbs at intervals of few days or weeks
♦ Lameness usually mild

Occurs in Osteodystrophia fibrosa in horses.

Limb action jerky

Clinical findings:
♦ Limb action jerky
♦ Sometimes limb locks into fixed position

Occurs in Joint luxation, subluxation, e.g. patellar luxation.

Limb advanced, crossed

Clinical findings:
♦ Affected limb held out in front of normal position, or across in front of opposite pair
♦ No weight taken

Occurs in:
♦ Severe pain, e.g. distal phalanx fracture

Limb deformity

See bone deformity, joint contracture.

Limb rested

Clinical findings:
♦ Limb held semiflexed
♦ Bears little weight

Occurs in:
♦ Pain in limb
♦ Peripheral nerve paresis, paralysis

Limbs splayed

Clinical findings:
♦ Limbs, usually fore limbs, abducted
♦ Chest and belly on ground

Occurs in:
♦ Pectoral muscle trauma
♦ Congenital splayleg in pigs

Limb weight shifted

Clinical findings Weight continually shifted between opposing limbs.

Occurs in Conditions with pain in all feet, e.g. laminitis.

Meningocele

See skull deformity, this section.

Muscle biopsy

Histopathological and histochemical information available from biopsy. Useful in differentiation of:
♦ Myositis
♦ Myopathy, especially degeneration

Muscle mass abnormal

Clinical findings:
♦ Size of the muscle mass varies from normal, often in same animal. May be:
  • Swollen, hot, painful – myositis, myopathy
  • Small – neurogenic atrophy, congenital arthrogryposis
  • Large – inherited double muscling (myofiber hyperplasia)
  • Asymmetric – idiopathic asymmetric hindquarters in pigs
♦ Muscle rigid – joint contracture

Muscle pain

Clinical findings On palpation in myositis.

Paresis, paralysis

In the absence of indications of neurological deficit plus signs of primary muscle involvement including:
♦ Pain, swelling, hardness of muscle mass

♦ History of trauma, violent effort, prolonged recumbency in one position, obese patient
♦ Elevated serum muscle enzymes (may be secondary changes from neurogenic, ischemic lesion)

Occurs in:
♦ Myasthenia
♦ Myopathy
♦ Myositis

Pelvis abnormality

Deformity in:
♦ Ischial tuberosity fracture
♦ Osteodystrophy
♦ Rickets
♦ Neoplasm

Excessive mobility in Sacroiliac dislocation.

Perineum swelling

Occurs in Udder edema.

Radiographic abnormality

Radiography used extensively to obtain reliable information about musculoskeletal tissues, especially limbs of adults, all tissues in young.

Recumbency

In musculoskeletal conditions, as well as those listed in nervous system diseases, include:
♦ General myaesthenia of toxemia, dehydration, anemia, starvation
♦ Generalized flaccid paralysis, e.g. botulism, milk fever
♦ Multiple joint disease, e.g. polyarthritis, congenital ankylosis, arthrogryposis
♦ Myopathy, downer cow syndrome
♦ Congenital limb defects, e.g. hemimelia, vestigial limbs, reduced phalanges, joint hypermobility, spina bifida
♦ Poisonings, e.g. tick paralysis

Rising with difficulty, this section.

See recumbency, this section.

Scapula protrudes dorsally

Occurs in Pectoral girdle muscles ruptured, paralyzed, degenerate, e.g. enzootic muscular dystrophy:
♦ Part of Jersey winged shoulder defect
♦ Local myopathy

Skull deformity

♦ Congenital skeletal deformity
  • Cranium domed in hydrocephalus
  • Cranium cleft in meningocele
  • Cyclopian defect in inherited prolonged gestation
  • Achondroplastic dwarfism
  • Inherited probatocephaly in cattle
  • Inherited prolonged gestation in Jerseys
  • Inherited cranium bifidum in pigs
  • Inherited craniofacial deformity in lambs
  • Inherited congenital osteopetrosis
♦ Osteodystrophia fibrosa
♦ Atrophic rhinitis

Spinal column rigidity

Occurs in Spondylosis.

Spinal vertebral deformity

Occurs in Spina bifida.

Stance rigid

Clinical findings Neck, limbs, and tail stiff, ears pricked.

Occurs in:
♦ Tetany
♦ Tetanus
♦ Meningitis
♦ Cerebellar disease
♦ Strychnine poisoning

Standing preferred

Clinical findings:
♦ Patient stands for long periods
♦ Evidence of visceral pain in some

Occurs in:
♦ Peritonitis
♦ Pleurisy
♦ Pneumonia

Tail abnormalities

♦ Congenital tail absence, deformity
♦ Anesthesia, paralysis in:
  • Cauda equina neuritis
  • Rabies
♦ Tail rigid in:
  • Tetanus
  • Tetany

♦ Tail held erect in – severe vaginal irritation
♦ Tail head elevated, damaged in – estrogen poisoning
♦ Idiopathic tail-tip alopecia
♦ Idiopathic tail-tip cellulitis

Tendon sheath distended, painful

Occurs in:
♦ Tenosynovitis due to tendon sprain
♦ Infection due to penetrating wound
♦ *Haemophilus somnus* in cattle
♦ *Streptococcus equi* in horse
♦ *Histophilus ovis* in sheep

Throat painful

Clinical findings:
♦ Dysphagia
♦ Anorexia
♦ Pain on palpation

Occurs in:
♦ Pharyngitis
♦ Laryngo-tracheitis
♦ Pharyngeal phlegmon
♦ Pharyngeal foreign body

Throat swollen

Occurs in:
♦ Goiter
♦ Pharyngeal phlegmon
♦ Lymphadenitis, e.g. strangles, tuberculosis, actinobacillosis
♦ Grass seed abscess
♦ Neoplasm metastases, e.g. ocular squamous cell carcinoma

Umbilicus swollen

Occurs in:
♦ Umbilical hernia
♦ Omphalitis (with suppuration)

DISEASES OF MUSCLES

MYAESTHENIA [VM8 p. 512]

Skeletal muscle weakness, usually incidental to primary disease. Usually reversible but in ischemic asthenia weakness initially, irreversible necrosis, paralysis terminally, due to:
♦ Ischemia, e.g.
  • Iliac thrombosis
  • Early stages of postrecumbency ischemic myonecrosis
♦ Toxemia
♦ Hypokalemia
♦ Hypocalcemia
♦ Possibly hypophosphatemia
♦ Hypomagnesemia
♦ Hypoglycemia
♦ Lactic acidemia, in grain engorgement
♦ Poisonous plants causing myopathy, myositis

MYOPATHY [VM8 p. 512]

Etiology

♦ Enzootic nutritional muscular dystrophy, all species
♦ Exertional rhabdomyolysis, including:
  • Equine paralytic myoglobinuria
  • Tying-up in horses
  • In sheep chased by dogs
  • Cattle after wild running
  • Capture myopathy in wildlife
♦ Outbreaks of idiopathic myoglobinuria in horses at pasture
♦ Porcine stress syndrome
♦ Inherited splaylegs
♦ Inherited diaphragmatic muscle dystrophy in Meuse–Rhine–Yessel cattle
♦ Poisonous plants including:
  • Cassia occidentalis
  • Karwinskia humboldtiana
  • Ixioloena spp.
  • Geigeria spp.
  • Lupinus spp.
♦ Enzootic calcinosis, with calcium deposits in all tissues but a syndrome of muscle damage
♦ Ischemic myonecrosis of recumbent cattle; downer cow syndrome
♦ Postanesthetic 'myositis'
♦ Neurogenic atrophy as in:
  • Akabane virus disease
  • Suprascapular nerve paralysis (sweeney)

Clinical findings

Nutritional and poisoning diseases often occur as outbreaks.

Basic syndrome
♦ Sudden onset
♦ Bright, alert, but anxious as if in pain

- Temperature high end of normal
- Tachycardia
- Heart action often irregular
- Reluctance to move, stiff gait, limb weakness, recumbency
- Acute heart failure causing
  - Sudden death, *or*
  - Acute pulmonary edema with profuse nasal froth, *or*
- Rapidly developing anasarca, ascites, engorged jugulars of congestive heart failure, *or*
- Dyspnea
- Red to dark brown urine common in horses, rare in other species
- Affected skeletal muscles may be hard, rubbery, enlarged *or* flabby
- Always bilateral, mostly hind limbs
- Many cases die, some as soon as 24 hours
- Less acute cases stiff gait, lethargy

Idiopathic myopathy in foals
- Foals with dams at pasture getting excessive exercise
- Basic syndrome plus firm swellings at base of mane, croup, salivation, hard masseter muscles; unable bend neck or suck
- Masseter muscle involvement may cause eye protrusion, trismus

Neurogenic atrophy
Nerve damage followed by flaccid paralysis, loss of reflexes, eventual atrophy of denervated muscle.

Diaphragmatic muscle dystrophy
- Recorded only in Meuse–Rhine–Yessel cattle
- Anorexia
- Recurrent bloat, reduced eructation
- Dyspnea, death from asphyxia

Clinical pathology

- Creatine kinase levels sharply elevated but decline quickly, normal in 3–4 days
- Serum glutamic oxaloacetic transaminase levels also elevated, stay high longer; not necessarily an indication of muscle damage
- Levels of both enzymes should be monitored to see if additional myopathic incidents occur
- Creatine kinase levels can rise significantly in:
  - Housed animals suddenly turned out to pasture
  - Animals recumbent for any reason
- Serum glutathione levels best indicator of selenium adequacy of diet

- Myoglobinuric urine is red to chocolate brown; differentiated from hemoglobin by spectrographic examination or orthotoluidine papers

Necropsy findings

- Affected muscles white, waxy like fish flesh in linear strips, distributed symmetrically
- Histopathologically lesions vary from hyaline degeneration to severe myonecrosis; muscle fibers replaced by connective tissue, calcification in some

Diagnosis

Resembles:
- Myositis
- Acute onset cardiac arrhythmia
- Acute heart failure due to other causes
- Congestive heart failure, developing quickly
- Equine babesiosis

Treatment

- Analgesia for relief of significant pain
- Slinging, proper bedding, frequent turning for recumbent patient
- Ensure adequate fluid, nutritional intake or administer parenterally or via stomach tube
- Intravenous isotonic fluids early if myoglobinuric nephrosis a potential threat
- Ensure diet adequate in vitamin E and selenium
- Ensure adequate training programs before serious physical exercise

MYOSITIS [VM8 p. 516]

Etiology

- Trauma by impact or strain
- Traumatic infection introduction, e.g. stake wound
- Intramuscular injections of infected or necrotizing material, e.g. escharotic iron preparations intended only for slow intravenous injection
- Inherited generalized myositis ossificans in pigs
- Blackleg
- Malignant edema
- Eosinophilic myositis
- Screw-worm infestation

Clinical findings

Acute

♦ Muscle pain and swelling
♦ Lameness
♦ Bacterial myositis has:
  • Fever
  • Tachycardia
  • Toxemia
♦ Fistulous tracts from foreign bodies, sequestra

Chronic

♦ Muscle atrophy, wasting
♦ Joint contracture
♦ Incomplete extension of joint

Clinical pathology

♦ Serum creatine kinase, glutamic oxalacetate transaminase levels elevated
♦ Leukocytosis, left shift in infection myositis
♦ Biopsy to establish lesion

Necropsy findings

♦ Bruising, hemorrhage in trauma
♦ **Acute** – edema, hemorrhage
♦ **Chronic** – atrophy, pallor
  • Fibrous adhesions between muscles (fibrotic myopathy)
  • Calcification in some (ossifying myopathy)

DISEASES OF BONES

OSTEODYSTROPHY [VM8 p. 517]

Etiology

♦ **Calcium, phosphorus, vitamin D** – absolute or relative (as imbalances) nutritional deficiencies cause:
  • Rickets in growing animals
  • Osteomalacia in adult ruminants
  • Osteodystrophia in adult pigs, horses
♦ Nutritional deficiency of **copper** can cause:
  • Osteoporosis in lambs
  • Epiphysitis in young cattle
♦ Nutritional deficiency of **protein** can cause **osteoporosis**
♦ **Horses** – osteodystrophia occurs on diets:
  • High in phosphorus, i.e. heavy grain, low roughage diets, especially high bran intake
  • High intakes of insoluble oxalates in poisonous plants causing a deficient calcium intake
  • Both are examples of **nutritional secondary hyperparathyroidism**
♦ **Pigs** – osteodystrophia is sequel to rickets, osteomalacia in pigs on diets low in calcium high in phosphorus

Other causes of osteodystrophic changes in bone include:

♦ Chronic parasitism in young ruminants
♦ Hypovitaminosis A and hypervitaminosis A in cattle and swine
♦ Prolonged high calcium diet in bulls
♦ Multiple mineral, vitamin nutritional deficiencies, cattle
♦ Poisonous plants including *Setaria sphacelata*, *Cenchrus ciliaris*, *Panicum maximum* var. *trichoglume*, osteodystrophia in horses
♦ Housing of pigs indoors on slatted or concrete floors
♦ Undesirable conformation, horses

Clinical findings

♦ First sign in racing horse is poor performance
♦ Stiff gait
♦ Moderate lameness, often shifting from limb to limb
♦ Arched back
♦ Crackling sounds in joint while walking
♦ Reluctant to move
♦ Disinclined to stand
♦ Recumbent
♦ Fractures common, especially long bones, pelvis, vertebrae, transverse processes, ribs
♦ Frontal bones soft to manual pressure
♦ Bone deformity, e.g. bowing long bones, pelvis collapse, especially young growing pigs
♦ Bone enlargement at epiphyseal plate, soft tissue swelling may be painful
♦ Easy detachment ligaments, tendons
♦ Terminal stages in pigs difficulty standing, eating; gross weight loss

Clinical pathology

♦ Radiographically:
  • Osteoporosis
  • Epiphyseal lines deformed, broadened
  • Unossified subperiosteal osteoid
♦ Serum calcium, phosphorus, alkaline phosphatase uninformative; feeding history,

- feed analysis better indicators of status of skeleton
- Non-invasive absorptiometric methods of bone analysis available

Necropsy findings

- Osteoporosis
- Soft bone, fibrous tissue thickening around enlarged ends of bones
- Collapse of subepiphyseal bone at pressure points
- Epiphyseal separation
- Healed fractures
- Bone ash determinations of calcium, phosphorus, magnesium standard procedure for confirming diagnosis

Diagnosis

May be mistaken for:
- Nutritional deficiency copper
- Weight-bearing leg weakness in swine raised indoors without exercise, on slatted or concrete floors
- Chronic fluorosis
- Chronic lead poisoning in sheep grazing old lead mine sites
- Bowie
- Inherited chondrodystrophies

Treatment

- Good response to diet correction is best diagnostic feature
- Oral administration of nutrient identified by analysis of bones and feed. (See sections on individual nutritional deficiencies)

HYPERTROPHIC PULMONARY
OSTEOARTHROPATHY (MARIE'S
DISEASE) [VM8 p. 521]

- Rare but occurs in horses, cattle, sheep
- Stiff gait, lame, reluctant to move
- Bilateral bone enlargements, usually long bones, painful, edematous in early cases
- Radiographically a shaggy periostitis with exostoses
- Associated with chronic pulmonary lesion, e.g. neoplasm, tuberculosis
- Treatment by removal of pulmonary lesion not usually attempted

OSTEOMYELITIS [VM8 p. 521]

Etiology

- Actinomycosis
- Brucellosis in pigs and cattle
- Necrotic rhinitis in pigs
- Atrophic rhinitis in pigs
- Non-specific infection introduced b[y] trauma, open fracture
- Extension from local arthritis
- Hematogenous spread, e.g. *Salmonell[a]* spp., *Actinomyces pyogenes*, *Escherich[ia] coli* mostly at the epiphysis

Clinical findings

- Lameness in limb bone involvement
- Local swelling, inflammation, cellulitis
- Pain on palpation
- Local muscle atrophy
- Pathological fracture common at site
- Draining fistula in many chronic cases
- Fever
- Toxemia
- **Jaw** involvement – teeth shed, dysphagia
- **Vertebral** involvement – spinal cord compression, paresis, paralysis
- **Cervical vertebrae 4–6 osteomyelitis i[n] horses** causes:
  - Stumbling, later stiff, gait
  - Inability to bend neck, kneels to graze
  - Pain on deep palpation affected vertebrae
  - Cervical muscle atrophy
  - Necropsy includes vertebral osteomyelitis, spinal cord compression
  - Treatment not attempted

Clinical pathology

- Radiographically – rarefaction at site, new bone growth locally, sequestrum in some

Necropsy findings

- Necrotic infected bone site
- Sequestrum often
- Foreign body in some

Diagnosis

Can be mistaken for:
- Fracture
- Traumatic ostitis, periostitis
- Bone tumor
- Nutritional osteodystrophy

Treatment

- Medical treatment alone rarely effective
- Surgical excision of affected tissue plus long-term, broad-spectrum treatment with antibacterial, preferably based on culture of organism from site. Anaerobic bacteria commonly involved

DISEASES OF JOINTS

ARTHROPATHY
(OSTEOARTHROPATHY,
DEGENERATIVE JOINT DISEASE)
[VM8 p. 522]

Etiology

Nutritional
♦ As part of:
  • Rickets
  • Osteomalacia
  • Osteodystrophia fibrosa
  • Bowie
♦ Nutritional copper deficiency in pigs and foals

Poisonings with:
♦ Chronic zinc
♦ Fluorine
♦ In enzootic calcinosis

Trauma as in:
♦ Acute injury to closed joints, e.g. cruciate ligaments of stifles in breeding bulls, femorotibial ligaments in horses
♦ Traction during difficult parturition
♦ Repeated subacute, e.g. heavy training in young horses, especially on hard running surfaces
♦ In unstable joints in aged animals

Inheritance including poor conformation:
♦ Osteochondrosis in young pigs, horses, and cattle; most commonly males; any limb joints may be affected
♦ Animals with straight limbs, maximizing percussive effects especially at fast gaits or in heavy animals; inherited conformation defects common in pigs
♦ Degenerative coxofemoral arthropathy inherited susceptibility in fast-growing, young beef bulls (9–24 months); secondary to hip dysplasia, congenital shallow acetabulum in a few
♦ Leg weakness of pigs

Age
♦ Young, fast-growing animals most susceptible
♦ Senior, high-producing cows an endangered group
♦ Degenerative joint disease in aged bulls, cows, as part of aging process

Corticosteroid-induced, intra-articular or prolonged parenteral injection.

Clinical findings

Basic syndrome
♦ Chronic, progressively worsening lameness
♦ Recumbency preferred, difficulty rising
♦ Reluctant to move
♦ Rests limb, shift weight from limb to limb
♦ Stiff gait, joints flexed little
♦ Breeding males can have excellent libido but disinclined to mate
♦ Milk yield declines
♦ Weight loss
♦ Muscle atrophy enhances moderate joint enlargement
♦ Crepitus during walk, passive movement
♦ Excessive movement in joint, most noticeable in hip

Femoral epiphysiolysis, young pigs:
  • Pigs 5 months to 1 year, sudden moderate lameness, one or both hind limbs
  • Progressive, recumbent in 7–10 days
  • Crepitus in hip joint in some
  • Radiographically epiphyseal separation evident

Epiphysitis, in rapidly growing yearling cattle fed intensively in confinement:
  • Severe lameness
  • Swelling of distal physes
  • Necrotizing epiphysitis radiologically

Epiphysitis in young foals:
  • Limb deviation in some cases
  • Enlargement distal physes radius, tibia, third metatarsal, metacarpal bones, proximal extremity first phalanx

Leg weakness, due to osteochondrosis and arthrosis in young pigs:
  • Carpal hyperflexion
  • Limb bowing
  • Adduction both fore limbs at carpus
  • Hyperextension of phalanges
  • Anterior curvature of carpus
  • Pronounced hindquarter sway with crossing of legs

Osteochondrosis in horses:
  • Intermittent, swinging limb, shoulder lameness
  • Pain on passive extension, flexion, abduction limb

Clinical pathology

♦ Radiographically – joint erosion, new bone formation, epiphyseal deformity
♦ Little change in synovial fluid

Necropsy findings

♦ Excessive sterile, brown fluid with floccules in joint cavity
♦ Cartilage patchy erosion, bone eburnation

- Ligament rupture, cartilage floating free or absent
- Epiphytes around joint edge
- Commonly tibial fractures in stifle disease
- Epiphysiolysis commonest at femoral head

Diagnosis

Needs to be differentiated from:
- Arthritis
- Sciatic nerve injury
- Hip dislocation

Treatment

- Responds poorly to standard treatments for arthritis
- Disease progress inexorable; meat animals should be sent for slaughter
- Many medical and surgical treatments are used for treatment of osteoarthritis in racing horses
- Prevention, rehabilitation require avoidance of known contributing causes listed above

ARTHRITIS [VM8 p. 527]

Etiology

Very young most susceptible; causes in them include septicemia, bacteremia in:

Young of all species
Non-specific infection from omphalophlebitis.

Calves
- Erysipelothrix insidiosa
- *Salmonella, Mycoplasma* spp.
- *Escherichia coli*

Lambs
- Erysipelothrix insidiosa
- Chlamydia spp.
- Tick pyemia

Foals
- Actinobacillus equuli
- Rhodococcus equi
- Salmonella abortivoequina
- Chlamydia spp.
- Immune-mediated polysynovitis

Piglets
- Erysipelothrix insidiosa

Adults of all species
- Traumatic joint perforation
- Spread from surrounding tissues
- Hematogenous spread

Cattle
- Haemophilus somnus
- Mycoplasma agalactia var. *bovis*
- Mycoplasma bovigenitalia
- Mycoplasma mycoides
- Brucella abortus
- Chlamydia spp.
- Ephemeral fever virus
- Bovine virus diarrhea virus

Sheep
- Corynebacterium pseudotuberculosis
- Melioidosis
- Mycoplasma spp. in serositis-arthritis

Pigs
- Erysipelothrix insidiosa
- Glasser's disease
- Mycoplasma spp.
- Brucella suis

Horses
- Strangles
- Immune-mediated polysynovitis, possibly

Clinical findings

Acute
- Sudden onset severe pain
- Severe lameness
- Recumbency preferred
- Joint swollen, hot, sore to touch
- Several joints in some cases
- Systemic reaction fever, toxemia in some

Chronic
- Persistent lameness
- Restricted joint movement
- Recumbency preferred, decubitus ulcers
- Joint may appear normal, commonly enlarged, cold, bony, not painful to touch

Clinical pathology

- Aseptically aspirated fluid contains leukocytes, somatic cells, especially acute cases; chronic cases may be normal
- Culture of fluid often negative
- Closed biopsy of synovial membrane offers no improvement in results over synovial fluid culture
- Serological results may indicate specific bacterial presence

Radiographic differentiation inflammatory versus degenerative lesion may be significant

Necropsy findings

Acute
- Synovial membrane thickened, inflamed
- Articular cartilage eroded
- Increased, serous to turbid to pus
- Some inflammation of periarticular tissues

Chronic
- Synovial fluid may be clear serous
- Proliferation of thickened synovial membrane
- Serious erosion and destruction of articular cartilage
- Plaques of inspissated necrotic material, fibrin float free
- Ankylosis, strong adhesions, fibrous tissue contracture in some

Diagnosis

Needs to be differentiated from:
- Degenerative joint disease
- Osteodystrophy with epiphysitis
- Osteomyelitis
- Myositis
- Tendon and ligament injuries
- Persistent recumbency due to:
  - Ischemic myopathy
  - Enzootic muscular dystrophy
  - Spinal cord injury, compression

Treatment

- Early antibacterial treatment essential
- Broad-spectrum antibacterial at heavy doses for up to 7 days recommended to start
- Culture of synovial fluid may give indication of better choice of drugs to use if initial treatment ineffective
- More intensive treatment includes:
  - Intra-articular injection of antibacterial plus
  - Lavage of joint
  - Surgical debridement of joint followed by frequent irrigation via a permanent drainage track
  - Surgical fusion of joint

TENOSYNOVITIS [VM8 p. 509t]

Inflammation of tendon sheath occurs in:
- Septic, due to:
  - Penetrating trauma with infection
  - Localization of systemic infection, e.g. *Haemophilus somnus* (cattle), *Streptococcus equi* (horse), *Histophilus ovis* (sheep)
- Traumatic due to sprain

Clinical signs include:
- Lameness
- Pain, heat, swelling of sheath
- Positive culture of aspirate in septic cases
- Infection of contiguous tissues
- Systemic fever, toxemia in some

BURSITIS [VM8 p. 509t]

Occurs in:
- Trauma
- Localization of systemic infection, e.g. brucellosis (cattle, horses)

DISEASES OF THE HOOF

PODODERMATITIS [VM8 p. 509, 510t]

Etiology

Cattle
- Footrot
- Stable footrot
- Interdigital papilloma (verrucose dermatitis)
- Interdigital fibroma
- Laminitis
- Sole abrasion
- Sole puncture wound

Sheep
- Footrot (interdigital dermatitis)
- Benign footrot (footscald)
- Foot abscess (infectious bulbar necrosis)
- Laminitis
- Shelly hoof

Pig
- Piglet sole abrasion
- Foot abscess (bush foot)
- Footrot

Horse
- Laminitis
- Canker

♦ Thrush
♦ Sole puncture wound

Clinical findings

Basic syndrome
♦ Severe lameness
♦ Compression, squeezing, percussion of hoof causes pain response
♦ Under-running of horn in some
♦ Pus exuding from coronet in some
♦ Foul odor if horn necrotic
♦ Many causative diseases occur as epidemics
♦ Extension to adjoining tendon sheaths, digital cushion rarely

Laminitis
♦ Often all four hooves, especially forelimbs
♦ Shuffling gait
♦ Refusal to move
♦ Terminal recumbency
♦ Rotation of third phalanx, penetration through sole
♦ Separation horn from sensitive laminae, rarely hoofs slough

Clinical pathology

Culture of pus from underneath horn critical for identification of infectious agent.

Necropsy findings

♦ Necrosis of soft tissue beneath horn
♦ Aggregations of pus in some cases
♦ Rarely inflammation, infection of adjoining tissue
♦ Vascular engorgement, separation of sensitive laminae, horn dehiscence in laminitis

SOLE ABRASION [VM8 p. 510t]

Etiology

♦ Hooves softened by continuous wetting, much walking, standing on concrete

♦ Non-slip, abrasive concrete
♦ Long, steep ramps into milking parlours especially with tight turns
♦ Excessive movement, e.g. heifers harassed by older cows, excessive mounting b nymphomaniac cows, buller steers in feed lots
♦ Newborn piglets raised on concrete expanded metal or slatted floors; durin, sucking thrusting movements of hindleg cause abrasion to sole, medial aspect claws carpal skin

Clinical findings

Basic syndrome
♦ Severe lameness; usually all four feet, often fore limbs or hinds worse depending o origin of abrasion
♦ Sole very flat
♦ Wall worn down to expose white line
♦ Sole bruised, tender to pressure
♦ Separation sole from wall in a few

Newborn piglets
♦ Piglets 1–8 days old
♦ Claws, accessory digits affected
♦ Sole swollen, erosion, cracking, peels,
♦ Medial aspect of sole worst
♦ Hind feet worst
♦ Skin over carpal joint abraded common

HOOF ABSCESS [VM8 p. 509t]

Etiology

♦ Sole abrasion
♦ Foot abscess (sheep)
♦ Under-run sole due to nail prick

Clinical findings

♦ Lameness
♦ Pain on compression or percussion
♦ Pus may leak at coronet
♦ Pus released by removal of horn
♦ Evidence of penetration in sole surface

CONGENITAL DEFECTS OF MUSCLES, BONES, AND JOINTS

DEFECTS OF MUSCLES

Myaesthenia [VM8 p. 533]

♦ Inherited hyperkalemic periodic paralysis in horses
♦ Inherited myotonia in goats

Myopathy [VM8 p. 533]

♦ Splayleg in pigs
♦ Inherited progressive muscle dystrophy in cattle
♦ Inherited spinal muscular atrophy in cattle

Muscle hyperplasia [VM8 p. 533]

♦ Inherited double muscling in cattle
♦ Creeper Pietrain pigs

DEFECTS OF BONES

Bone absence [VM8 p. 533]

♦ Taillessness in calves
♦ Reduced phalanges in calves
  • Hemimelia in calves
  • Amputates in calves
  • Peromelia in kids
♦ Agnathia in lambs

Bone deformity [VM8 p. 533]

♦ Achondroplastic dwarfism in calves
♦ Miniature calves
♦ Bulldog calves
♦ Tail kinked in calves
♦ Vestigial limbs
♦ Arachnomelia in cattle and sheep
♦ Congenital thickleg in piglets
♦ Osteopetrosis in calves
♦ Displaced molar teeth, mandibular prognathism in calves
♦ Corkscrew claw in calves
♦ Multiple exostoses in foals
♦ Craniofacial deformity in sheep
♦ Cranium bifidum in pig
♦ Cyclopian deformity, inherited, poisoning by *Veratrum californicum*

DEFECTS OF JOINTS

Congenital articular rigidity (CAR) [VM8 p. 532]

Calves
♦ Inherited CAR in:
  • With cleft soft palate
  • With normal soft palate
  • arthrogryposis

• Multiple tendon contracture
• Multiple ankylosis
♦ Environmental CAR
  • Akabane virus intra-uterine infection
  • Lupin poisoning
  • *Astragalus, Oxytropis* spp. *poisoning*
  • *Sorghum* spp. *poisoning*
  • *Nutritional deficiency of manganese*

Lambs and kids
♦ Inherited CAR, merinos
♦ Akabane virus infection in utero
♦ Astragalus, Oxytropis spp. poisoning
♦ Parbendazole, cambendazole poisoning

Piglets
♦ Inherited CAR
♦ Nutritional deficiency vitamin A
♦ *Conium maculatum, Prunus serotina, Datura stramonium*, tobacco wastes, poisoning

Foals
♦ Idiopathic 'contracted' foals in USA, contractures limbs, vertebral column, thin or absent ventral abdominal wall
♦ CAR in foals from mares fed hybrid sudan grass
♦ Sporadic occurrence mild tendon contracture distal limbs; most recover spontaneously

Congenital joint hypermobility [VM8 p. 533]

♦ Inherited joint hypermobility in cattle
♦ Inherited osteogenesis imperfecta in cattle
♦ Hyperelastosis cutis
♦ Dermatosparaxia
♦ Ehlers–Danloss syndrome
♦ Inherited patellar subluxation in cattle and horses

14 DISEASES OF SKIN, CONJUNCTIVA AND EXTERNAL EAR

The first decision in the diagnosis of a case of 'skin disease' is to determine whether it is primarily a disease restricted in its occurrence to the skin, or secondary to some other principal disease affecting other organs. This chapter deals with the general diseases of the skin and refers the reader to the specific diseases in other chapters.

CLINICAL INDICANTS

The principal clinical signs, clinicopathological findings and special examination techniques on which clinical diagnoses of skin are based include the following.

Absence or loss of skin

♦ Necrosis, gangrene
♦ Congenital absence
  • Epitheliogenesis imperfecta
  • Epidermolysis bullosa
  • Inherited redfoot

Alopecia

See hair abnormality, this section.

Anhidrosis

See sweating absent, this section.

Coloration of skin abnormal

Seen best in mucosae except in white pigs.
♦ Jaundice
♦ Erythema
♦ Pallor
♦ General lack of skin pigment; albinism, pseudoalbinism
♦ Local skin pigment lack; vitiligo

Conjunctiva inflamed

Clinical findings:
♦ Eye discharge
♦ Blepharospasm
♦ Sequels keratitis, corneal opacity, ulceration

Occurs in:
♦ Conjunctivitis
♦ Keratoconjunctivitis

Conjunctival mass

♦ Bovine ocular squamous cell carcinoma
♦ Equine ocular squamous cell carcinoma
♦ Congenital dermoid cysts

Cords connecting nodes

Lymphangitis

Corneal lesions

Include sequels to chronic conjunctivitis, e.g.
♦ Corneal **opacity**
♦ Corneal **ulcer**
♦ Chronic **vascularization**
♦ Congenital mass of dermoid cyst

ar swollen

early photosensitization

ar exudate

Clinical findings:
Smelly discharge in depths
Frequent head-shaking

Occurs in Otitis externa

ar gangrene

Occurs in:
Late stages photosensitization
Ergot toxins

ye discharge

Serous, purulent in conjunctivitis, keratitis

Eyeball anterior chamber hemorrhage in (hyphaema)

Occurs in:
Head trauma
Hemorrhagic disease

Eyeball anterior chamber, pus in (hypopyon)

Occurs in:
Secondary to bacteremia, septicemia, especially neonates
Penetrating wound to cornea

Eyeball deformed

♦ Sporadic **anophthalmia**
♦ Cyclopian defect in
  • Inherited prolonged gestation
  • *Salsola tuberculata* poisoning
♦ Sporadic, inherited microphthalmia

Eyelid spasm (blepharospasm)

In conjunctivitis, keratitis

Eyelid swollen

Occurs in:
♦ Anasarca
♦ Photosensitization

Greasy skin exudate

Seborrhea

Hair abnormality

♦ Complete deficiency – alopecia
♦ Partial deficiency – hypotrichosis
♦ Hairiness (hirsutism)
♦ Color abnormality:
  • Pigment absence, achromotrichia
♦ Specific coloration:
  • Fleece rot
  • Mycotic dermatitis
♦ Curly, excessive in inherited cardiomyopathy
♦ Singed in fire injury, electrocution
♦ Fibers broken in ringworm, metabolic wool break

Hoof diseases

See musculoskeletal system.

Horn diseases

♦ Absence in inherited epidermal dysplasia
♦ Mass at base indicates horn cancer

Hyperelasticity

♦ Inherited defects
  • Ehlers–Danlos syndrome
  • Dermatosparaxia
  • Hyperelastosis cutis
  • Epidermolysis bullosa

Hypotrichosis

See hair abnormality, above.

Lesions, discrete

Definitions in Table 14.1
♦ Dermatitis
♦ Impetigo
♦ Urticaria

Nodules, papules

Occur in:
♦ Dermatitis
♦ Folliculitis
♦ Panniculitis
♦ Lymphangitis
♦ Granuloma
♦ Neoplasms

Phlegmon

Clinical findings:
♦ Diffuse subcutaneous swelling
♦ Local swelling
♦ Part painful, tense, rarely hot

Table 14.1 Terms used to identify skin lesions

Name of lesion	Nature of lesion	Relation to skin surface	Skin surface
		Diffuse lesions	
Scales	Dry, flaky exfoliations	On surface, no penetration of skin	Unbroken
Excoriations	Traumatic abrasions and scratches	Penetration below surface	Variable skin surface damage – depends on severity
Fissures	Deep cracks	Penetrate into subcutis	Disrupted
Dry gangrene	Dry, horny, black avascular, shield-like	Above skin, usually all layers affected	Removed
Early moist gangrene	Blue, black, cold, oozing serum	In plane of skin or below	Complete depth of subcutis
Keratosis	Overgrowth of dry horny keratinized epithelium	Above skin	Undamaged; stratum corneum is retained
Acanthosis	Like keratosis but moist, soft	Above skin	Prickle cell layer swollen; is really part of skin
Hyperkeratosis	Excessive overgrowth of keratinized epithelium-like scab	Above skin	Skin surface unbroken
Parakeratosis	Adherent to skin	Above skin	Cells of stratum corneum nucleated and retained; really part of skin
Eczema	Erythematous, itching dermatitis	Superficial layer of epidermis affected	Weeping, scabby disruption of surface

	Discrete lesions		
Vesicle, bleb, bullae, blister	Fluid (serum or lymph)-filled blister 1–2 cm diameter	Above surface, superficial	Unbroken, but will slough
Pustule	Pus-filled blister, 1–5 mm diameter	Above, superficial	Will rupture
Wheals	Edematous, erythematous swellings, transitory	Above; all layers affected	Undamaged
Papules (pimples)	Elevated, inflamed, necrotic center; up to 1 cm diameter	Above surface, all layers affected	Points and ruptures
Nodules, nodes	Elevated, solid, up to 1 cm diameter acute or chronic inflammation. No necrotic center	Above surface; all layers affected	Surface unbroken
Plaque	A larger nodule, up to 3–4 cm diameter	All layers affected; raised above surface	Unbroken surface
Acne	Used synonymously with pimple, but strictly means infection of sebaceous gland	Above surface of skin; all layers affected	May point and rupture
Impetigo	Flaccid vessicle, then pustule, then scab, up to 1 cm diameter	Raised above skin. Very superficial	Upper layers destroyed
Scab	Crust of coagulated serum, blood, pus and skin debris	Raised above skin	Disrupted, depth varying with original lesion

Occurs in Sporadic local infection

Pigment deficient, skin

Occurs in Vitiligo

Pruritus (itchiness)

Indicated by scratching, rubbing; difficult to differentiate from insect 'worry'.

Occurs in:
♦ External parasite infestations:
  • Lice
  • Itch mite
  • Ticks
  • Ked
  • Harvest mite
  • Mosquitoes
  • Midges
  • Flies
♦ Urticaria
♦ Allergy
♦ Angioedema
♦ Dermatitis
♦ Photosensitization
♦ Folliculitis
♦ Specific diseases, e.g.:
  • Scrapie in sheep
  • Aujeszky's disease in cattle
  • Citrinin poisoning

Pustules

Occur in Impetigo.

Scaly skin

Occurs in Pityriasis.

Sweating excessive (hyperhidrosis)

Occurs in:
♦ General
  • Anaphylaxis
  • Hyperthermia after violent exercise
  • Endotoxic shock
  • Severe pain
  • Dinitrophenol poisoning
♦ Local excessive sweating:

• Peripheral nerve injury
• Spinal cord compression, injury

Sweating absent (anhidrosis)

Occurs in Non-sweating syndrome.

Swelling, cutaneous, subcutaneous

Occurs in:
♦ Diffuse
  • Anasarca
  • Angioedema
  • Emphysema, subcutaneous
  • Hemorrhage (hematoma)
  • Suppurative in phlegmon
♦ Discrete (see also nodules, papules)
  • Abscess
  • Cyst
  • Dermoid cyst
  • Granuloma
  • Lymphangitis
  • Neoplasm
  • Naevus, vascular

Tents easily

Clinical findings:
♦ Skin dry, lacking turgor
♦ Tents easily, return to normal delayed

Occurs in Dehydration.

Thickening, skin

Occurs in:
♦ Hyperkeratosis
♦ Pachydermia
♦ Parakeratosis
♦ Chronic lymphangitis

Wheals

Occur in Urticaria.

White skin lesions only

Occurs in Photosensitization.

DISEASES OF EPIDERMIS AND DERMIS

PITYRIASIS (DANDRUFF) [VM8 p. 539]

Clinical findings:
- Thin, dry, bran-like scales of epithelial cells on skin surface
- Dry, lustreless hair coat
- **Test** by skin scraping for arthropod parasites, or fungal hyphae and spores

Occurs in:
- Hypovitaminosis A
- Hypovitaminosis B complex in pigs
- Iodine poisoning
- Highly chlorinated naphthalene poisonings
- Louse and mite infestations
- Ringworm

Differentiate from:
- Hyperkeratosis
- Parakeratosis

PARAKERATOSIS [VM8 p. 540]

Clinical findings:
- Thick greasy scales of epithelial cells free or accumulated as crusts on skin surface
- Lesions crack and fissure; raw undersurface
- Mostly in limb joint flexures
- **Test** by biopsy

Occurs in:
- Chronic inflammation
- Nutritional deficiency of zinc
- Inherited bovine Adema disease
- Inherited porcine dermatosis vegetans
- Porcine pityriasis rosea

Differentiate from Pityriasis, hyperkeratosis.

Treat by vigorous washing plus keratolytic ointment.

HYPERKERATOSIS [VM8 p. 540]

Clinical findings:
- Most of skin surface intact but patches of thick, corrugated, hairless, scaly, sometimes fissured
- **Test** by biopsy

Occurs in:
- Highly chlorinated naphthalenes poisoning
- Chronic arsenic poisoning

- Inherited bovine ichthyosis (fish-scale disease)
- Persistent local compression

Differentiate from Pityriasis, parakeratosis.

Treat Primary cause.

PACHYDERMA [VM8 p. 541]

Clinical findings:
- Local areas thick, inelastic, tough skin with sparse hair, intact surface
- Includes **scleroderma**

Occurs in Chronic, non-specific inflammation, e.g. lymphangitis.

Differentiate from Parakeratosis, hyperkeratosis.

Treat by:
- Excision small, chronic areas
- Local cortisone to new lesions

IMPETIGO [VM8 p. 541]

Clinical findings:
- Small vesicles surrounded by erythema
- To pustules
- Rupture to form scabs
- **Test** by culture of vesicle fluid

Occurs in:
- Demodectic mange
- Bovine udder impetigo
- Contagious pyoderma of piglets

Differentiate from Cow pox, swine pox

Treat by:
- Penicillin injection
- Antibacterial ointment or wash

URTICARIA [VM8 p. 542]

Clinical findings:
- Sudden appearance, multiple 0.5–5.0 cm dia. wheals without skin discontinuity
- Itchiness
- After contact with plants or insects
- Spontaneous recovery in hours to several days
- Dermatographism in some

Occurs in:
- Insect stings
- Plant stings
- Food allergy
- Reaction to penicillin injection
- Warble fly death in tissues
- Milk allergy
- Transfusion reaction
- Equine upper respiratory infection
- Swine erysipelas

Differentiate from angioedema.

Treat with Antihistamine.

DERMATITIS [VM8 p. 543]

Etiology

All species
- *Dermatophilus congolensis*
- *Ringworm*
- *Photosensitization*
- Chemical contact
- Arsenic poisoning
- Mite infestation – mange, trombidiforms
- *Stephanofilaria* spp.
- *Strongyloides* spp.
- *Besnoitia* spp.

Cattle
- Udder impetigo
- Cowpox
- Ulcerative mammillitis
- Lumpy skin disease
- Foot-and-mouth disease
- Vesicular stomatitis
- Rinderpest
- Bovine virus diarrhea
- Bovine malignant catarrh
- Sweating sickness
- Mushroom poisoning
- Potato poisoning
- Vicia spp. poisoning
- Flexural seborrhea
- Bovine exfoliative dermatitis

Sheep and goats
- Strawberry footrot
- Staphylococcal dermatitis
- Sheep pox
- Contagious ecthyma
- Ulcerative dermatosis
- Rinderpest
- Peste des petits ruminants
- Bluetongue
- Fleece rot
- Mycotic dermatitis

- Itch-mite
- Blowfly infestation
- Cockle
- Elaeophoriasis
- Ovine atopic dermatitis
- Caprine idiopathic dermatitis

Pigs
- Infectious pyoderma
- Ulcerative pyoderma
- Exudative epidermitis
- Pig pox
- Swine vesicular disease
- Vesicular exanthema of swine
- Foot and mouth disease
- Parsnip, celery (moldy) poisoning
- Sunburn
- Porcine necrotic ear syndrome
- B vitamin nutritional deficiency
- Pityriasis rosea

Horses
- *Staphylococcal dermatitis*
- *Greasy heel*
- *Horse pox*
- *Viral papular dermatitis*
- *Vesicular stomatitis*
- *Sporotrichosis*
- *Ringworm*
- *Pythiosis*
- *Scald*
- *Queensland itch*
- *Eosinophilic dermatitis*
- *Pemphigus*
- *Lupus erythematosus*
- *Erythema multiforme*
- *Molluscum contagiosum*
- *Linear hyperkeratosis*
- *Nodular necrobiosis*
- *Ear plaque*
- *Uasin gishu*
- *Cutaneous habronemiasis*
- *Tropical lichen*
- *Hydrotoea* spp. *infestation*
- *Trombidiosis*

Clinical findings

Syndromes include:
- Erythema, weeping, gangrene
- Vesicles, pustules, scabs
- Erythema, weeping, scab
- Pruritus, excoriation, pachydermia
- Dandruff, crust, depilation

Individual dermatitides include:

ovine exfoliative dermatitis
VM8 p. 544]
In sucking neonates
Scaling, hair loss
Spontaneously recover

vine atopic dermatitis [VM8
 544]
Recurrent summer excoriation
Alopecia on woolless parts

aprine idiopathic dermatitis
VM8 p. 544]
In pygmy goats
Alopecia, exudation

orcine necrotic ear syndrome
VM8 p. 544]
Probably bite trauma

Porcine recurrent idiopathic
dermatitis [VM8 p. 544]
Pigs in particular farm or pen
Papular dermatitis on white skin

Equine staphylococcal dermatitis
VM8 p. 544]
♦ Mostly under harness
♦ Small, painful nodules
♦ Shed scab leaving small ulcer
♦ Meager pus
♦ New lesions ensure lengthy course

Chronic equine eosinophilic
dermatitis [VM8 p. 544]
♦ Acanthosis
♦ Hyperkeratosis
♦ Eosinophilic granulomas in internal organs

Equine nodular necrobiosis [VM8
p. 544]
Small nodules contain eosinophils

Molluscum contagiosum in horses
[VM8 p. 544]
♦ Chronic hairless lesions
♦ Bleed easily during grooming
♦ Intracellular inclusions resemble pox virions

Systemic lupus erythematosus
(SLE) [VM8 p. 544]
♦ Chronic, extensive, scaly, crusty, depilated dermatitis
♦ Local subcutaneous edema, lymphadenopathy
♦ Oral mucosal ulcers

♦ Weight loss
♦ Fever
♦ Arthropathy, lameness
♦ Necropsy lesions include glomerulonephritis
♦ Diagnosis confirmed by antinuclear antibody test

Discoid lupus erythematosus
[VM8 p. 545]
♦ Similar to SLE
♦ Lesions only on skin

Erythema multiforme [VM8
p. 545]
♦ Self-limiting, annular or crescent-shaped bullous skin lesions
♦ Arranged symmetrically on body

Pemphigus [VM8 p. 545]
♦ Vesicles followed by ulcers on skin and mucosae
♦ Sometimes weight loss

Pemphigus foliaceous, goats,
horses [VM8 p. 545]
♦ Lesions at coronets, mucocutaneous junctions, or in mouth or vulva
♦ Temporary relief with corticosteroids

Equine ear plaque [VM8 p. 545]
Papilloma-like plaques inside pinna

Equine tropical lichen [VM8
p. 545]
♦ Recurrent in summer
♦ Irritating lesion containing microfilaria at mane and tail head
♦ Similar to Queensland itch
♦ Dramatic response to ivermectin

Equine linear keratosis [VM8 p.
545]
♦ Scaly lumps arranged in line coalesce forming hairless, hyperkeratotic ridge
♦ Persist for life
♦ Common in Quarterhorses

Clinical pathology

♦ Scrapings, swabs, impression smears and biopsies, with microbiological, parasitic

and histopathological examinations essential for complete examination
♦ Autoimmune diseases need serological analysis

Necropsy findings

♦ Dermatological lesions may be an expression of systemic disease
♦ Necropsy necessary in fatal dermatitis cases

Diagnosis

Similar to:
♦ Impetigo
♦ Photosensitization
♦ Folliculitis
♦ Seborrhea
♦ Necrosis, gangrene
♦ Absence, loss of skin
♦ Granulosa
♦ Tumors
♦ Dermatosis vegetans
♦ Epitheliogenesis imperfecta

Treatment

Specific Depends on accurate diagnosis of specific cause.

Supportive Includes corticosteroids, non-steroidal anti-inflammatory drugs, antihistamines and autogenous vaccines systemically, and astringent or emollient topical applications, as appropriate.

PHOTOSENSITIZATION [VM8 p. 546]

Etiology

Exogenous plant photodynamic agents:
♦ Dianthrone derivatives:
  • **Hypericin** in *Hypericum* spp.
  • **Fagopyrin** in *Polygonum, Fagopyrum* spp.
♦ Furanocoumarins in:
  • *Ammi, Cymopteres* spp., *Thamnosma texana*
  • *Apium graveolens* (celery) and *Pastinaca sativa* (parsnip) infested with fungi
  • **Steroidal saponins** causing crystal-associated cholangiohepatopathy in:
♦ *Agave lecheguilla, Narthecium ossifragum, Tribulus terrestris, Panicum* spp., etc.

Endogenous PDAs due to:

♦ Faulty porphyrin metabolism in inherited bovine porphyria
♦ Hepatic insufficiency causing phylloerythrin accumulation in many fungal, bacterial and plant poisonings, e.g.:
  ♦ *Pithomyces chartarum* (facial eczema), *Microcystis* spp. (water bloom), *Phomopsis leptostromiformis* (lupinosis), *Lantana camara, Myoporum* spp., *Crotalaria* spp., *Senecio* spp., etc.
♦ Inherited congenital photosensitivity

Unidentified PDAs, e.g.:
♦ Corticosteroids, phenanthridium
♦ Ingestion of *Medicago denticulata* and its resident aphid, *Brassica* spp., *Trifolium* spp. *Erodium* spp.

Clinical findings

♦ Dermatitis of unpigmented, lightly haired skin, mucosa, and conjunctiva
♦ Only when patient exposed to direct sunlight
♦ Intense irritation within few hours of exposure to sun
♦ Sequence of skin erythema, edema (ear droop), exudation, gangrene (death common at this stage)
♦ Sloughing of skin or mucosa in survivors
♦ Severest lesions on muzzle, around eyes (puffy eyelids, lacrimation), white skin or dorsum, sides, lateral aspects of teats, coronets, buccal surface of lips, ventral tongue surface (salivation)
♦ Conjunctivitis on lateral cornea in some
♦ Death in many due to shock or hepatic failure

Clinical pathology

♦ Identify liver damage by marked elevation in serum levels of liver enzymes in acute cases.

Necropsy findings

♦ Hepatitis
♦ Brown color of teeth and bones in porphyria
♦ Skin gangrene only in exogenous PDA poisoning
♦ Recommended specimens – drinking water containing algae, poisonous plants, mouldy feed, ruminal contents for botanical or chemical analysis

Diagnosis

Differentiation necessary from:
Mycotic dermatitis
Bovine malignant catarrh, epidemic form
Fire injury

Treatment

♦ Move from current feed and water but toxicity usually of short duration
♦ Remove from solar exposure
♦ Test subsequent toxicity with trial group

DISEASES OF THE HAIR, WOOL, FOLLICLES, SKIN GLANDS, AND HORNS
N.B. Diseases of hooves are in musculoskeletal system, Chapter 13

ALOPECIA AND HYPOTRICHOSIS
[VM8 p. 548]

Etiology

Follicles absent or non-functional
♦ Inherited hypotrichoses
♦ Inherited epidermal dysplasia (baldy calves)
♦ Adenohypophyseal hypoplasia
♦ Congenital hypothyroidism
♦ Congenital infection by bovine virus diarrhea, border disease viruses
♦ Peripheral nerve damage
♦ Skin scars
♦ Alopecia areata

Loss of preformed fibers
♦ Ringworm
♦ Mycotic dermatitis
♦ Metabolic alopecia; weakness of section of fibers due to disease or nutritional stress (**break in wool**)
♦ Trauma, scratching
♦ Thallium poisoning
♦ Leucaena leucocephala poisoning
♦ Idiopathic tail switch hair loss in well-fed beef bulls
♦ Folliculitis
♦ Wool slip

Clinical findings

♦ In congenital defects:
  • Skin thin, shiny
  • Coarse tactile hairs usually present
♦ In diseases with fiber loss:
  • Hair stumps visible
  • Evidence of infection, or trauma

Alopecia areata
♦ Circular lesions of non-scarring alopecia
♦ Lymphocyte aggregations around follicles
♦ Disappears spontaneously

Clinical pathology

♦ Biopsy determines state of follicles
♦ Microbiological/fungal examination advisable

ACHROMOTRICHIA [VM8 p. 549]

Clinical findings

♦ Pigment absent from colored skin fibers, complete or in bands
♦ Deficiency may be partial, e.g. black hair may go gray, dark red goes to washed out red

Occurs in

♦ Copper nutritional deficiency
♦ Molybdenum nutritional excess, both in ruminants
♦ Idiopathic vitiligo or **snowflakes** as patches of premature graying
♦ Idiopathic patchy depigmentation of skin in horses on undersurface of tail, prepuce, perineum resembles vitiligo
♦ Application of super-cooled appliances, as in freeze branding, X-irradiation or physical pressure

SEBORRHEA [VM8 p. 549]

Clinical findings and basic syndrome

♦ Excessive greasiness of skin covered by slippery film or dried crust
♦ No damage to skin unless secondarily infected

Occurs in

♦ Porcine exudative epidermitis
♦ **Greasy heel** in cattle and horses:

- Swelling of skin at back of pastern
- Deep, horizontal fissures (called **scratches**)
- Seborrhea
- Lame, often all four feet
♦ Flexural seborrhea in heavy milking cows:
  - Lesions in axilla, groin, and between udder halves
  - Lameness
  - Necrotic odor
  - Early treatment by warm detergent wash plus astringent lotion, keeping part kept dry effective

ACNE AND FOLLICULITIS [VM8 p. 550]

Clinical findings

♦ Inflammation of coat fiber follicles
♦ Includes **acne, sycosis, boils, furuncles**

DISEASES OF THE SUBCUTIS

SUBCUTANEOUS EDEMA (ANASARCA) [VM8 p. 551]

Clinical findings:
♦ Widespread accumulation edema fluid in subcutaneous tissue
♦ Visible or palpable, pitting, painless swelling
♦ Usually of submandibular space, brisket, ventral abdomen

Occurs in:
♦ **Increased vascular resistance**:
  - Congestive heart failure
  - Vascular compression by tumor or fetus
  - Congenital lymph node absence
♦ **Vascular damage**:
  - Purpura hemorrhagica
  - Angioedema
  - Endothelial damage in equine infectious anemia
  - Dourine
  - Horses bedded on shavings of *Juglans nigra* (black walnut)
♦ **Hypoproteinemia**:
  - Nephrosis
  - Renal amyloidosis
  - Protein-losing enteropathy, e.g. in lymphosarcoma
  - Intestinal nematodiasis
  - Protein starvation; inflammatory edema

♦ Itchy or painful nodules around hair base
♦ Later pustules, then crusts, shedding of hair

Occurs in

♦ Equine staphylococcal dermatitis
♦ Demodectic mange
♦ Bovine sterile eosinophilic folliculitis

Test

Nodules filled with eosinophils, culture sterile.

Treatment

♦ Disinfectant rinse plus local antibacterial ointment standard treatment
♦ Systemic antibiotic for extensive cases
♦ Autogenous vaccine in chronic cases
♦ Disinfection of gear, clothing, grooming kits

♦ *Clostridium* spp. infections
♦ *Bacillus anthracis* in swine and horses
♦ Myxedema – in porcine goiter

Resembles Infiltration of belly wall by urine in male urethral rupture.

Treatment With diuretics enhances treatment of primary cause.

ANGIOEDEMA (ANGIONEUROTIC EDEMA) [VM8 p. 552]

Clinical findings:
♦ Sudden onset, usually transient
♦ Extensive but discrete, areas subcutis, painless, itchy edema.
♦ Mostly affects head causing salivation, nasal discharge, head-shaking, rubbing
♦ Eyes causing puffy eyelids, protruding nictitating membrane lacrimation
♦ Local swellings on perineum, teats, udder, lower limbs from knees or hocks to coronets

Resembles:
♦ Subcutaneous hemorrhage
♦ Purpura hemorrhagica
♦ Equine viral arteritis
♦ Equine infectious anemia
♦ Dourine

Treatment:
♦ Change of environment may separate patient from assumed allergen
♦ Antihistamines standard treatment

EMPHYSEMA [VM8 p. 553]

Clinical findings:
♦ Fluctuant, diffuse swellings anywhere on body, mostly along back
♦ Crepitate on palpation
♦ Skin normal
♦ Swellings may impede respiration, limb movements

Occurs in:
♦ Cutaneous wound
♦ Lung puncture by fractured rib
♦ Internal penetrating wound of trachea, reticular wall and through diaphragm
♦ Rumen gases from rumenotomy incision or trocarization penetration
♦ Extension from primary pulmonary emphysema

Treatment Multiple incision if life-threatening.

Resembles Gas gangrene due to *Clostridium* spp. infection.

LYMPHANGITIS [VM8 p. 553]

Clinical findings:
♦ Chronic inflammation, enlargement lymph vessels and nodes due to local infection
♦ Corded, fibrous, tortuous lymphatics; focal abscesses, ulcers along their course
♦ Local obstruction edema in some
♦ Long-standing lesions cause local subcutis inflammatory tissue causes skin thickening
♦ Lesions usually on limbs, ventral abdomen
♦ Acute cases cause extensive local inflammatory edema

Occurs in:
Horse
♦ Glanders
♦ Epizootic lymphangitis
♦ Sporadic lymphangitis
♦ Ulcerative lymphangitis
♦ Aberrant strangles
Cattle
♦ Skin farcy
♦ Cutaneous tuberculosis (mycobacteriosis)
♦ **Lechiguana** (Brazil), multiple dense subcutaneous granuloma containing *Pasteurella granulomatis*

Treatment
♦ Acute cases – hot fomentations, systemic antibiotics
♦ Chronic cases – surgical excision

PANNICULITIS [VM8 p. 554]

Clinical findings:
♦ Diffuse inflammation of subcutaneous fat
♦ Multiple, firm, deep-seated, painless nodules on neck sides
♦ Spontaneous variation in size
♦ May disappear permanently
♦ Transitory response to corticosteroids

Occurs in Young horses.

HEMORRHAGE [VM8 p. 554]

Clinical findings:
♦ Acute onset diffuse, fluctuating, swellings
♦ May be accompanying hemorrhages of mucosa, or hemorrhagic anemia
♦ Confirmed by closed aspiration; opening a swelling not recommended especially if clotting defect possible

Occurs in:
♦ Trauma
♦ **Coagulation defect** as in:
  • Dicoumarol poisoning
  • Hemophilia
♦ **Endothelial damage** as in purpura hemorrhagica

Treatment Surgical; may require blood transfusion.

NECROSIS AND GANGRENE [VM8 p. 554]

Clinical findings:
♦ Gradual loss or total slough of part
♦ Initial lesion may be swollen, raised, discolored red and hot on palpation, *or*
♦ In **gangrene**
  • Lesion blue to black, cold
  • Margin of lesion separates, slough dry and hard
  • Underlying surface raw tissue

Caused by:
♦ Pressure sores, e.g. saddle, girth galls, carpal and tarsal necrosis in recumbent patients

- Caustic chemicals
- Fire injury
- β-irradiation
- Infections including:
  - Porcine salmonellosis
  - Erysipelas
  - Bovine staphylococcal mastitis
  - Ulcerative mammillitis
  - Ovine pasteurella mastitis
  - Mycotoxins including ergotamine in:
    - *Claviceps purpurea*
    - *Aspergillus terreus*
    - *Fusarium equiseta*
    - *Balansia epichloe*
- Bacterial emboli causing vessel obstruction
- Severe dermatitis as in:
  - Photosensitization
  - Flexural seborrhea
  - Screw-worm infestation

SUBCUTANEOUS ABSCESS [VM8 p. 555]

Clinical findings:
- Acute, painful, or chronic, cold, sub-cutaneous enlargements, yielding pus on aspiration or lancing
- Similar to suppurative lymphadenitis

Occur in:
As part of a systemic infection with **hematogenous spread** in:
- *Corynebacterium pseudotuberculosis* equine pectoral abscesses
- *Rhodococcus equi* infection of foals
- *Pasteurella pseudotuberculosis*
- *Histophilus ovis;* extension from folliculitis etc,
- Penetration by plant awns; **grass seed abscess:**
  - *Hordeum jubatum*
  - *Stipa* spp.
  - *Agrostis* spp.

Treatment If required, is surgical drainage or excision.

CUTANEOUS CYSTS [VM8 p. 555]

Clinical findings:
- Smooth, round bodies, fluctuating-to-hard in consistency
- Sometimes leak mucoid contents to exterior
- May be:
  - **Congenital**, sometimes inherited, *or*
  - **Acquired** as a result of injury

- May be:
  - Epidermoid (lined with skin)
  - Dermoid (containing differentiated tissues such as bone), or
  - Dentigerous (containing tooth elements)
- Acquired cysts may be
  - Apocrine
  - Sebaceous
  - Keratinaceous
- **Developmental** cysts occur in the:
  - Neck (branchial)
  - False nostril, or
  - Base of the ear of horses
  - In the wattles of goats
- Cysts may be confused with dermoid teratoma

GRANULOMATOUS LESIONS OF THE SKIN [VM8 p. 556]

Clinical findings:
- Chronic tumor-like masses of granulation tissue in skin as nodules or plaques, ulcers
- Often with lymphangitis and lymphadenitis

Causes include:
Cattle
- *Mycobacterium* spp.
- *Nocardia farcinicus*
- *Actinobacillus lignieresi*
- *Onchocerca* spp.
- *Hypoderma* spp. larvae
- *Mucor* spp. fungi in hard, cutaneous nodules on back of udder
Sheep
- Strawberry footrot
- Ecthyma
- *Actinobacillus lignieresi* ulcers of lower jaw and dewlap
Pig
- Udder skin granuloma caused by:
  - *Actinomyces* spp
  - *Borrelia suilla*
Horse
- **Tumorous calcinosis** containing calcified material, near joints, tendon sheaths
- **Botryomycosis**, usually on ventral abdomen, containing foreign body, discharge yellow granules in pus
- **Equine eosinophilic granulomas**, nodules containing many eosinophils
- Cutaneous farcy (glanders)
- Mycetomas (containing *Actinomadura* spp. and *Nocardia braziliensis*)
- *Histomonas farcinicus* (Epizootic lymphangitis)

- *Corynebacterium pseudotuberculosis* (ulcerative lymphangitis)
- *Habronema megastoma*

- *Pythium insidiosum* (swamp cancer, pythiosis)
- *Onchocerca* spp. (onchocercosis)

CUTANEOUS NEOPLASMS

PAPILLOMA AND SARCOID [VM8 p. 556]

Discrete nodular growths of viable epithelial, connective tissue described under papilloma, sarcoid.

SQUAMOUS-CELL CARCINOMA
[VM8 p. 556]

Occur as:

- **Cancer-eye** of horses and cattle; invasive lesions commence on eyelid, nictitating membrane or cornea, with metastases to local lymph nodes
- **preputial, penile malignant tumors** of old male horses requiring early penile amputation; squamous papillomata, habronemiasis, epithelial hyperplasia cause similar lesions
- **Vulvar tumors** of cows, goat does and Merino ewes; in ewes a high incidence is related to the use of the radical Mules operation for blowfly prophylaxis; bilateral swelling of ectopic mammary tissue in the vulvar wall may be mistakenly confused with squamous-cell carcinoma
- **Horn core cancer** in aged, white colored Indian breeds of cattle and in goats, causing head-shaking, holding the head down, and nasal bleeding, eventually shedding of the horn and exposure of the tumor mass
- **Ear cancer** at a high incidence in some flocks of sheep and in goats

Treatment of horn cancer Not usually undertaken because of high incidence of metastases but immunotherapy is used; excision by cryotherapy or radiofrequency hyperthermia of eye cancer widely practiced

MELANOMA [VM8 p. 557]

Clinical findings:
dense, black, smooth, sometimes ulcerated, single or multiple cutaneous tumors.

Occur in:
- Rare benign cases in dark skinned cattle, sheep, and goats

- High incidence in young Duroc–Jersey pigs
- Spontaneously regressing tumors in Sinclair miniature pigs
- Common in aged gray horses, mostly at root of tail, metastasize widely

Treatment With cimetidine may halt growth.

CUTANEOUS ANGIOMATOSIS
[VM8 p. 557]

- Recurrently hemorrhagic, single, small, granuloma-like lesions on back of dairy cows. Excision effective
- **Juvenile angiomatosis** causes similar lesions in many organs, including skin of calves

LYMPHOMATOSIS [VM8 p. 557]

- Subcutaneous nodules or diffuse skin thickening are lesions in cases of bovine viral leukosis
- Similar malignant lesions, consisting largely of immature lymphocytes in the skin in horses

MAST CELL TUMORS
(CUTANEOUS MASTOCYTOMA)
[VM8 p. 557]

Cattle
- Multiple, intradermal nodules
- Recur widely intradermally after excision
- Commonly ulcerate
- Remission after levamisole treatment

Horse
- Single cutaneous lesions in adults
- Multiple in neonates
- May regress spontaneously then recur, excision recommended

NEUROFIBROMATOSIS [VM8 p. 558]

- High incidence in neonates of pied European cattle
- Benign, flat, round tumors on face

HISTIOCYTOMA [VM8 p. 558]

♦ Rare tumor in ruminants
♦ Spontaneously regressing, single or multiple nodules or plaques

HEMANGIOMA [VM8 p. 558]

Horses
♦ Small, round, benign hemangiomas bleed easily
♦ Resemble vascular naevi in neonates
♦ Common in yearlings

Pigs
Similar lesions on scrotum of mature boars.

HEMANGIOSARCOMA [VM8 p. 558]

♦ In adult horses
♦ Large subcutaneous masses
♦ Commonly accompanied by internal lesions, likely to bleed spontaneously, fatally

RETICULUM CELL SARCOMA [VM8 p. 558]

Multiple subcutaneous masses in horses and cattle.

LIPOMA [VM8 p. 558]

Large subcutaneous masses, easily removed surgically.

CONGENITAL DEFECTS OF THE SKIN [VM8 p. 559]

Most are inherited and detailed elsewhere. They include the following.

Cattle
♦ Parakeratosis (Adema disease)
♦ Congenital ichthyosis (fish-scale disease)
♦ Inherited epidermal dysplasia (baldy calves)
♦ Inherited hypotrichosis and alopecia
♦ Epitheliogenesis imperfecta; lesions commonly at coronet; hooves may be absent
♦ Acantholysis; skin shed at carpus, coronet
♦ Dermatosparaxia, hyperelastosis cutis, Ehlers–Danlos syndrome; loose skin, hypermobile joints.

Sheep
♦ Epidermolysis bullosa; skin, horn and mucosa shed in neonates

♦ Inherited redfoot; similar lesions to epidermolysis
♦ Mild form of dermatosparaxia

Pigs
♦ Dermatosis vegetans
♦ Epitheliogenesis imperfecta
♦ Congenital skin gangrene in *Fusarium* spp. poisoning

Horses
♦ Rare dermatosparaxia
♦ Non-inherited defects include:
  • Vascular naevus on lower limbs of foals; pink, irregular shaped masses, bleed easily, composed entirely of blood vessels. Surgical excision recommended
  • Dermoid cysts on neck or in mouth

DISEASES OF THE CONJUNCTIVA

CONJUNCTIVITIS AND KERATOCONJUNCTIVITIS [VM8 p. 559]

Etiology

Inflammation of the covering membrane (conjunctivitis) and the deeper layers of the cornea (keratoconjunctivitis).

Specific conjunctivites
Cattle
- Moraxella bovis
- M. bovis plus infectious bovine rhinotracheitis virus
- Neisseria catarrhalis
- Mycoplasma spp.
- Chlamydia spp.

Sheep
- Rickettsia conjunctivae
- Neisseria catarrhalis
- Mycoplasma conjunctivae
- Acholeplasma conjunctivae
- Chlamydia spp.

Goats
- Rickettsia conjunctivae

Pigs
- Rickettsia spp.

Horses
Moraxella equi

Specific keratites
Cattle
- Thelazia spp.
- Onchocerca spp.

Sheep and goats
Elaeophora schneideri

Horses
- Thelazia spp.
- Habronema spp.

Secondary conjunctivites

Cattle
- Bovine viral diarrhea
- Bovine malignant catarrh
- Rinderpest
- Infectious bovine rhinotracheitis
- Viral pneumonia (several viruses)

Sheep
Bluetongue

Pigs
- Swine influenza
- Inclusion body rhinitis

Horses
- Equine viral arteritis
- Equine viral rhinopneumonitis

Non-specific conjunctivites
- Foreign body
- Exposure, e.g. when recumbent or eyelid paralysis
- Ant-bite when recumbent
- Congenital entropion

Clinical findings

- Blepharospasm
- Watery lacrimation followed by mucopurulent, purulent discharge

Sequels Include corneal under-running with pus, vascularization, opacity, white scarring.

CONGENITAL DEFECTS OF THE EYELIDS AND CORNEA

DERMOID CYSTS [VM8 p. 560]

- Firm, skin-covered teratomas on cornea, eyelid, nictitating membrane, medial canthus
- Contain elements of skin
- Obstruct vision in calves and foals
- Inherited in Hereford cattle
- Ablation recommended

DISEASES OF THE EXTERNAL EAR

SQUAMOUS-CELL CARCINOMA
[VM8 p. 560]

♦ Common in some sheep flocks
♦ Commences along free edge of ear
♦ Terminates as cauliflower-shaped mass

OTITIS EXTERNA [VM8 p. 560]

♦ *Rhabditis bovis, Raillietia auris* cause high incidence in range cattle
♦ Frequent head-shaking
♦ Dysphagia
♦ Smelly discharge

Treatment Ivermectin, topical antibiotic.

PART TWO

SPECIAL MEDICINE

15 MASTITIS

The principal clinical signs, clinicopathological findings, special examination techniques, and the basic syndrome on which clinical diagnoses of udder disease are based include the following.

BASIC SYNDROME [VM8 p. 563]

Clinical findings Mastitis is inflammation of the mammary parenchyma characterized by the following indicants:

♦ **Constant** – elevated somatic cell count, and chemical tests dependent on the cell count
♦ **Variable:**
  • Presence of a pathogen in the milk
  • Watery milk
  • Clots or flakes in milk (blood is not an indicator)
  • Reduced milk yield
  • Swelling (acute, hot, or chronic cold; edema not an indicator)
  • Atrophy of gland in long-standing cases
  • Lumps of scar tissue in the gland
  • Gangrene of part or whole of a quarter

Caused by:
♦ Bacteria, most commonly
♦ Viruses, only as part of a major disease
♦ Fungi, rarely
♦ Algae, very rarely
♦ Chemical agents, including intramammary infusions of irritant substances and toxins ingested in poisonous plants, including estrogens

INDIVIDUAL CLINICAL INDICANTS

Milk clotted

Occurs in Mastitis.

Milk orange, thick

Occurs in:
♦ Colostrum, some cattle breeds
♦ Acute leptospirosis
♦ anthrax

Milk pink, brown, red, contains blood clots

Occurs in Blood in milk.

Milk purulent

Occurs in Mastitis.

Milk somatic cell count elevated

Occurs in Mastitis.

Milk watery

Occurs in:
♦ Normal cows at end of lactation
♦ Chronic mastitis

Milk watery with flakes

Occurs in Acute *Escherichia coli* mastitis.

Milk yield nil

Occurs in:
♦ Agalactia
♦ Mastitis–metritis–agalactia (MMA) in sows

Milk yield sudden drop

Occurs in:
♦ Many severe acute diseases, e.g. intestinal obstruction, traumatic reticuloperitonitis
♦ Milk drop, summer slump

Teats edematous

Occurs in Udder congestion, edema.

Teat skin lesions

Clinical findings:
♦ Focal, discrete lesions in most
♦ Complete covering with scabs

Occurs in:
♦ Udder, teat dermatitis
♦ Black spot
♦ Udder impetigo
♦ Lacerations
♦ Chapped cracks

Teat skin reddened, thickened laterally

Occurs in Photosensitization.

Teat slack, udder filled

Occurs in Congenital closure milk cistern sphincter.

Teat sphincter blocked

Clinical findings:
♦ Teat distended with milk
♦ Milk cannot be expressed
♦ Squeezing teat causes discomfort

Occurs in:
♦ Congenital teat defect
♦ Mastitis clots
♦ Blood in milk
♦ Black spot
♦ Teat end sore
♦ Corpora amylacea

Teat swollen, painful

Occurs in Thelitis.

Teat tip sore

Clinical findings:
♦ Milking obstructed
♦ Milking very painful; cups kicked off
♦ Mastitis a common sequel

Occurs in:
♦ Black spot
♦ Overmilking with machine
♦ Abrasive teat necrosis in piglets

Udder drops away from abdominal wall

Occurs in:
♦ Udder suspensory ligament rupture
♦ Ventral abdominal hernia

Udder edematous

Clinical findings:
♦ Anasarca udder and teats
♦ Perineum, ventral abdominal wall may be affected

Occurs in:
♦ Udder congestion, edema
♦ Udder suspensory ligament rupture
♦ Ventral abdominal hernia

Udder enlarged

Clinical findings:
♦ Udder edematous, congested, milk normal, e.g. udder congestion, edema, hard udder (indurative mastitis)
♦ Udder hot, hard, painful, milk watery, contains clots, flakes, pus – acute mastitis
♦ Udder uniformly hard or contains many large, hard masses, cold, not painful, milk may be watery, otherwise normal – chronic mastitis

Udder flaccid

Occurs in:
♦ Dry cows
♦ Milking cow with severe disease causing anorexia, or starvation

Udder gangrene

Occurs in Peracute staphylococcal mastitis.

Udder, hard masses in

Occurs in:
♦ Chronic mastitis
♦ Udder neoplasms

Udder hard, possibly hot, painful

See udder enlarged, this section.

Udder small

Occurs in Agalactia.

BOVINE MASTITIS [VM8 p. 563]

Etiology

Bacterial mastitis
Major infectious mastitides Infections persisting in the udder, the source of infection:
♦ *Streptococcus agalactiae*
♦ *Staphylococcus aureus*

Major environmental mastitides Infection persists in environment, the source of infection:
♦ *Escherichia coli*
♦ *Streptococcus dysgalactiae*
♦ *Streptococcus uberis*

Other bacterial infections occurring infrequently:
♦ *Corynebacterium (Actinomyces) pyogenes*
♦ *Klebsiella* spp.
♦ *Pasteurella multocida, P. hemolytica*
♦ *Pseudomonas pyocyaneus*
♦ *Mycoplasma* spp.
♦ *Nocardia* spp.
♦ and many others, some anaerobic species

Minor pathogens Low pathogenicity, constant mammary infections, no inflammation:
♦ *Corynebacterium bovis*
♦ *Staphylococcus epidermidis, S. hyicus*

Special note Leptospira hardjo and *L. pomona* cause systemic disease damage to blood vessels in mammary gland, simulating mastitis.

Fungal infections
♦ *Aspergillus, Trichosporon, Pichia* spp.
♦ *Candida, Cryptococcus, Saccharomyces* spp.

Algal infection
♦ *Prototheca* spp.

Epidemiology

Occurrence
♦ Universal in machine milking dairy herds
♦ Average infection prevalence in herds not practicing control, 40% cows, 25% quarters
♦ Quarter infection rate in herds practicing control 10%
♦ Sporadic similar incidence beef herds.

Pastured herds Streptococcus agalactiae common cause acute clinical mastitis; *Staphylococcus aureus* common cause subclinical and chronic cases.

Housed or penned herds Escherichia coli other environmental infections also prominent.

Case fatality rate Nil, except immediate postparturient *S. aureus, E. coli*, dry cow *C. pyogenes.*

Source and transmission
Infectious mastitis Milk from infected quarter via hands, milking machine liners, udder towels, wash water.

Environmental mastitis Infected bedding, infusion material, wash water, dirty teats; spread via direct contact and during milking.

Risk factors
♦ Existing high prevalence in herd
♦ Unhygienic, inefficient milking
♦ Unclean bedding
♦ Poor stall design and size
♦ Increasing age
♦ Early lactation
♦ High-yielding cows
♦ Teat lesions common in herd
♦ Complete sterilization of quarters, especially minor pathogens

Importance
♦ Few deaths
♦ Loss of milk production 15% for lactation
♦ Eventual loss of quarter as producing unit causes high culling rate, reduced longevity

Clinical findings

Vary with pathogen and stage of lactation.

Peracute Systemic reaction (fever, tachycardia, depression, anorexia), usually marked swelling, pain and hardness of quarter, severe milk abnormality (clots, flakes, bad odor).

Acute As for peracute without systemic reaction.

Subacute Mild swelling, milk abnormality, clots, wateriness persisting through milking.

Chronic Lumps in gland, or atrophy; milk watery at beginning of milking, persisting for long period.

Subclinical High cell count or similar positive test, without clinical signs.

Clinical pathology

Tests to detect mastitis
California mastitis test Cow-side test based on cell count; time-consuming, interpretation difficulties.

Milk electrical conductivity Cow-side appliances too variable; sophisticated sensors incorporated into milking machines show promise.

Laboratory tests Based on cell count (NAGase, direct capture ELISA tests), or serum leakage from damaged mammary epithelium (chloride, bovine serum albumin, antitrypsin tests).

Laboratory cell counts Individual quarter, individual cow, bulk herd count, performed electronically; individual quarter counts too expensive so composite samples usual; threshold is 250 000 cells/ ml for individual cow counts, 300 000 for bulk milk counts (500 000 cells/ml adequate in most situations).

Total bacterial count On sample of bulk milk; undependable; >50% violations of quality code are due to unhygienic milking practices.

Tests to identify causative agent
♦ Milk culture of sample from bulk tank
♦ Composite cow sample collected for fat test or similar
♦ Individual quarter (more commonly composite sample) collected specifically for culture examination

Recommended culture procedure includes:
♦ Individual quarter preferred to composite sampling if infection rate low (e.g. 10%)
♦ Cows reacting positively to indirect test but negatively to culture, considered positive for treatment purposes
♦ Disregard infections with **minor pathogens**
♦ Collect sample from **dry**, alcohol-rubbed, third and fourth streams; most accurate is to collect also, last few streams
♦ **Augmented culture technique** includes pre-culture incubation, followed by freezing, and large inoculum

Test program for continuing surveillance
Periodic (usually monthly) bulk milk cell count or similar; when cell count exceeds 300 000/ml a mastitis problem exists.

Test program for herd with mastitis problem
Alarm raised by:
♦ High bulk milk cell count, or
♦ High bulk milk bacterial count on culture
♦ High incidence of clinical mastitis cases
Requires individual cow examination of all or sample of herd by:
♦ Screening indirect test (CMT, cell count, NAGase test, etc.), plus
♦ Culture, and possibly antibiotic sensitivity, of cows positive to screening test

Test for individual cow with mastitis problem
♦ Complete physical examination of quarter, teat and milk
♦ Indirect test to ensure identity of cellular reaction
♦ Culture, preferably of milk containing no antibiotic

Recommended response to positive test in individual cows
♦ Clinical cases always treated at once
♦ Positive cows (or quarters) in early lactation treated at once

Positive cows in mid to late lactation treated in next dry period, except
▶ Positive cows with fibrosed udders, aged cows, cows with bad prior history, to be culled

Necropsy findings

Not a usual examination method in mastitis; see under each bacteriological type of mastitis.

Diagnosis

Mastitis unlikely to be confused with other disease except:
♦ Toxemic, recumbent cow with *Escherichia coli* mastitis resembles milk fever, acute diffuse peritonitis or other severe puerperal endotoxemia
♦ Lameness due to gangrenous *Staphylococcus aureus* mastitis resembles blackleg
♦ For differentiation of bacteriological types of mastitis see Table 15.1.

Treatment

Details of treatment for individual bacteriological types in Table 15.1. General principles include the following.

Peracute and acute cases
Evacuate quarters by massage, frequent milking, even pituitary extract
♦ Supportive anti-endotoxemia parenteral fluids and electrolytes
♦ Parenteral treatment with potentiated sulfonamide or broad-spectrum antibiotic in cases with systemic reaction, or badly swollen quarter
♦ Supplement parenteral treatment with intramammary infusion, unless quarter being frequently milked, or use as sole treatment; infusion should maintain adequate level antibiotic in quarter for six days
♦ Anti-inflammatories when required but avoid immunosuppression
♦ Recommended intramammary treatment, in the absence of information about the specific infection and its sensitivities are:
  • Mixture of aminoglycoside (framycetin or neomycin) + a penicillin
  • Ampicillin
  • Amoxycillin
  • Third generation cephalosporin
♦ Remind farmers of obligation to allow withdrawal time before sending milk for sale for human consumption

Withdrawal times, lactating cows:
♦ Udder infusion, quick release base – 72 hours
♦ One parenteral injection – 36 hours
♦ Series parenteral injections – 72 hours
♦ Parenteral injection long-acting preparation – 10 days
♦ Intra-uterine tablet – 72 hours

Withdrawal times, dry cows Intramammary infusion at least 4 weeks before calving – 96 hours after calving.

Subacute and chronic cases – dry period treatment
♦ Consider recommendation to cull
♦ Restrict treatment to dry period
♦ Treat in accordance with laboratory tests of sensitivity
♦ Use long-acting base
♦ One treatment at drying off, second 4–6 weeks before calving. Common usage is one infusion at drying off
♦ Recommended infusions:
  • Cloxacillin
  • Nafcillin
  • Cephalosporins

THE CONTROL OF BOVINE MASTITIS [VM8 p. 601]

The following recommended program is aimed at the control of the common infectious causes of bovine mastitis, *Streptococcus agalactiae* and *Staphylococcus aureus*. Its intensity may be slackened if the prevalence before control is much less than 15% quarter infection rate, 30% cow infection rate. It will need to be vigorously implemented if:
♦ The prevailing infection is with an environmental or atypical bacteria

♦ The herd has a problem with:
  • A high prevalence of clinical cases, *or*
  • A high rate of repeat clinical episodes in the same cows, *or*
  • A high bulk milk cell count, *or*
  • A high quality violation rate at the milk-receiving depot
in spite of what the farmer believes is a control program. (See below for Recommended Procedures for Problem Herds.)

Table 15.1 Differentiation of bovine mastitis

(See p. 252 for descriptions of standard cases of peracute, acute, chronic, subclinical mastitis and their diagnosis, treatment and control. Only notable features that facilitate diagnosis are listed here.)

Etiological agent (alphabetical)	Type (acute, chronic etc.)	Clinical and clinical pathology features	Epidemiological features	Response to treatment and control procedures
Actinomyces pyogenes [VM8 p. 583]	Peracute suppurative in late pregnant or fresh cows	Putrid odor in milk. Abscesses rupture at teat base, other bacteria, including anerobes in culture	Sporadic cases in housed cattle or summer outbreaks in dry cattle at pasture. 'Summer mastitis' of Europe	Poor response, quarter lost cow survives. Parenteral – potentiated sulfonamide or tetracyclines. i/mam broad-spectrum antibiotic. Dry period, every 3 wks cloxacillin and ampicillin i/mam. Fly control
Algae. (*Prototheca trispora*, *P. zopfii*) [VM8 p. 600]	Chronic	Pyogranulomatous lesion	Environmental mastitis. Sporadic cases. Rare outbreak	Poor response. Cull cow
Bacillus spp. *B. cereus*, *B. subtilis* [VM8 p. 599]	Peracute, acute hemorrhagic in fresh cows	Red serous secretion. Some gangrenous	Environmental mastitis. Sporadic cases. Due to teat injury, contaminated i/mam infusion	Poor response. Quarter lost, case fatality rate high
Campylobacter jejuni [VM8 p. 599]	Subclinical	Transient swelling, fine clots. High cell count	Possible public health hazard. Rare	No information
Clostridium perfringens A [VM8 p. 599]	Peracute gangrenous	Thin brown secretion contains gas. Subcutis emphysema	Rare	Successful if early. Broad-spectrum antibiotic intramammary infusion
Escherichia coli (Coliform mastitis) [VM8 p. 584]	Peracute, toxemic in fresh cows. Rarely acute or subclinical	Peracute recumbent, very toxic. Milk is thin serous fluid with flakes. Short course 24–48 hours	Environmental mastitis. Sporadic cases, high prevalence associated with dirty bedding, dirty teats	Response poor. High mortality rate. Supportive anti-endotoxemia treatment essential for survival. i/mam and parenteral gentamicin or tetracyclines. Bedding and teat hygiene

254

Organism		Gross in udder		
Fungi and yeasts (Trichosporon spp) [VM8 p. 600]	Acute			Spontaneous recovery or severe damage leads to culling
Cryptococcus neoformans [VM8 p. 600]	Acute	Viscid, gray-white secretion	Contaminated infusions	Spontaneous recovery. Few granuloma, chronic abscess. Antifungal agents e.g. miconazole etc. as i/mam infusion
Candida spp, etc. [VM8 p. 600]	Acute	Lymph node swelling. Lesion in milk system wall	Contaminated infusions or teat cup liners	Poor response to broad-spectrum antibiotics
Fusobacterium necrophorum [VM8 p. 598]	Chronic	Viscid, clotty, stringy secretion. Little fibrosis	Rare herds with high incidence	Nil
Haemophilus somnus [VM8 p. 600]	Peracute gangrenous, acute or chronic	Nil	Nil	Poor response to penicillin but bacteria sensitive
Listeria monocytogenes [VM8 p. 600]	Subacute or subclinical	Normal milk, production decreases, high cell count	Persistent infection. Public health importance	
Mycobacterium spp. e.g. M. lacticola, M. fortuitum, M. smegmatis [VM8 p. 500]	Chronic / Acute	Gross hypertrophy of gland, clots in discolored milk. Mild form in self terminating outbreaks also occur. Cases with M. fortuitum respond positively to mammalian tuberculin	Environmental mastitis. Infection in oil-based i/mam infusions or watery infusion followed by oil	No treatment effective. Case dies or culled because of udder damage in M. fortuitum infection
Mycoplasma bovis and other Ureaplasma spp [VM8 p. 596]	Acute	Often all quarters simultaneously. Dramatic milk yield decline. Milk separates to turbid watery supernatant over flaky, floccular deposit. Smooth, painless hypertrophy. Very high cell counts	Infectious mastitis outbreaks in large herds with poor hygiene after introduction of new cows. In herds using common syringe for bulk i/mam treatments	Poor response because damage severe. i/mam tylosin and tetracyclines. Cull isolate infected cows. Intense hygiene at milking and i/mam infusion
Nocardia asteroides, N. braziliensis, N. farcinicus [VM8 p. 595]	Peracute (rarely). Acute, subacute	Extensive udder granulomas. Grayish, viscid secretion, small white particles. Gross gland enlargement, may discharge via sinuses	Environmental mastitis. Contaminated soil infects via teat. In udder infusion or infected chlorhexidine teat dip	Poor response to miconazole, erythromycin, neomycin for 1–2 wks. Intense hygiene required at milking and i/mam infusion

Table 15.1 (Cont'd)

Etiological agent (alphabetical)	Type (acute, chronic etc.)	Clinical and clinical pathology features	Epidemiological features	Response to treatment and control procedures
Pasteurella multocida, P. hemolytica [VM8 p. 594]	Peracute, toxemic	May affect all 4 quarters together. Red, watery, secretion plus flakes. Recumbent	Rare. Sporadic cases. Some in 'summer mastitis' outbreaks	Poor. Cow usually survives, quarter lost with tetracycline i/mam and parenteral
Pseudomonas aeruginosa [VM8 p. 598]	Peracute, often fresh cows after dry period treatment	Culture difficult and may be few organisms. Clotted discolored milk	Rare. Contaminated i/mam infusion or contaminated udder wash water plus poor milking technique	Poor. Case fatality rate high in some outbreaks. Quarter function loss. Third generation cephalosporins (cefoperazone) recommended
Serratia marcescens, S. liquefaciens [VM8 p. 599]	Mild chronic	Periodic clots in milk	Environmental mastitis due to infection from contaminated bedding. Rare, outbreaks	Neomygecin i/mam and parenteral effective
Staphylococcus aureus (coagulase positive) [VM8 p. 579]	Peracute (gangrenous) in fresh cows. Acute, subclinical	Gangrenous cases, lame, severe pain, gangrene of udder quarter and teat. Subclinical cases have high cell counts, major cause of lost production, high culling rate, ELISA and Rapid Lab Test System available	Commonest infectious mastitis. Source is infected quarters. Insidious spread	Penicillin-nitrofurazone, erythromycin, spiramycin, ampicillin and cloxacillin. Lactating cows 3 i/mam × 24 hrs; Dry cow 1 i/mam infusion in long-acting base. Strict application of standard control program effective. Some deaths. Quarter always lost in gangrenous form. Acute and chronic case 60% recover
Staphylococcus epidermidis (coagulase negative) [VM8 p. 579]	Minor pathogen. Rarely even subclinical	Elevated cell count. No clinical effect	Elimination may increase susceptibility to environmental pathogens	None recommended

Organism	Type	Clinical features	Epidemiology	Treatment / response
Streptococcus agalactiae [VM8 p. 574]	Acute. Subacute. Chronic	Spreads quickly, many clinical cases. High cell counts. CAMP test on culture standard diagnostic procedure. Available now Latex agglutination test, ELISA	Infectious mastitis. Source is an infected quarter	Excellent response. Lactating cows two penicillin i/mam infusions 72 hrs apart. Penicillin and neomycin common i/mam infusion. Dry cows, cloxacillin single infusion
Streptococcus dysgalactiae, S. uberis [VM8 p. 577]	Acute	Outbreaks or sporadic clinical cases. Rapid Lab Test System available	Environmental mastitis infection from bedding plus teat injury, rough milking procedure	Good response to parenteral + i/mam infusion penicillin or erythromycin. Intensive bedding and teat hygiene. Dry period treatments, one at drying off, one 6 wks before calving
Traumatic mastitis mixed infectious [VM8 p. 601]	Acute	Intractable, suppurative, often with toxemia	Sporadic cases. Teat lacerations or treads	Poor. Many environmental bacteria present
Leptospira hardjo, L. pomona [VM8 p. 590]	Not a mastitis. Systemic disease with endothelial damage in udder	All 4 quarters affected. Thick, yellow or blood-tinged milk. No gland change	Associated with outbreak of leptospirosis	Treat systemic disease

Program adoption

Encouraged by:

♦ Milk depot paying a premium or refusing to handle milk on basis of bulk milk cell count
♦ Voluntary move by farmer cooperative
♦ Presentation of practicality and profitability reasons by veterinarian

Program objectives

♦ Limitation of infection rate, not complete eradication
♦ Avoid elimination of minor pathogens (*Corynebacterium bovis*) which help maintain resistance to infection
♦ Detect, cure or cull all clinical cases early
♦ Detect and eliminate all infected quarters as sources of infection
♦ Prevent new infections by spread from other cows or the environment by hygiene at milking time
♦ Reduce susceptibility by gentle milking technique
♦ Monitor mastitis prevalence

Detection of infected quarters

♦ Detection clinical cases by hand-held or floor insert strip plate
♦ Detection subclinical cases, on advice that bulk milk cell count too high, by individual cow cell count, or indirect, e.g. NAGase or CMT test
♦ Culture cows (quarters) with high cell count (or other test)

Treatments

Specific treatments for each infection are also in Table 15.1.

Lactating cows

♦ Of clinical cases as they occur until signs eliminated, not less than 2 infusions 72 hours apart, or equivalent, and withdraw milk from sale; forbid use of long-acting dry cow preparations
♦ Of subclinical cases deferred until dry period except option to treat *Streptococcus agalactiae* infection during early lactation, in high producing cows when herd infection rate high

Dry cows

♦ Blanket treatment all quarters if infection rate high; variable but say over 15%
♦ Selective treatment infected quarters if identity known and incidence less than a variable but say 15%

♦ Infusion **immediately** after last milking ensures protection for only 25 days; in problem herds or where environmental infections predominate administer second infusion in last 6 weeks of pregnancy but ensure no carry-over of antibiotic into lactation
♦ Intensive teat sterilization at dry period infusions
♦ Suitable infusion components – benzathine cloxacillin, cephalonium, cephapirin benzathine, nifuraquine, or procaine penicillin + furaltodone, or neomycin, or novobiocin
♦ Soluble polymer teat sealant recommended for use at drying off

All cows

♦ Intensive hygiene of alcohol scrub and dipping teat in commercial dip before and after infusion
♦ For choice of antibiotic see Table 15.1.
♦ In repeat cases, early lactation heavy-producing cows, or systemic reaction combine standard intramammary infusion with same or complementary/compatible antibiotic parenterally

Culling chronic cases

In high-prevalence herds maintain high culling rate of repeat cases and lumpy udders

Milking procedure – hygiene

♦ **Pre-wash teat stripping** valuable in reducing new infection rate if rate already high
♦ **Pre-milking washing and drying teats** valuable principally for milk quality effect; thorough drying with single use towel essential; valuable if teamed with teat disinfection routine
♦ **Pre-milking teat disinfection** with dilute (0.1–0.25% iodine) iodophor dip or spray should reduce bacterial count of milk but has little reliable effect on mastitis infection; low concentration needed to avoid iodine residues in milk
♦ **Post-milking teat disinfection** one of the critical features of the control program especially for the infectious mastitides; iodophor solutions containing 1% available iodine, or chlorine preparations containing 4% free chlorine satisfactory; chlorhexidine (0.3% solution or 0.5% in polyvinyl pyrrolidone) widely used but ineffective against *Nocardia asteroides*); iodine dips banned in some countries because of residues in milk; many other preparations have excellent early reputations.

Chapping is a serious side-effect with many dips in some herds; additives to reduce chapping may reduce bactericidal efficiency

Post-milking teat cup disinfection or back-flush valuable if infection rate high and heifers milked amongst cows; often omitted because of time required; rinse then dip in chemical disinfectant or 80°C water but 15 second cold water back-flush best suited to automated milking

Milking procedure – machine operation

♦ Machine design innovations reduce new infection rate – automatic cup removers reduce overmilking; teat cup deflector shields reduce impact of infected milk on teat orifices; reduction of cross-flow of milk between cows achievable by very long milk lines; one way valves in milk lines reduce reflux between quarters
♦ Reduction of trauma to mammary and teat tissues promised by hydraulic milking system
♦ Excessive vacuum pressure (>50 kPa or 37.5 cm hg) likely to cause injury; leads to red, prominent teat end with eversion of lining, possibly sores, leading to mastitis
♦ Vacuum stability – random acute changes in vacuum pressure increase infection rate; liner slip due to badly moulded teat cup liners, causes vacuum instability
♦ Inadequate vacuum reserve in high-line milking machines causes reverse milk flow and spreads infection
♦ Frequent cleaning and changing of teat cup liners prevents infection transmission and liner slip

Milking technique

Good milking practice avoids overmilking and excessive vacuum pressure and includes:
♦ Gentle machine stripping
♦ Gentle cup removal after vacuum release
♦ Cups removed as soon as milk ceases to flow
♦ Average milking time per cow 4–6 minutes
♦ Number of machine clusters per milker 4–6

Milking order

To reduce infection transmission between cows:
♦ Milk heifers before young, mastitis-free cows, before heavy-yielding mastitis-free cows, before mastitis cows, and subclinical before clinical cases

♦ Introduced cows milked in quarantine until mastitis status known

Drying-off

♦ In low mastitis prevalence herds, abrupt cessation of milking is satisfactory
♦ Mastitis flare-ups may result when many subclinicals in herd; milk once daily, reduce feed and water, for one week

Selection criteria for genetic protection against mastitis

Teat characteristics which increase chances of mastitis:
♦ Cylindrical versus funnel-shaped teats
♦ Wider teat canals, i.e. fast milkers, leak milk between milkings
♦ Inverted, funnel-shaped, or recessed plate-like, ends
♦ Deep udders with low back quarters
♦ Widely placed teats, rear teats too far back, short wide teats

Housing

Mastitis-enhancing features of barn or pen housing:
♦ Slippery floors, narrow stalls encouraging teat trauma
♦ Inadequate manure/bedding removal, leads to soiled teats and environmental mastitis

Miscellaneous

Aids to preventing mastitis:
♦ Prevent calves sucking each other
♦ Only feed mastitic milk to calves if formalin- or antibiotic-treated
♦ Special observation of cows close to and right after calving to avoid recumbency, teat injury and soiling
♦ Intramammary devices have little demonstrable value, attract an amorphous deposit and are easily colonized by *Corynebacterium pyogenes*
♦ Special attention to rapid cure of teat chapping, sores and cuts
♦ Hand disinfection where hand-stripping or hand-milking practiced
♦ Valuable breeding cows with a persistently infected quarter can have quarter permanently dried off
♦ Fly control by automatic sprays at feeding points necessary where 'summer mastitis' prevalent

Control techniques requiring special attention in herds with environmental mastitis problem

♦ Identification of causal organism
♦ Correct poor bedding hygiene
♦ Eliminate bulk mastitis treatments using one syringe
♦ Check microbiology of intramammary infusions, especially home-made bulk infusions
♦ Check microbiology of wash water, wash cloths, teat dip
♦ Keep environment dry and clean
♦ Dry teats before milking

Monitoring mastitis incidence

♦ Periodic (monthly in herds with consistently good cell counts, weekly when mastitis a problem) bulk milk somatic cell count (<500 000/ml essential, <300 000 preferred) or bacterial count (<100 000 bacteria/ml) or in-line electrical conductivity test
♦ Periodic individual cow cell counts on milk samples collected for butter fat test if selective drying off practised (target is <10% infected quarters)

Problem herds

Protocol for examination of a problem herd includes:

♦ Examination of environment looking for deep mud in gateways, narrow or short beds, stall beds, and dirty, wet bedding
♦ Examination of milking machine for dirty faulty teat cup liners, too small vacuum reserve
♦ Examine sample of cows by physical palpation, teat end examination, cell count CMT or similar, microbiological culture
♦ Observe milking technique and milking machine operation, especially teat liner slip and random fluctuation in vacuum pressure

Checklist of common faults in mastitis control program

♦ Teat dip too dilute or inefficient or insufficient used in spray
♦ Wash water infected
♦ Infusion material contaminated
♦ Resistant strains of bacteria
♦ Lactating cow treatments inadequate usually because of too few or too small infusion doses
♦ Teat disinfection at udder infusion inadequate
♦ Drying-off treatment inadequate
♦ Culling pressure insufficient
♦ Order of milking to milk infected cows last not maintained
♦ Pre-milking teat sanitization and drying inadequate

PORCINE MASTITIS [VM8 p. 624]

MASTITIS–METRITIS–AGALACTIA
SYNDROME IN SOWS [VM8 p. 618]

Etiology

Mastitis due to *Escherichia coli*, *Klebsiella pneumoniae* the only significant cause.

Epidemiology

♦ Sometimes occurs in sporadic outbreaks
♦ Heavy (up to 80% mortality) wastage of piglets from starvation, secondary diseases
♦ Sow mortality less than 2%

Risk factors
♦ Individual sows more susceptible, but disease does not recur
♦ Mostly in mature sows farrowed indoors in crates
♦ Sows with large litters
♦ Overfeeding, especially sudden change in feed close to farrowing

Clinical findings

♦ In sows farrowed 12–48 hours
♦ Anorexia, drinks little
♦ Lethargy

- Sow disinterested in piglets; will not suckle them; restless, tramps on piglets
- Fever >40°C
- Swollen, warm, painful mammary glands, often with subcutaneous edema around them
- Teats empty
- Milk in severe cases may be watery, contain flakes
- Agalactia
- Large, flaccid uterus in many
- Constipation, but common in normal sows in group
- Vaginal discharge, clear mucus containing white material common in normal sows for 3 days after farrowing
- Poor milk ejection tested manually
- Piglets restless, noisy, thirsty

Clinical pathology

- Often not a significant diagnostic aid
- Severe leukopenia with degenerative left shift in bad cases; shift regenerative in milder cases
- Milk pH increased to 7.8; somatic cell count >2 million/ml; bacteria cultivable from most affected glands

Necropsy findings

- Focal or diffuse mastitis in some individual mammary gland segments in most sows
- Mastitis varies from mild catarrhal to severe purulent, necrotizing mastitis

Diagnosis

Resembles:
- Other causes of agalactia:
  - Primary agalactia
  - Mammary hypoplasia
  - Greater than normal mammary congestion, edema
  - Failure of milk ejection reflex
- Eclampsia, responding to calcium, magnesium therapy
- Farrowing fever, with minimal changes in mammary glands
- Sow hysteria, characterized by full mammary glands without letdown reflex; responds dramatically to ataractic drug

Treatment

- Most recover with combination of **antimicrobials, oxytocin, and corticosteroids**
- Broad-spectrum antibacterial for 3 days
- Oxytocin (30–40 units I/M or 20–30 units I/V, plus warm-water massage) repeated hourly till milk flow commences; may need to be repeated
- Dexamethazone (20 mg/day I/M for 3 days) a suitable corticosteroid
- Piglets need supplementary feeding, e.g. with 50 ml warm cows milk by stomach tube hourly for 500 ml daily intake; or porcine gamma globulin-fortified canned milk, diluted 1:1, or balanced electrolytes plus 5% glucose

Control

- Disinfect farrowing crates
- Wash sow clean, disinfect mammary area
- Sow into crate 7 days before due date
- Continue gestation diet without any change; with possible exception of substituting bran for up to half of ration, or lucerne meal up to 15%
- Feeding sulfonamides 3–5 days before farrowing is used
- Induction of parturition with prostaglandins gives inconsistent results

SOW MASTITIS DUE TO
MISCELLANEOUS CAUSES [VM8
p. 624]

Etiology

- *Escherichia coli* and other gram-negative bacteria
- Coagulase-positive *Staphylococcus aureus*
- *Streptococcus agalactiae, S. dysgalactiae, S. uberis*

Clinical findings

- Sporadic cases in recently farrowed sows
- Inflamed gland
- Anorexia, recumbency, fever, agalactia
- Piglet mortality
- Abscesses discharging through sinuses in some cases

OVINE MASTITIS [VM8 p. 624]

EWE PASTEURELLA MASTITIS
[VM8 p. 624]

Etiology

Pasteurella hemolytica

Epidemiology

Close to parturition or after weaning.

Risk factors
♦ Infection of bedding grounds at pasture
♦ Vigorous sucking by big, strong lambs
♦ Teat abrasions on rough barn floors
♦ Infection on bedding or floors in housing

Clinical findings

♦ Fever, toxemia
♦ Lameness on affected side
♦ Swelling, gangrene of udder, belly wall
♦ Watery red secretion with clots
♦ Ewe dies or recovers with udder slough in 7 days

Diagnosis

Resembles mastitis caused by *Staphylococcus aureus, Pseudomonas aeruginosa*.

Treatment and control

♦ Potentiated sulfonamide or broad-spectrum antibiotic
♦ Autogenous vaccine plus bedding hygiene

MINOR SPECIES MASTITIS

EWE MASTITIS [VM8 p. 625]

Etiology

Mostly *Staphylococcus aureus*, few *Streptococcus agalactiae, Pasteurella hemolytica*, rarely *Escherichia coli, Histophilus ovis*.

Epidemiology

High prevalence in ewes in commercial milk producing units.

Clinical findings

♦ Acute or subacute forms as in cows
♦ Recently lambed brood ewes tend to gangrenous mastitis caused by *Staphylococcus aureus, Pasteurella hemolytica* or rarely *Clostridium perfringens A, Histophilus agni, Actinobacillus lignieresi*
♦ *Mycoplasma* spp. agalactia is dealt with separately (p. 362)
♦ Ewes with clostridial mastitis may show hemolytic anemia, with hemoglobinuria, jaundice and anemia

Clinical pathology

♦ Milking ewes have high milk cell counts (>300 000/ml)
♦ Positive CMT and NAGase tests

Diagnosis

Udder lesions common in **caseous lymphadenitis** but no involvement of mammary tissue.

Treatment

Standard cow intramammary infusions.

Control

♦ Streptococcal and staphylococcal mastitis transmitted as in cows by hands, teat cup liners, udder cloths
♦ Standard bovine control program effective
♦ Ewes with sloughed quarters or draining sinuses must be culled

CAPRINE MASTITIS [VM8 p. 626]

Etiology

♦ Specific infectious diseases having mastitis as part of syndrome – infection with *Mycoplasma agalactiae, M. mycoides* var. *mycoides*
♦ Other causes rare, include:
  • Coliforms
  • *Pseudomonas* spp.
  • *Staphylococcus aureus*
  • *Actinomyces pyogenes*
  • *Nocardia asteroides*

Clinical findings

♦ As in cows
♦ Streptococcal, staphylococcal mastitis appear as peracute gangrenous, acute, chronic, subclinical; milk often misleadingly normal
♦ *Actinomyces pyogenes* as suppurative
♦ Pseudomonas and pasteurella mastitis are peracute, gangrenous mastitis

Clinical pathology

♦ High cell counts in clinically normal quarters; cell count threshold is >1 million cells/ml
♦ NAGase, other indirect tests also undependable in goat milk

Treatment and control

♦ Streptococcal, staphylococcal mastitis highly infectious as in cows; treatment, control measures, as recommended for cow mastitis, apply

MARE MASTITIS [VM8 p. 627]

Etiology

Corynebacterium pseudotuberculosis, Pseudomonas aeruginosa, Streptococcus zooepidemicus, S. equi, S. pyogenes, Staphylococcus aureus, Escherichia coli, Klebsiella and *Neisseria* spp. all recorded.

Epidemiology

♦ Rare
♦ Occurs any time in lactation, some in nonlactating mares

Clinical findings

♦ Swollen, painful gland
♦ Mild fever in some
♦ Gangrene uncommon
♦ Milk may appear normal
♦ Both halves often affected
♦ Foal will not feed and may attract attention to mare

Treatment

♦ Broad-spectrum antibiotic needed because of frequency of coliforms as cause
♦ Intensive parenteral, systemic therapy recommended
♦ Hot fomentations plus frequent stripping

MISCELLANEOUS ABNORMALITIES OF THE UDDER AND TEATS [VM8 p. 614]

Dermatitis of udder and teat skin – specific diseases

Cows
♦ Cowpox
♦ Pseudocowpox
♦ Bovine ulcerative mammillitis
♦ Papillomatosis
♦ Udder impetigo
♦ Mycotic dermatitis
♦ Bovine malignant catarrh
♦ Foot and mouth disease
♦ *Stephanofilaria* spp. larval invasion

Sows
♦ Swine vesicular disease
♦ Vesicular exanthema

Ewes
♦ Ecthyma
♦ Ulcerative dermatosis

Thelitis in cows

Due to:
♦ Trauma
♦ Burns from grass fire
♦ Of lateral aspects of teat due to photosensitization
♦ Due to administration corticosteroids
♦ Alpine nodular thelitis of multicentric tuberculoid granulomas containing mycobacteria

Teat necrosis of piglets

Abrasion on rough floor leads to occlusion of teat end.

Blood in milk of fresh cows

Due to blood vessel rupture. Often all 4 quarters. Treat with parenteral coagulants or calcium borogluconate if it persists beyond 48 hours.

Udder edema and congestion

♦ Edema of fresh cows and mares includes teats, belly wall, perineum persisting beyond 2 days after parturition
♦ Congestion of skin of udder floor may lead to permanent scleroderma. Treat with acetazolamide, chlorothiazide, hot fomentations, massage
♦ Hard udder a feature of caprine arthritis/encephalitis

Udder suspensory ligament rupture

Acutely at parturition, or over period of years. Udder drops markedly, teats point laterally; impossible to milk by machine

Parturient agalactia

Complete or almost complete absence of milk at parturition

Occurs in:
♦ Mastitis–metritis–agalactia in sows
♦ Poor letdown due to piglet sharp teeth
♦ Inverted nipples of sows
♦ Teat duct occlusion, e.g. after nipple abrasion in piglet
♦ Endocrinal failure of letdown in gilts, heifers, with full udder; treated effectively with pitocin
♦ Sow hysteria induced letdown failure
♦ *Claviceps fusiformis* ergot poisoning in sows.

Midterm agalactia due to free electricity

Due to static electricity build-up or intermittent shorting to interconnected metal parts of milking machine and stanchions, especially in defective earthing installation or drought time fall in ground water table. Cows restless, no milk letdown. Voltage of 0.5–1.5 volts.

Antibiotic residues in milk

After treatment for mastitis.

'Milk drop'

Precipitate fall in herd milk yield caused by:
♦ *Acremonium coeniaphilum* poisoning (summer slump)
♦ *Leptospira hardjo* infection.

Milk fat depression

Herd average falls precipitately to below 3%, often below 1% in presence of good feed. Due to <17% fiber in ration.

Black spot

Black, tenacious scab on sore at teat sphincter caused by rough teat cup removal before vacuum release. Teat duct obstructed, very painful causing no milk letdown. Cured by correction of milking technique.

Udder impetigo

Thin-walled, 2–4 mm dia. pustules on skin of teats and lower udder, transmitted by milking. *Staphylococcus aureus* isolated and outbreak terminated by autogenous vaccine. Transmissible to milker's hands. May lead to flexural seborrhea.

Udder neoplasms

Occur as:
♦ Bovine papillomatosis, rarely develop to squamous-cell carcinoma
♦ Nearby fibrosarcoma
♦ Primary teat fibroma and fibrosarcoma in cows
♦ Rare malignant mammary carcinoma in mares and goat does

Corpora amylacea

Inert, wheat-grain-sized amyloid mass, blocks teat duct.

Teat and udder congenital defects

Include:
♦ Supernumary teats
♦ Fused teats
♦ Aplasia of teat canal, sinus, mammary gland
♦ Inverted teats in sows
♦ Insufficient mammary glands in sows
♦ Misplaced teats in sows (too far anteriorly)

16 DISEASES CAUSED BY BACTERIA – I

Examination of a disease problem thought to be caused by an infectious agent should pay some attention to the following points:

♦ A history of introductions to the farm of animals, animal products or materials from an animal environment, e.g. feeding utensils
♦ Seasonal influences, e.g. high rainfall, heavy insect populations likely to encourage disease spread
♦ Examination of neighboring or local farms for evidence of the disease
♦ Vaccination history on the subject farm
♦ Proximity of wild animals likely to be carriers
♦ Clinical examination when appropriate
♦ Serological examination for evidence of past or present infection; repeat visits to observe seroconversions and movement in titers
♦ All examinations should include as many clinical cases, and suspect past cases as possible, plus an adequate number of apparent normals
♦ Regional abattoir surveillance
♦ Success or otherwise of treatment

DISEASES CAUSED BY *STREPTOCOCCUS* spp. [VM8 p. 629]

SEPTICEMIA [VM8 p. 629]

♦ *Streptococcus zooepidemicus* causes sudden death in 12–48 hours in adult sows, piglets, up to 90% mortality in lambs, kids
♦ *Streptococcus pneumoniae* causes sudden death in calves
♦ *Streptococcus suis* causes bacteremia with lesions in all organs in ruminants

ENTERITIS [VM8 p. 629]

Streptococcus durans causes diarrhea in foals.

PNEUMONIA [VM8 p. 629]

♦ *Streptococcus zooepidemicus* causes pneumonia, fibrinous pleuritis, pericarditis in lambs
♦ *Streptococcus pneumoniae* causing pneumonia in calves may be contracted from human attendants; in horses may be combined with a virus or *S. zooepidemicus*

MENINGOENCEPHALITIS [VM8 p. 630]

♦ *Streptococcus suis* type 2 causes meningoencephalitis in weaned pigs (10–14 wks old) and feeder pigs (5–6 months old); course a few hours, pigs often found dead

STREPTOCOCCAL LYMPHANGITIS [VM8 p. 630]

S. zooepidemicus a cause in horses, 6 months to 2 years.

STREPTOCOCCAL ARTHRITIS [VM8 p. 630]

Streptococcus faecalis a cause, with pericarditis, in foals, yearlings.

DERMATITIS [VM8 p. 630]

♦ Unidentified streptococci and staphylococci in pustules caused by bites, scratches from piglet needle teeth (contagious pyoderma)

STREPTOCOCCAL METRITIS [VM8 p. 630]

S. zooepidemicus a cause in mares, plus abortion and sterility, and neonatal infection in foals.

- β-hemolytic streptococci cause abortion in sows
- Unidentified streptococci a cause in sows

STRANGLES (DISTEMPER) [VM8 p. 630]

Etiology

- *Streptococcus equi*, all international isolates identical
- Capsule-deficient variant causes mild, atypical disease

Epidemiology

Occurrence
- Universal
- Most common where large horse congregations move around, in studs with visiting mares, polo matches
- Commonest in foals, yearlings
- Morbidity 10–100%
- Case fatality rate 10% without treatment, 1% with treatment

Transmission
- Ingestion, inhalation of nasal discharge from active case
- Infectivity usually 4 weeks but infected horses may act as carriers up to 8 months
- Organism resistant in environment

Risk factors
- Horses, burros only
- Immunity after an attack lasts 6 months

Importance
Disrupts training and racing calendar.

Clinical findings

Horse
- Incubation period 1–3 weeks
- Fever, anorexia, depression
- Copious serous then purulent nasal discharge
- Mild conjunctivitis
- Dysphagia, some regurgitate feed, water through nostril
- Painful cough
- Swollen, painful throat, head extended
- Submandibular lymph nodes swollen, rupture, discharge pus at 10 days
- Respiration noisy, dyspnea
- Course 3 weeks to 3 months

Sequels:
- Pneumonia
- Extensive suppurative lymphangitis
- Localization in any organ

Burro
Prolonged, debilitating disease, weight loss.

Clinical pathology

- Nasal swabs, abscess discharge cultured for *Streptococcus equi*
- Leukocytosis, left shift; anemia

Necropsy findings

- Extensive suppuration any or all organs
- Extensions to body cavities in some

Diagnosis

In early stages, mild cases resemble:
- Equine viral rhinopneumonitis
- Equine viral arteritis
- Equine viral influenza
- Equine rhinovirus infection
- Equine adenovirus infection
- Guttural pouch disease
- Sinusitis

In severe cases resemble:
- S. zooepidemicus lymphangitis
- S. faecalis arthritis

Treatment

- Isolate for 8 months
- Treat early cases intensively with parenteral penicillin, large intravenous dose first, then daily for 7 days; or 5 days after signs disappear
- Cases with severe lymphadenitis improve but recur
- Final recovery only after nodes rupture
- Irrigate sinuses with povidone/iodine

Control

- Quarantine introduced horses
- Clean up stables, feed troughs
- Isolate clinical cases
- Prophylactic penicillin injections young horses
- Vaccinate all exposed horses; annual boosters to all horses older than 3 months in high-risk situations
- Strangles vaccination causes severe local reactions in some

- Immunity brief, e.g. killed, young culture, 3 injections causes 12 months immunity
- Part-cell vaccines, including M protein, the protective antigen of *S. equi*, avoid adverse reactions, produce more durable immunity

NEONATAL STREPTOCOCCAL INFECTION [VM8 p. 634]

Etiology

- *Streptococcus genitalium (S. pyogenes equi)*, the common pathogen in foals
- Streptococci in Lancefield's groups C, E, L cause sporadic cases in pigs
- *S. equisimilis* in piglets
- *S. faecalis*, group C streptococci in lambs
- *S. pyogenes* in calves

Epidemiology

- Important horse disease; sporadic cases only in other species
- Foals infected via the umbilicus from environment contaminated by uterine discharges from mare, *or* discharges from other cases
- *Or* infection via palatine tonsil or skin
- Screw-worm (*Cochliomyia americana*) can be carrier
- Stressed neonates, or one which did not receive colostrum very susceptible
- Potent cause of abortion in mares in same herds
- Affected foals commonly die; survivors have permanent damage in joints, heart valves
- Some outbreaks in pig herds with high morbidity, with infection originating from sow

Clinical findings

Foal

- Foals less than a week old, acute, fatal septicemia
- Navel swelling at 2–3 weeks
- Purulent discharge from the navel in some
- Patent urachus a common accompaniment
- Moderate fever
- Lameness causes recumbency most of time
- Fails to suck; becomes emaciated, dehydrated
- Joints, knee, hock, stifle most commonly, swollen, painful; some with extension to cause local tenosynovitis
- Hypopyon in one or both eyes in some

Sequels:

- Joints rupture, ankylose
- Endocarditis
- Meningoencephalitis
- Euthanasia due to emaciation, bed sores

Pigs

- Arthritis at 2–6 weeks
- Meningitis causes stiff gait, piglet standing on tip toe, hindquarter sway
- Ears retracted against head
- Blindness
- Tremor
- Lose balance, recumbency
- Paddling convulsions
- Piglets with endocarditis usually found comatose or dead
- Most die

Sheep

- Outbreaks 2–3 days after birth or docking
- Sudden onset, severe lameness, then swollen joints, then rupture in many
- Some die, many recover with little residual joint damage

Calves

- Polyarthritis; lameness, chronic without toxemia
- Meningitis; fever, hyperesthesia, rigidity
- Ophthalmitis; hypopyon, blindness
- Omphalophlebitis

Clinical pathology

- Organism in culture from discharges, possibly dam's uterine discharge, blood culture; identification desirable for best treatment choice

Necropsy findings

- Suppuration at navel, surrounding tissues
- Suppurative arthritis
- Multiple abscesses in internal organs
- Valvular endocarditis, especially in piglets, lambs
- Turbidity of cerebrospinal fluid, meningeal inflammation in meningitis; liquefaction necrosis of nervous tissue in some

Diagnosis

In foals resembles infection with:

- *Escherichia coli*
- *Actinobacillus equuli*
- *Salmonella abortivoequina*

In piglet resembles arthritis caused by:

♦ *Mycoplasma hyorhinis*
♦ Glasser's disease
♦ *Erysipelothrix insidiosa*

In calves, lambs, and piglets resembles arthritis caused by:
♦ *Actinomyces pyogenes*
♦ *Fusobacterium necrophorum*
♦ *Erysipelothrix insidiosa*

Resembles meningitis caused by:
♦ *Pasteurella multocida* in calves
♦ *Streptococcus suis* type 2 in older, 10–14 week pigs

Treatment

♦ Penicillin (20 000 units/kg body weight, once daily for 3 days) effective if given early; combinations of short-acting and long-acting penicillins advised
♦ When suppuration present, prolong treatment to 7–10 days
♦ Treat all litter mates

Control

♦ In horses, treat dam to prevent environmental contamination
♦ Mixed bacterins used widely in mares; no evaluation available
♦ On farms with high prevalence, dose foals prophylactically with long-acting penicillin
♦ Use movable pens, disinfect pens, stalls, and clean surroundings generally for birthing to prevent navel infection
♦ Docking, vaccination to be done in clean surroundings
♦ Docking instruments sterilized between patients
♦ Disinfect navel at birth
♦ Repel flies, screw-worm flies, chemically

STREPTOCOCCUS SUIS
INFECTION OF YOUNG PIGS [VM8 p. 636]

Etiology

♦ *Streptococcus suis* types 1 and 2 the originally identified types causing the disease; many more capsular types since identified; type 2 the most important
♦ Significant differences in virulence between strains have biochemical bases

Epidemiology

Occurrence

♦ Disease of piglets 2–22 weeks old
♦ Wherever pigs are raised
♦ Most cases just after weaning associated with stresses of moving, overcrowding, poor ventilation
♦ Morbidity rates as high as 15%; case fatality rates up to 9%

Source and transmission

♦ The organism occurs in palatine tonsils and other tissues of 50–75% of pigs
♦ Hysterectomy-derived pig, pigs in specific-pathogen-free herds free of infection
♦ Transmission occurs within a few days of mixing infected and non-infected pigs
♦ Organism can persist in clinically normal, infected pigs for over a year
♦ Persists in a herd by transmission from sows to young

Importance
A zoonosis

Clinical findings

♦ Occurs as outbreaks of arthritis or meningitis or both together
♦ Sudden death of a few pigs may be first sign

Meningitis Fever, anorexia, depression
♦ Fever
♦ Stiff gait
♦ Standing on toes
♦ Swaying hindquarters
♦ Ears retracted against head
♦ Blindness
♦ Tremor
♦ Lateral recumbency, paddling convulsions
♦ Death after a course of a few hours unless treated

Endocarditis Coma or found dead without premonitory signs.

Arthritis:
♦ Swollen, hot, painful joints
♦ Often several joints affected in the one pig
♦ Severe lameness
♦ Reluctant to stand; lateral recumbency

Clinical pathology

Streptococcus suis cultivable from tonsils, joint fluid, blood, cerebrospinal fluid.

Necropsy findings

One or more of the following:
♦ Fibrinous, purulent polyserositis

♦ Fibrinous, hemorrhagic bronchopneumonia
♦ Purulent meningitis with liquefaction necrosis of nervous tissue
♦ Vegetative valvular endocarditis

Diagnosis

In pigs resembles:
♦ *Mycoplasma hyorhinis* arthritis
♦ Erysipelas
♦ Glasser's disease
♦ Viral encephalitides

In calves resembles infections with *Pasteurella multocida* meningitis.

In all species resembles infections with:
♦ *Actinomyces pyogenes*
♦ *Fusobacterium necrophorum*

Treatment

♦ Penicillin most widely used but sensitivity of all strains should not be assumed
♦ Infection susceptible to ampicillin, with some exceptions, to trimethoprim/sulfamethoxazole, resistant to gentamicin, nitrofuran, tetracycline

Control

♦ Hygiene, stress-reducing management, early treatment of sick animals the only procedure likely to be effective
♦ Medicated early weaning combined with specific-pathogen-free (SPF) procedures effective in producing pigs free of infection
♦ Eradication by depopulation, repopulating with SPF pigs, avoidance of any importations
♦ To reduce risk of deaths in an infected population use mass medication at danger periods, either by injection of all pigs at the same time, or by feed medication with potentiated sulfonamides or phenoxymethyl penicillin; tiamulin in drinking water also effective

STREPTOCOCCAL LYMPHADENITIS OF SWINE (JOWL ABSCESSES, CERVICAL ABSCESS)
[VM8 p. 640]

Etiology

♦ β-hemolytic streptococci of Lancefield's group E type IV
♦ *Pasteurella multocida*, *Escherichia coli*, *Actinomyces pyogenes* also present in many cases

Epidemiology

♦ Commonest in fattening, postweaning pigs
♦ Infection thought to be via pharyngeal mucosa from infected feed, water
♦ Persistence in herds thought due to survival of infection in carrier sows
♦ Importance is loss of rejected pigs at abattoirs; much lower now than previously

Clinical findings

Throat lymph nodes, especially submandibular nodes, enlarged.

Clinical pathology

Microtitration test available.

Necropsy findings

Suppurative lymphadenitis in throat; rarely in other locations.

Diagnosis

Resembles infection with:
♦ Mycobacterium spp.
♦ Rhodococcus equi

Treatment

Not undertaken.

Control

♦ Vaccination with an injected bacterin, or a pharyngeal spray reported effective
♦ Mass medication, e.g. with chlortetracycline, in the feed appears to control spread of infection

DISEASES CAUSED BY *STAPHYLOCOCCUS* spp. [VM8 p. 641]

Listed elsewhere:
♦ Bovine mastitis

♦ Bovine udder impetigo
♦ Equine staphylococcal pyoderma

♦ Porcine exudative epidermitis

Minor diseases are as follows.

NEONATAL STAPHYLOCOCCAL SEPTICEMIA [VM8 p. 641]

For example, lambs; infection via navel or marking wounds; many deaths due to myocardial lesions

STAPHYLOCOCCAL DERMATITIS [VM8 p. 641]

♦ Ulcerative facial of adult sheep, caused by *Staphylococcus aureus*
♦ Facial folliculitis in lambs
♦ Of lower limbs of sheep
♦ Dermatitis of horse, donkey, on neck, back characterized by scabs, alopecia, pruritus caused by *Staphylococcus hyicus*

TICK PYEMIA OF LAMBS (ENZOOTIC STAPHYLOCOCCOSIS) [VM8 p. 641]

Etiology

The rickettsia *Cytoecetes phagocytophila* transmitted by *Ixodes ricinus* plus *Staphylococcus aureus*.

Epidemiology

♦ Occurs only in United Kingdom hill country inhabited by *Ixodes ricinus*
♦ Spring and summer disease
♦ Morbidity averages 5%; may be 30%
♦ In 2–10 week lambs; most die or are unprofitable

Clinical findings

♦ Arthritis; lame, joints painful, swollen, hot
♦ Meningitis; fever, limb rigidity, recumbency

Clinical pathology

Lymphocytopenia, neutropenia, thrombocytopenia.

Necropsy findings

♦ Suppurative meningitis, arthritis
♦ Abscesses in skin, muscles, tendon sheaths, joints, viscera

Diagnosis

Resembles other neonatal infections of lambs, e.g. *Streptococcus zooepidemicus*

Treatment

Antibiotic treatment of established cases of limited value.

Control

♦ Long-acting antibiotics the main instrument
♦ Benzathine penicillin injected at 3 weeks old; long-acting tetracyclines (2 injections, at 2 and 6 weeks old) also have effect on rickettsia
♦ Tick control by 3-weekly dipping in organophosphate insecticide also effective; pour-ons also effective

EXUDATIVE EPIDERMITIS (GREASY PIG DISEASE) [VM8 p. 642]

Etiology

Staphylococcus hyicus (S. hyos).

Epidemiology

♦ Most affected pigs are less than 1 week old, some up to 6 weeks; rarely groups up to 3 months old affected
♦ Morbidity within litters 20–90%; case fatality rate 50–75%
♦ Source of infection probably carrier dams; organism also survives in environment
♦ Environmental stress, e.g. sow agalactia, intercurrent infection, may predispose
♦ Lesions commonly commence on face, due possibly to bites from uncut needle teeth

Clinical findings

♦ Acute, generalized, seborrheic dermatitis in week-old pigs
♦ Lesions painful; piglets squeal a lot
♦ Anorexia, dehydration, weakness, death in 24–48 hours
♦ All of skin wrinkled, reddened, covered with greasy gray-brown exudate, in some places in thick clumps
♦ In older pigs exudate dries to form scales on face, behind ears, skin tick, wrinkled, with thick scabs which crack along flexion lines; some have ulcerative glossitis, stomatitis

Clinical pathology

Culture of organism from skin.

Necropsy findings

Skin lesions
Degenerative lesions in renal tubular epithelium, ureteral blockage

Diagnosis

Resembles:
Swine pox
Skin necrosis at pressure points, anterior carpus, fetlock, hock, elbow, coronet, anterior 2–3 pairs of teats in piglets on abrasive flooring
● Facial dermatitis
● Allergic dermatitis due to Tyroglyphus spp. infestation

◆ Sarcoptic mange
◆ Dermatosis vegetans
◆ Pityriasis rosea
◆ Zinc nutritional deficiency

Treatment

◆ Early administration of combination of:
 • Parenteral cloxacillin
 • Topical cloxacillin (10 000 units/g lanolin, plus 1% hydrocortisone)
◆ Skin wash with disinfectant soap

Control

◆ Cleaning, disinfection of accommodation before next sow admitted
◆ Isolation affected litter and sow
◆ Wash dam with disinfectant soap

DISEASES CAUSED BY *CORYNEBACTERIUM* spp.

Actinomyces pyogenes is a major cause of bovine mastitis in calves, of sheep viral pneumonias, and sheep foot abscess.

Minor corynebacterial diseases are as follows.

ACTINOMYCES PYOGENES INFECTION [VM8 p. 645]

◆ Ubiquitous organism in environment, on skin, in intestines, on tonsils normal ruminants in pigs, but rarely in horses
◆ Gains entry via wounds, insect bites
◆ Causes subcutaneous abscess, *or*
◆ Proceeds to draining lymph nodes to body generally as bacteremia
◆ Specific occurrences include:
 • Frontal sinusitis after dehorning
 • Injection site abscess
 • Surgical wound contamination
 • Extensive cellulitis in buller cattle in feed lot
 • Endocarditis
 • Spinal abscess accompanying tail biting in pigs
 • Intracranial abscess in male deer associated with velvet shedding and antler casting
◆ Treatment results poor, although organism sensitive *in vitro*

METRITIS AND ABORTION [VM8 p. 645]

◆ *Actinomyces pyogenes, Fusobacterium necrophorum, Bacteroides melaninogenicus* common inhabitants of bovine postpartum metritis, leading to infertility, possibly abortion
◆ Infection commoner after retained placenta
◆ Sequels include:
 • Chronic endometritis with vaginal discharge
 • Subsequent infertility
 • Pyometritis
 • Abortion

PERINATAL DISEASE [VM8 p. 645]

Recorded as causing death in many neonatal lambs and calves.

ARTHRITIS AND BURSITIS [VM8 p. 645]

Corynebacterium pseudotuberculosis causes non-suppurative arthritis, bursitis in lambs.

PERIODONTAL DISEASE (CARA INCHADA) [VM8 p. 645]

Corynebacterium pyogenes, Bacteroides melaninogenicus found in periodontal lesions in Brazilian cattle.

CHRONIC PECTORAL AND
VENTRAL MIDLINE ABSCESS IN
HORSES [VM8 p. 646]

♦ Multiple chronic abscesses in North American horses due to *Corynebacterium pseudotuberculosis*
♦ Horses of all ages, related to high insect populations, only a few horses per farm
♦ Abscesses in any subcutaneous site but most along underline from chest to pelvis
♦ During 1–4 weeks abscesses grow up to 20 cm dia.
♦ local swelling, lameness, painful to palpate, local edema, dermatitis, depression, fever, rupture
♦ Treat by surgical drainage, systemic antibiotic

CONTAGIOUS BOVINE
PYELONEPHRITIS [VM8 p. 646]

Etiology

♦ *Corynebacterium renale*, up to 4 serotypes; all cross-react with *Mycobacterium johnei*
♦ *Corynebacterium pilosum*, *C. cystitidis* commonly found in association with *C. renale* but thought to have no pathogenic role
♦ Many other bacteria also isolated in field cases of pyelonephritis
♦ Stagnation in part of the urinary tract a significant risk factor

Epidemiology

♦ Sporadic cases only but some herds have enzootic problem
♦ Adult cows most affected, bulls very rarely
♦ Most cases in early lactation
♦ Infection via vulva; source probably carrier cows; prepuce of clinically normal bulls
♦ Transmission venereally, by contaminated catheter
♦ Disease usually fatal

Clinical findings

♦ Blood-stained urine
♦ In some a transient episode of renal colic:
  • Tail-swishing
  • Treading with hind feet, kicking at abdomen
  • Straining to urinate
♦ More commonly slow onset of:
  • Fluctuating fever
  • Capricious appetite

• Weight loss
• Milk yield decline
♦ Diagnostic urinary tract signs often intermittent, not observed:
  • Blood, pus, tissue debris, particularly la part of urination
  • Urination frequent or dribbling, wit straining, dysuria
  • In late stages bladder shrunken, thick walled, painful on palpation, ureter thickened, left kidney enlarged, painful
♦ Terminal **uremia** after a course, usually c several months

Clinical pathology

♦ Blood, protein in urine
♦ Pyuria
♦ *Corynebacterium renale* identified in urine
♦ Elevated serum creatinine, blood urea i uremic stage

Necropsy findings

♦ Kidney(s) often enlarged, with light colored necrotic areas
♦ Pus, blood, mucus in renal pelvis, ureters
♦ Bladder, urethra thick-walled, mucosa hemorrhagic, edematous, eroded

Diagnosis

Resembles:
♦ Non-specific cystitis, including polypoi cystitis
♦ Acute intestinal obstruction
♦ Enzootic hematuria
♦ Chronic cases may resemble traumatic reti culoperitonitis

Treatment

Procaine penicillin (15 000 units/kg body weight daily for 3 weeks; recovery if treated early; most cases unobserved until too late and relapse after a brief improvement.

Control

♦ Isolation of infected animals
♦ Destruction of infected bedding
♦ Hygiene during insemination, introduction catheters, uterine catheters, obstetrical instruments
♦ Artificial insemination if natural breeding practiced

CYSTITIS AND PYELONEPHRITIS
OF SOWS [VM8 p. 648]

Etiology

Eubacterium suis.

Epidemiology

* Occurs in postpubertal sows after remating
* Sometimes as outbreaks
* Organism a common inhabitant of normal prepuce or diverticulum, not in female tract
* Transmitted venereally, often amongst sows bred to a particular boar
* Also spread from environment and from boar to boar; more common in sows in intensive housing
* Usually ends fatally
* A significant form of loss in most pig industries

Clinical findings

* Clinical signs appear in sows 3–4 weeks after mating
* Boars may suffer brief intermittent hematuric episodes

Acute disease
* Unwilling to rise
* Profound depression
* Circulatory failure
* Death within 12 hours

Chronic disease
* Depression, anorexia
* Mild fever
* Arched back, dysuria in some
* Frequent urination, turbid, blood-stained urine
* Blood-stained vaginal discharge, emanating from bladder
* Thickened bladder wall palpable in very large sows
* Death within 2–5 days
* Case fatality rate high; survivors develop chronic renal failure with polyuria or polydipsia

Clinical pathology

* Urine contains blood, leukocytes, bacteria, has a high protein level
* *Eubacterium suis* identifiable
* Advanced cases show elevated blood levels of urea, creatinine, potassium, N-acetyl-B-D-glucosaminidase, and low levels of sodium

Necropsy findings

* **Acute** – bladder wall thick, edematous, hyperemic; diffuse tubular damage, interstitial nephritis
* **Chronic** – erosions, ulcerations in bladder wall; pyelonephritis

Diagnosis

Acute disease resembles:
* Acute heart failure due to endocarditis
* Acute intestinal accidents
* Septicemia
* Hemorrhagic bowel syndrome

Chronic cases resemble:
* Cystitis caused by other infection
* Hematuria due to *Stephanurus dentatus* infestation

Treatment

* Penicillin, ampicillin, lincomycin daily, 3–5 days successful in early cases
* Supplementary oral treatment with fluids, electrolytes advised
* Long-standing cases may respond temporarily, then relapse

Control

* During outbreaks attempts to disinfect boars' prepuces with daily tetracycline infusions, use artificial insemination
* Avoid vaginal trauma at mating by careful boar management
* Sows showing pain or blood from the vagina after mating, or farrowing treated prophylactically with broad-spectrum antibiotic
* Hygiene by cleaning pens, washing sow perineum before mating

ENZOOTIC POSTHITIS (PIZZLE
ROT, SHEATH ROT
BALANOPOSTHITIS) [VM8 p. 650]

Etiology

* *Corynebacterium renale*, the causative organism of contagious bovine pyelonephritis
* Also isolated from prepuces of bulls,

Angora goat wethers with posthitis, ewes with vulvitis

Epidemiology

Occurrence

♦ Principally Merino wethers, older than 3 years
♦ May extend to young wethers in bad seasons; also young rams; may be unable to mate subsequently
♦ Enzootic, with 40% morbidity, where pasture plentiful and has high legume content; worst in spring/fall when pasture growth most profuse
♦ Transmission of infection between wethers not identified
♦ Importance is serious production loss, mortality, inability to run wethers on productive land

Risk factors

♦ Encouraging growth of external lesion:
  • High urinary alkalinity causing inflammation of lesions
  • High estrogen intake in pasture causing preputial congestion, swelling
♦ Promoting extension to internal lesion include:
  • Wetness around preputial orifice due to preputial hair removal at shearing
  • High calcium/low phosphorus diet
  • Ingestion of large volumes alkaline bore water
  • Close adherence penile to preputial lining in castrates, immature entires
♦ Associated vulvitis in ewes commingled with affected wethers probably venereal infection with C. renale

Clinical findings

Wethers

♦ Initial small, thick, tenacious skin scab dorsal to preputial orifice; may persist for long period
♦ Spread to internal lesion causes scabbing of orifice:
  • Restlessness, kicking at belly
  • Dribbling urine
  • Swollen prepuce
  • Blowfly strike of site
  • Scabs, adhesions cause inability to protrude penis
♦ Some deaths due to uremia, toxemia
♦ Many sheep affected with external lesions not observes, recover spontaneously

Ewes

♦ Scabs and ulcers on vulvar lips
♦ Prelude to blowfly strike

Bulls

♦ Usually only external lesion
♦ May persist for long periods with extensive lesions

Clinical pathology

Isolation of *Corynebacterium renale* from prepuce.

Necropsy

♦ Local lesions in most cases
♦ Rarely urinary retention, hydronephrosis uremia

Diagnosis

♦ In **wethers** resembles obstructive urolithiasis
♦ In **ewes** and **rams** resembles ulcerative dermatosis
♦ In **bulls** resembles infectious pustular vulvovaginitis

Treatment

♦ Restriction to feed subsistence requirements for several days halts progress of disease
♦ Regular inspection; wool shorn around prepuce if wet, lesions treated with 10% copper sulfate ointment on external lesions; testosterone implant helps
♦ Sheep with internal lesions need twice-weekly 5% copper sulfate irrigation; penicillin systemically or locally also useful but lesions may relapse
♦ Severe cases with adhesions and compromised urine flow need surgical relief by opening the prepuce back to the penis tip

Control

♦ Restrict diet intake; avoid legumes
♦ Testosterone propionate 60–90 mg subcutaneous implant very successful prevention, persisting 3 months; useful also in treatment; fringe benefit is better weight gain; usually administered just before bad season commences
♦ Short-scrotum lambs (testicle pushed into inguinal canal, scrotum removed with rubber ring) have very low incidence

◆ Shear around preputial orifice, vulva (called 'ringing')

CASEOUS LYMPHADENITIS OF SHEEP AND GOATS [VM8 p. 652]

Etiology

Two biotypes of *Corynebacterium pseudotuberculosis*: ovine/caprine, and equine/bovine.

Epidemiology

◆ Organism persists for long period in environment
◆ Major infection source is pus from discharging abscesses, or nasal discharge from pulmonary cases
◆ Entry via skin wound or through intact skin
◆ Transmission in sheep largely by shearing wounds and equipment, through infected dip, enhanced by close contact during these procedures, and by absence of protective effect of wool
◆ Concentration in goats of lesions on head, neck, brisket suggest transmission by butting, on browse and via neck collars
◆ Peak incidence in adults due to longer exposure period; often 50% morbidity in adult sheep, 20% in goats
◆ Importance is in value depreciation of meat from infected flocks
◆ Rarely a zoonosis by infection of skin wounds in shearers

Clinical findings

◆ Palpable, hard enlargement peripheral lymph node(s)
◆ Nodes rupture, discharge thick, green pus
◆ Hematogenous spread with local abscesses may cause:
 • Chronic pneumonia
 • Pyelonephritis, embolic nephritis
 • Ataxia, paraplegia
 • Chronic emaciation as in **thin ewe syndrome**
◆ Mammary lymph node abscesses may spread to mammary tissue

Clinical pathology

◆ Culture of *C. pseudotuberculosis* in needle biopsy sample
◆ Many serological tests trialled to enable infected, carrier animals to be identified but have not matched necessary standards of specificity

Necropsy findings

◆ Caseous, yellow-green pus in peripheral lymph nodes, and any internal tissues
◆ May extend to a diffuse bronchopneumonia

Diagnosis

Resembles:
◆ Melioidosis
◆ Suppurative lymphadenitis due to *Pasteurella multocida*, lambs
◆ **Morel's disease** caused by gram-positive micrococcus, in sheep

Treatment

Not attempted.

Control

◆ Identify affected animals at shearing (not without error), and cull
◆ Hygiene at lambing, docking to include:
 • Instrument disinfection
 • Disinfection of surgery location, *or*
 • Temporary pens in open fields
 • Clean up spilt pus
 • Disinfection of wounds
◆ Avoid contaminating dip fluids, add disinfectant to fluid
◆ Vaccines with good reputations in terms of good protection against infection and abscess development in sheep, commercially available
◆ Little protection provided for goats by commercial vaccines
◆ Vaccination recommended in sheep only after 10 weeks old because of interference provided by passive intake of maternal antibodies in colostrum

ULCERATIVE LYPHANGITIS OF HORSES AND CATTLE [VM8 p. 655]

Etiology

Corynebacterium pseudotuberculosis.

Epidemiology

◆ Mildly contagious, sporadic disease of horses, but only rarely of cattle

♦ Commonest in horses in crowded, unhygienic stalls, pens
♦ Infection via injuries to lower limbs
♦ Important because of long course, interference with work ability

Clinical findings

Horse
♦ Pastern swollen and painful
♦ Lameness, may be severe
♦ Subcutaneous nodules around fetlock,
sometimes extensive spread
♦ Nodules enlarge to 5–7 cm dia.; rupture,
discharge creamy green pus, form ulcers
♦ Lesions heal in 1–2 weeks; fresh crops for
up to 12 months

Cattle
♦ Similar pattern to horse except
  • Lymph nodes may be involved
  • Discharge from ruptured node is clear,
  gelatinous

Clinical pathology

C. pseudotuberculosis isolatable from pus.

Diagnosis

Resembles other diseases affecting equine
lower limbs:
♦ Glanders
♦ Epizootic lymphangitis
♦ Sporotrichosis
♦ Swamp cancer
♦ Greasy heel
♦ Chorioptic mange
♦ Similar lesions caused by non-specific
streptococci, staphylococci, Rhodococcus
equi, Pseudomonas aeruginosa

Treatment

♦ Parenteral penicillin, tetracycline injections
♦ Local antibacterial treatment for ulcers

Control

♦ Hygiene in stables
♦ Careful protection injuries

CONTAGIOUS ACNE OF HORSES
(CANADIAN HORSE POX,
CONTAGIOUS PUSTULAR
DERMATITIS) [VM8 p. 656]

Etiology

Corynebacterium pseudotuberculosis.

Epidemiology

♦ Uncommon disease; causes inconvenien
interference with horse working
♦ Spread by contaminated grooming utensils, harness

Clinical findings

♦ Groups of painful nodules turning to 1.0–
2.5 cm pustules
♦ Pustules discharge green-tinged pus, form
scab
♦ Lesions heal within a week but successive
crops of lesions may prolong case to 4
weeks plus

Clinical pathology

C. pseudotuberculosis in pus.

Diagnosis

Resembles:
♦ Some forms of ringworm
♦ Staphylococcal dermatitis
♦ Cutaneous pythiosis
♦ Cutaneous habronemiasis

Treatment

♦ Parenteral antibiotics in severe cases
♦ Local disinfectant skin wash plus antibiotic
ointment on lesions

Control

Isolate infected animals, disinfect grooming
equipment.

RHODOCOCCUS
(CORYNEBACTERIUM) EQUI
PNEUMONIA OF FOALS [VM8
p. 656]

Etiology

Rhodococcus equi.

Epidemiology

♦ Sporadic cases up to 15% morbidity on
enzootic farms
♦ Only foals less than 5 weeks old susceptible
to infection
♦ Disease appears only in young foals, 2
weeks to 6 months old; in older horses only
if immunosuppressed

♦ Source of infection is soil; infection can persist more than 12 months
♦ Transmission by inhalation, ingestion, umbilical contamination; especially inhalation in dusty surroundings causes pneumonia; ingestion of soil-contaminated feed leads to intestinal infection

Clinical findings

Many bad cases are subclinical, or develop signs only after massive lesions present.

Pneumonic form in young foals, about one month old
♦ Acute pneumonia
♦ Sometimes acute polyarthritis
♦ Fever, anorexia

Pneumonic form in older foals
♦ Slowly developing, subacute pneumonia
♦ Cough
♦ Deep respiration proceeding to dyspnea in late stages
♦ Loud crackling sounds on auscultation, especially after coughing or having foal rebreathe in a bag
♦ Temperature normal
♦ Foal keeps sucking
♦ Emaciation
♦ Diarrhea in some
♦ Death after 2 week course

Intestinal form
Acute, chronic or intermittent diarrhea.

Clinical pathology

♦ Radiographic demonstration of lung cavitation, consolidation lymphadenopathy
♦ Leukocytosis, neutrophilia, monocytosis
♦ Plasma fibrinogen levels elevated
♦ *Rhodococcus equi* in transtracheal swabs
♦ Serological tests of limited value

Necropsy findings

♦ Suppurative pyogranulomatous pneumonia
♦ Multiple abscesses along ventral lung border, bronchial lymph nodes
♦ Ulcerative enterocolitis in many
♦ Mesenteric lymph node abscessation
♦ Subcutaneous lymph nodes in some
♦ Suppurative arthritis in some

Diagnosis

Resembles:
♦ Equine herpesvirus-1
♦ Equine viral arteritis
♦ Strangles
♦ Foals with septicemias, e.g. those caused by *Actinobacillus equuli*, *Escherichia coli*, *Streptococcus zooepidemicus*, *Salmonella* spp. may develop arthritis but pneumonia is unusual

Treatment

♦ Usually unsuccessful unless early
♦ Combination of erythromycin (25 mg/kg body weight 3 times daily), rifampicin (5 mg/kg 2 times daily), all administered orally, for 30 days, monitoring efficiency with plasma fibrinogen concentration
♦ Trimethoprim–sulfadiazine may also be effective
♦ Non-steroidal anti-inflammatory drugs, plus bronchial dilators, mucolytics recommended support therapy

Control

♦ Ensure adequacy of colostral transfer of colostral immunoglobulins
♦ Reduce dust in areas frequented by young foals
♦ In enzootic herds frequent auscultation young foals to detect early lung changes plus early vigorous treatment
♦ Hyperimmune serum to foals during first month of life

DISEASES CAUSED BY *LISTERIA* spp.

LISTERIOSIS [VM8 p. 660]

Etiology

Listeria monocytogenes with 13 serovars of widely differing genetic makeup, virulence and geographical distribution.

Epidemiology

Occurrence
♦ A disease of temperate climates; uncommon in tropical, subtropical climates
♦ Principally a disease of ruminants, especially sheep; occasional cases of horses and pigs, but infection occurs in all species; causes a serious human disease
♦ Occurs as outbreaks, usually of either encephalitis or abortion; not the two together
♦ Septicemia usually occurs in newborn associated with abortion outbreak
♦ Mostly a winter disease
♦ All ages

Source
Infection very widespread, including many feedstuffs, feces of many animals, especially winter.

Transmission
♦ In septicemic, abortion forms transmission is by ingestion
♦ In encephalitic form transmission by infection of trigeminal nerve endorgans through oral mucosal abrasions

Risk factors
♦ Animals carry infection in ingesta without harm for long periods
♦ Invasion occurs when:
  • Infection pressure of organism is high, usually due to feeding poorly fermented grass or corn silage in which the organism proliferates
  • Resistance lowered by poor nutrition
  • Sudden changes in and change to very wet, cold weather
  • Late pregnancy, parturition
  • Possibly ingestion of *Pinus ponderosa* foliage

Importance
♦ Morbidity usually low, sporadic up to 10%, but can be 35%
♦ Case mortality very high in encephalitic, septicemic forms and is main cause of loss

♦ Biggest problem is difficulty of dealing with large amounts of silage and large groups of animals feeding on it when the disease appears

Clinical findings

The following syndromes occur separately; very rarely septicemia, abortion, encephalitis have occurred in a sheep flock.

Listerial encephalitis, in sheep and cattle
♦ Fever up to 42°C (107°F) early but normal when nervous signs appear
♦ Depression to somnolence, separation from flock
♦ Hunched stance
♦ Incoordination, fall easily if disturbed
♦ Head deviation or tilt, circling, retroflexed or ventroflexed; returns to former position if moved passively
♦ Unilateral facial hypalgesia, paralysis (ear, eyelid, lip droop)
♦ Exposure keratitis, ulceration in affected eye
♦ Strabismus or nystagmus in some
♦ Panophthalmitis, hypopyon one or both eyes, common in cattle
♦ Jaw muscle paresis, jaw droop, saliva drools, prehension ineffective,
♦ Terminal recumbency
♦ Death due to respiratory failure after course of 2–4 days in sheep and goats, 1–2 weeks in cattle

Listerial abortion
♦ Usually sporadic in cattle, outbreaks in sheep, goats, rare in pigs
♦ May recur each year
♦ **Cattle** abort or stillbirth during last trimester, retain placenta with metritis, fever
♦ **Sheep** and **goats** abort after 12th week of pregnancy, retain placenta, bloody vaginal discharge, dam may die of septicemia if fetus retained

Septicemic listeriosis
♦ Mostly ruminant neonates; rarely adult ruminants
♦ Depression, weakness, fever, diarrhea, weight loss
♦ Calves show corneal opacity, dyspnea, nystagmus, opisthotonus, death in 12 hours

Mastitis

Single quarter
Chronic
Unresponsive to standard treatments
Milk has high cell count, normal appearance

Spinal myelitis

Hind limbs knuckle, then paralysis
Front limbs affected in some

Clinical pathology

◆ Hematology uninformative
◆ Cerebrospinal fluid contains inflammatory cells, high protein, culture rarely positive
◆ Serological tests inconclusive
◆ Culture of relevant fluids attempted in abortion, from blood, tissues in septicemia

Necropsy findings

◆ Macroscopic findings not marked
◆ May be cloudy cerebrospinal fluid, meningeal congestion, panophthalmitis in some cattle
◆ Diagnostic lesion is microabscesses in brain stem (encephalitis) or spinal cord (myelitis); submit half brain for culture, half for histopathology
◆ In septicemia multiple necrotic foci in liver, spleen, myocardium
◆ In aborted lambs small, yellow, necrotic foci in liver, abomasal erosions, yellow–orange meconium, fetuses usually edematous
◆ Dams of aborted fetuses have placentitis, endometritis

Diagnosis

Meningoencephalitis resembles:
◆ Pregnancy toxemia
◆ Acetonemia
◆ Polioencephalomalacia
◆ Brain abscess
◆ Otitis media
◆ Otitis interna
◆ Coenurosis
◆ Rabies

Abortion resembles:
◆ Brucellosis due to *Brucella abortus, B. melitensis*
◆ Other causes of infectious abortion
◆ Abortion, stillbirth due to *Listeria ivanovii* sporadic in cattle and sheep

Treatment

◆ Pointless if clinical signs severe; must treat early
◆ Chlortetracycline 10 mg/kg body weight, I/V, daily for 5 days reasonably effective for cattle, less so for sheep
◆ Penicillin (44 000 units/kg, I/M daily for 7–14 days) also recommended

Control

In silage-fed groups:
◆ Introduce silage slowly
◆ Limit amount fed
◆ Reject spoiled ensilage or silage with pH > 5
◆ Low level tetracycline feeding
◆ Avoid soil contamination of ensilage
◆ Additives to promote fermentation
◆ Vaccination practiced but not highly regarded

DISEASES CAUSED BY *ERYSIPELOTHRIX RHYSIOPATHIAE (INSIDIOSA)* [VM8 p. 666]

ERYSIPELAS IN CATTLE [VM8 p. 666]

◆ Isolated outbreaks septicemia
◆ Calf polyarthritis:
  • Lameness
  • Recumbency
  • Fluctuating joint capsules
  • Rapid emaciation

ERYSIPELAS IN SHEEP [BR. 666]

◆ Sheep resistant, generalized infection unlikely
◆ Recorded diseases:
  • **Polyarthritis** (acute, chronic)
  • **Post-dipping laminitis**
  • Valvular endocarditis
  • Skin infections
  • Septicemia
  • Pneumonia

♦ Acute non-suppurative polyarthritis:
  • Begins 14 days after docking or birth (infection via umbilicus)
  • Lameness, minor joint swelling
  • Chronic, slow recovery
  • Responds to penicillin if given early
  • Control by hygiene at marking or birthing
  • Vaccination not recommended
  • Up to 50% morbidity
  • 5% of affected lose weight, have permanently swollen joints
  • High rejection rate at abattoirs
♦ Chronic non-suppurative polyarthritis:
  • In 2–6 months lambs
  • Infection by soil of umbilical or docking wounds
  • Morbidity up to 30%
  • Poor response to treatment, most sent for slaughter
  • Lame, often in all limbs
♦ Post-dipping laminitis:
  • After dipping in heavily contaminated fluid containing inadequate disinfectant
  • Also if sheep exposed to contaminated mud without access to dip
  • Infection via skin abrasion, localizes in sensitive laminae of feet without joint involvement
  • Morbidity about 25%, deaths rare
  • Severe lameness 2–4 days after exposure
  • One limb to all four
  • Heat, swelling coronet to below knee, hock
  • Local hair falls out
  • Serious weight loss
  • Most recover spontaneously, penicillin hastens recovery
  • Prevented by inclusion 0.04% copper sulfate in dip fluid

ERYSIPELAS IN SWINE [VM8 p. 667]

Etiology

♦ *Erysipelothrix insidiosa*, great variation in virulence between strains; avirulent strains used in vaccine production
♦ 22 serotypes, only 2 of them associated with clinical disease

Epidemiology

Occurrence

♦ Wastage due to pig deaths, carcase rejection at abattoirs, the heavy costs of control or eradication
♦ Morbidity, mortality, carcase rejection rate very variable

♦ In unvaccinated pigs morbidity rate i acute disease 10–30%, case fatality rate u to 75%
♦ Susceptible age group varies:
  • Virulent strain – all ages including ne nates susceptible
  • Low virulence strain – adults only, esp cially puerperal sows

Source and transmission

♦ Continuous soil reinfection by carriers, c use of slurry as fertilizer the main infectio source
♦ Persistence of infection in soil very variabl but organism generally resistant to en vironmental influences
♦ Invasion via skin abrasions, alimentar tract

Clinical findings

Acute

♦ Incubation period 1–7 days
♦ High fever
♦ Prostration, anorexia, thirst, vomiting i some
♦ Marked red to purple discoloration jow ventral abdomen skin
♦ Reluctant to rise
♦ Incoordination
♦ Ocular discharge
♦ Some pigs will have diamond, red urticaria 2–5 cm square plaques on skin of belly inside thighs, on throat, neck, ears
♦ Recovery or
♦ Terminal diarrhea, dyspnea, cyanosis
♦ Death on day 2–4
♦ Skin form is acute disease with mild sign other than skin lesions
♦ Most survive after course of about 10 days
♦ Skin lesions may coalesce to form a shiel over back; hardens, separates at edge, lift off but hangs on

Chronic

♦ Swollen joints; hot, painful at first, ther cold, hard
♦ Lameness, stiff gait
♦ Recumbency in some due to intervertebra joint involvement
♦ Alopecia, sloughing of tips of ears, tail cutaneous hyperkeratosis of back shoulders, legs
♦ **Endocarditis** usually characterized by:
  • Sudden death, *or*
  • Exercise intolerance, emaciation; dyspnea, cyanosis with exercise

- Heart murmur, cardiac thrill, large cardiac impulse, tachycardia

Clinical pathology

- Blood culture, repeated at short intervals, usually necessary for identification
- Leukocytosis early in acute disease, then leukopenia, marked monocytosis
- Agglutination tests adequate only for herd diagnosis
- Complement fixation and enzyme immunoassay tests available

Necropsy findings

Acute
- Diffuse, purple edema of belly wall
- Large ecchymotic hemorrhages in all tissues, especially under kidney capsule, pleura, peritoneum
- Venous infarction stomach wall
- Swollen, hemorrhagic mesenteric lymph nodes

Chronic
- Non-suppurative proliferative arthritis
- Long-standing lesions are fibrosed, ankylosed
- Large, crumbly lesions on heart valves in some pigs
- Infarcts in kidney
- *Erysipelothrix insidiosa* isolated from endocardial lesions; many joints sterile and special techniques used to culture the organism

Diagnosis

Acute erysipelas resembles:
- Salmonellosis
- Swine fever

Chronic erysipelas resembles:
- Streptococcal arthritis and endocarditis
- Glasser's disease
- *Mycoplasma hyorhinis* infection
- *Mycoplasma hyosynoviae*
- Rickets

- Chronic zinc poisoning
- Footrot of pigs
- Chronic osteoarthritis
- Leg weakness

Treatment

Acute
- Penicillin plus antierysipelas serum is standard treatment for virulent strains
- Penicillin alone; (50 000 units/kg procaine penicillin for 3 days is adequate for cases caused by strains of mild virulence
- Chronic cases with badly compromised joints may make a temporary recovery, then relapse

Chronic
No specific treatment of any value.

Control

- Eradication impossible because of ubiquitous distribution and possible long survival in ground
- Specific-pathogen-free pigs on new land may remain clear but infection is highly likely
- Immunization in common use:
  - Antierysipelas serum provides good protection for a few days; valuable during an outbreak or in neonates in herds where disease frequent
  - Vaccination with bacterin or attenuated or avirulent live cultures but much variation in virulence and protective capacity between strains
  - Vaccination reduces prevalence of acute polyarthritis but does not eliminate mild arthritis
  - Some outbreaks of the disease result from vaccination using commercial vaccines
  - Two vaccinations 2–4 weeks apart, starting at 6–10 weeks, recommended for market pigs; first injection postponed when dam has been vaccinated during pregnancy
  - In endemic herds gilts and sows need to be vaccinated at 6 month intervals, preferably 3–6 weeks before farrowing

DISEASES CAUSED BY *BACILLUS* spp.

ANTHRAX [VM8 p. 671]

Etiology

♦ *Bacillus anthracis*
♦ Avirulent strains exist; lack lethal factor, possess protective antigen, edema factor of virulent strain
♦ Special strain in pigs in Papua-New Guinea not transmissible to other species.

Epidemiology

Occurrence

♦ Worldwide in **anthrax belts**, enzootic areas where bacilli multiply in soil
♦ Most common in rich soil in tropical and subtropical heavy rainfall areas
♦ Outbreaks every year in tropics to 30 year intervals in subtropics
♦ Sudden simultaneous occurrence of outbreaks in separate locations
♦ Most outbreaks in warm weather with heavy rainfall, in animals confined to small areas.
♦ Morbidity high, variable, case fatality rate 100%

Source

♦ Soil contamination by discharges of sick animals
♦ Cut open dead animals
♦ Tannery effluent
♦ Hides, bone meal
♦ Possibly inert wild animal carriers
♦ Persists indefinitely in soil as spores

Transmission

♦ Ingestion mostly, inhalation, percutaneous possible
♦ Biting insects suspected of passive transfer

Risk factors

♦ All species susceptible, commonest cattle and sheep, then goats, horses and pigs
♦ Dwarf pigs and Algerian sheep totally resistant

Importance

♦ Transmissible to humans
♦ Heavy death losses
♦ Interference with normal trading due to quarantine

Clinical findings

Incubation period 1–3 weeks.

Ruminants

♦ Early cases found dead without premonitory signs
♦ Depression
♦ Fever
♦ Dyspnea
♦ Tachycardia
♦ Mucosae congested, petechiated
♦ Anorexia
♦ Ruminal stasis
♦ Milk yield drops precipitately
♦ Milk blood tinged
♦ Diarrhea, dysentery
♦ Edema of tongue, throat, brisket, perineum, flanks
♦ Collapse, dies after terminal convulsions
♦ Blood discharges from mouth, nostrils, anus, vulva
♦ Course 1–48 hours

Pigs

♦ Fever, dullness, anorexia
♦ Hot inflammatory edema throat, face; obstructs respiration swallowing
♦ Blood-stained froth at mouth
♦ Dysentery
♦ Course 12–36 hours
♦ Baby pigs develop lobar pneumonia due to inhaling spores

Horses

♦ Spore ingestion causes septicemia, enteritis, colic
♦ Insect transmission causes fever, edema of throat, neck, ventral area chest, abdomen, prepuce, udder, dyspnea in some
♦ Death in 48–96 hours

Clinical pathology

♦ Organism visible in stained smear of blood or edema fluid from live animal
♦ Culture of organism
♦ Experimental transmission to laboratory animals used to identify the infection
♦ Available serological tests include ELISA and EITB (electrophoretic immunotransblots)

Necropsy findings

♦ No rigor mortis, rapid decomposition and gassy swelling

♦ Characteristic sawhorse attitude
♦ Blood not clotted
♦ Dark tarry blood from all orifices
♦ DO NOT OPEN CARCASE. Collect blood or edema fluid by needle, for smear to lab for staining
♦ Decomposed carcase, send ear to laboratory; large, black, pulpy spleen

Diagnosis

Resembles:
♦ Lightning stroke
♦ Electrocution
♦ Cyanide poisoning
♦ Peracute blackleg
♦ Bacillary hemoglobinuria
♦ Peracute lead poisoning
♦ Acute hypomagnesemic tetany
♦ Acute bloat

Treatment

♦ Oxytetracycline or procaine penicillin combined with streptomycin, streptomycin alone, ampicillin, methicillin, erythromycin are effective
♦ Very large doses, twice daily for at least five days
♦ Only early cases respond
♦ Too early withdrawal of treatment causes relapse

Control

♦ Quarantine of farm essential
♦ Vaccinate clinically normals
♦ Hygienic disposal discharges, unopened carcases
♦ Long-acting tetracycline to in-contacts
♦ Special disinfection techniques for clothing, shoes, wool, hides, sites where sporulation has occurred, soil, etc.
♦ Special care needed to select correct vaccine to give maximum protection without causing anthrax in patient

♦ Avirulent, living, spore vaccines probably best
♦ Annual revaccination in enzootic area
♦ Milk not suitable for sale for 72 hours after vaccination

TYZZER'S DISEASE [VM8 p. 676]

Etiology

Bacillus piliformis.

Epidemiology

Rare, in 1–5 week old foals and calves.

Clinical findings

♦ Sudden onset, high fever, terminal coma, death in 2 days
♦ jaundice, diarrhea in some

Clinical pathology

♦ Severe leukopenia
♦ Serum levels of liver enzymes increased

Necropsy findings

♦ Miliary necrotic foci
♦ Necrotizing colitis
♦ Bacteria in smear, ELISA test

Diagnosis

Resembles:
♦ Shigellosis
♦ *Rhodococcus equi* infection
♦ Adenovirus pneumonia of foals with combined immunodeficiency

Treatment

Tetracycline.

17 DISEASES CAUSED BY BACTERIA – II

DISEASES CAUSED BY *CLOSTRIDIUM* spp.

TETANUS [VM8 p. 677]

Etiology

♦ *Clostridium tetani*
♦ Spores resistant to disinfectants, heat, persist in soil

Epidemiology

Occurrence
♦ Universal, especially intensely cultivated, closely settled areas
♦ Sporadic cases mostly
♦ Occasional outbreaks sheep, rarely cattle, after contaminated surgery, navel
♦ Case fatality rate 100% horses, 80% young cattle, sheep, goats and pigs; more than 50% adult cattle patients survive

Source and transmission
♦ Soil-borne infection
♦ Wound contamination, especially puncture wound of sole in horses, or uterus, possibly gut, by infected soil
♦ Significant number of cases, often in outbreaks, have no identifiable portal

Risk factors
♦ Any age, either sex, all species
♦ Horses most susceptible, cattle least
♦ Commonest at pasture, in recently castrated, dehorned, docked animals, or those recently calved with placenta retention and contaminated manipulation

Importance
Wastage due to deaths and long-term nursing care of survivors.

Clinical findings

Incubation period 1–3 weeks usual, rarely 3 days, up to 2 months.

Constant signs
♦ Generalized spasticity
♦ Sawhorse posture
♦ Exaggerated, spastic response to touch or sound
♦ Stiff gait, passive limb flexion not possible
♦ Tremor
♦ Third eyelid prolapse
♦ Trismus (locked jaw)
♦ Eating impeded
♦ Tail rigid
♦ Bloat in cattle but strong ruminal movements

Variable signs
♦ Regurgitation through nostrils
♦ Recumbency
♦ Tetanic convulsions
♦ Sweating
♦ Opisthotonus
♦ Dyspnea, nostril dilation
♦ Ear rigidity
♦ Constipation
♦ Urination – large volumes infrequently
♦ Saliva drools
♦ Spinal curvature, tail deviation

Course
♦ In sheep, pigs, horses 3–5 days for fatal outcome
♦ Adult cattle may recover after 1–2 months

Clinical pathology

Dubious significance of tetanus antitoxin levels in serum.

Necropsy findings

♦ Location of entry site, e.g. nail prick in hoof, often impossible
♦ Check for bacteria in tissue

Diagnosis

Resembles:

Polioencephalomalacia
Lactation tetany in mares
Strychnine poisoning
Acute laminitis in horses
Lactation tetany of cows
Whole milk tetany of calves
Enterotoxemia of lambs
Enzootic muscular dystrophy

Treatment

Systemic antibiotic to destroy tetanus bacilli. Any of the penicillins, tetracyclines, cephalosporins, macrolides especially erythromycin

- Limited value unless infection site located, debrided and treated
- Tetanus antitoxin, horses 300 000 units every 12 hours for 3 injections; 20 000 units into cerebrospinal fluid has some support. Similar doses for cattle, but ruminants not usually treated. Limited value of treatment in other species
- Reduce hypersensitivity with acetyl promazine twice daily
- Keep quiet and in dark

Control

- Short-term prevention after injury or surgery, tetanus antitoxin, 200 iu lambs, 3000 iu horse, plus toxoid vaccination, plus treatment dose antibiotic
- Ensure clean surroundings sterile instruments for bulk surgery, e.g. tail-docking lambs
- High-risk flocks, 2 vaccinations at 2 months intervals
- High-prevalence areas, 2 vaccinations at 2 month intervals then annually
- To protect neonates, vaccination of dams in late pregnancy

BOTULISM [VM8 p. 680]

Etiology

Preformed toxin of one of 5 serotypes (A,B,C,D,E) Clostridium botulinum.

Epidemiology

Occurrence
- Sporadic outbreaks all countries
- Morbidity variable, case fatality rate approximates 100%

Source and transmission:
- Ingestion of preformed toxin in decayed animal or plant organic matter
- Possibly implantation Cl. botulinum in tissue (toxoinfectious botulism)

Risk factors
- Persistence of infection in soil ensured by spore formation
- Presence of carcases in pasture
- Dead rodents in hay
- Poultry litter containing carcases as feed in feedlots, or fertilizer on pasture
- Feeding spoiled potatoes, other vegetable industrial waste
- Mouldy, damp hay, haylage, high moisture grain, brewers' grains
- Water pollution by toxin from cadavers, especially birds in wetlands
- Nutritional deficiency of phosphorus or protein encourages ingestion of carrion (bone-chewing)
- Cattle, sheep, horses susceptible; pigs resistant
- Most outbreaks in drought when cadavers likely to be eaten

Clinical findings

Cattle and horses
- Signs appear 3–17 days after access to toxin
- Peracute cases die without signs other than not taking feed or water
- Common **acute** syndrome is progressive paralysis of limbs, jaw, throat, head and neck
- Sensation, consciousness retained.
- Severe tremor, often shaking a limb
- Restless, anxious
- Stumbling, knuckling, unable to rise, or lift head
- Sternal recumbency with head on ground or in flank
- In some cases tongue paralysis, unable to chew or swallow, drools saliva, or may eat till just before death
- Terminally abdominal respiration
- Death on day 1–4

Subacute cases in cattle are affected for 3–4 weeks, then convalescence up to 3 months:
- Same, but milder syndrome as acute
- Recumbent most of time
- Some prehension difficulty
- Roaring sound with each respiration in a few

♦ Survive or euthanized because of work involved in maintaining care

Sheep

♦ Stiff gait, incoordination
♦ Head held to one side or bobbed up and down
♦ Salivation
♦ Nasal discharge
♦ Tail-switching
♦ Abdominal respiration
♦ Eventual recumbency, death

Pig

♦ Very rare
♦ Staggery gait
♦ Recumbency, flaccid paralysis
♦ Vomiting, no feed or water taken
♦ Pupillary dilation

Toxoinfectious botulism (see below)

Clinical pathology

♦ No test available for patient
♦ Assay of serum antitoxin in subacute cases or normal animals in group which may be survivors
♦ Culture of suspect feed
♦ Supply feed, or infusion of it as drinking water, to experimental animals but feed often polluted in very small locations, e.g. around a rodent carcase

Necropsy findings

♦ No specific lesions
♦ May be suspicious material in stomach
♦ Toxin in liver accepted as diagnostic
♦ Filtrate of intestinal contents fed to experimental animals

Diagnosis

Resembles:
♦ Milk fever in cows
♦ Periparturient hypocalcemia in ewes
♦ Paralytic rabies
♦ Equine herpesvirus-1 encephalomyelitis
♦ Nigropallidal encephalomalacia
♦ Hepatic encephalopathy in horses
♦ Phalaris aquatica poisoning in sheep

Treatment

♦ Purgative or gastric lavage
♦ Nervous system stimulants
♦ Sling horses feed by nasogastric tube
♦ Vaccinate remaining animals immediately

Control

♦ Correct nutritional deficiency
♦ Cease feeding suspect feed
♦ Remove carcases
♦ Vaccinate with specific serotype toxoid o combined vaccine, immunity persists 2 years

SHAKER FOAL SYNDROME
(TOXOINFECTIOUS BOTULISM)
[VM8 p. 683]

Etiology

Probably *Clostridium botulinum* type A or E toxin from bacteria implanted in tissues.

Epidemiology

♦ Only 3–8 week foals
♦ Mostly sporadic cases but recurs regularly on some farms
♦ Recorded in standardbred and thoroughbreds
♦ Most cases fatal

Clinical findings

♦ Sudden onset of recumbency
♦ Gross muscle tremor if held up
♦ Periods of being able to rise but gross tremor, stiff gait, toes dragged
♦ Sucks milk but drools from mouth
♦ Feed regurgitated from nostrils if eating attempted
♦ Always constipated
♦ Pupils dilated, sluggish light reflex
♦ Respiratory failure terminally
♦ Death at about 72 hours

Necropsy findings

♦ Contracted colon, small, hard, dry feces
♦ Liver enlarged
♦ Fibrinous pericardial exudate

Diagnosis

Resembles:
  Grass sickness
  Equine herpesvirus-1 encephalomyelitis

Control

Vaccinate pregnant mares with *Cl. botulinum* type B vaccine.

BLACKLEG [VM8 p. 684]

Etiology

Clostridium chauvoei (= *Cl. feseri*).

Epidemiology

Occurrence
♦ Usually as outbreaks, on farms where soil contains spores of *Cl. chauvoei*
♦ Morbidity variable, case fatality rate approximates 100%

Source and transmission
♦ Soil-borne infection, acquired by **cattle** probably by ingestion with spores localizing in muscle and other sites
♦ In **sheep** a wound infection at shearing, lamb docking, vulva at lambing, head by rams fighting, fetal lambs after pregnant ewes exposed to infection

Risk factors

Cattle Mostly 6 months to 2 years old growing cattle on good nutritional plane.

Sheep Any age, high protein diet increases susceptibility.

Importance
Severe death losses unless vaccination carried out.

Clinical findings

Cattle
♦ Severe lameness
♦ Hot, painful (later cold, painless, with edema, emphysema), swelling of upper part of limb
♦ Rarely lesion at tongue base, brisket, udder, or internally
♦ Depression
♦ Anorexia
♦ Rumen stasis
♦ Fever
♦ Tachycardia
♦ Death at 12–36 hours

Sheep
♦ Cases with limb lesions show same signs as cattle except local edema, emphysema not features
♦ Local lesions cause swelling of vulva, udder or head
♦ Severe toxemia as in cattle

Horse
♦ Stiff gait, incoordination
♦ Pectoral edema

Clinical pathology

Bacteriological examination of needle aspirate.

Necropsy findings

Cattle
♦ Characteristic posture at death, on side with affected limb stuck up in air
♦ Rapid bloating, decomposition
♦ Blood-stained froth from nostrils and anus
♦ Dark, discolored, swollen tissue with metallic sheen on incision, exudes excess thin, sanguineous fluid containing gas, rancid smell
♦ Lesion may be small, easily missed
♦ Excess fibrinous, blood-stained fluid in all body cavities

Sheep
♦ Similar to cattle but less gas and fluid, smaller lesions
♦ In pregnant ewes, entire fetus may be decomposed and cause abdominal distension with blood-stained, fibrinous fluid
♦ Proper bacteriological examination requires early necropsy, before invasion from gut over-runs tissue microbiology

Diagnosis

Resembles:
♦ Malignant edema
♦ Anthrax in pigs and horses
♦ Bacillary hemoglobinuria
♦ Limb bone fracture

Treatment

♦ Massive parenteral antibiotic therapy, usually penicillin intravenously, required

because of extensive lesion and the highly fatal toxin
* Intralesional injection also advisable if accessible

Control

Cattle
* On enzootic farms annual vaccination (formalin-killed, alum-precipitated bacterin) all animals 6 months to 2 years just before expected danger period
* Vaccinate calves at 3 weeks in bad areas
* During outbreak move herd from field, vaccinate all animals over 3 weeks immediately and inject treatment dose of penicillin; cases still occur for 14 days after vaccination

Sheep
* Vaccinate ewes 3 weeks before lambing
* In subsequent years only maiden ewes vaccinated
* Supplementary vaccination usual before danger period, e.g. fighting, lambing
* Vaccination breakdowns usually due to inadequate content of appropriate antigen
* Polyvalent clostridial vaccines popular at little extra cost

MALIGNANT EDEMA (GAS GANGRENE) [VM8 p. 686]

Etiology

* *Clostridium septicum* the principal pathogen
* Also *Cl. chauvoei, Cl. perfringens, Cl. sordelli, Cl. novyi, Cl. fallax*

Epidemiology

Occurrence
* Universally as sporadic cases, rarely outbreaks
* All animal species
* Highly fatal without treatment

Source and transmission
* Soil-borne, spores confer long-term survival
* Dirty environment encourages wound or umbilical cord contamination

Risk factors
* Intramuscular injection without skin disinfection
* Parturition causing vulvar, vaginal laceration
* Dipping in contaminated dip immediately after shearing
* Castration, docking wounds
* Crows picking at weak lambs
* Head fight wounds in young rams run as a band

Importance
Significant death losses now rare with better hygiene.

Clinical findings

* Incubation period 12–48 hours
* Soft, painful, doughy swelling at site, local erythema
* Later dark colored, taut, emphysema with frothing from wound in some
* Fever
* Depression
* Tremor
* Lame, stiff gait
* Mucosae congested, dry, poor capillary refill
* Peri-parturient cases show vulvar discharge with swelling extending to all pelvic tissues
* Death at 24–48 hours

Clinical pathology

Aspirated fluid cultured for early identification of bacteria

Necropsy findings

* Skin gangrene at site, inflammatory, sometimes gelatinous, fluid in subcutaneous, intermuscular connective tissue planes; emphysema in some
* Subserous hemorrhages
* Serosanguineous fluid in body cavities
* Rapid postmortem invasion of tissues from gut

Diagnosis

Resembles:
* Blackleg

♦ Cl. sordelli infection
♦ Anthrax in pigs and horses

Treatment

♦ Emergency treatment large doses crystal-line penicillin or broad-spectrum antibiotic I/V, every 6 hours
♦ Some injected direct into site
♦ Incision, irrigation with hydrogen peroxide in late cases

Control

♦ Hygiene at parturition, shearing, castration, tail docking, injection
♦ Vaccination in high-risk areas with combined vaccine of local bacteria, formalin-killed bacterin
♦ Prophylactic penicillin injection, wound disinfection after trauma

Clostridium sordelli infection
[VM8 p. 677]
Can cause:
♦ Fatal myositis similar to that caused by *Cl. welchii* or *Cl. septicum*
♦ Fatal hepatitis in newborn lambs
♦ Enteritis with hemorrhagic diarrhea in calves
♦ Convulsive disease with opisthotonus similar to that caused by *Cl. perfringens* type D

BRAXY (BRADSOT) [VM8 p. 688]

Etiology

Clostridium septicum.

Epidemiology

Occurrence
♦ In weaner, yearling sheep
♦ In midwinter during heavy frosts, snow
♦ Low incidence; case fatality rate about 50%

Clinical findings

♦ Sudden onset acute toxemia
♦ Separation from group
♦ Depression
♦ Complete anorexia
♦ High fever
♦ Abdominal pain, abdomen distended with gas in some
♦ Recumbency, coma
♦ Death after a course of a few hours

Clinical pathology

No antemortem indicants.

Necropsy findings

♦ Local areas edema, congestion, necrosis, ulceration of abomasal wall
♦ *Clostridium septicum* in smears of abomasal lesions or culture of heart blood
♦ Specimens for culture must be collected within an hour of death

Diagnosis

Resembles:
♦ Carbohydrate engorgement
♦ Infectious necrotic hepatitis

Treatment

None of value.

Control

♦ Yard sheep at night, fed hay before letting out to pasture
♦ Vaccination with a formalin-killed whole culture, 2 injections, 2 weeks apart, effective

INFECTIOUS NECROTIC HEPATITIS (BLACK DISEASE) [VM8 p. 689]

Etiology

An acute toxemia caused by toxins elaborated by *Clostridium novyi* in damaged liver tissue, e.g. that caused by *Fasciola hepatica*.

Epidemiology

Occurrence
♦ Commonest in well-nourished 2–4 year old sheep
♦ Sporadic losses in cattle; rare in pigs at pasture
♦ Seasonal variation in occurrence due to seasonality of liver fluke invasion, i.e. commonest summer and fall, cease when frosts start
♦ Outbreaks when sheep grazed on swampy land
♦ Morbidity usually 10–30%, up to 50% in worst environment
♦ Factors enhancing snail multiplication, e.g. pasture irrigation, increase black disease prevalence

Source and transmission
♦ Sheep infected from soil-borne infection via ingestion
♦ Soil infected by feces of carrier animals, cadavers of animals dying of disease

Clinical findings

Sheep
♦ Usually found dead
♦ Segregate from flock
♦ Go down if driven
♦ Fever, later hypothermia
♦ Rapid, shallow respiration
♦ Sternal recumbency; may die sitting up
♦ Course of a few hours

Cattle
♦ Longer course; 1–2 days
♦ Sudden onset of severe depression
♦ Reluctant to move
♦ Transient fever early; hypothermia, skin cold
♦ Rumen sounds absent
♦ Heart sounds soft, muffled
♦ Abdominal pain, especially on palpation over liver
♦ Feces semifluid
♦ Periorbital edema in some

Pigs
Sudden death.

Horses
♦ Depression
♦ Reluctant to walk
♦ Pain on abdominal palpation
♦ Frequent straining
♦ Recumbency
♦ Death after course of about 72 hours

Clinical pathology

♦ Little information available
♦ Abdominal paracentesis fluid in horses shows great increase in inflammatory cells

Necropsy findings

♦ Rapid putrefaction of carcase
♦ Marked engorgement of subcutaneous vessels, some subcutaneous edema
♦ Underside of skin becomes very dark on drying, hence **black disease**
♦ 1–2 cm dia. areas of yellow necrosis surrounded by red hyperemic zone under liver capsule on diaphragmatic surface of liver or deep in liver
♦ Evidence of recent fluke invasion

♦ Blood-stained serous fluid in all body cavities
♦ Many subepicardial, subendocardial petechiae
♦ *Clostridium novyi* in necrotic lesion identified by culture, or fluorescent antibody, or toxin by ELISA test on intestinal contents

Diagnosis

Resembles:
♦ Acute fascioliasis
♦ Enterotoxemia
♦ Blackleg
♦ Malignant edema
♦ Bacillary hemoglobinuria
♦ Anthrax

Treatment

♦ No effective treatment available for sheep
♦ Very early cases in cattle may respond to heavy doses penicillin, tetracyclines

Control

♦ Control liver fluke
♦ Vaccination with toxoid before danger period with annual booster subsequently in danger areas

BACILLARY HEMOGLOBINURIA
[VM8 p. 691]

Etiology

Clostridium hemolyticum (Cl. novyi type D)

Epidemiology

♦ Uncommon disease
♦ Occurs principally in cattle
♦ Peak occurrence in summer and autumn
♦ Losses on infected farms may be 25%
♦ Case fatality rate 100%
♦ Precipitated by liver fluke migration in liver
♦ Organism persists in soil for long periods, up to 1 year

Clinical findings

♦ Acute onset of anorexia
♦ Cessation of milk flow
♦ Rumen stasis
♦ Disinclination to move
♦ Arched back
♦ Grunt on walking, percussion over liver
♦ Respiration shallow, labored, dyspnea terminally

- Pulse rapid, weak
- Fever early, soon hypothermia
- Brisket edema common
- Feces dark, may be diarrhea, dysentery
- Urine red
- Moderate jaundice
- Abortion
- Death after course of 12 hours to 4 days

Clinical pathology

- Hemoglobinuria
- Blood levels hemoglobin, erythrocytes reduced severely
- Variable degrees of leukocytosis
- *Cl. hemolyticum* agglutinins markedly elevated in survivors

Necropsy findings

- Rapid rigor mortis
- Subcutaneous gelatinous edema
- Extensive subcutaneous, subserous hemorrhages
- Jaundice
- All body cavities contain excessive amounts serous to blood-stained fluid
- Hemorrhagic abomasitis, enteritis
- **Ischemic infarct in liver**
- Red urine
- *Cl. hemolyticum* visible in hyperemic area around infarct by use of fluorescent antibody test on impression smear

Diagnosis

Resembles:
- Postparturient hemoglobinuria
- Poisoning by Brassica spp.
- Babesiosis
- Chronic copper poisoning in sheep
- Causes of hematuria

Treatment

- Immediate parenteral injection large doses of penicillin, tetracycline in febrile cattle on an enzootic farm
- Supportive treatment with fluids, blood transfusions if necessary

Control

- Control of liver fluke, elimination other causes of liver damage
- Vaccination with formalin-killed whole culture 4–6 weeks before danger season; black disease vaccine a satisfactory alternative

- Annual vaccination all animals over 6 months of age on enzootic farm
- Careful destruction all cadavers

ENTEROTOXEMIA CAUSED BY
CLOSTRIDIUM PERFRINGENS
TYPE A [VM8 p. 693]

Diseases in which *Clostridium perfringens* type A may play an etiological role include:
- **Equine intestinal clostridiosis**
- Acute, profuse watery diarrhea
- High case fatality rate
- Large numbers of the bacteria in intestine at necropsy
- Has occurred in horses which:
  - Collapsed/died during exercise
  - Had hemorrhagic cecitis/colitis like colitis-X
- **Hemorrhagic enteritis** in calves and adult cattle
- Identical with syndrome caused by *Cl. perfringens* B, C
- In adults usually in puerperal calves
- Antiserum, or formalized vaccine protective
- **Acute hemolytic enterotoxemia** in foals
- **Fatal hemolytic disease** in cattle and sheep characterized by:
  - Acute onset severe depression, collapse
  - Mucosal pallor, jaundice
  - Dyspnea
  - Abdominal pain
  - Hemoglobinuria
  - Fever in some
  - Most die, short course a few hours, rarely several days
  - **Necropsy** – pallor, jaundice, hemoglobinuria
  - Small intestinal necrosis
  - Large amounts of toxin, large numbers clostridia in gut

ENTEROTOXEMIA CAUSED BY
CLOSTRIDIUM PERFRINGENS
TYPES B, C AND E [VM8 p. 694]

Etiology

Clostridium perfringens types B, C and E cause hemorrhagic enteritis in young animals of several species, known as specific diseases:
- **Lamb dysentery** – *Cl. perfringens* type B in lambs up to 3 weeks old
- **Struck** – *Cl. perfringens* type C in adult sheep on abundant pasture
- **Hemorrhagic enterotoxemia** – *Cl. perfr-*

ingens type C in young lambs, piglets, foals up to 1 week old, and goats; type B in calves up to 10 days old and foals up to 1 week old
♦ **Necrotic hemorrhagic enteritis** in calves – *Cl. perfringens* type E
♦ Bacteria form spores which survive for long periods in soil, found in gut of normal animals
♦ Disease caused by rapid multiplication of bacteria stimulated by several risk factors

Epidemiology

♦ Sporadic occurrence; lamb dysentery enzootic some areas
♦ Patchy occurrence due to limited occurrence of the several types of the bacteria
♦ **Lamb dysentery** in lambs born to densely grouped ewes in contaminated surroundings when feed plentiful in cold weather. Case fatality rate 100%
♦ **Hemorrhagic enterotoxemia (type C)** in **piglets** occurs as outbreaks affecting a number of litters; case fatality very high, morbidity may be 80%; sudden death in piglets less than 1 week old; older ones live longer. In **lambs** and **kids** occurs in densely housed groups at lambing; fatality rate 100%, up to 20% morbidity. In **foals** single cases only

Clinical findings

Lamb dysentery
♦ Lambs up to 2 weeks old
♦ Sudden death, *or*
♦ Anorexia
♦ Severe abdominal pain
♦ Fluid, brown feces, some with blood
♦ Tenesmus
♦ Recumbency, coma
♦ Death after 24 hour course, *or*
♦ Chronic **pine** in older lambs on enzootic farms
  • Chronic abdominal pain
  • Refuses to suck
  • No diarrhea
  • Responds to antiserum treatment

Struck
♦ In adult sheep
♦ A few cases show abdominal pain, convulsions
♦ Most cases found dead

Hemorrhagic enteritis and enterotoxemia in calves
♦ Outbreaks of diarrhea dysentery mostly in calves up to 10 days old, some up to 10 weeks.

♦ Acute abdominal pain, bellowing, frenzied running, tetany, opisthotonus
♦ Death in few hours up to 4 days

Hemorrhagic enteritis and enterotoxemia in piglets
♦ Sudden death in very young
♦ Older piglets show fluid diarrhea, dysentery, reddening of anus
♦ Dullness, depression
♦ Death after 24 hour course

Foal enterotoxemia
♦ Severe depression
♦ Marked abdominal pain
♦ Bloody diarrhea in some
♦ Hypothermia
♦ Dyspnea
♦ Tachycardia
♦ Death within 24 hours

Clinical pathology

♦ Diagnosis usually made on autopsy material
♦ Large numbers of clostridia in fecal smear
♦ Specific serum antitoxins detectable by ELISA in recovered patients, cases with longer courses

Necropsy findings

♦ Hemorrhagic enteritis; ulceration in some; extensive lesions in small intestine
♦ Excess serous fluid in peritoneal cavity
♦ In **struck** peritonitis evident, muscles may resemble malignant edema
♦ Culture of intestinal contents, examination for toxins, desirable to confirm diagnosis

Diagnosis

In neonates resembles:
♦ Colibacillosis
♦ Salmonellosis
♦ Actinobacillus equuli infection
♦ Porcine transmissible gastroenteritis

Treatment

♦ Hyperimmune sera the only treatment likely to be of value
♦ Oral antibiotics may prevent further bacterial proliferation in cases with longer courses

Control

Vaccination with type-specific toxoid, bacterin preferred but need is for speed; good cross-protection between vaccines composed of either types B or C, *Clostridium perfringens*

In an outbreak vaccinate all pregnant animals, requires 2 weeks for antibody production. Specific antiserum for short-term protection

Depot amoxycillin, benethamine penicillin at birth, repeated through danger period

In enzootic herds, flocks vaccination of pregnant dams, 2 injections 1 month apart first year, then single annual injection subsequent years

ENTEROTOXEMIA CAUSED BY
CLOSTRIDIUM PERFRINGENS
TYPE D (PULPY KIDNEY) [VM8
p. 697]

Etiology

Clostridium perfringens type D; rapid proliferation in intestine produces potent exotoxins, especially *epsilon* toxin.

Epidemiology

Occurrence
♦ Worldwide distribution
♦ Prevalence limited in most countries because of widespread vaccination
♦ Commonest in lambs, especially sucking lambs aged 3–10 weeks and weaned, feeder lambs up to 10 months, important in calves, especially 1–4 month vealers, adult goats and kids; rare in adult cattle; causes focal symmetrical encephalomalacia in adult sheep
♦ Worst in fat lamb flocks practising intensive nutrition; feedlots
♦ Morbidity up to 10%; case fatality 100%

Source and transmission
♦ *Cl. perfringens* type D a common, short-term inhabitant of soil contaminated by feces, and of intestine of animals grazing over it; transmission assumed to be by ingestion
♦ Factors, including good bodily condition of lambs, feed supply excellent, e.g. high grain diets, lush pasture, cereal crops, promote rapid multiplication of bacteria, production of lethal quantities of toxins

Clinical findings

Lambs
♦ Short, fatal course; 2–12 hours
♦ Dullness, depression, yawning
♦ Facial twitches
♦ Anorexia
♦ Severe clonic convulsions with opisthotonus, mouth frothing
♦ Green pasty diarrhea
♦ Staggery gait
♦ Recumbency
♦ Temperature normal

Adult sheep
♦ Similar syndrome, up to 24 hours duration, plus tremor, bloat, in a few, *or*
♦ Focal symmetrical encephalomalacia

Calves
♦ Some found dead without evidence of struggling
♦ Most start with bellowing, mania violent convulsions
♦ Death after 2 hour course
♦ A few subacute cases quiet, docile, anorexia, blind actions but menace reflex present; recover after 2–3 days

Goats
♦ Peracute cases abdominal pain, dysentery, fever, convulsions, death after 4–36 hours
♦ Acute cases diarrhea most prominent sign, abdominal pain, death or survival at 2–4 days
♦ Subacute cases with anorexia, severe intermittent diarrhea, dysentery for several weeks
♦ Chronic cases with anemia, chronic wasting

Clinical pathology
♦ Hyperglycemia (150–200 mg/dl, glycosuria in sheep; occurs also in other diseases
♦ Large numbers clostridia, specific toxins, in feces

Necropsy findings
♦ No gross lesions in some
♦ Excess clear, straw-colored, gelatinous fluid in pericardial sac, pulmonary edema
♦ Rapid decomposition, purple discoloration skin, wool easily plucked; soft pulpy kidneys

- Fibronecrotic, hemorrhagic enterocolitis in goats
- Symmetrical, focal, degenerative brain lesions in subacute cases in sheep
- Many clostridia in gut segments; accompanied by toxin which can be filtered off and used to test mice for presence of specific toxin
- Identification of presence of toxin now performed using ELISA test or counter-immunoelectrophoresis

Diagnosis

In lambs resembles:
- Acute pasteurellosis
- Hypocalcemia-hypomagnesemia
- Hemophilus agni septicemia
- Carbohydrate engorgement

In adult sheep and calves resembles:
- Rabies
- Lead poisoning
- Hypomagnesemia
- Pregnancy toxemia
- Louping-ill

Treatment

- Course too short for effective treatment in lambs
- If course 2–3 days use antiserum plus oral sulfonamide

Control

- Reduce feed intake; not too sharply to cause hypoglycemia, acetonemia or major setback in lamb growth, *plus*
- Vaccination with activated alum-precipitated toxin of:
  - Pregnant ewe plus revaccination at 1 month old or
  - Newborn animal at 3 days with a repeat at 1 month
  - Revaccination at 6 month intervals
- Fat lamb flocks and in feedlots need special vaccination programs suited to their risk seasons
- Vaccination may precipitate attacks of blackleg
- Multiple clostridial vaccines (enterotoxemia, blackleg, tetanus, braxy) are popular, effective
- Vaccination of goats unreliable, and antiserum may precipitate attacks of anaphylaxis
- Toxoid vaccines likely to cause blemishes

in tissue; careful selection of vaccination sites recommended

FOCAL SYMMETRICAL ENCEPHALOMALACIA [VM8 p. 701]

Etiology

Clostridium perfringens type D.

Epidemiology

Occurrence
- Lambs, weaners, mature sheep, and possibly calves
- Morbidity about 15%, case fatality high

Clinical findings

- Many found dead
- Segregate from flock
- Appear blind, aimless wandering, gait incoordination
- Unable to eat, drink
- Worst cases show lateral recumbency, opisthotonus, paddling convulsions
- Death or euthanasia
- Course varies from 1–14 days

Clinical pathology

No significant changes.

Necropsy findings

Soft, hemorrhagic foci in internal capsule, thalamus, cerebellar peduncles.

Diagnosis

Resembles polioencephalomalacia.

Treatment and control

- No treatment
- Cases cease after vaccination with *Cl. perfringens* type D vaccine

ENTEROCOLITIS ASSOCIATED WITH *CLOSTRIDIUM DIFFICILE*
[VM8 p. 701]

Epidemiology

Foals less than 3 days old.

Clinical findings

+ Severe diarrhea, dehydration, metabolic acidosis
+ Abdominal pain
+ Leukopenia, degenerative left shift, lymphopenia
+ Death within 12 hours
+ Resembles foal enterotoxemia due to *Cl. perfringens* type C

Necropsy findings

+ Diffuse hemorrhagic enteritis
+ Segmental mucosal erosions, necrosis
+ *Cl. difficile* isolated with difficulty; may be missed by standard procedures

18 DISEASES CAUSED BY BACTERIA – III

DISEASES CAUSED BY *ESCHERICHIA COLI*

ACUTE UNDIFFERENTIATED DIARRHEA OF NEWBORN FARM ANIMALS [VM8 p. 703]

Syndrome of acute diarrhea in neonates before an etiological diagnosis available.

Etiology

See Table 18.1.

Epidemiology

Risk factors
Factors which enhance the incidence of calf diarrhea include **management factors**:
♦ Dam nutrition, colostrum quality, quantity
♦ Exposure to cold, dampness, draughts, windy weather
♦ Increased population density in housing, calving pens
♦ Poor drainage in outdoor pens
♦ Mixing heifers, adult cows in calving groups
♦ Quality of husbandry
Pathogen factors that influence which infection will predominate:
♦ Infection rate of each of the pathogens, and the mix of them in the population
♦ Each pathogen has its predilection for an age group of calves
♦ Each pathogen responds differently to management risk factors
Host factors
♦ Immaturity of calf
♦ Lack if vigor at birth
♦ Hypoxemia, acidosis due to a long, difficult birth
♦ Failure to acquire sufficient colostral antibody to protect against bacterial and viral pathogen

Clinical findings

♦ In calves younger than 30 days, piglets, lambs, and foals younger than 7 days

♦ Sudden onset profuse watery diarrhea
♦ Progressive dehydration, acidosis
♦ Death, usually in a few days, some sooner

Necropsy findings

♦ Dehydration
♦ Emaciation
♦ Fluid-filled intestine
♦ Some, e.g. salmonellosis, clostridiosis, coccidiosis have significant lesions of the enteric mucosa

Treatment

♦ Oral and/or parenteral fluid, electrolytes as indicated (Tables 2.2 and 2.5)
♦ Broad spectrum antibacterials, parenterally, orally for not more than 3 days, on the assumption that all acutely sick calves will have a bacterial disease and will be septicemic or bacteremic
♦ Treatment on a scientifically logical basis requires definition of the exact cause, determined by:
  • Necropsy examination of all affected animals that die
  • Laboratory examination of fecal samples, cadavers, in search for identity of the pathogen
  • Serological examination in survivors to defect antibodies to the significant pathogens

Control

♦ Check for, and correct where possible, risk factors especially quantity of colostrum fed, quality, and amounts fed, of milk replacer used
♦ Late pregnant cows moved to a low-risk venue
♦ Vaccinate late pregnant cows

Table 18.1 Possible causes of septicemia and acute neonatal diarrhea in farm animals [VM8 p. 716]

Septicemia

Calves	Piglets	Lambs and kids	Foals
E. coli	E. coli	E. coli	E. coli
Salmonella spp.	Streptococcus spp.	Salmonella spp.	Actinobacillus equuli
Listeria monocytogenes	Listeria monocytogenes	Listeria monocytogenes	Salmonella abortivoequina
Pasteurella spp.		Erysipelas insidiosa	Salmonella typhimurium
Streptococcus spp.			Str. pyogenes
Pneumococcus spp.			Listeria monocytogenes

Acute neonatal diarrhea

Calves	Piglets	Lambs and kids	Foals
Enteropathogenic and enterotoxigenic E. coli	Rotavirus	Coronavirus	Salmonella spp.
Rotavirus Coronavirus	Enteropathogenic E. coli	Cryptosporidium	Eimeria spp.
Cryptosporidium	Salmonella spp.	Cl. perfringens type C	Foal-heat diarrhea
Salmonella spp.	Transmissible gastroenteritis virus	Rotavirus	Rotavirus
Eimeria spp. (calves at least 3 weeks of age)	Cl. perfringens type C	Caprine herpesvirus	Cl. perfringens type B
Cl. perfringens type C	Rotavirus		
	Isospora spp.		

COLIBACILLOSIS OF NEWBORN
FARM ANIMALS [VM8 p. 707]

Etiology

Specific pathogenic serotypes of *Escherichia coli* some of which cause septicemic colibacillosis, others cause diarrhea and dilation of isolated loops of intestine

Epidemiology

Occurrence
♦ Worldwide, in all species
♦ **Dairy calves** – morbidity usually 30%, may reach 70% in intensively farmed herds, case fatality rate 10–50%
♦ **Beef calves** – morbidity 10–50%, case fatality 5–25%
♦ **Piglets** – very variable but colibacillosis accounts for 50% of losses due to gastroenteritis in the preweaning period
♦ **Foals** – 25% septicemias due to colibacillosis

Source and transmission
♦ Infected animals the main source
♦ Transmission mostly by ingestion from contaminated skin of dam, feeding utensils; can occur via navel or nasopharynx
♦ Spread between herds by introduction of infected animals

Risk factors
♦ **Age of young** – most cases in calves less than 4 days old, rarely in older calves, never in adults
♦ **Age of dam** – offspring of heifers, gilts more susceptible than those from adult dams
♦ **Colostrum intake** – newborn farm animals are agammaglobulinemic at birth; passive protection against *E. coli* depends on ingestion and absorption of adequate quantities (3–4 liters) of colostrum containing high levels of immunoglobulins soon after birth (maximum absorption in calves at 6–12 hours)
♦ Factors reducing colostral intake include:
  • Immaturity of dam
  • Misshapen teats or udder
  • Weak calf, e.g after prolonged birth
  • Poor maternal attention to calf
  • Cold, wet, windy weather
♦ Environmental contamination
  • Overcrowding
  • Failure to move puerperal cows to clean surroundings
♦ Concurrent disease

• Dietary diarrhea contributed to by:
  • Poor quality milk replacers
  • Irregular feeding regime
• Presence of pathogenic viruses; facilitate development of colibacillosis in calves older than 4 days
♦ Virulence of specific *E. coli* serotypes
  • Geographical location of specific enterotoxigenic *E. coli* serotypes patchy
♦ Inheritance – resistance to *E. coli* inherited in piglets

Clinical findings

Septicemic colibacillosis in calves
♦ Depression, weakness, no suck reflex
♦ Tachycardia
♦ Fever early, soon hypothermic
♦ Recumbency, coma, moribund
♦ Oral mucosae cold, dry
♦ Diarrhea, dysentery rarely
♦ Death in most by 24–96 hours
♦ Survivors at 1 week show one or more of –
  • Arthritis
  • Meningitis
  • Panophthalmitis
  • Pneumonia

Enterotoxigenic colibacillosis in calves
Occurs in two forms:
♦ **Enteric toxemia:**
  • Severe weakness, recumbency
  • Coma, hypothermia, cold clammy skin
  • Pale mucosae, wetness around mouth
  • Superficial veins collapsed
  • Slow, irregular heart
  • Mild convulsive movements
  • Periodic apnea
♦ Diarrhea:
  • Feces watery to pasty, pale yellow to white, occasional blood streaks, foul-smelling
  • Frequent, effortless defecation
  • Buttocks smeared, tail soiled
  • Appetite indifferent but may take some milk
  • Dehydration
  • In early stages abdomen slightly distended, fluid splashing on succussion
  • Spontaneous recovery in about 80%
  • Others worsen during 3–5 day course, die of dehydration

Acidosis
♦ Calves and kids recovered from diarrhea become weak, ataxic, recumbent, comatose, respond quickly to intravenous

treatment with sodium bicarbonate solution

Lambs

- Most cases peracute, septicemic
- 2 age groups: 1–2 days, 3–8 weeks
- Found dead, *or*
- Recumbent, comatose
- Occasionally meningitis with stiff gait, hyperesthesia, tetanic convulsions
- Survivors have chronic arthritis

Piglets – septicemic form

- In piglets 24–48 hours old
- Some found dead
- Some or all of litter affected
- Weak to comatose
- Cyanotic
- Cold, clammy, hypothermic
- Usually no diarrhea
- Most die

Piglets – diarrheic form

- The common form
- 12 hours to 3 days old
- May be entire litter
- Puddles of thin, yellow diarrhea on floor
- Gradual loss of appetite
- Tails straight, wet; buttocks soiled
- Temperature normal to subnormal
- Dehydration, weakness, lateral recumbency, paddling
- Die after 24-hour course

Clinical pathology

- Blood and fecal culture for identification of organism, antibiotic sensitivity
- Most reliable information from fresh necropsy specimen
- Total, differential leukocyte counts to determine existence of septicemia or serious intestinal injury
- Dehydration, electrolyte imbalance, acidosis detected in blood chemistry examination
- Serum immunoglobulin estimations, e.g. by use of zinc turbidity test, will indicate adequacy of colostrum intake

Necropsy findings

- Culture of organism and definition of antimicrobial sensitivity from heart blood, mesenteric lymph nodes, gut contents from freshly dead untreated piglet dead after typical illness

- Virulence determinants assessed by DNA gene probes or ELISA
- Detection of enterotoxin in intestine

Septicemic colibacillosis

- No lesions in many
- Subserous, submucosal petechiae
- Some enteritis, gastritis
- Fibrinous exudate in joints, serous cavities, omphalophlebitis, peritonitis, meningitis in a few

Enteric colibacillosis – piglets

- Flaccid, fluid-filled intestines, clotted milk-filled stomach
- Intestinal mucosa may be hyperemic, mesenteric lymph nodes edematous
- Villous atrophy
- Dehydration

Enteric colibacillosis – calves

- Similar to piglets
- Pseudomembranous ileitis, mucohemorrhagic colitis, proctitis in cases infected with highly virulent serotypes

Diagnosis

(See Table 18.1.) The major problem is to differentiate infectious causes of diarrhea from dietary diarrhea.

Treatment

- In dairy calves replace milk with fluid-electrolyte mixtures for the period of diarrhea then fed small amounts milk increasing to normal over several days; beef calves, piglets are left with dam and supplemented with oral fluids containing antibacterials
- Parenteral **fluid therapy** (see Chapter 2, and Tables 2.2 and 2.5). Oral fluid and electrolyte therapy are still effective in the presence of hypersecretion caused by enterotoxigenic E. coli, provided the solution contains glucose as well as sodium and chloride. Fluids should be given separately to any milk being fed and can be administered by nipple bottle or esophageal feeder. Up to 2 liters are given at a time; more may cause abdominal pain
- A poor response to fluid therapy is often due to failure to correct the acidosis present
- **Antibacterial, immunoglobulin therapy:** Single substance preparations and mixtures, are routinely used in very large amounts in calf scours. Commonly used commercial products given orally include neomycin, tetracyclines, sulfonamides,

trimethoprim-sulfonamide mixtures, nifuraldezone, ampicillin; their use should be discontinued after 3 days
- For calves and piglets with suspected septicemic colibacillosis, trimethoprim–sulphonamide combinations or broad spectrum antibiotics are administered parenterally
- Routine prophylactic medication via milk replacers or other feeds discouraged because of the possible creation of antibiotic-resistant bacteria
- Intravenously administered bovine gammaglobulin is rational therapy in hypo-gammaglobulinemic calves but dose rates need to be high and costs prohibitive

Miscellaneous treatments
- Blood transfusions
- Antimotility drugs
- Intestinal protectants have no discernible effect on outcomes

Management
- Isolate affected animals
- New neonates housed-penned separately and hygienic precautions to avoid spread; beef cows and calves moved to a new pasture; piglets treated and left with sow
- Treat all new cases immediately
- Dead animals necropsied

Control

General recommendations set out in Chapter 3. Special recommendations include the following.

Dairy calves housed indoors
- If calf a vigorous sucker leave with cow; others encouraged to suck or separated from cow, fed colostrum 50 ml/kg body weight minimum; if colostrum pooled, preserved feed 3–4 liters
- Leave with cow 2 days, or remove to single stall, force feed harvested colostrum
- Post-colostral feeding, into single pen, feed fermented colostrum for first 3 weeks; feed regularly, by same person if possible

Beef calves
- Assist calves at birth to avoid early weakness
- Calves that do not suck before 2 hours need help by assisting to suck, or stomach tube dosing of harvested colostrum
- Constant surveillance of bedding yards to observe difficult parturitions, mismother-

ing, twins, ensure calf sucks colostrum early, avoid overcrowding,

Lambs
- Attempt to provide about 200 ml colostrum/kg body weight during first 18 hours
- Supplement twins or lambs of low milk producing ewes with stored colostrum

Piglets
- Surveillance of birth to ensure no piglets stuck
- Ensure piglets close to udder soon after birth to salvage ejected milk
- Farrowing pen floor needs to be well drained, non-slip
- Disinfect farrowing pen between sows
- Warm water/soap wash sow's udder and perineum before birth
- Dry, warm creep area

Vaccination
- Parenteral vaccination pregnant cows with purified E. coli K99$^+$ pili or whole cell preparation containing sufficient K99$^+$ antigen reduces colibacillosis prevalence in calves
- Oral or parenteral vaccination of pregnant sows and ewes with 3 antigen types of pili confers protection against colibacillosis caused by homologous enteropathogenic E. coli in piglets, lambs

ESCHERICHIA COLI INFECTIONS IN WEANED PIGS [VM8 p. 724]

- Includes edema disease, coliform gastroenteritis and cerebrospinal angiopathy
- The two former are serious diseases but edema disease much reduced in prevalence now compared with 30 years ago
- The two major diseases are caused by E. coli hemolytic serotypes, and occur under similar management systems; angiopathy is thought to be caused by E. coli

EDEMA DISEASE (BOWEL EDEMA, GUT EDEMA, ENTEROTOXEMIA) [VM8 p. 724]

Etiology

Proliferation of hemolytic E. coli in intestine producing an identified toxin known as the edema disease principle.

Epidemiology

- The specific serotypes responsible for the disease are introduced into the piggery
- Cause the disease when stimulated to proliferate excessively in intestine
- Mostly in 6–14 week pigs, especially the largest, fastest-growing ones
- Occurs as outbreaks after stress factor introduced, e.g. diet change, affecting up to 50% of pigs
- Outbreak sudden, lasts about 8 days, rarely more than 15 days
- Does not spread to other contiguous groups

Clinical findings

- Sudden outbreak affecting a number of pigs within a short time
- Transient diarrhea first in some
- Incoordination, especially hind limbs
- Stiff gait, stringhalt-like gait in fore or hindlimbs
- Paresis, sways, sags, difficulty getting up
- Some show tremor, aimless wandering, clonic convulsions
- Edema of eyelids, cornea, face, ears but only in some and not a gross lesion
- Blindness, hoarse voice to inaudible in some
- Illness lasts 6–36 hours
- Flaccid paralysis terminally
- Few survivors usually have gait defect

Clinical pathology

- Excessive numbers hemolytic *E. coli* in feces
- The edema disease principle cytotoxic to Vero cells

Necropsy findings

- Subcutaneous edema head, throat, stomach wall, colonic mesentery
- Excess fluid in body cavities
- Pale skeletal muscles
- Hemolytic *E. coli* cultivable from alimentary tract
- Histopathological lesions are hyaline degeneration, fibrinoid necrosis in arteries, arterioles and encephalomalacia

Diagnosis

Resembles:
- Mulberry heart disease

- Encephalomyocarditis virus infection
- Salt poisoning
- *Amaranthus, chenopodium* spp. poisoning

Treatment

- Immediately reduce feed supply
- Melperone 4–6 mg/kg body weight recommended as a tranquilizer in early cases
- Purgative to clean out alimentary tract
- Oral antibiotic in feed, drinking water to restrain the coliform's growth

Control

- Gradual change from creep feed to production ration, introduced later than usual
- Dilute production ration with inert feed e.g. rice hulls

POSTWEANING DIARRHEA
(COLIFORM GASTROENTERITIS)
[VM8 p. 726]

Etiology

- Associated with proliferation specific, enterotoxin-producing serotypes *E. coli* usually hemolytic
- Rotavirus infection may contribute

Epidemiology

- Predominantly in pigs 3–10 days after weaning
- Rapid spread within group
- Morbidity rate commonly 80% within a few days; case fatality rate 30%; survivors have a slow growth rate
- Other groups become affected as they are weaned

Clinical findings

- Post-weaning growth rate reduction, without diarrhea for 10–14 days considered to be the simplest form of the disease
- Severest cases found dead
- Average case show depression, diarrhea
- Anorexic but still drink
- Feces very watery, yellow, often unsuspected
- Severe dehydration, weight loss
- Pink under the belly
- Voice loss, incoordination in final stages

♦ Outbreak lasts 7–10 days
♦ Survivors show growth retardation

Clinical pathology

Excessive numbers hemolytic *E. coli* in feces

Necropsy findings

♦ Dehydrated
♦ Mild skin discoloration along belly
♦ Mesenteric hemorrhages
♦ Intestines dilated with yellowish or blood-stained liquid
♦ Hemorrhagic areas, congestion of intestinal mucosa
♦ Hemolytic *E. coli* in intestine in large numbers

Diagnosis

Resembles:
♦ Salmonellosis
♦ Swine dysentery
♦ Erysipelas
♦ Pasteurellosis
♦ *Hemophilus parahemolyticus* infection

Treatment

♦ Clinically abnormal pigs to be treated urgently, intensively
♦ All others in group to receive prophylactic treatment in drinking water
♦ Neomycin, neofurans, tetracyclines, sulfonamides, trimethoprim-potentiated sulfonamides, ampicillin the preferred drugs; treatment for 2 days after treatment stops, usually total of 5–7 days

Control

♦ Complete withholding of post weaning creep feed until after weaning appears to restrain the disease, *or*
♦ Alternatively introduce the production ration to the pigs as early as 10 days old with all subsequent feed changes being made gradually
♦ Litters kept separate for immediate post weaning period; merging of litters to be arranged so that pigs of equal size move in together
♦ Prophylactic antibiotic feeding for 20 days after weaning practised but has implications for development of drug-resistant strains

CEREBROSPINAL ANGIOPATHY
[VM8 p. 730]

Etiology

Likely to be a sequel to chronic edema disease

Clinical findings

♦ Sporadic cases in recently weaned pigs, up to 5 weeks after weaning
♦ Only 1 or 2 cases per litter
♦ Incoordination, blindness, hypoesthesia generally
♦ Aimless wandering, circling
♦ Rapid, severe emaciation
♦ Subject to savaging by pen mates

Necropsy findings

Angiopathy similar to that in chronic edema disease.

Diagnosis

Resembles:
♦ Viral encephalomyelitides
♦ Spinal cord abscess
♦ Brain abscess

Treatment

Recovery unlikely in any circumstances.

DISEASES CAUSED BY *SALMONELLA* spp.

SALMONELLOSIS (PARATYPHOID)
[VM8 p. 730]

Etiology

♦ The *Salmonella* spp. serotypes that commonly cause diseases in farm animals include:

• Cattle – *S. typhimurium, S. dublin, S. newport*
• Sheep and goats – *S. typhimurium, S. dublin, S. anatum*
• Pigs – *S. typhimurium, S. choleraesuis*
• Horses – *S. typhimurium, S. anatum, S. newport, S. enteriditis, S. heidelberg, S. arizona, S. angona*

Epidemiology

Occurrence
♦ Worldwide in all animal species
♦ Earlier high prevalence in pigs reduced by better hygiene, less saleyard selling, less garbage feeding
♦ Recent increased prevalence in cattle due to intensification of farming
♦ Present increase in occurrence of unusual serotypes due to feeding exotic feeds containing animal or fish products
♦ Prevalence in dairy herds likely to be about 20% in countries with intensive dairy industries
♦ Occurs as sporadic cases or outbreaks with morbidity up to 50%; case fatality rates are high, up to 100% without treatment

Source and transmission
♦ Fecal contamination of feed, pasture, water, utensils, and troughs; infected bone and meat meal, fish meal, milk, pooled colostrum; grain contaminated by rodent feces
♦ Factors increasing pasture contamination include continued wetness, irrigation with slurry of manure from yards, milking parlour, irrigation with human sewage
♦ Carrier animals, latent or active, are common with *S. dublin*; they maintain the infection in a herd; *S. typhimurium* occur widely in many species but tend not to persist in carriers for long periods
♦ Introduction carrier animals onto a farm, or mixing animals in transport vehicles, in rail or sale yards, at shows, fairs, races, in veterinary hospitals, wildlife access to pasture, water holes
♦ Transmission by fecal or oral contamination

Risk factors
♦ Infection alone does not cause clinical disease
♦ Stressors which precipitate attacks of clinical disease include transport, cold, wet weather, intercurrent disease, vaccination reaction, anesthesia and surgery, feed or water deprivation, concentration of livestock on small sections of pasture e.g. during drought, flood, **parturition**

Importance
♦ Varies with serotype, e.g. *S. dublin* persists in a herd, causing serious losses; *S. typhimurium* is as dangerous to individual cows but tends not to persist and is usually of minor importance in cattle

♦ Animal salmonellosis is now a serious zoonosis

Clinical findings

Septicemia
♦ Common in neonatal foals, calves, pigs up to 4 months old
♦ Depression, recumbency
♦ High fever
♦ Skin red discoloration in pigs
♦ Survivors may develop enteritis, arthritis
♦ Most die after 24–48 hour course

Acute enteritis
♦ Common syndrome adults, all species
♦ High fever
♦ Profuse, fluid diarrhea
♦ Feces contain mucus, sometimes blood, epithelial shreds, casts; putrid smell
♦ Severe dehydration, weight loss
♦ Complete anorexia; some will drink
♦ Tachycardia
♦ Hyperpnea
♦ Mucosae congested
♦ Abortion
♦ Recumbency, death after 3–5 day course
♦ Case fatality 75%

Chronic enteritis
♦ Common in pigs, occasional cases in calves and horses
♦ Often succeeds initiating attacks acute enteritis
♦ Intermittent or persistent moderate diarrhea
♦ Occasional blood spots, patches mucus, firm intestinal casts
♦ Intermittent, moderate fever
♦ Weight loss to emaciation

Bovine salmonellosis
♦ Sporadic cases endemically on farm with *S. dublin* infection
♦ Outbreaks when herd subjected to severe nutritional stress
♦ With *S. typhimurium* single or several cases at one time; in calves point outbreak or succession of newborn calves or puerperal cows
♦ Septicemic disease in neonates, some with nervous signs e.g. incoordination, nystagmus
♦ Calves older than a week and adults usually have acute enteritis (dysentery, clots of blood, abdominal pain, rolling, flank kicking, pain on rectal, agalactia) followed by abortion, polyarthritis, gangrene of extremities in survivors

- Abortion without prior enteritis common in *S. dublin* infection
- Chronic enteritis after acute enteritis or initially

Ovine and caprine salmonellosis

- Acute enteritis in sheep flock with some cases septicemia; some abortions with *S. dublin*
- Goats; septicemia in newborn, acute enteritis, similar to cattle disease, in older goats

Pig salmonellosis

- Septicemia with purple belly skin, cutaneous petechiation
- Tremor, weakness, convulsions, paralysis, very high case fatality rate common
- Also acute enteritis with secondary pneumonia, occasionally encephalitis
- Rectal stricture a sequel in enteric salmonellosis (*S. typhimurium*) in feeder pigs

Equine salmonellosis

- Mostly single sporadic cases
- Outbreaks or series in neonates, transported or hospitalized horses
- Variable syndromes:
  - Asymptomatic shedding salmonella
  - Subacute enteric disease (fever, depression, anorexia, soft porridge-like feces, neutropenia with left shift)
  - Common syndrome is fulminating enteritis (diarrhea, fever, dehydration, neutropenia, colic, often severe)
  - Foals a few days old, fatal septicemia; survivors have polyarthritis, meningoencephalitis etc.

Clinical pathology

- Valuable in diagnosis, monitoring sick animal
- Bacterial culture using blood, feces, milk because bacteria difficult to find, present for short period only; results improved by serial culture, or pinch biopsy of rectal mucosa; test feces of other animal species, plus drinking water, suspect feeds, when *S. typhimurium* present in sick animals
- Identifying carrier animals requires fecal sample culture all cows at 2 week intervals, especially on day of calving, including calf; of value only when cows are tied in barns; at pasture too many are passive carriers. Procedure difficult, expensive, inaccurate
- DNA probes
- Serological tests; species-specific agglutinins appear in serum of survivors 2 weeks after attack; many normal animals

in herd will also carry modest titers. Serum ELISA also available
- Indirect evidence by leukopenia, neutropenia, severe degenerative left shift; marked hyponatremia, high fecal leukocyte counts in horses

Necropsy findings

Septicemia
Eextensive subserous, submucosal petechiation.

Acute enteritis

- Varies from mucoenteritis to hemorrhagic enteritis in small, large intestines, with abomasitis in *S. dublin* infection; necrotic enteritis in ileum, large intestine in *S. typhimurium* infection; diphtheritic pseudomembrane in long-standing cases
- Intestinal contents watery, contain mucus, tinge of blood or blood clots, putrid odor
- Mesenteric lymph nodes enlarged, edematous, hemorrhagic
- Gallbladder wall thickened, inflamed
- Subserous, especially subepicardial, petechiation; very obvious in pig kidney, hence 'turkey-egg kidney'
- Pneumonia, purpling of skin or circumscribed, scabby lesions all marked in pig salmonellosis

Chronic enteritis

- Discrete area of necrosis in cecum, colon wall, especially button ulcers around ileocecal valve in pigs
- Chronic pneumonia in some
- **Culture of salmonellae** from gut contents, mesenteric lymph nodes, gall bladder, liver, heart blood in acute forms, only in gut in chronic disease

Diagnosis

Resembles:
- Colibacillosis in neonates
- Ccoccidiosis in young
- Acute intestinal obstruction
- Winter dysentery
- Mucosal disease
- Bracken poisoning
- Arsenic poisoning
- Molybdenum poisoning
- Johnes disease
- Heavy stomach fluke infestations

Sheep
- *Campylobacter* spp.
- Coccidiosis
- Heavy worm infestation

Horses
- *Escherichia coli, Actinobacillus equuli* infections in foals
- colitis-X

Pigs
- Hog cholera
- Coliform gastroenteritis
- Pasteurellosis
- Erysipelas
- Swine dysentery
- Streptococcal meningitis

Treatment

- Consideration needs to be given to the risk of creating carriers of salmonellosis by treatment of clinic cases, then moving survivors into herds where salmonellosis may not occur
- Mass treatments via feed or drinking water may produce antibiotic resistant strains of salmonellae but their epidemiological or economic significance appears not to attract much attention
- Oral treatment with antibacterials is standard for salmonellosis in pigs and ruminants but is inclined to cause or prolong a severe diarrhea in horses
- Choosing the best antibacterial for any situation should be based on isolation of the causative organism and identifying its antibacterial sensitivities; common usage is:

Calves with S. dublin infection:
- Trimethoprim with sulfadoxine or sulfadiazine, parenterally daily, *or*
- Ampicillin, amoxicillin parenterally; orally in preruminant calves

Foals, septicemic salmonellosis Systemic and oral treatment 6-hourly ampicillin or gentamicin.

Horses (adults) Ampicillin or potentiated sulfonamide combinations.

Pigs, septicemia Trimethoprim-sulfadoxine, combined with chlortetracycline and sulfamezathine by mass medication.

Supportive treatments
See enteritis, and fluid and electrolyte therapy (Tables 2.2, 2.5).

Control

Introductions

- Calves and feeder pigs are a big risk if purchased very young; usually impossible to purchase guaranteed free of disease or from disease-free farm; vaccinated animals are best
- Avoid processing bought-in animals through communal facilities, e.g sale-yards; at least avoid more than a minimal stay there
- Provide some quarantine initially from resident population

Restraining spread within herd or flock
- Sterilize or cull carriers; difficulty in identifying them
- Prophylactic medication of entire herd via drinking water not highly successful
- Identify infected groups; avoid moving infected groups to contact other groups
- All drinking water to be via troughs with no chances of fecal contamination
- Where possible an all-in, all-out policy with vigorous disinfection between groups when animals housed or closely confined in pens
- Proper design of housing to minimize contamination by feces
- Slurry disposal as fertilizer restricted to crops, not pasture
- Carcase disposal of salmonella cases burned, not converted to bone meal

Animals on transports
- Animals to be transported should be penned and fed hard feed for 5 days before shipping, in high risk situations prophylactic feeding of antibacterials
- Unloaded, exercised, fed, and watered every 24 hours
- Vehicles clean, disinfected between shipments

Vaccination
- Valuable as an auxiliary provided density of salmonella population restrained to reasonable levels
- Good commercial vaccines not generally available
- Live, attenuated or lowly virulent strains much superior to killed vaccines
- Autogenous vaccines popular but have limited efficiency and some inclination to cause anaphylactic response
- Best results are with living vaccine used to vaccinate pregnant dams with immune offspring as the objective

ABORTION IN MARES AND
SEPTICEMIA IN FOALS CAUSED BY
SALMONELLA ABORTIVOEQUINA
[VM8 p. 746]

Etiology

Salmonella abortivoequina often in association with other unidentified filterable agents.

Epidemiology

♦ Rarely reported nowadays
♦ Sources are infected carrier mare, possibly stallion
♦ Transmission by ingestion pasture contaminated by uterine discharges, aborted fetuses; possibly venereal

Clinical findings

♦ Abortion at 7–8 month
♦ No illness but may be dystokia
♦ Placenta, metritis common sequelae; subsequent fertility normal
♦ Foal from infected mare may develop fatal septicemia during first days, or polyarthritis at 2 weeks
♦ Stallion may show fever, edema prepuce, scrotum, epididymitis, orchitis

Clinical pathology

♦ Organism in placenta, uterine discharge, aborted fetus, joints
♦ High titer salmonella agglutinins 2 weeks after abortion

Necropsy findings

♦ Aborted placenta edematous, hemorrhagic, patchily necrotic
♦ Septicemia in very young foals, polyarthritis in foals 2 weeks old

Diagnosis

Mare abortions more commonly caused by –
♦ Equine herpesvirus-7
♦ Equine viral arteritis
♦ *Streptococcus zooepidemicus*
Foal septicemia, polyarthritis more commonly caused by:
♦ *Escherichia coli*
♦ *Actinobacillus equuli*
♦ *Streptococcus zooepidemicus*
♦ *Salmonella typhimurium*

Treatment

Ampicillin, amoxycillin, trimethoprim-sulfonamide combinations, gentamicin.

Control

♦ Hygienic disposal of fetuses
♦ Isolation infected mares, stallions
♦ Vaccination with killed bacterin was popular; 3 injections a week apart after end of breeding season on enzootic farms
♦ Widespread use of vaccine credited with virtual disappearance of disease

ABORTION IN EWES CAUSED BY
SALMONELLA ABORTUSOVIS
[VM8 p. 747]

Etiology

Salmonella abortusovis

Epidemiology

♦ Enzootic some areas
♦ Source is infected carrier animals that do not abort
♦ Transmission probably by ingestion; venereal transmission does not occur in spite of infection in rams

Clinical findings

♦ Occurs as abortion storms, 10% of ewes abort, 6 weeks before lambing
♦ Few ewe deaths due to metritis
♦ Some lamb deaths due to weak lambs or pneumonia at 2 weeks

Clinical pathology

♦ *S. abortusovis* in large numbers in aborted fetus, placenta, uterine discharge
♦ Positive agglutination tests in ewes for 8–10 weeks after abortion

Necropsy findings

♦ Septic metritis in ewes
♦ Septicemia, pneumonia in lambs

Diagnosis

Abortion also caused by infection with:
♦ *Brucella ovis*
♦ *Campylobacter fetus*

- Enzootic abortion due to *Chlamydia* spp.
- *Listeria monocytogenes*
- *Salmonella dublin*
- *Salonella ruiru*
- *Salomonella typhimurium*
- *Toxoplasma gondii* (New Zealand type 2)
- Virus of Rift Valley fever, Wesselbrons disease

Treatment

Ampicillin, amoxycillin, gentamicin, trimethoprim–sulfonamide combinations

Control

Vaccines available but not extensively field tested

DISEASES CAUSED BY *PASTEURELLA* spp.

Diseases caused by *Pasteurella* spp. but listed at other locations include
- Pasteurella mastitis
- Atrophic rhinitis
- Versiniosis

Miscellaneous sporadic diseases caused by *Pasteurella* spp. include the following:

Calf and yearling meningoencephalitis [VM8 p. 747]

Etiology P. multocida.

Clinical findings:
- Tremor
- Opisthotonus
- Eyeball rotation
- Coma, death within few hours

Horse, donkey, and mule meningoencephalitis [VM8 p. 747]

Etiology P. haemolytica.

Clinical findings:
- Incoordination
- Tremor
- Blindness
- Tongue paralysis
- Death after 1–7 days

Lamb lymphadenitis [VM8 p. 749]

Etiology P. multocida.

Clinical findings:
Submandibular, cranial, cervical, prescapular lymph node enlargement.

Horse, donkey septicemia [VM8 p. 747]

Etiology P. multocida.

PASTEURELLOSIS [VM8 p. 748]

Includes:
- Septicemic pasteurellosis – *P. multocida* type 1 (B)
- Bovine pneumonic pasteurellosis – *P. haemolytica* biotype A, serotype 1, and *P. multocida* biotype A
- Porcine pasteurellosis – *P. multocida*. Pneumonic disease
- Ovine and caprine pasteurellosis – *P. haemolytica*. Pneumonic disease, some septicemias especially in lambs

BOVINE SEPTICEMIC PASTEURELLOSIS (HEMORRHAGIC SEPTICEMIA, BARBONE) [VM8 p. 748]

Etiology

P. multocida type 1(B), occasionally type 4(D), type E.

Epidemiology

Occurrence
- Chiefly southeast Asia; recorded in USA
- Water buffalo, cattle, camels, yaks, rarely pigs, horses, bison
- In low-lying, wet areas exposed to chilly weather
- Animals exhausted by heavy work
- Morbidity, case fatality rates 50–100%, higher in buffalo; very heavy death losses, long convalescence in survivors

Source and transmission
- Organism persists on tonsils, nasopharyngeal mucosa of carriers
- Large numbers bacteria in saliva
- Spread by ingestion contaminated feed
- Organism on pasture survives less than 24 hours

Clinical

Cattle and pigs
- Sudden onset of high fever
- Severe depression
- Profuse salivation
- Submucosal petechiation
- Warm, painful swellings at throat, dewlap, brisket, perineum
- Throat swelling may cause severe dyspnea
- Death after 24 hour course

Sequels Survivors may develop diarrhea, pneumonia

Clinical pathology

- Organism cultivable from saliva, blood stream
- Rapid ELISA available for identification of serotypes

Necropsy findings

- Generalized petechiae, especially subserosal
- Lung and lymph node edema
- Subcutaneous aggregations gelatinous fluid
- Enteritis, pneumonia in survivors from septicemia
- *P. multocida* in spleen and blood

Diagnosis

Resembles:
- Anthrax
- Blackleg
- Acute leptospirosis

Treatment

Tetracyclines, potentiated sulfonamides extensively used

Control

- Vaccine of killed organisms in an adjuvant base very effective; immunity lasts 12 months
- Recent vaccines include endotoxin-free capsular antigen, mutant avirulent strains

UNDIFFERENTIATED BOVINE
RESPIRATORY DISEASE [VM8
p. 749]

Any serious respiratory disease problem in cattle before an etiological diagnosis has been made.

Etiology, Clinical signs, and Clinical pathology

For descriptions of the diseases that are likely to be present, singly or in combination, in a clinical situation that can only be identified initially as **undifferentiated bovine respiratory disease**. Individual descriptions of the large number of diseases which may be involved, singly or in combination, can be found in the lists entitled:
- Pneumonia
- Aspiration pneumonia
- Lung abscess
- Caudal vena caval thrombosis
- Pulmonary congestion, edema
- Pulmonary hypertension
- Pulmonary emphysema
- Rhinitis
- Laryngitis, tracheitis, bronchitis

Treatment

- Careful, three times daily surveillance of group for signs of illness
- Immediate treatment of all febrile animals, assuming they are early cases of the target disease
- Patients with toxemia assumed to have bacterial infection will need parenteral broad-spectrum antibacterial injection
- Patients without toxemia assumed to have viral infection, but likely to develop secondary bacterial infection, will need same treatment but as prophylaxis
- Recommended 3 day courses of treatment include:
  • Oxytetracycline 10 mg/kg body weight I/M, *or*
  • Procaine penicillin G 30 000–45 000 iu/kg I/M, *or*
  • Trimethoprim–sulfadoxine 3 ml/45 kg body weight I/M, *or*
  • Tilmicosin 10 mg/kg body weight S/C
- Prophylactic treatment to remainder of the group by:
  • Mass medication in water or feed widely used but lacks experimental support; a matter for the individual veterinarian in each situation
  • Individual treatments to in-contacts

recommended when morbidity rate high enough (6–10%) to suggest a major loss about to occur; long acting tetracycline 20 mg/kg I/M or tilmicosin 10 mg/kg S/C
♦ Failure to respond to treatment for 3 days probably due to:
• Late or wrong diagnosis, or treatment; prognosis bad
• severe viral infection; prognosis fair

Control

Principles include:
♦ Accurate determination of cause at the earliest possible time
♦ Mixing groups of young cattle from different origins creates a hazard
♦ High frequency of excellent quality surveillance of suspect groups essential
♦ Avoidance of stress by overcrowding, exposure to inclement weather, dietary mismanagement; indoors stress of bad ventilation
♦ Putting cattle through communal saleyards, long-distance, long duration transport increases exposure to infection, adds physical stress
♦ Mass medication on entry to a feedlot or other hazardous situation is widely practiced; recommended procedures include:
• Long-acting tetracycline 20 mg/kg I/M or tilmicosin 10 mg/kg S/C injection on arrival
• Mass medication in feed; chlortetracycline (1–4 g/head daily for 2 weeks after arrival) appears beneficial
♦ **Vaccination** is widely practiced but results are sufficiently variable to make a general recommendation hazardous; local experience with local vaccines containing *Pasteurella*, *Haemophilus* and *Mycoplasma* spp., and the respiratory viruses and the virus of bovine virus diarrhea is probably as good a guide as is available

PNEUMONIC PASTEURELLOSIS OF CATTLE (SHIPPING FEVER PNEUMONIA) [VM8 p. 758]

Etiology

♦ Usually *Pasteurella haemolytica* (biotype A, serotype 1), occasionally *P. multocida*, possibly aided by the simultaneous infection with a virus or mycoplasma.

Epidemiology

Occurrence

♦ A common disease in North America, UK, and continental Europe
♦ Commonest form is of young beef cattle recently introduced (first 3 weeks) to feedlots
♦ Herd morbidity up to 35%, case fatality rate 5–10%
♦ Clustering of cases occurs in particular drafts of cattle, particular truck-loads, and particular pens in the lot

Source and Transmission
♦ Nasal discharge of clinical cases, infected animals, possibly carriers
♦ Inhalation; spread can be very rapid in poorly ventilated housing

Risk factors
♦ All ages; peak losses in 6 months to 2 years old
♦ Mixing of calves from different origins, of different ages
♦ Stress of transportation, infection opportunities in communal sale, rail yards
♦ Stress of feed shortage, water deprivation
♦ Communal summer grazing
♦ Vaccination on arrival at feedlots
♦ Drafty, humid indoor housing

Importance
Major cause of loss by death or by prolonged stay in fattening unit.

Clinical findings

♦ Depression
♦ Rapid shallow respiration
♦ Increased loudness breath sounds, over increasing area with time, progressing to crackles, wheezes
♦ Pleuritic friction sounds for a short period, early in disease; later grunting with each expiration
♦ Dyspnea in terminal stage
♦ Fever
♦ Cough, increased by walking
♦ Anorexia, gaunt abdomen, may drink
♦ Mucopurulent nasal discharge, crusty nose
♦ Eye discharge
♦ Course 2–4 days, responds well to treatment

Sequels
♦ Lung abscess
♦ Chronic pleurisy
♦ Pericarditis
♦ Congestive heart failure due to cor pulmonale

Outbreak history

◆ In feedlots outbreaks last 2–3 weeks unless additional susceptible cattle added.

Clinical pathology

◆ Bacteriological findings based on nasal or pharyngeal swabs undependable as a guide to bacteriology of alveoli
◆ Hematological findings vary from neutrophilia to neutropenia

Necropsy findings

◆ Marked consolidation of anteroventral parts of lungs with serofibrinous exudate accumulation in interlobular spaces
◆ Lung cut surface shows red or gray consolidation
◆ Catarrhal bronchitis, bronchiolitis, serofibrinous pleurisy with accumulation large quantities pleural fluid, plus fibrinous pericarditis in some
◆ Chronic cases – bronchopneumonia, pleural adhesions, lung abscess
◆ *P. haemolytica* associated with fibrinous pleuropneumonia; *P. multocida* with bronchopneumonia with little fibrin exudation

Diagnosis

Resembles other diseases listed under:
◆ Pneumonia
◆ Pulmonary congestion, edema, emphysema
◆ Rhinitis
◆ Laryngitis, tracheitis, bronchitis

Treatment

◆ Most cases recover within 24 hours after a single treatment with oxytetracycline, trimethoprim–sulfadoxine, penicillin or tilmicosin (see bovine respiratory disease)
◆ Poor response due usually to complicated etiologies or late treatment; these need daily treatment for 3–5 days
◆ Complete failure to respond due usually to lung abscess, bronchioectasis, pleurisy, or non-bacterial cause

Control

Preconditioning

◆ Calves prepared for sale and move to feedlots by
  • Weaning 2 weeks before moving

  • Vaccinations for all the high-risk diseases in the feedlot
  • Deworming
  • Castration, dehorning, branding where applicable
  • Watering, feeding in a feedlot with standard feedlot feed mixes
◆ Recommended for creation of quality product; doubts as to its economic viability

Management

◆ Wean before bad weather arrives
◆ Begin feeding hay, possibly grain in a creep, 2 weeks before weaning
◆ Careful surveillance for signs illness
◆ Do not ship sick cattle
◆ Avoid long transport hauls without rest
◆ Avoid sale, rail yards; proceed directly from farm to feedlot
◆ Allow a breaking-in period of 2–3 weeks gradual reduction of roughage before introduction of heavy grain diets

Vaccination

Much is carried out but the results are marginal; vaccination on arrive at the feedlot with a modified live-virus vaccine may actually increase mortality

Chemoprophylaxis

◆ Mass medication of all animals on arrival at the feedlot is practiced (see bovine respiratory disease)
◆ Mass medication in feed may reduce mortality but will have little effect on morbidity; number of advanced cases may increase because surveillance intensity diminishes

PASTEURELLOSIS OF SHEEP AND GOATS [VM8 p. 770]

Etiology

◆ *Pasteurella haemolytica* (biotypes A, T with many serotypes); *P. multocida* uncommon as a respiratory pathogen in sheep
◆ Adenovirus, parainfluenza-3 viruses predispose

Epidemiology

◆ *P. haemolytica* a normal inhabitant of ovine nasopharynx
◆ Infection persists in flock, passes from flock to flock via carrier sheep

♦ **Pneumonic pasteurellosis** due to biotype A; occurs most parts of world
♦ Losses due to deaths and failure to gain weight
♦ In all ages but young lambs, puerperal ewes worst affected, most cases in spring and summer
♦ Most due to climate, nutrition, management stress
♦ Occurs in sheep at pasture but much faster spread in feedlot lambs
♦ Not unusual for it to occur with septicemic pasteurellosis in lambs
♦ Sheep and goats similar morbidity 5%, case fatality up to 20%
♦ Septicemic pasteurellosis
♦ Only young lambs up to 2 months old, most at 2–3 weeks
♦ Often apart of pneumonic pasteurellosis outbreak
♦ **Systemic pasteurellosis:**
♦ Due to biotype B; in lambs 5–12 months old, following stressful episode including move from dry, poor feed to rich, lush pasture
♦ Population mortality may reach 5%
♦ **Pasteurella mastitis** – caused by *P. haemolytica* biotype A

Clinical findings

Pneumonic pasteurellosis
♦ Dyspnea, exaggerated by exercise
♦ Slight mouth-frothing
♦ Cough
♦ Nasal discharge
♦ Fever
♦ Depression
♦ Anorexia
♦ Loud breath sounds, some gurgling
♦ Death after 1–3 day course
♦ Survivors have chronic pneumonia, ill-thrift

Systemic pasteurellosis
♦ Short course, 6 hours; many found dead
♦ Dullness, recumbency,
♦ Frothy, bloody nasal discharge terminally

Clinical pathology

♦ No examinations practicable; the dead sheep afford a more realistic appraisal.

Necropsy

Pneumonic pasteurellosis
Lung consolidation, large quantities serous pleural fluid, organisms present in large numbers.

Systemic pasteurellosis
♦ Subcutaneous hemorrhages over neck, thorax
♦ Trachea, bronchi contain blood-stained froth
♦ Lungs edematous with subpleural ecchymoses but no pneumonia
♦ Ulceration, necrosis pharynx, esophagus
♦ Tonsils, pharyngeal lymph nodes enlarged
♦ Small necrotic ulcers on tips of abomasal folds
♦ Organisms in large numbers in tonsils, pharynx, esophagus

Diagnosis

♦ **Pneumonic pasteurellosis** commonly secondary to chronic progressive ovine pneumonia. Resembles:
  • Parasitic pneumonia
  • Jaagsiekte
  • Maedi
♦ **Septicaemic pasteurellosis** resembles – *Haemophilus agni septicemia*

Treatment

♦ Many dead without clinical illness observed
♦ Recommended 3 day courses of treatment, as for cattle, include:
  • Oxytetracycline 10 mg/kg body weight I/M, *or*
  • Procaine penicillin G 30 000–45 000 iu/kg I/M, *or*
  • Trimethoprim-sulfadoxine 3 ml/45 kg body weight I/M, *or*
  • Tilmicosin 10 mg/kg body weight S/C

Control

♦ Avoidance of climatic, nutritional, managerial stress where possible
♦ Long-acting tetracycline for in-contacts during outbreak (20 mg/kg body weight every 4 days)
♦ Mass medication in feed also available for feedlot lambs
♦ Vaccines available but usefulness marginal

PASTEURELLOSIS OF SWINE
[VM8 p. 774]

Two forms of the disease:
♦ Porcine pneumonic pasteurellosis
♦ Porcine septicemic pasteurellosis

PORCINE PNEUMONIC PASTEURELLOSIS [VM8 p. 774]

Etiology

◆ *Pasteurella multocida*, serotypes A, D common isolates from pneumonic pig lungs, including enzootic pneumonia caused by *Mycoplasma hyopneumoniae*, *Actinobacillus pleuropneumoniae*
◆ Not considered to be a primary pathogen

Epidemiology

◆ Source is tonsils, nasopharynx of carrier pigs
◆ Transmission by inhalation, direct nose-to-nose contact

Clinical findings

◆ Fever
◆ Anorexia
◆ Recumbency
◆ Dyspnea
◆ Death after 4–7 day course
◆ Survivors have chronic pneumonia, ill-thrift, recurrent acute attacks of pneumonia

Necropsy findings

Chronic bronchopneumonia, lung abscess; pleuritis, pericarditis in some.

Diagnosis

Resembles:
◆ Enzootic swine pneumonia
◆ *Actinobacillus pleuropneumoniae* pleuropneumonia
◆ Septicemic salmonellosis

Treatment

◆ Chlortetracyclines, but sensitivity testing of bacterial isolates recommended because of variability in antibiotic sensitivity

Control

◆ Control of primary disease
◆ Avoidance of managemental, climatic, feeding stress

PORCINE SEPTICEMIC PASTEURELLOSIS [VM8 p. 775]

Etiology

P. multocida.

Epidemiology

◆ Occasional outbreaks in baby pigs, or adults, or grower pigs
◆ Up to 40% herd mortality

Clinical findings

◆ Fever
◆ Dyspnea
◆ Throat, lower jaw swelling
◆ Death within 12 hours

Necropsy findings

◆ Subserosal hemorrhages
◆ Vascular damage with thrombus formation
◆ Bacteria in all tissues

Treatment

Tetracycline effective.

TULAREMIA [VM8 p. 775]

Etiology

Francisella tularensis; 2 types: A is *F. tularensis* var. *tularensis*, occurs in rabbits; B is *F. tularensis* var. *palaearctica*, occurs in waterborne diseases of rodents.

Epidemiology

Occurrence
◆ Most northern hemisphere countries
◆ Seasonal, mostly in spring
◆ Primarily a disease of wild animals, birds; rarely transmits to domestic animals, usually pigs, sheep, calves
◆ A rare disease but morbidity in sheep flocks may be up to 40%, case mortality 50%

Source, transmission
◆ Hares, rabbits, wild rodents
◆ Transmitted mostly by tick bite (*Dermacentor andersoni*, *Haemaphysalis otophila*); infestation must be massive, continuous
◆ Organism persists over a year in water, mud; infection in humans can occur through skin

Importance Minor disease in farm animals; serious zoonosis.

Clinical findings

Sheep
♦ Heavy tick infestation
♦ Gradually developing stiff gait, head dorsiflexion, hunched hindquarters
♦ Lags behind
♦ Fever, tachycardia, hyperpnea
♦ Dark, fetid diarrhea
♦ Urination small amounts, frequently
♦ Recumbency after several days; patient struggles
♦ Death after course of few days to 2 weeks
♦ Survivors shed fleece

Pigs
♦ Latent disease in adults
♦ Fever, depression, dyspnea, profuse sweating in piglets
♦ Course 7–10 days

Horses
♦ Fever
♦ Stiff gait
♦ Limb edema
♦ Foals worst affected; show additionally:
  • Incoordination
  • Dyspnea

Clinical pathology

♦ Diagnostic agglutination test available
♦ Positive serum agglutinates brucella antigen

Necropsy findings

♦ Care needed because of transmissibility to humans through skin
♦ Heavy tick infestation, areas of congestion on skin undersurface marks tick attachment sites
♦ Lymph node enlargement draining tick bite sites
♦ Congestion, hepatization lung; pulmonary edema
♦ Abscessation head lymph nodes, pleurisy, pneumonia in pigs
♦ *F. tularensis* in lymph nodes, spleen, ticks

Diagnosis

In sheep resembles:
♦ Tick paralysis
♦ *Pasteurella haemolytica* septicemia
♦ *Escherichia coli* septicemia

♦ *Hemophilus agni* septicemia
♦ Tick-borne fever

Treatment

Oxytetracycline preferred to penicillin, streptomycin.

Control

Tick control and avoidance.

YERSINIOSIS [VM8 p. 777]

Etiology

♦ *Yersinia pseudotuberculosis, Y. enterocolitica*, both with many serotypes, some biovars. Closely related to and cross-reacts with, *Brucella* spp.
♦ *Y. pseudotuberculosis* the important infection associated with farm animal disease; *Y. enterocolitica* less common

Epidemiology

♦ *Y. pseudotuberculosis* common gut inhabitant of all domestic and many feral, mammals and birds
♦ *Y. enterocolitica* carried in large numbers in tonsils of healthy pigs
♦ Fecal/oral transmission via water or pasture
♦ Disease only with heavy infection pressure in debilitated animals stressed by bad weather, starvation, capture trauma, transport

Clinical findings

♦ Watery diarrhea
♦ Mucus, blood in feces in some cases
♦ Chronic illthrift as sequel or independent syndrome in sheep

Clinical pathology

♦ Neutrophilia with left shift
♦ Patient often hypoproteinemic, anemic
♦ Organism isolatable from feces

Necropsy findings

♦ No gross findings except liquid feces, thickened small intestinal mucosa, enlarged lymph nodes in some sheep
♦ Characteristic segmental suppurative,

erosive enterocolitis in histopathology, especially in jejunum and ileum

Diagnosis

In cattle resembles:
♦ Salmonellosis
♦ Winter dysentery
♦ Arsenic poisoning

In sheep resembles:
♦ Weaner illthrift
♦ Nutritional deficiency cobalt

Treatment

Long-acting tetracyclines preferred to sulfonamides.

Control

Maintenance of good nutritional status, a difficult program in times of flood or drought, the usual provoking circumstance.

ATROPHIC RHINITIS [AR,
TURBINATE ATROPHY OF SWINE
[VM8 p. 779]

Etiology

Initial infection with *Bordetella bronchiseptica* followed by infection with toxigenic strains of *Pasteurella multocida*.

Epidemiology

Occurrence
♦ Worldwide where pigs raised intensively
♦ Common disease of pigs; morbidity variable because of variation in criteria and assessment methods

Source and transmission
♦ Infected pigs the source and mode of transmission between herds
♦ Direct contact, inhalation means of within-herd spread
♦ Infected carrier sow infects litter
♦ Cross-litter infection when litters of weaner pigs mixed
♦ *Brucella bronchiseptica* ubiquitous between piggeries, infection rate in a piggery may reach 90% incidence but soon eliminated from respiratory tract most pigs. *Pasteurella multocida* occurs only in some piggeries, those with progressive AR Litters

infected from sows. These infections often persist

Risk factors
♦ **Age** – piglets infected after 10 weeks develop no lesions; worst lesions are in non-immunes affected in first week of life
♦ **Immunity** – piglets from immune sows less likely to develop serious lesions
♦ **Bacterial virulence** – the toxigenic factor produced by the strains of *Pasteurella multocida* capable of causing turbinate atrophy and the nasal deformity is an osteolytic toxin
♦ **Housing** – overcrowding, poor ventilation, unsanitary conditions, exert an influence on prevalence of AR because of their influence on spread of infection

Importance
Evidence on the effects of atrophic rhinitis on feed conversion efficiency and rate of gain are conflicting.

Clinical findings

Non-immune piglets 3–9 weeks old, acute stage
♦ Sneezing, coughing
♦ Small amount serous to mucopurulent nasal discharge
♦ Transient uni- or bilateral epistaxis
♦ Rubbing snout on ground or objects
♦ Watery ocular discharge with mud streaks on face
♦ Decreased growth rate in some
♦ Many completely recover

Older piglets, mostly 8–10 weeks, chronic stage
♦ Dyspnea, cyanosis
♦ Thicker nasal discharge
♦ Severe facial deformity; facial dishing, bulging, snout deviation if condition asymmetrical
♦ Malocclusion, especially incisors, interference with prehension, mastication

Clinical pathology

Detection of carrier animals by special swab-collection and transport technique; series of 3 swabs gives 77% accuracy

Necropsy findings

♦ Lesions only in nasal cavity, adjoining facial bones
♦ Acute turbinate inflammation early

Characteristic lesion is late stage of –
nasal mucosal atrophy
- Turbinate decalcification, atrophy turbinates, ethmoids; complete disappearance in some
- Extension of inflammatory, atrophic changes to facial sinuses in some
- Standard evaluation of change is by viewing skull cross sectioned at second premolar tooth

Diagnosis

Acute phase resembles:–
- Swine influenza
- Inclusion body rhinitis

Chronic phase resembles:
- Necrotic rhinitis
- Normal inherited prognathic jaw some pig breeds
- Snout compression caused by constant pushing of snout against fixed equipment e.g. feed hopper bars, nipple drinkers

Treatment

- Only effective in very early stages, not after deformity; parenteral administration, single injection every 3–7 days for 3 injections of:
  - Tylosin 20 mg/kg body weight
  - Oxytetracycline 20 mg/kg
  - Trimethoprim–sulfadoxine 16–24 mg/kg
  or creep feed supplement for 3–5 weeks of:
  - Sulfamezathine 200 mg/kg feed
  - Tylosin 100 mg/kg feed
- Injection of individual pigs too labor intensive; creep feed supplementation too inaccurate

Control

- Aim is control/elimination of toxigenic strains of *Pasteurella multocida*
- Must include method of monitoring facial deformity

Eradication
By depopulation for 4 weeks, repopulation with specific-pathogen-free stock, or similar; expensive, high relapse rate

Infection reduction
For example, by:
- Allowing average age of sow herd to increase
- Also raising litters of old sows in separate establishment
- Culling affected (clinically or radiographically) and infected (positive nasal swabs for *P. multocida*) pigs; neither procedure practicable commercially
- Reduction of environmental infection, provocative influences by conversion to all-in, all-out system, elimination of dust, overcrowding, high humidity, inadequate ventilation

Mass medication
- Medication commences 2 weeks before farrowing, continued through lactation, included in creep feed for suckers, starter feeds for weaners with:
  - Sulfamezathine 450–1000 mg/kg feed
  - Carbadox 55 ppm plus sulfamezathine 110 ppm

Vaccination
- Conflicting evidence about efficiency of *B. bronchiseptica* vaccine
- A recombinant *P. multocida* toxin derivative vaccine given to gilts before and after farrowing more protective to piglets

Nutrition
Ensure adequate intake pregnant and young pigs:
- Calcium 1.2% of ration (requires additional zinc in diet – up to 100 mg/kg total diet)
- Phosphorus 1.0% of ration

DISEASES CAUSED BY *BRUCELLA* spp.

BRUCELLOSIS CAUSED BY
BRUCELLA ABORTUS (BANG'S
DISEASE) [VM8 p. 787]

Etiology

Brucella abortus

Epidemiology

Occurrence
- Widespread most countries
- Highest prevalence in dairy cattle, rare in other species than cattle

- In horses found in chronic bursal enlargements (fistulous withers, poll evil), has caused mare abortions
- Occurrence in pigs, sheep, horses, and dogs is a potential, not necessarily real, threat to cattle eradication program
- Infection in wild ruminants not known to be infection source for cattle
- Virtual eradication achieved in most developed countries

Source and transmission
- Aborted fetuses, placenta, infected live calves, uterine discharges from infected cows main source
- Infected, clinically normal carrier cows, discharging infection with normal calf, in placenta, uterine discharges
- Potential source in infected other species (above)
- Transmission within a herd by:
  - Ingestion contaminated water, feed (bacteria survives on pasture 100 days in winter, 30 days in summer in temperate climate)
  - Penetration intact skin, conjunctiva (e.g. by tail swipe)
  - Contamination teats during milking
- Transmission between herds:
  - Introduction infected cow, possibly a clinically normal carrier
  - On inanimate objects, boots, feed, etc., but possibility low
  - Venereal from infected bull highly improbable; infected semen used by artificial insemination transmits infection
- Embryo transfer a safe method of salvaging genetic material from infected animals

Risk factors
- Infection occurs at any age, persists only in sexually mature animals; small proportion of intrauterine infections persist in calves passively immune via colostral intake; such calves should not be bred
- Stage of pregnancy; the later the pregnancy at exposure the greater the probability of infection occurring

Importance
- Milk production and calf replacement lost due to abortion
- A serious zoonosis

Clinical findings

Cows
- Abortion principally in last trimester
- Subsequent pregnancies carried to full term

in most cows but 2nd, 3rd pregnancy abortions may occur
- Placental retention, metritis common sequels; rarely metritis septicemic, sometimes fatally, or chronic causing infertility

Bulls
- Orchitis, epididymitis; acute, painful swelling, one or both scrotal sacs, testis painful may be swollen; subsequently atrophies may regain fertile status after acute stage in one testicle unaffected

Either sex
Non-suppurative synovitis causing hygromatous swellings at carpus, progressive erosive arthritis of stifle.

Herd history
- Infection occurs after introduction of infected cow, rarely a bull or horse with fistulous withers
- In unvaccinated herds storm of abortions lasting one calving season followed by herd immunity stage with abortions occurring only in heifers

Horses
- High proportion of horses running with cattle herd become infected, are seropositive
- Rare cases have systemic reaction with fever, lethargy, stiff gait; others have distended bursae, fistulous withers, navicular bursa causing lameness; mares may abort.

Clinical pathology

- Culture of the organism unpopular because of zoonotic hazard; nucleic acid probe assay may be available
- Serological tests the basis for diagnosis but:
  - Some latent infections serologically negative
  - Tests tend to become negative at calving or abortion
  - Long lead time between infection and positive titer, especially in non-pregnant cow
  - Infected bulls often negative; bulls in infected herds should be regarded as suspicious regardless of serology, and not used for artificial insemination

Recommended usage of serological tests
- Screening test to determine herd status:
  - Buffered plate antigen test or

- Indirect enzyme immunoassay test
♦ Confirmatory test when high specificity required:
  - Complement fixation test or
  - Indirect enzyme immunoassay
♦ For detection of latent infections in serologically negative patients – anamnestic reaction test (one injection K45/20A vaccine causes high titers complement fixation antibodies)
♦ For monitoring herds:
  - Milk ring test, preferably 3 tests per year, or
  - ELISA
♦ Suspected false positives, i.e. cattle remaining serologically positive over a period in a brucellosis-free herd; difficulty differentiating cross-reactions to other organisms, e.g. *Yersinia*, *Francisella*, *Pseudomonas*, *Vibrio* spp. and persistent titers due to Strain 19 calfhood vaccination

Necropsy findings

♦ Necrotising placentitis
♦ Disseminated inflammatory reactions in aborted fetal tissues
♦ *B. abortus* isolated from:
  - Pregnant cow – mammary lymph node best; other nodes, uterine caruncles, cotyledons, fetal tissues
  - Heifers – mandibular lymph node
  - Bulls – mandibular, cervical, subiliac, scrotal lymph nodes

Diagnosis

Other causes of bovine abortion include:
♦ Leptospirosis
♦ Infectious bovine rhinotracheitis
♦ Listeriosis
♦ Mycotic abortion
♦ *Pinus* spp. poisoning
♦ Trichomoniasis
♦ Vibriosis (*Campylobacter fetus*)
♦ Epizootic abortion (a borrelia-like spirochete)

A large proportion of abortions are not diagnosed as being any of the above causes. To assist in the resolution of this fault a protocol for the examination of all abortions in cattle is proposed.

Recommended protocol for examination of a herd abortion problem

♦ Age the fetus by examination; check by breeding records

♦ Serological tests for brucellosis, leptospirosis, listeriosis, infectious bovine rhinotracheitis
♦ Immediate microscopic examination fetal fluids, fetal abomasal fluid, for trichomonads
♦ Culture fetal fluids, fetal abomasal fluid for *B. abortus*, *Campylobacter fetus*, *Listeria* spp., fungi
♦ Examine urine for *Leptospira* spp.
♦ Placenta in formalin for placentitis
♦ All examinations should be carried out on all cases

Treatment

♦ Treatment is relatively unsuccessful and not undertaken in cattle
♦ Horses with fistulous withers treated with *B. abortus* strain 19 vaccine, 3 injections 10 days apart; chloramphenicol 1 g/100 kg daily by injection for 12–20 days also used

Control

Ultimate eradication is the objective, now virtually eradicated in many developed countries

Herd control

♦ In herds with a low incidence test and slaughter all reactors, repeat at 3 month intervals until all tests negative for 2 consecutive tests, then annual tests
♦ In herds with high prevalence vaccinate all calves at 4–8 (optimum 5) months with strain 19 *B. abortus* vaccine until incidence low enough (<4%) to undertake test and slaughter program; vaccination at younger ages does not provide strong enough immunity; vaccination at older ages causes too many persistent titers and interferes with interpretation of testing program
♦ In herds in which the disease is spreading rapidly and heavy losses are imminent, adult vaccination has been widely used; abortion is prevented but the cows are serologically positive for life

Area control

♦ Undertaken when area incidence 5% or less
♦ Herds to be tested selected by screening test
♦ Quarantine of infected herds marked for eradication, depopulation of farms where incidence too high to make eradication cost-effective
♦ Special quarantine and testing procedures need to be put into effect in countries free of

the disease but seeking to import live cattle from countries where brucellosis persists
♦ Test and slaughter of reactors in quarantined herds

Hygiene
♦ Infected cows to calve in quarantine
♦ Aborted fetuses, uterine discharges effectively disposed of
♦ Chlorhexidine or similar disinfectant used by veterinarian or farmer to avoid between cow transmission

BRUCELLOSIS CAUSED BY
BRUCELLA OVIS [VM8 p. 803]

Etiology

Brucella ovis.

Epidemiology

Occurrence
♦ Worldwide; sheep only; British breeds more susceptible than merinos; flock prevalence 75%, up to 60% rams infected before control program begun
♦ Infection in ewes transient, 1 or 2 estrus cycles
♦ Most important in flocks practicing multi-sire breeding
♦ If rams infected >10% flock fertility decreased

Source and transmission
♦ Source is penis of infected rams; infected rams secrete bacteria in semen permanently
♦ Transmission venereal:
  • Ram to ram passively via ewe bred to infected ram during same estrus cycle
  • Directly ram to ram during homosexual activity, sniffing, licking genitalia

Risk factors
♦ All ages susceptible; prevalence increases with age
♦ Transmission greatest during breeding season

Importance
♦ Ram relative infertility; more rams needed to settle standard number of ewes; lambs per hundred ewes reduced 15–30%
♦ In ewes few abortions, stillbirths; some outbreaks abortion recorded

Clinical findings

♦ Enlargement, firmness, pain, heat of scrotum in early cases
♦ Fever, depression, hyperpnea
♦ In late cases testicle usually atrophic, epididymis enlarged, hard, scrotal tunics thick, hard
♦ Libido normal

Clinical pathology

♦ Semen reduces in quality, contains increased leucocyte numbers, *Brucella ovis*
♦ Serological tests in use include complement fixation test, ELISA
♦ Both used as basis of control program

Necropsy findings

♦ Acute cases – inflammatory edema in scrotal fascia
♦ Chronic cases – testicular tunics thick, fibrous with adhesions, epididymis enlarged, testicle shrunken, *B. ovis* isolatable
♦ Placenta thick, edematous in parts; intercotyledonary yellow-white plaques
♦ *B. abortus* in fetus, placenta

Diagnosis

In ram resembles suppurative epididymitis. In ewe resembles abortion caused by:
♦ *Campylobacter fetus, C. jejuni*
♦ *Chlamydia psittaci*
♦ *Listeria monocytogenes*
♦ *Salmonella abortusovis*
♦ *Salmonella* spp., e.g. *S. dublin*
♦ *Toxoplasma gondii*
♦ Rift Valley fever
♦ *Coxiella burnetii*
♦ Border disease virus

Treatment

♦ Rarely attempted because of the improbability of complete cure
♦ Can improve ram fertility if treated very early, before lesions palpable, with long-acting oxytetracycline every 4 days plus daily streptomycin, both for 24 days; impracticable except in valuable rams

Control

♦ Young rams isolated from adult rams, and ewes mated to adult rams
♦ Vaccination and/or test and slaughter of

positive reactors; vaccination best strategy for high incidence situations, test and slaughter for chronic, stable situation; usually both used, with vaccination first, followed by test and slaughter when rapid spread phase is over

♦ **Vaccination** of all yearling rams at least 3 months before joining with one of the following:
  • Single injection of killed *B. ovis, B. abortus* in adjuvant base: can cause systemic reaction, temporary infertility, some cases osteomyelitis
  • Two injections killed *B. ovis*
  • Live vaccines containing *B. melitensis* Rev 1, an avirulent *B. suis* also used

plus culling all rams with palpable testicle/epididymis lesions, replacement rams all young, maiden, vaccinated at 4–5 months old

♦ Ewe vaccination has no apparent effect on disease spread but may improve ratio of lambs

♦ **Test and slaughter** of all rams each year before mating using complement fixation test or ELISA; physical palpation is insufficiently accurate

BRUCELLOSIS CAUSED BY
BRUCELLA SUIS [VM8 p. 807]

Etiology

Brucella suis, 3 biovars infect pigs.

Epidemiology

Occurrence –
♦ Most continents but an uncommon disease in domestic and feral pigs; some biovars occur only in wildlife
♦ Pathogenic only in pigs and humans; recorded also in cattle and horses
♦ Occurs in all ages; prevalence higher in adults; most infection occurs after weaning
♦ Morbidity up to 66%; piglet mortality up to 80%

Source and transmission
♦ Introduced by infected pig, communal use of boar, use of infected semen, sharing range with feral pigs; has been spread from horses to pigs
♦ Within herd spread by –
  • Ingestion
  • Coitus
♦ Outbreak occurs when disease introduced; then health problems subside, affecting only introduced pigs

♦ No prolonged herd resistance, disease recurs

Importance
♦ Wastage due to
  • Reduced piglets reared per litter
  • Culling of infertile adults
  • Sporadic paralysed pigs
♦ Biovars 1 and 3 serious zoonoses in farm workers, veterinarians and consumers of infected meat and infected cow milk when pigs and cattle share common range

Clinical

♦ High incidence of clinically inapparent infections
♦ Common syndrome of temporary sow infertility with:
  • Abortions, mostly in third month; low incidence
  • Low piglet per litter numbers
  • Irregular estrus
  • Stillbirths, neonatal mortality during first day
♦ Boar – swelling, necrosis one or both testicles, sterility
♦ Lameness, incoordination, posterior paralysis common

Clinical pathology

♦ No really satisfactory serological test, so culture of organism, usually from dead piglets, the definitive test
♦ For herd diagnosis satisfactory agglutination, complement fixation, ELISA tests available

Necropsy findings

♦ Chronic arthritis
♦ Nodular thickening, abscessation in uterus wall
♦ Testicular necrosis, epididymitis, seminal vesiculitis
♦ Vertebral arthritis, osteomyelitis in paralysed, incoordinate pigs
♦ Lymphadenopathy, nodular splenic enlargement

Diagnosis

Abortion syndrome resembles:
♦ Leptospirosis
♦ SMEDI viruses
♦ Parvovirus
♦ Pseudorabies
♦ Swine fever

Piglet mortality syndrome resembles other causes perinatal piglet disease (p. 45).

Posterior paralysis syndrome resembles:
♦ Vertebral fracture due to osteodystrophy
♦ Hypovitaminosis A

Treatment

♦ No commercially practicable treatment available or anticipated.

Control

♦ No vaccine available
♦ High-incidence stud herds' and commercial herds' best procedure is depopulation with farm left 6 months before restocking; restocking only from certified free herds
♦ Stud herds with low incidence can attempt two-herd program where existing pigs considered infected, serologically negative piglets at weaning go into new quarters, retested before mating, gilts farrowed in isolation and her piglets used as foundation stock

BRUCELLOSIS CAUSED BY
BRUCELLA MELITENSIS
[VM8 p. 810]

Etiology

Brucella melitensis

Epidemiology

Occurrence
♦ Widespread but many countries free; commonest where goats prevail as domestic ruminants
♦ Significant cause of brucellosis in sheep and goats but can infect most species
♦ Can be high incidence in cattle where they share pasture with goats
♦ Occurs as abortion storms in naive flocks, subsequently abortion only in introduced animals
♦ Infected ewes excrete organism for only brief periods, disease can be self-limiting in self-contained sheep flocks

Source and transmission
♦ Infected ewes and does contaminate pasture with uterine discharges after abortion or normal parturition
♦ Infection probably by ingestion

♦ Transmission between flocks by introduced, infected females

Importance
♦ A serious zoonosis transmitted mostly by infected milk used for drinking

Clinical findings

♦ Abortion in late pregnancy, mostly in last two months
♦ Abortion storms in naive flocks
♦ No clinical mastitis
♦ Orchitis, often unilateral
♦ Uncommon systemic syndrome in goat includes:
  • Fever, depression
  • Weight loss
  • Diarrhea
  • Mastitis
  • Lameness, hygroma

Clinical pathology

♦ Agglutination and complement fixation tests available but satisfactory only as flock tests
♦ Definitive diagnosis in individuals is blood culture in early cases, isolation of organism from aborted fetus, vaginal discharge, milk

Necropsy findings

♦ No characteristic lesions
♦ Organisms most cultivable from spleen, lymph nodes and udder

Diagnosis

Other causes of abortion in does include:
♦ *Campylobacter fetus, C. jejuni*
♦ *Chlamydia psittaci*
♦ *Listeria monocytogenes*
♦ *Salmonella abortusovis*
♦ *Salmonella* spp., e.g. *S. dublin*
♦ *Toxoplasma gondii*
♦ Rift Valley fever
♦ *Coxiella burnetii*

Treatment

No practicable treatment available or anticipated.

Control

♦ Hygiene at kidding, lambing to include:
  • Individual, disinfected birthing stalls
  • Early weaning of kids and lambs, removal to clean environment
  • Disposal of fetuses and placenta discharged

♦ High-incidence flocks should be depopulated

♦ Disposal infected or reactor animals

♦ **Vaccination** – Elberg's Rev 1 universally recommended for goats and sheep; a living vaccine of attenuated bacteria not to be used in pregnant animals nor for one month before mating – interferes with test and slaughter program causing prolonged high brucella titers

♦ Other vaccines available, including one dispensed in drinking water, for difficult management situations

DISEASES CAUSED BY *HAEMOPHILUS* spp. AND *MORAXELLA* spp.

HISTOPHILUS OVIS INFECTION
[VM8 p. 813]

Etiology

Exact identity of *H. ovis* uncertain; probably related to *Hemophilus* spp.

Clinical findings

Recorded as a cause of:
♦ Ram epididymitis
♦ Lamb polyarthritis
♦ Ewe mastitis, abortion

SEPTICEMIA CAUSED BY *HAEMOPHILUS PARAINFLUENZAE* [VM8 p. 817]

Clinical

Fatal septicemia in 1–2 week old piglets.

Treatment

Responds well to streptomycin.

INFECTIOUS KERATITIS OF CATTLE (PINKEYE, BLIGHT)
[VM8 p. 813]

Etiology

♦ Hemolytic *Moraxella bovis* initiates lesions; other participants enhance severity, e.g.:
  • Rickettsia
  • Chlamydia
  • Mycoplasma, acholeplasma

  • Viruses, e.g. infectious bovine rhinotracheitis virus
  • Solar radiation
  • Flies
  • Dust
♦ *Moraxella ovis* (syn. *Neisseria ovis, Branhamella ovis*) also recorded as cause

Epidemiology

Occurrence
♦ Worldwide
♦ Common in summer and autumn
♦ Epizootics in feedlots, cattle at pasture some years
♦ Rarely in cattle closely confined in winter
♦ Young most susceptible
♦ Morbidity up to 80%; no deaths; some culled for blindness

Source and transmission
♦ Carried over from year to year on nasal mucosa carrier animals
♦ Source is ocular discharge affected animals carried by flies, dust, and grass
♦ Infection portal is conjunctiva

Risk factors
♦ Higher prevalence in *Bos taurus* compared with *Bos indicus*
♦ Less pigmented eyes more susceptible
♦ High prevalence summer and autumn when flies and dust are worst and grass longest
♦ Heavy face fly (*Musca autumnalis*) population enhances prevalence; infection survives in flies several days
♦ Previous infection confers immunity for the year; recurrent attacks clinically mild

Importance

♦ Some production loss, time, money in treatment
♦ Rarely culled for blindness
♦ Esthetically unattractive; a nuisance disease

Clinical findings

Initially:
♦ One or both eyes affected
♦ Incubation period 2–3 days
♦ Corneal vessel injection
♦ Conjunctival edema
♦ Copious, watery eye discharge
♦ Blepharospasm, photophobia
♦ Mild fever, anorexia, milk yield fall in some

Two days later:
♦ Small corneal opacity either recovers spontaneously, or
♦ Becomes elevated, ulcerates, spreads to cover as much as entire cornea
♦ Opacity white to deep yellow (when conjunctive underrun by pus)
♦ Eye discharge lessens, becomes purulent, opacity shrinks
♦ Complete recovery at 3–5 weeks

Sequels

♦ Small white, central scar in many
♦ Eye develops conical shape, due to accumulation yellow pus under conjunctiva, intense vascularization and erythematous zone around lesion
♦ Ulceration at center of lesion may lead to eye rupture
♦ Complete, permanent corneal opacity rarely

Clinical pathology

♦ M. bovis cultured from conjunctival swabs; identified by modified gel precipitin diffusion test or fluorescent antibody technique

Diagnosis

Resembles:
♦ Infectious bovine rhinotracheitis
♦ Photosensitive dermatitis
♦ Thelaziasis
♦ Pasteurella multocida rarely
♦ The keratitis of bovine malignant catarrh, rinderpest, bovine virus diarrhea

Treatment

♦ Early, acute cases respond quickly to ophthalmic ointments and solutions applied into upper and lower conjunctival sacs, a sprays, dusts containing:
  • Furazolidone
  • Oxytetracycline
  • Penicillin and streptomycin mixtures
  • Benzathene cloxacillin persists longest in sac
♦ Once daily application customary but times daily would be better
♦ Patient better off in dark; alternative i glued-on eye patch, lifted up for ointmen application
♦ Severe cases with extensive vascularisatio need subconjunctival (bulbar) injection of:
  • Dexamethazone 1 mg
  • Penicillin and streptomycin or similar Recovery may take 3–4 weeks; repea injections may be necessary
♦ Systemic treatment also used; maintain level equal to that in serum with:
  • Sulfadimidine 100 mg/kg body weigh daily for 3 days
  • Single injection long acting oxytetra cycline 20 mg/kg
♦ Surgical creation of temporary eye fla sutured across eye, e.g. third eyelid, for 7-10 days, aids healing in severe, slow healing eyes

Control

♦ Fly control, e.g. repellent impregnated ea tags, can reduce prevalence
♦ Vaccines are widely used but evidence fo their efficiency lacking
♦ Most herds rely on close surveillance, early treatment

SEPTICEMIA CAUSED BY
HAEMOPHILUS AGNI
(HISTOPHILUS OVIS) [VM8 p. 816]

Etiology

The closely related bacteria Haemophilus agni and Histophilus ovis.

Epidemiology

♦ Occurs in 4–7 month old lambs
♦ Sporadic cases
♦ Morbidity averages 10%; case fatality rate 100%

Clinical findings

High fever, depression, disinclination to move
Muscle stiffness
May die within 12 hours

Survivors for more than 24 hours develop
Severe arthritis
Muscle stiffness, pain on palpation

Clinical pathology

Complement fixation test available.

Necropsy findings

◆ Multiple hemorrhages through carcase
◆ Focal, hepatic necrosis surrounded by hemorrhage zone
◆ Basically a disseminated vascular thrombosis leading to severe focal vasculitis
◆ Patients surviving more than 24 hours have:
  • Fibrinopurulent arthritis
  • Basilar meningitis
  • Pulmonary congestion, edema causes fatal asphyxia
◆ Definitive diagnosis is culture of organism

Diagnosis

Resembles:
◆ *Escherichia coli*
◆ *Pasteurella hemolytica*
◆ Enterotoxemia due to *Clostridium perfringens* type D
◆ *Haemophilus parainfluenzae* septicemia in 1–4 week old lambs

Treatment

Streptomycin effective if given early.

Control

Vaccination should be effective; immunity after field attack solid

HAEMOPHILUS SEPTICEMIA OF CATTLE (*HAEMOPHILUS SOMNUS* DISEASE COMPLEX) [VM8 p. 817]

Etiology

Hemophilus somnus

Epidemiology

Occurrence
◆ Principally a disease of feedlot cattle in North America
◆ Many clinically inapparent infections
◆ Morbidity usually 2%, up to 10%; case fatality rate 90% unless treated early
◆ When disease first appeared most cases had meningoencephalitis; nowadays the majority have pleuritis, myocarditis, and pneumonia

Source and transmission
◆ Both unclear; the organism occurs widely on most mucosae and in most secretions in a high proportion of cows and bulls in herds with the infection
◆ Dam considered to be a major source for calf
◆ Transmission probably contact with infective respiratory, reproductive secretions by immediate or aerosol contact

Risk factors
◆ Climate – most cases in autumn and winter
◆ Age – 6–12 months, the age they go into the feedlots
◆ Most cases within a few weeks after entering feedlots
◆ Respiratory disease often precedes *H. somnus* septicemia
◆ Possible interspecies transmission with sheep

Clinical findings

Meningoencephalitis
◆ Commonly a number of cases at the same time
◆ Stumbling gait, fetlock knuckling, fall easily, difficulty rising
◆ Recumbent
◆ Fever in most
◆ Depression, eyelids drooped giving a sleeping impression
◆ May be blindness in one eye
◆ Recumbent cows have tremor, opisthotonus, nystagmus, occasionally convulsions
◆ Otitis media rarely
◆ Ocular lesions are focal retinal hemorrhages
◆ Conjunctivitis in some
◆ Ear droop in some
◆ Joint capsule distension with lameness only in a few
◆ Rapidly fatal in 6–12 hours unless treated

Respiratory disease

Syndrome not described, but standard syndrome of suppurative bronchopneumonia includes cough, loud, crackling respiratory sounds, dyspnea.

Clinical pathology

♦ Neutropenia, leukopenia in severe cases, neutrophilia with left shift in mild cases
♦ Neutrophilia, leukocytosis, positive Pandy globulin test on cerebrospinal fluid and synovial fluid
♦ *H. somnus* in body fluids and tissues, but transport and culture need special media
♦ Complement fixation test positive from 10–50 days after infection; an immunoblot procedure performs well experimentally

Necropsy findings

♦ Multiple necrotic infarcts in any part of brain or spinal cord
♦ Focal or diffuse cerebral meningitis
♦ Cerebrospinal fluid turbid, yellow
♦ Petechial hemorrhages in most tissues
♦ Edematous, petechiated synovial membranes
♦ Fibrinopurulent bronchopneumonia especially antero-ventral parts
♦ Fibrinous, serofibrinous peritonitis, pericarditis, pleuritis in more than 50% of cases; focal ulceration, pseudodiphtheritic membranes from pharynx into trachea
♦ Characteristic histopathological lesion is vasculitis, thrombosis

Diagnosis

Meningoencephalitis syndrome resembles:
♦ Polioencephalomalacia
♦ Listerial meningoencephalitis
♦ Bovine spongiform encephalopathy
♦ Hypovitaminosis A
♦ Lead poisoning
♦ Mercury poisoning
♦ Ammoniated hay poisoning
♦ Nervous acetonemia
♦ Hypomagnesemic tetany
♦ Hepatic encephalopathy
♦ Sporadic bovine encephalomyelitis
♦ *Clostridium perfringens* type D enterotoxemia
♦ Brain abscess, injury
♦ Rabies
♦ Pseudorabies
♦ Coccidiosis, nervous form

Pneumonic form resembles:
♦ Pneumonia
♦ Aspiration pneumonia
♦ Lung abscess
♦ Caudal vena caval thrombosis
♦ Pulmonary congestion, edema
♦ Ppulmonary hypertension
♦ Pulmonary emphysema

Treatment

♦ Good response if treatment (oxytetracycline 20 mg/kg body weight I/V daily for 3 days) provided while patient still standing
♦ Other antibiotics likely to be effective penicillin G, ampicillin, colistin, novobiocin
♦ Careful surveillance, early treatment of remainder, *or* mass medication in feed and water

Control

♦ Standard procedure is to maintain close surveillance and treat as the cases occur
♦ Vaccination with a bacterin practiced with good results but cost-efficiency not established

INFECTIOUS POLYARTHRITIS
(GLASSER'S DISEASE, PORCINE
POLYSEROSITIS) [VM8 p. 822]

Etiology

♦ *Hemophilus suis, H. parasuis* both cause the disease; at least 5 serovars of *H. parasuis*, some occur only in SPF herds, some only in conventional herds

Epidemiology

Occurrence

♦ A rare disease
♦ Sporadic outbreaks in weaning to 4 months old pigs
♦ SPF pigs very susceptible
♦ Morbidity low except in naive herds when disease introduced
♦ Case fatality rate high without treatment

Source and transmission

♦ probably respiratory carrier state with disease initiated by stress
♦ In piglets which have lost maternal immunity but not yet acquired active immunity

Risk factors
Outbreaks within 7 days after stress of chilling, transport, weaning, moving to another pen.

Clinical findings

- Sudden onset high fever, anorexia
- Rapid, shallow respiration with
- Anxious expression, head extended, mouth breathing
- Cough in some
- Severe lameness, shuffling gait
- All joints swollen and painful
- Tendon sheaths swollen
- Some cases develop meningitis with signs of:
  - Tremor
  - Paralysis
  - Convulsions
- Red–blue skin discoloration terminally
- Death in most after course of 2–5 days

Sequels
- Survivors develop arthritis
- Intestinal obstruction due to adhesions

Clinical pathology

- Organism cultivable from joint fluid and pleural exudate
- Serology includes complement fixation test

Necropsy findings

- Fibrinous pleurisy, pericarditis, peritonitis in all cases
- Pneumonia in some
- Arthritis, turbid joint fluid
- Fibrinopurulent meningitis in some
- SPF pigs may have minimal lesions; sudden deaths

Diagnosis

Resembles:
- Erysipelas
- Streptococcal arthritis
- Mycoplasma arthritis
- Streptococcal meningitis
- Porcine viral encephalomyelitis (Teschen disease)

Treatment

- Penicillin, trimethoprim–sulfadoxine, oxytetracycline effective if patients treated early

- Mass medication via drinking water for pigs at risk

Control

- In enzootic herds:
  - Avoid stress
  - Prophylactic dosing at shipping, usually via feed, drinking water on arrival
- Formalin-killed, whole culture bacterin effective

PLEUROPNEUMONIA OF PIGS
CAUSED BY *ACTINOBACILLUS
(HAEMOPHILUS)
PLEUROPNEUMONIAE*
[VM8 p. 824]

Etiology

Actinobacillus pleuropneumoniae, previously classified as *Haemophilus pleuropneumoniae*; up to 12 serovars.

Epidemiology

Occurrence
- Worldwide; increasing prevalence in intensive husbandry systems; majority of herds seropositive
- Many subclinical infections
- Morbidity 30–50%; case fatality rate up to 50%
- Affects predominantly 2–6 months old pigs
- Spreads rapidly through piggery, then subsides to sporadic cases as herd immunity develops

Source and transmission
- Source is infected pigs, clinical cases or inapparent respiratory carriers
- Transmission by inhalation

Risk factors
- Serovars vary in pathogenicity, sensitivity to antibiotics, have patchy spread
- Possible interaction between *A. pleuropneumoniae*, *Pasteurella multocida* to cause severe pneumonia
- Overcrowding
- Lack of previous exposure to the infection
- Ventilation system failure
- Dramatic ambient temperature change

Importance
♦ Wastage due to sudden deaths, variable delays in reaching market weight, costs of medication.

Clinical findings

♦ Sudden onset
♦ Some sudden deaths, some cases with acute dyspnea
♦ Anorexia, fever, disinclined to move,
♦ Dyspnea characterised by jerky abdominal component – **thumps**
♦ Cyanosis
♦ Blood stained froth from nose, mouth in many
♦ Death after course of a few hours, usually 1–2 days

Sequels
♦ Survivors likely to be subclinical carriers
♦ Some chronic cases persist with moderate dyspnea, cough
♦ Abortion

Clinical pathology

♦ When an outbreak develops diagnosis by necropsy preferred
♦ Diagnostic serological tests include complement fixation, a 2-mercaptoethanol tube agglutination test as an alternative, an ELISA
♦ Because of the importance of identifying the serotype involved in any infection, serological tests capable of determining the serotype are also widely used
♦ All of the tests are effective as agents for herd diagnosis but none is sufficiently accurate to guarantee protection against the introduction of the disease into a susceptible herd by an individual pig

Necropsy

♦ Pleuropneumonia with a tendency to sequestration in chronic cases
♦ Peracute cases have firm, swollen lungs with interlobular septal edema
♦ Less acute case have focal black or red, raised areas of pneumonia, later encapsulated in chronic cases, fibrinous pleurisy; fibrinous pericarditis in some cases

♦ Organism cultivable only from respiratory system
♦ Pleuritic adhesions, necrotic sequestra in chronic cases

Diagnosis

Resembles:
♦ Glasser's disease
♦ Enzootic pneumonia
♦ Pasteurellosis
♦ Swine influenza

Treatment

♦ Results disappointing because of disease's severity and persistence of chronic cases as sick animals and as carriers
♦ Clinical cases, in-contact pigs treated parenterally with lincomycin (10 mg/kg body weight I/M for 3 days), then oxytetracycline (500 g/tonne) in feed or sulfathiazole 28 g/gallon) or tiamulin (to deliver 23 mg/kg body weight) in drinking water for 12 days recommended
♦ In-contact pigs to be on the medicated feed or water
♦ Other effective antibiotics include oxytetracycline, penicillin, spectinomycin, trimethoprim-sulfonamide mixtures
♦ When disease confirmed in a herd, twice daily injection of approved antibiotic, based on sensitivity tests, recommended to avoid losses

Control

♦ Persistence of chronic carriers and rapid spread of disease make containment of this disease almost impossible in fattening units that buy in their pigs
♦ All-in, all-out management least wasteful of losses
♦ Aim for purchases from herds free of disease
♦ Availability of a simple accurate serological test would be a great advantage
♦ Imported breeding stock quarantined and tested twice before admission
♦ Young stock reared separately from adults
♦ No safe, effective vaccine available

19 DISEASES CAUSED BY BACTERIA – IV

DISEASES CAUSED BY *MYCOBACTERIUM* spp.

TUBERCULOSIS CAUSED BY *MYCOBACTERIUM BOVIS*
[VM8 p. 830]

Etiology

Mycobacterium bovis

Epidemiology

Occurrence
Worldwide, but virtual eradication in most developed countries.

Source
Infected animals with some persistence in fomites e.g. feces and contaminated pasture infective 6–8 weeks.

Transmission
+ Mostly inhalation in housed cattle
+ Ingestion in pastured cattle, goat, pig herds
+ Infected milk from tuberculous cow, especially fostered foals
+ Feces and contaminated water supply a risk

Host risk factors
+ All species but mostly cattle
+ Zebu breeds more resistant than European breeds
+ Common in pigs only if local cattle badly infected; tuberculosis due to *M. avium* common in pigs
+ Rare in sheep and horses due to natural resistance and lack of exposure
+ Problems in eradication in countries with tuberculosis in wild animals, e.g. possums in New Zealand, badger in UK

Pathogen risk factors
M. bovis moderately resistant to heat, dryness, disinfectants, may survive weeks in shaded, moist, warm locations

Importance
+ Transmissible to humans
+ Slaughter policy for eradication means heavy losses for individual farmer
+ Presence of disease in a country a barrier to international trade in animal products

Clinical findings

Cattle
Many badly affected cattle clinically normal.
+ **Generalized infection** syndrome – docility, weight loss, capricious appetite, intermittent fever, rough coat
+ **Pulmonary** syndrome – cough, abnormal breath sounds on auscultation, dyspnea terminally
+ **Alimentary tract** syndrome – dyspnea, respiratory stertor, dysphagia due to retropharyngeal lymph node enlargement, chronic bloat due to mediastinal lymphadenitis, rarely chronic diarrhea due to intestinal ulcer
+ **Bacteremia** syndrome – multifocal lymph node enlargement
+ **Tuberculous metritis** – failure to conceive, abortion, chronic, yellow, purulent discharge
+ **Tuberculous mastitis** – induration, hypertrophy in upper parts of glands. Fine floccules in amber fluid in last strippings

Pigs
+ Mostly subclinical
+ Rare generalised infections similar to cows

Horses
Cervical vertebral osteomyelitis commonest syndrome. Stiff, painful neck, unable eat off ground

Sheep and goats
+ **Pulmonary syndrome** as in cows
+ **Alimentary tract** syndrome in goats, similar to cows

Clinical pathology

Tuberculin tests in cattle

Injection of purified extracts of cultures of M. bovis or M. tuberculosis into infected animals produces a sensitivity response

Problems Include low sensitivity in pre- and immediate postparturient cows, early cases, and advanced cases with extensive lesions.

♦ For expected low-sensitivity cases use short thermal or Stormont tests
♦ For possible Johne's disease or avian tuberculosis use comparative test

Single intradermal test:

♦ Most widely used
♦ Injection intradermal in caudal tail fold or cervical skin fold
♦ Positive reaction is diffuse swelling at site 72–96 hours later
♦ In final stages of an eradication program, poor specificity of test results in excessive no-visible-lesion reactors.

Alternative tests in late stages Include:

♦ **Short thermal test** – subcutaneous injection of tuberculin causes fever peak 6–8 hours later
♦ **Stormont test** – single intradermal injection plus second injection same site 7 days later; read at 24 hours, positive reaction >5 mm thickening at site
♦ **Comparative test** – single intradermal tests using mammalian, avian tuberculin 25 cm apart on neck; greater reaction indicates type of infection

Tuberculin tests

Pigs Single intradermal test, base of ear, read at 24–48 hours.

Horse Anaphylactic reaction may occur, use only 0.1 ml tuberculin intradermal; many false positives

Sheep and goats As for cattle, into skin fold medial thigh.

Serological tests

Recommended for final stages of campaign to detect anergic non-reactor carriers to single intradermal. Best results with **interferon gamma assay (IFN-8) test**.

Necropsy findings

♦ Culture of organism from lesions
♦ Identification of *Mycobacterium bovis*

now possible by DNA and immunologic techniques

Cattle, sheep and goats

♦ Tuberculous granulomas in any lymp node, especially bronchial, mediastinal miliary abscesses any organ, especiall lungs
♦ Chronic lesions contain caseated pu sometimes calcified, surrounded by fibrou capsule, acute lesions contain semi-liqui pus; pus characteristically yellow–orange

Pig

♦ Rarely generalized, with miliary abscesses
♦ Mostly enlarged internal lymph node containing white caseous material i fibrous capsule

Horse

Firm lesions resembling neoplastic tissu in intestinal wall, mesenteric lymph nodes skeleton, especially cervical vertebrae.

Diagnosis

Resembles:

♦ Mycobacterioses due to M. *avium*, M. *afri canum*, M. *tuberculosis*
♦ Aspiration pneumonia
♦ Traumatic reticulitis
♦ Contagious bovine pleuropneumonia
♦ Actinobacillosis of pharyngeal lymph nodes
♦ Allergic rhinitis
♦ Enzootic nasal granuloma
♦ Bovine viral leucosis

Treatment and control

♦ Treatment not an option
♦ Eradication a universal goal

Test and slaughter

♦ The only acceptable herd control method
♦ Quarantine, single intradermal test al cattle over 3 months old
♦ Slaughter positive reactors
♦ Repeat suspicious tests with more sensitive test
♦ Retest whole herd every 3 months till clear
♦ Then tests at 6 months; if clear retest annually till area clear
♦ Then 3 year intervals till country clear

♦ If too many **no-lesion reactors** – use more specific or comparative test

Hygiene
♦ Disinfect or destroy feed troughs, water holes and troughs
♦ Only tuberculosis free milk to calves
♦ Introduced cattle to be from tested herds

Area control
♦ Education about plan first
♦ Test and slaughter commencing in low incidence areas
♦ Develop accredited herds, then areas
♦ Increase inter-test intervals
♦ Monitor prevalence at abattoirs with traceback procedure
♦ **BCG vaccination** used if slaughter losses not sustainable
♦ Vaccinates positive to tuberculin test

Problems in eradication program
♦ High **no-lesion-reactor** rate – use interferon gamma assay, or other more specific test
♦ Lack of **traceback** procedure at abattoirs
♦ Failure to ensure testing all herds, all cattle in each herd due to malpractice or extensive management procedures
♦ Tuberculosis in local wildlife

Control in pigs
♦ Eradicate disease in local cattle
♦ Check sources of feed and test animal sources
♦ Test and slaughter program used but inefficient

MYCOBACTERIOSIS CAUSED BY
M. AVIUM (AVIAN TUBERCULOSIS)
[VM8 p. 838]

Etiology

Mycobacterium avium

Epidemiology

♦ Not a fatal disease
♦ Importance is in false positive tuberculin tests and condemnations at abattoirs
♦ Infection from birds or bird-contaminated fomes, possibly inter-pig transmission

Clinical findings

Cattle Rarely generalized, lymph node induration, chronic metritis, abortion.

Sheep and goats Not recorded in sheep; occasional flock outbreaks in goats.

Pigs No clinical signs, only necropsy lesions

Horses Very rare generalized cases; rare cervical vertebral osteomyelitis.

Clinical pathology

♦ Sensitive to intradermal tuberculin test
♦ Comparative test identifies

Necropsy findings

♦ Enlarged lymph nodes, firm tissue resembling neoplastic tissue.

MYCOBACTERIOSIS CAUSED BY
ATYPICAL MYCOBACTERIUM
[VM8 p. 839]

Etiology

Mycobacterium intracellulare, M. kansasii, M. fortuitum, M. aquae, M. scrofulaceum, M. cookii, other unidentified species.

Epidemiology

♦ Commonest in pigs, rarely cattle
♦ Commonest in deep litter management systems

Clinical findings

Symptomless.

Clinical Pathology

Cause false positive tuberculin reactions.

Necropsy findings

Lymph node enlargement, induration, some calcified, rarely arthritis.

TUBERCULOSIS CAUSED BY
*MYCOBACTERIUM
TUBERCULOSIS* [VM8 p. 840]

♦ Rare, symptomless cases in pigs
♦ False positive tuberculin test reactors

♦ Reactions disappear when infected human removed
♦ May be minor lymph node lesions

'SKIN TUBERCULOSIS' [VM8 p. 840]

Etiology

♦ Unidentified acid-fast organisms in lesions.

Epidemiology

♦ Mostly housed cattle
♦ Prevalence on lower limbs and ventral abdomen suggests infection of cutaneous wounds or tick bites
♦ Rarely sequel to aluminium adsorbed vaccine
♦ Sensitize cattle to tuberculin tests

Clinical findings

♦ Small, long-term, cutaneous lumps, single or in chains connected by thin tissue cords
♦ Mostly on limbs but also ventral abdomen with spread up sides
♦ Some lumps discharge thick yellow pus

Clinical pathology

♦ React positively to tuberculin test
♦ Biopsy shows fibrous tissue surrounding caseated, sometimes calcified, pus

Diagnosis

Resembles:
♦ Bovine farcy
♦ Ulcerative lymphangitis

Treatment

♦ In rare cases surgical excision performed for aesthetic reasons.

PARATUBERCULOSIS (JOHNE'S DISEASE) [VM8 p. 841]

Etiology

Mycobacterium paratuberculosis (three strains and some variants); the organism is closely related to *M. avium*.

Epidemiology

Occurrence

♦ In most countries
♦ Primarily a cattle disease; increasingly important disease of sheep and goats; inevitably fatal in cattle, many sheep recover spontaneously
♦ A sheep strain causes serious disease in Iceland sheep
♦ Occurs in many wild ruminants
♦ Transmissible experimentally to pigs and horses
♦ Mostly in temperate climates; also some tropical areas
♦ Morbidity low, case fatality rate 100%, infection rate can be high, e.g. 50% with an annual population mortality rate of 5%

Source and transmission

♦ Feces of infected animal infect feed and water
♦ Transmission between countries and herds by importation of infected animal
♦ Long incubation period; infected animals commonly excrete organisms in feces for 15–18 months before signs appear
♦ Many animals living in a contaminated environment become clinically normal carriers
♦ Bacteria occur in semen, vaginal washings of infected animals but venereal transmission not recorded
♦ Transmission to fetuses in utero occurs commonly, usually in heavily infected dams
♦ Infected cows also excrete the organism in their milk

Risk factors

♦ *M. paratuberculosis* survives in pasture under the right conditions of moisture, shadow, acidity for over a year
♦ Infected, clinically normal cattle may develop clinical disease in the following circumstances:
  • Movement from pasture on an acid to an alkaline one
  • Parturition
♦ Transport
♦ Nutritional deficiencies or excesses

Importance

♦ Recurrent production loss over a long period in each cattle patient
♦ Negligible salvage value of carcase
♦ Costs of control, including loss of culled adult animals, can be very high in stud herds

Clinical findings

Cattle
- No signs before 2 years old; peak clinical cases 2–6 years old, sporadic cases only
- Emaciation
- Submandibular edema; fades as diarrhea develops
- Fall in milk yield; often before diarrhea appears
- No fever or toxemia, appetite good, thirst excessive
- Diarrhea commences; thin like thick pea soup, homogeneous, no odor; no blood, epithelial shreds, mucus
- Diarrhea continuous or intermittent, may improve in late pregnancy or on dry ration
- After course of weeks or months terminates in euthanasia because of emaciation and weakness

Sheep and goats
- Emaciation
- Weakness
- Fleece shedding in sheep
- Lose weight for up to 4 months
- Feces soft, lose pelleted form in late stages, often intermittent
- Depression and dyspnea may be evident in goats

Clinical pathology

- Control aimed at detecting the subclinical carriers (incubating and intermediate cases)
- Available tests include:

Tests in feces
- **Standard fecal culture**, the most reliable index of infection; can detect infected cattle up to 2 years before clinical illness; slow, cumbersome, requires minimum of 8 weeks
- **Microscopic examination** of fecal smear stained with Ziehl–Neelsen; smear or rectal pinch biopsy

Serological tests
- **Complement fixation test**; false positives due to infection with *Mycobacteria* spp., *Actinomyces* spp., *Dermatophilus* spp., *Nocardia* spp., *Streptomyces* spp., or *Corynebacterium* spp.
- False negatives due to anergy, usually in terminal stages of clinical disease
- **Agar gel immunodiffusion** (AGID) test most suitable test for clinical cases ; limited to use in tuberculosis-free herds
- **ELISA and LAM-ELISA**

Cell-mediated immunity tests
All suffer from lack of specificity and are useful only as herd tests:
- Single intradermal johnin test
- Double intradermal avian tuberculin test
- Intravenous avian tuberculin test

In vitro cell-mediated immunity tests
For example lymphocyte stimulation test, accurate and recommended.

Recommended test profiles
For all species surgical biopsy of terminal ileum or ileocecal lymph node the definitive diagnosis. Less traumatic, more commonly used tests include:

Cattle No single test sufficiently accurate. Combination of three tests used, e.g. fecal culture or stained smear (or pinch biopsy), plus complement fixation (or AGID or ELISA), plus single intradermal johnin (or avian tuberculin or intravenous avian tuberculin) test or lymphocyte stimulation test

Sheep D-AGID or LAM-ELISA test.

Goat ELISA.

Necropsy findings

Definitive diagnosis based on microscopic lesions *plus* culture of organism

Cattle and goats
- Intestinal wall thickened to 3–4 times normal thickness from terminal small intestine, through cecum to first part of colon
- In bad cases, lesion stretches from duodenum to rectum
- Mucosa corrugated
- Ileocecal valve red-lipped to edema, gross thickening, corrugated later
- No ulceration
- Mesenteric, ileocecal lymph nodes enlarged, edematous
- Gross lesions may be negligible in clinical cases; but have significant microscopic lesions in intestinal wall plus lymphangitis of intestinal vessels
- No lesions in placenta, fetus but organism isolatable
- Arteriosclerosis

Sheep
♦ Intestinal wall deep yellow pigmented
♦ Wall may be thickened, rarely corrugated
♦ Mesenteric, ileocecal lymph nodes enlarged, necrotic, caseated, calcified

Diagnosis

In cattle resembles:
♦ Salmonellosis
♦ Coccidiosis
♦ Helminthiasis
♦ Secondary copper deficiency (molybdenum poisoning)

In sheep and goats resembles:
♦ Caseous lymphadenitis
♦ Helminthiasis
♦ Caprine arthritis/encephalitis
♦ Ovine progressive pneumonia
♦ Nutritional deficiency cobalt
♦ Nutritional deficiency copper
♦ Dental disease

Treatment

No treatment of more than transitory value.

Control

Eradication impossible without total depopulation because of long incubation period and absence of accurate test to locate heavy shedding, clinically normal, carriers.

Herd eradication

Test and slaughter method:
♦ Quarantine herd
♦ Identification of carriers by clinical pathology tests (above) and sold for slaughter; best single test probably absorbed-ELISA
♦ Retest residual animals at 6 month intervals till 2 consecutive negative herd tests
♦ Success rate poor, but may keep losses of valuable stud animals low
♦ Non-infected cows lost because of false positive sensitivity tests

Culture and cull method:
♦ Feces of all cows cultured every 6 months
♦ Cows with positive cultures, and their offspring culled
♦ Reduces pasture contamination

♦ Intermittent shedders likely to go undetected

Three herd scheme:
♦ Non-infected herd
♦ Infected cows
♦ Progeny of infected cows

Total depopulation:
♦ All cattle, sheep, and goats sold off
♦ Farm left unstocked for 3 years

Hygiene:
♦ Avoid fecal contamination of water and feed troughs
♦ Fencing marshes and ponds
♦ Close up infected pastures for 3 years
♦ Avoid strip grazing
♦ Piped water instead of ditches
♦ Pasture harrowing to break up dung pats
♦ Manure applied only to crop fields
♦ Rear calves separately from each other and from dams
♦ Keep late pregnant cows separate from milking herd
♦ Calves fed colostrum for 1 day only
♦ No sucking on dams or nurse cows
♦ Rear on milk substitutes
♦ Calves from clinical cases not reared as herd replacements

Vaccination:
♦ With Vallee's vaccine – live M. *paratuberculosis* in paraffin oil and pumice stone adjuvant, *or*
♦ Sigurdsson's vaccine contains killed organisms
♦ In **cattle** herds may reduce number of clinical cases but vaccinants are temporarily sensitive to tuberculin, johnin
♦ Recommended in heavily infected, tuberculosis-free herds in areas where tuberculosis eradication completed or not contemplated
♦ Excellent results in **sheep** flocks

Area eradication
♦ Rarely contemplated because of high risk of reinfection from introduced cattle not able to be fully guaranteed to be free from infection, and
♦ Prevalence and losses rarely sufficiently great over significant areas to warrant expensive eradication program
♦ Most countries settle for a program to encourage, even subsidize, farmers to maintain a low level of clinical cases

DISEASES CAUSED BY *ACTINOMYCES* spp., *ACTINOBACILLUS* spp., *NOCARDIA* spp., AND *DERMATOPHILUS* spp. [VM8 p. 850]

Uncommon diseases caused by these infections include:

Painless, cutaneous granulomas (mycetoma) caused by *Nocardia brasiliensis*, *Actinomadura* spp. [VM8 p. 850]

Actinomyces actinoides as secondary invader in enzootic calf pneumonia, seminal vesiculitis [VM8 p. 850]

* *A. bovis* in equine fistulous withers, poll evil [VM8 p. 850]

* *Actinobacillus equuli* in equine peritonitis. Two syndromes: colic, pain, tenseness on palpating abdominal wall, fever, intestinal stasis; or chronic weight loss, ventral edema, pleurisy, mucosal pallor. Clear paracentesis fluid has high white cell count; excellent response to penicillin/streptomycin or ampicillin [VM8 p. 850]

* *A. equuli* in calf diarrhea [VM8 p. 850]

* *Actinobacillus suis* causing septicemia, arthritis in pigs [VM8 p. 850]

* *Actinobacillus seminis* and *A. actinomycetemcomitans* in ram epididymitis, orchitis; infection after in virgin rams; causes some fertility loss but major importance is interference with diagnosis of brucellosis [VM8 p. 850]

* *Histophilus ovis* causes septicemia, synovitis, multiple abscessation in lambs, *or* lamb neonatal mortality [VM8 p. 850]

* *A. seminis* in lamb polyarthritis [VM8 p. 850]

ACTINOMYCOSIS (LUMPY JAW)
[VM8 p. 851]

Etiology

Actinomyces bovis

Epidemiology

* Widespread; enzootic to particular herds but sporadic cases only
* Common only in cattle
* Rare cases pigs and horses

Source and transmission

* Infection from discharging sinuses on pasture, feed troughs
* Invasion via oral mucosal lesions, erupting teeth sockets, or laceration reticular, intestinal mucosa by sharp foreign body

Importance

* Affected animals usually euthanised
* Zoonosis

Clinical findings

Cattle – Head form
* Commences as painless, immovable, bony swelling on mandible, maxilla at central molar teeth
* Swelling diffuse or discrete
* May be mostly on medial aspect of mandible, in intermandibular space
* Enlarge over weeks or months
* Become painful, open, discharge sticky, honey-like fluid pus, containing minute, hard, yellow–white granules, onto skin
* Sinuses may heal, then break out in new site
* May spread to surrounding soft tissues
* Teeth in lesion malaligned, painful, cause difficult mastication
* Dyspnea when throat obstructed
* Weight loss
* Euthanasia after course of months to a year

Cattle – soft tissue lesions
* Impaired digestion, diarrhea, chronic bloat, pica when lesions involve esophagus, reticulum
* Orchitis
* Trachea causing dyspnea
* Brain abscess
* Lung abscess

Pigs
* Wasting due to visceral lesions
* Extensive cutaneous granuloma, especially over mammary glands

Clinical pathology

Gram-positive filaments in granules in pus.

Necropsy findings

* Bone rarefaction
* Loculi, sinuses, containing gritty granules in thin clear pus, in extensive fibrous tissue reaction, spreading to surrounding tissue, or
* Granulomatous lesions lower esophagus, esophageal groove, reticular wall, spreading to local peritonitis

♦ Characteristic **club colonies** containing bacteria in sections, pus
♦ No involvement of local lymph nodes

Diagnosis

Jaw lesions resemble:
♦ Grass seed abscess
♦ Foreign bodies or feed jammed between cheek and teeth

Visceral lesions resemble –
♦ Chronic peritonitis
♦ Peritoneal abscess

Cutaneous lesions in sows resemble *Borrelia suilla* in porcine ulcerative granuloma.

Treatment

♦ Sulfonamides, penicillin–streptomycin, tetracyclines all used
♦ Iodides parenterally (sodium iodide 1 g/12 kg body weight in 10% solution I/V, repeated twice at 2 week intervals) or potassium iodide orally (6–10 g daily for 7–10 days as a drench); transitory iodism (anorexia, dandruff, lacrimation, coughing) may develop with either treatment
♦ Lesion may stop growing, discharging but bony lesion remains
♦ Isoniazid 10–20 mg/kg body weight orally for 30 days prevents further growth

Control

♦ Isolate patients especially those with draining sinuses
♦ culling commercial cattle most cost-effective strategy

ACTINOBACILLOSIS (WOODEN TONGUE) [VM8 p. 852]

Etiology

Actinobacillus lignieresi ·

Epidemiology

Occurrence
♦ Cattle disease worldwide; sporadic occurrence on individual farms
♦ Some outbreaks when cattle graze pasture on sharp pumice gravel, or when spiky plants in feed, e.g. *Opuntia* spp. (prickly pear)

♦ Lesions at site of nose grip or venepuncture injury
♦ Sheep disease recorded most countries uncommon, sporadic, enzootic some farms
♦ One case recorded in a horse

Source and transmission
♦ *A. lignieresi* a normal inhabitant of ruminant oral cavity, rumen
♦ Tongue abscesses infecting saliva, pasture and other feed
♦ Organism survives up to 5 days on hay
♦ Invasion via mucosal, cutaneous injury
♦ Many subclinical lesions found in tongue at abattoirs

Clinical findings

Cattle
♦ Acute onset inability to eat for 48 hours
♦ Saliva drools
♦ Gentle chewing movements continuously
♦ Base of tongue swollen, hard, painful to touch; tip may be normal; nodules, ulcers on sides; often an ulcer at front of dorsum
♦ Weeks later shrunken, fibrous, unable to prehend
♦ Parotid, submandibular retropharyngeal lymphadenitis in some; may be no associated tongue lesion; may rupture, discharge pus
♦ Retropharyngeal lymph node enlargement causes loud, snoring respiration, difficulty swallowing, coughing up food; palpable per os in adults
♦ Granulomatous, easy bleeding skin lesions on eyelid, at nostril edge, rarely generally over body, may be up to several centimeters diameter; contain small, caseated foci (cutaneous actinobacillosis)

Sheep
♦ Granulomatous lesions, up to 8 cm dia., discharging thick, yellow–green pus containing small granules through small openings on lower jaw, face, nose, or skin folds down front of neck
♦ Lips thick, scabby in some
♦ Bilateral discharge with lesions in nasal cavities
♦ Cranial and cervical lesions abscessed
♦ Rarely tongue lesions; multiple hard nodules
♦ Difficult eating, cud-dropping in some, green staining around lips (**tobacco chewers**), weight loss, starve to death

Clinical pathology

Actinobacillus in pus, especially in club colony granules.

Necropsy findings

- Necropsy not a usual examination
- Sheep lesions granulomas containing abscesses filled with thick, tenacious, yellow–green pus
- Lymphangitis, abscesses in draining lymph nodes

Diagnosis

Resembles:
- Tuberculosis
- Bovine viral leucosis
- Grass seed abscess

Treatment

Dramatic improvement in acute cases with:
- Iodides parenterally (sodium iodide 1 g/12 kg body weight in 10% solution I/V, repeated twice at 2 week intervals) or potassium iodide orally (6–10 g daily for 7–10 days as a drench); transitory iodism (anorexia, dandruff, lacrimation, coughing) may develop with either treatment
- Isoniazid 10–20 mg/kg body weight orally for 30 days
- Sulfonamides
- Penicillin
- Streptomycin
- Broad-spectrum antibiotics

Control

- Isolation, intensive, early treatment clinical cases, especially those with discharging lesion
- Disinfect contaminated troughs
- Keep livestock away from mucosal lacerating pasture

GLANDERS [VM8 p. 854]

Etiology

Pseudomonas (Actinobacillus) mallei.

Epidemiology

Occurrence
- Eradicated from most developed countries; persists elsewhere
- Solipeds, especially horses, mules, and donkeys; rarely in sheep, goats; carnivores eating infected meat
- Obligate parasite; organism survives only few weeks in environment

Source and transmission
- Clinical cases discharging pus, recovered carriers
- Ingestion contaminated feed mostly; rarely inhalation, skin contact

Importance
- Fatal zoonosis
- Mostly fatal in animals, long convalescence in survivors

Clinical findings

Acute
- High fever
- Cough
- Nasal discharge
- Dyspnea
- Nasa mucosal ulcers
- Skin nodules lower limbs, ventral abdomen
- Death due to septicemia after course of few days

Chronic
- **Lung lesions** cause chronic cough, dyspnea, epistaxis
- **Nasal mucosal lesions** commence as 1 cm dia. nodules, then ulcerate, coalesce, discharge serous, later bloody, purulent, submandibular lymph nodes enlarged;
- Healed ulcers replaced by characteristic stellate scars
- **Skin lesion** are subcutaneous nodules 1–2 cm dia.
- Ulcerate, discharge pus like dark honey, or deeper lesions that discharge through fistulous tracts
- Thickened, fibrous lymph vessels connect nodules
- Draining lymph nodes abscess, drain externally
- Lesions anywhere on body; most common on medial aspect hock
- Most die after course of several months; some survive, act as carriers

Clinical pathology

- Intradermopalpebral mallein test positive reaction 48 hours after mallein injection in lower eyelid is edematous swelling, blepharospasm, severe conjunctivitis

♦ Complement fixation test; may be cross reaction with *P. pseudomallei*
♦ Other tests include indirect haemagglutination, dot ELISA
♦ Identification of organism in pus by culture or intraperitoneal injection into guinea-pigs

Necropsy findings

Acute glanders
♦ Generalized petechiation
♦ Severe catarrhal bronchopneumonia
♦ Bronchial lymph node enlargement

Chronic glanders
♦ Miliary nodules in lung
♦ Nasal, laryngeal, tracheal, bronchial mucosal ulcers
♦ Limb skin, subcutis nodules, ulcers; limbs enlarged
♦ Draining lymphatics, lymph nodes contain purulent foci
♦ *P. mallei* in tissues

Diagnosis

Acute glanders resembles:
♦ Strangles
♦ Equine pleuropneumonia

Chronic glanders resembles:
♦ Epizootic lymphangitis
♦ Sporotrichosis
♦ Ulcerative lymphangitis
♦ Swamp cancer
♦ Greasy heel
♦ Chorioptic mange

Treatment

♦ Sulfonamides, with or without mallein or formolized *P. mallei*, reported to be effective.

Control

♦ Complete quarantine of affected farm
♦ Euthanasia all clinical cases
♦ Euthanasia of positive reactors to mallein test
♦ Repeat mallein test at 3 week intervals until negative test
♦ Vigorous disinfection of premises and troughs

BOVINE FARCY [MYCOTIC LYMPHANGITIS, BOVINE NOCARDIOSIS) [VM8 p. 856]

Etiology

Mycobacterium farcinogenes or *M. senegalese*, possibly also *Nocardia farcinicus*

Epidemiology

Occurrence
♦ Tropical countries
♦ Adult cattle
♦ Probably soil-borne infection of lower limb wounds
♦ Soil infected by wound discharges

Clinical findings

♦ Slowly progressive, small, round, hard subcutaneous swellings
♦ Enlarge and coalesce to form indurated subcutaneous swellings, lesions along thickened lymphatics, in lymph nodes
♦ Lesions rupture discharge thick gray or yellow granular or cheesy pus through sinus, from indolent ulcer
♦ Lesions principally at prescapular, precrural, or cranial nodes, at shoulder joint, all limbs, axilla, crutch, base of ear, and at site of any tick bite

Clinical pathology

Organisms in pus.

Necropsy

Small lung or mammary gland nodules in rare fatal cases.

Diagnosis

Resembles:
♦ Skin tuberculosis
♦ Ulcerative lymphangitis
♦ Lumpy skin disease
♦ Tuberculosis

Treatment

♦ Sodium iodide solution parenterally 1 g/12 kg body weight in 10% solution I/V, repeated twice at 2 week intervals) or
♦ Potassium iodide orally (6–10 g daily for 7–10 days as a drench)

Control

Isolation, early treatment of clinical cases.

MYCOTIC DERMATITIS (CUTANEOUS STREPTOTHRICOSIS, SENKOBO, KIRCHI, SARIA DISEASE, LUMPY WOOL OF SHEEP) [VM8 p. 857]

Etiology

♦ *Dermatophilus congolensis* plus either skin penetration or maceration caused by continuous skin-wetting
♦ Organism is dimorphic, growing as branched filamentous mycelia containing dormant zoospores
♦ Zoospores transformed by moisture to infective coccal stage
♦ May be combined with **demodicosis** to form Senkobo disease

Epidemiology

Occurrence –

♦ Epizootics in tropical, subtropical countries; morbidity 15% in enzootic herds, 100% in epizootics
♦ Sporadic in temperate climate countries; significant prevalence in sheep in special circumstances
♦ All species, especially sheep (lumpy wool), goats, and cattle, uncommon in horses
♦ All ages

Source and transmission

♦ Organism can survive in dry, detached scabs for several months
♦ Most transmissions occur by direct contact with infected sheep, often non-clinical carriers, carrying infective, motile zoospores
♦ Organism not very invasive; requires prior skin damage
♦ Primary lesion in sheep commonly on face, lower limbs; spread from there by nuzzling each other and scratching
♦ Primary lesion in cattle often backs and sides due to injuries during mounting while on heat

Risk factors

♦ Hot, humid weather
♦ Long rain spell sufficient to wet though fleece to skin; macerates skin, activates motile zoospores
♦ Frequent, protracted jetting, spraying, dipping for external parasite control

♦ Sheep with open fleece, low wax, high suint content most susceptible
♦ Amongst Merinos, strong, medium-woolled strains most susceptible
♦ Dipping in infected dips
♦ Frequent, tight yarding
♦ Heavy fly tick populations may assist transmission by mechanical transport, in ticks by skin bite wounds

Importance

♦ Deaths of cattle in epizootics; mostly an inconvenience, some hide damage
♦ Significant loss of fleece and skin value in sheep
♦ Interference with shearing causes major inconvenience
♦ Deaths in lambs during spring lambing; may force lambing to less profitable autumn timing
♦ Significant risk of infection to humans handling infected animals

Clinical findings

Cattle

♦ Lesions on neck and body, especially along back, back of udder; may extend down sides, limbs, and ventral abdomen
♦ Thick, horny, cream to brown, 2–5 cm dia. crusts; may be confluent, forming mosaic
♦ Crusts difficult to remove initially; shed later but held in place by fibers
♦ Granulation, some pus under scabs initially

Calves

♦ Hair loss
♦ Dandruff without crust formation
♦ Skin thickened
♦ Lesions around muzzle; may extend to neck, rarely to lungs

Sheep

♦ Primary lesions on face, wool-less limbs, scrotum
♦ Secondary principal lesions are in sheep fleece; pyramid shaped, thick, up to 3 cm, circular, often pigmented crusts; wool often discolored also
♦ Spontaneous recovery in 3 weeks in most sheep
♦ Heavy losses in very young lambs covered all over with scabs
♦ Blowfly maggot infestation often secondary
♦ Fatal secondary pneumonia in some

Goats

♦ Lesions commence on external ear; heavy crusts may block ear canal
♦ Also at external nares
♦ Extend along dorsal midline
♦ Inside thighs

Horses

♦ Usually begin at muzzle, up face to around eyes; may be lacrimation, profuse mucopurulent nasal discharge, *or*
♦ Commence on lower limbs, behind pastern, around coronet, anterior aspect hind cannon bones, may extend to belly
♦ Lesions are exudative dermatitis with matted hair, leaving raw ovoid lesion if removed
♦ No itching but lesions sore, horse may be lame

Clinical pathology

♦ Typical, branching organisms in scrapings, biopsy, impression smear of acute lesion
♦ Satisfactory identification of infection by serological tests including:
  • Fluorescent antibody
  • ELISA
  • Counterimmunoelectrophoresis

Necropsy findings

♦ Only occasional deaths in most circumstances
♦ Extensive dermatitis
♦ Secondary pneumonia in a few
♦ Frequently fatal intercurrent disease

Diagnosis

Resembles:
♦ Photosensitive dermatitis
♦ Fleece rot
♦ Cockle in sheep
♦ Congenital ichthyosis in calves
♦ unspecified dermatitis

Treatment

♦ Individual treatment with broad spectrum antibacterial, e.g.
  • Long-acting tetracycline, one injection
  • Heavy doses penicillin–streptomycin mixture (70 mg streptomycin, 70 000 units penicillin G/kg body weight)
  • Large doses of antibiotics are not favored for horses in training, topical applications of suitable antibacterials are required

Alternative treatment for sheep is:
♦ Shear when scabs lifted
♦ Dip or spray in zinc sulfate (0.2–0.5%) solution
♦ Dip in 1% potassium–aluminium sulfate (alum) solution or 57% dust in inert carrier
♦ For manual application to individual lesions use 0.2% cooper sulfate or 1:200 solution quaternary ammonium compound after prior removal of scabs, if practicable
♦ Response may be poor in wet weather

Control

♦ Disease disappears spontaneously in many cases in dry weather
♦ Common practice is to cull sheep which do not respond to treatment
♦ Tick control
♦ Prophylactic dipping, spraying in zinc sulfate or alum solution (as above) or magnesium fluosilicate after shearing
♦ No vaccine available

STRAWBERRY FOOTROT
(PROLIFERATIVE DERMATITIS)
[VM8 p. 861]

Etiology

Dermatophilus congolensis.

Epidemiology

♦ Commonest in lambs
♦ Summer disease, disappears in winter
♦ Thought to be transmitted by soil infection of injuries to lower limbs
♦ Organisms in dried crusts infectious for long periods
♦ Morbidity may be 100%
♦ Losses due to failure to make good weight gain

Clinical findings

♦ Cases appear usually 2–4 weeks after sheep moved onto pasture
♦ Small, heaped scabs on limbs from coronet to knee or hock
♦ Enlarge to 3–5 cm dia. wart-like lesions
♦ Hair lost from lesion
♦ Scabs coalesce
♦ Under scabs is bleeding, fleshy mass (like a fresh strawberry) in a shallow ulcer
♦ No itching, lameness unless lesions in interdigital space

⇒ Lesions heal in 5–6 weeks
⇒ Occasional cases persist for 6 months

Clinical pathology

Causative bacteria under scabs.

Diagnosis

Resembles:
♦ Contagious ecthyma lesions
♦ Sheep pox

Treatment

♦ None listed; treatments recommended for
  mycotic dermatitis should be effective.

Control

♦ Quarantine infected bands of sheep
♦ Rest paddocks where infected sheep have
  been

ACTINOBACILLOSIS IN PIGS [VM8
p. 862]

Actinobacillus spp., other than *A. pleuropneumoniae* cause several diseases in pigs.

Sporadic, late term abortions
Septicemic sudden death in piglets up to 3
months old:
♦ Piglets surviving 24 hours show signs of:
  • Lethargy
  • Fever
  • Petechiae or cyanosis in skin of belly, ears
  • Lameness, recumbency, swollen joints
    due to polyarthritis
♦ Necropsy lesions include:
  • Widespread petechiation
  • Focal necrosis in liver
  • Polyarthritis
  • Endocarditis
  • Focal pneumonia
♦ Organism susceptible to most antibiotics
♦ Treatment may be largely prophylactic to
  in-contacts because of acute nature of dis-
  ease

Erysipelas-like disease in minimal disease
herds:
♦ All ages
♦ Raised, round, oval or rhomboid, ery-
  thematous skin lesions
♦ Fever
♦ Treatment with benzathine penicillin
  halted the clinical disease

SHIGELLOSIS OF FOALS (SLEEPY
FOOD DISEASE) [VM8 p. 862]

Etiology

Actinobacillus equuli.

Epidemiology

Occurrence
♦ Only in horses
♦ Foals mostly; rare in older horses
♦ Intra-uterine infection possible but infec-
  tion via navel the common route of
  infection
♦ Mare clinically normal; infection in uterus
  short-lived
♦ Infection route to mare unknown
♦ Sporadic cases only; case fatality rate
  100%
♦ Important cause of foal deaths in most
  countries
♦ Infection in same mare in successive years
  so disease recurs on same farm in successive
  years

Clinical findings

♦ Sick at birth or within a few hours, few up
  to 3 days old
♦ Fever
♦ Few show acute abdominal pain early
♦ Prostration, lethargy (sleepy foals)
♦ Diarrhea, dysentery in a few
♦ Dyspnea
♦ Ceases to suck
♦ Death after 24 hour course
♦ Survivors develop swollen joints, lameness,
  recumbency within 1–2 days
♦ Death after 2–7 day course

Clinical pathology

♦ Blood cultures
♦ Serum antibody levels checked to test col-
  ostral transfer efficiency
♦ Culture from cervical swabs of mares

Necropsy findings

Acute deaths
♦ Septicemic petechiae
♦ Severe enteritis

Subacute deaths
♦ Arthritis, synovitis; fluid sanguineous to
  purulent

♦ Diagnostic pinpoint abscesses in renal cortices
♦ *A. equuli* in tissues

Diagnosis

Resembles septicemia caused by:
♦ *Escherichia coli*
♦ *Salmonella typhimurium*
♦ *S. abortivoequina*
♦ Neonatal maladjustment syndrome
♦ Idiopathic myopathy

Treatment

♦ Ampicillin parenterally is effective
♦ Streptomycin and tetracyclines also reported to give good result

Control

♦ Cull or treat and clear of infection infected mares
♦ Hygiene at foaling
♦ Treat foals of carrier mares prophylactically from birth

20 DISEASES CAUSED BY BACTERIA – V

DISEASES CAUSED BY *FUSOBACTERIUM* AND *BACTEROIDES* spp.

Common *Fusobacterium necrophorum* secondary infections:
- Navel-ill
- Hepatic necrobacillosis
- Calf pneumonia
- Necrotic enteritis of pigs
- Rhinitis of pigs
- Vulvitis, vaginitis, and metritis
- Granulocytopenic disease of calves
- Endocarditis
- Osteomyelitis

NECROBACILLOSIS OF THE LIVER
[VM8 p. 865]

Etiology

Hepatic localization of *F. necrophorum*, *Actinomyces pyogenes*, unspecified streptococci from infection in rumen wall or navel.

Epidemiology

- Mostly secondary to rumenitis in feeder cattle or lambs on heavy grain ration
- Dirty surroundings contaminated by infection from a clinical case is main source of infection
- Rejection of livers at abattoirs is main cause of loss

Clinical findings

Most cases subclinical

Acute
- Fever
- Anorexia
- Hyposensitivity
- Milk yield depression
- Pain on palpation over right costal arch
- Arched back
- Reluctant to lie down
- Grunting with each breath in some

Chronic
- Anorexia
- Weight loss
- Low milk yield

Newborn
- Ill at about 7 days
- Omphalophlebitis accompanies

Clinical pathology

- Severe leukocytosis and neutrophilia
- Blood sialic acid levels elevated

Necropsy findings

- May be primary rumenitis, omphalophlebitis
- Multiple hepatic abscesses, mostly on diaphragmatic surface with extensions to diaphragm or renal tissue in some
- Suppurative peritonitis a sequel
- Caudal esophageal lesion in some lambs

Diagnosis

Resembles:
- Bacillary hemoglobinuria
- Traumatic reticuloperitonitis

Treatment

- Course of potentiated sulfonamide or broad-spectrum antibiotic gives good response in acute cases
- Relapse common

Control

- Avoid rumenitis in feedlot cattle
- Low-level antibiotic feeding widely used but effectiveness varies

BOVINE INTERDIGITAL
NECROBACILLOSIS (FOUL IN THE
FOOT, FOOTROT) [VM8 p. 867]

Etiology

♦ *Fusobacterium necrophorum* (A biotype)
♦ Possibly in association with *Bacteroides melanogenicus* or *B. nodosus* as initiators by setting up a preliminary inflammation

Epidemiology

Occurrence

♦ Commonest in adults, also young calves, rarely bulls
♦ Zebu type breeds more resistant
♦ Worst in high rainfall seasons, small fields, high soil pH

Source and transmission

♦ Soil contaminated by infected feet
♦ Entry through abrasions on continually wet skin
♦ Introduction of infected cattle onto farm

Clinical findings

Acute

♦ Sudden onset severe lameness
♦ Mild fever in some
♦ Milk yield drops temporarily
♦ Coronet swollen
♦ Claws spread
♦ Pain on local palpation
♦ Swollen-edged, necrotic fissure at top of interdigital cleft has characteristic rancid smell
♦ Rapid response to treatment in most

Chronic

♦ Few, especially untreated, very lame, swollen claws at coronet, due to infection spread to joints, tendons, or
♦ Wart-like mass, **interdigital fibroma**, at anterior end of cleft, causes chronic mild lameness

Clinical pathology

♦ Culture of pus from cleft yields *Fusobacterium necrophorum* with or without *Bacteroides* spp.

Necropsy findings

Suppuration in flexor ligaments and interphalangeal joints in worst cases.

Diagnosis

Resembles:
♦ Traumatic injury
♦ Sole puncture
♦ Laminitis
♦ Sole wear by rough concrete in yarded cattle or slats in housing
♦ Flexor tendon contracture in housed cattle due to collateral ligament strain as hoof rolls into slots in grating
♦ Double sole due to hoof wall overgrowth and curling over sole trapping debris
♦ **Stable footrot** at heels with under-running and necrosis of sole, penetrating odor due possibly to *B. nodosus* infection
♦ **Verrucose dermatitis**, proliferative inflammatory lesion at back of pastern down onto heels due to constant wetting; often all four feet painful and lame; *F. necrophorum* in large numbers; rapid response to drying and parenteral broad-spectrum antibiotic
♦ **Interdigital papillomatosis** (digital dermatitis) due to invasive spirochete; usually on one hind limb just above horn-skin junction; superficial erythematous, then hyperkeratinized round, painful lesion; patient lame, restless, stands on toe and wears it down

Treatment

♦ Parenteral potentiated sulfonamide or broad-spectrum antibiotic early after lameness commences
♦ Excellent recovery in 2–4 days
♦ Treatment may need to be repeated several times in bad cases
♦ Local treatment for chronic lesions requires heavy sedation, paring, debriding necrotic material, application of 5% copper sulfate lotion or antibiotic ointment, bandage and keeping foot dry
♦ Joint, tendon sheath lesions respond moderately to claw amputation
♦ Daily walk through footbath of 10% copper sulphate in slaked lime or 5% copper sulfate solution prevents reinfection

Control

♦ Daily foot-bathing, as above, recommended
♦ Feeding low-level antibiotics or organic

iodides, and vaccination with *Fusobacterium necrophorum* or *B. nodosus* widely used but value moderate only
♦ Daily dosing with zinc sulfate no value

INFECTIOUS FOOTROT OF SHEEP
[VM8 p. 870]

Etiology

♦ *Dichelobacter (Bacteroides) nodosus*; benign, intermediate, virulent strains depending on keratolytic capacity
♦ *Spirochaeta penortha* and a motile fusiform bacillus commonly present also but disease can occur in their absence

Epidemiology

Occurrence
♦ Worldwide in warm, wet climates; not in arid or semi-arid areas
♦ In sheep, goats, and wild ruminants
♦ Morbidity up to 75%; case fatality rate nil but many are culled for slaughter

Source and transmission
♦ Discharges from infected feet of chronic, acute cases of footrot in sheep; rarely infection from cattle
♦ Bacteria survives up to 2 weeks separate from host
♦ Infection persists indefinitely in chronic lesions in about 10% of infected feet
♦ Disease introduced to farm in sheep with infected feet, *or*
♦ On healthy feet of sheep passing through transports or yards used by infected sheep in immediate past
♦ Spread within flock facilitated by flocking habits of sheep, concentration of animals around water and feeding points

Risk factors
♦ Wet, warm weather encourages survival of bacteria on pasture, transmission between sheep, susceptibility of feet to infection; duration of wetness has to be of the order of several months of persistent rain in summer or fall, with daily mean temperature greater than 10°C (50°F), and provide free surface water
♦ Irrigated improved pasture
♦ Housed sheep affected when standing in wet straw or feces
♦ Packing sheep together
♦ Merino sheep most susceptible; British breeds, especially Romney, more resistant; susceptibility probably genetically determined
♦ Skin penetration favored by injury, infestation with *Strongyloides* spp. larvae
♦ Virulence of infecting strain

Importance
♦ Serious loss of weight, wool production, disruption of farm routine, costs of labor, treatment, costs of eradication programs.

Clinical findings

Virulent footrot
♦ Swelling, moistness of interdigital cleft skin, parboiled, pitted appearance of thin horn at skin/horn junction
♦ Lameness, increasing as horn under-run, commencing at axial site spreading to abaxial, sole locations; may be detectable only with a knife blade
♦ Both claws affected; often more than one hoof affected
♦ Severe lameness in multiple feet may lead to the patient walking on its knees or being recumbent
♦ Small volume evil-smelling exudate at lesion; no abscess formation
♦ Extensive under-run can be pared off in sheets
♦ Fever, anorexia in a few patients
♦ Complications include secondary bacterial invasion, fly strike, hoof sloughing
♦ Recumbent patients become emaciated, may need to be euthanized

Intermediate footrot
♦ Poorly defined milder disease with less severe under-running, less tendency to persist as carriers
♦ Occur in same flocks as virulent footrot

Chronic footrot
♦ Symptomless carriers persisting for periods up to 3 years
♦ Hoof misshaped, horn under-run with pockets of infection, *or*
♦ Less commonly moist skin between claws without horn involvement
♦ Acute footrot may develop when patient exposed to wet, warm weather

Goats
Severe interdigital dermatitis, some horn under-running at axial surface but not extending to sole, abaxial surface.

Cattle
- Severe interdigital dermatitis
- Severe lameness
- Fissuring, hyperkeratosis of interdigital skin, pitting, erosion of thin horn at skin/horn junction in cleft
- Minimal horn underrunning at heel

Clinical pathology

- Culture of swabs of pus necessary for complete identification of footrot; quicker, less accurate decision often based on examination of gram-stained smear, or one stained with fluorescein-stained antibody
- Serological evidence of infection detectable 2 weeks after disease commences, persists for several months
- *Fusobacterium necrophorum* a common finding in the pus of virulent footrot

Necropsy findings

Examination not usually performed.

Diagnosis

Resembles:
- **Ovine interdigital dermatitis** (footscald); clinically silent, spontaneously resolving
- **Benign footrot**, with no horn underrunning, caused by invasion by an avirulent strain of *D. nodosus*
- Foot abscess
- Strawberry footrot
- Contagious ecthyma
- *Strongyloides papillosus* infestation
- Trombiculid mite infestation
- Metabolic laminitis
- Laminitis caused by *Erysipelothrix insidiosa*
- Ulcerative dermatitis
- Bluetongue
- **Shelly hoof,** a common problem in Merinos; abaxial hoof wall separates from sole, space impacted with dirt under crumbly dry horn

Treatment

Topical
- Labor intensive
- Difficult to apply, less effective during wet weather
- The only effective program includes:
  - Complete paring of all under-run horn
  - Parings burned
  - Application of antibacterial to lesions by paint brush, spray, ointment of:

- 10% chloramphenicol in methylated spirits, propylene glycol
- 5% oxytetracycline in methylated spirits
- 20% cetrimide in alcohol
- 10% solution zinc or copper sulfate
- 10% dichlorophen in alcohol
- Footbathing in solutions containing a surfactant and:
  - 5% copper sulfate
  - 5% formalin
  - 10% zinc sulfate

Treated sheep must be kept on dry ground for a few hours after treatment.

With all treatments, feet to be examined 21 days later and persistent cases retreated or culled.

Preferred retreatment procedure is to stand patients in footbath containing 20% zinc sulfate, 2% sodium lauryl sulfate for 1 hour; repeat in 5 days, check 21 days later.

Parenteral antibiotic treatment
- No need to pare feet
- Not thwarted by wet conditions underfoot but response best if kept on dry surface for 24 hours after treatment
- Single I/M injection of 70 000 units procaine penicillin G plus 70 mg streptomycin/kg body weight effective, *or*
- Single injection 5 mg/kg lincomycin plus 10 mg/kg body weight spectinomycin I/M also effective
- Check treated sheep at 21 days, cull or retreat those not recovered

Vaccination
- Therapeutic effect varies widely
- Best results when associated with hoof-paring and foot-bathing
- Hastens healing, prevents relapses and reinfection

Control

Eradication principles based on:
- Removal of infection source by treatment, culling infected sheep
- Leaving pasture unstocked for at least 14 days
- Eradication in a flock best undertaken in dry times
- Area eradication requires quarantine, inspection powers to ensure all farms in area comply with eradication program
- Carriage of infection by cattle, goats may breach quarantine barrier

On farm, eradication routine includes:
- Inspection all feet of all sheep

Foot-bathing of all clean sheep, pass to rested clean pasture

Treating all affected feet by individual antibiotic, or footbathing (repeated at 1 week), or vaccination

Inspect at 3 weeks; clean sheep to clean pasture; resistant sheep culled or retreated with 20% zinc sulfate foot bath (see above)

Prevention of introduction onto farm

Introduce sheep from only footrot-free premises

Vaccination as prophylaxis too variable for blanket recommendation; major problem is protection provided only against strains included in the vaccine; also high level of antibodies required necessitates use of adjuvants in vaccine causing serious local reactions, especially in British breeds; duration of protection limited to 4–12 weeks

Outbreak control

♦ During wet season eradication impossible because reinfection occurs too quickly
♦ Isolate infected flocks
♦ Prophylactic footbaths
♦ Isolate, treat clinical cases with parenteral antibiotics

FOOT ABSCESS OF SHEEP
[VM8 p. 877]

Etiology

Fusobacterium necrophorum; other bacteria commonly found in chronic lesions include *Escherichia coli* and *Actinomyces pyogenes*.

Epidemiology

♦ Commonest in wet seasons
♦ On stony ground and abrasive stubble
♦ Only adult sheep, especially rams, late pregnant ewes
♦ Morbidity low
♦ Worst when sheep crowded together because of limited housing or tight flocking habit, e.g. young rams in muddy yards

Clinical findings

♦ Usually one foot, one claw; rarely severe outbreaks with all four feet
♦ Affected digit hot, painful on pressure
♦ Severe lameness

Toe abscess
♦ Pus under-runs horn at toe
♦ Front hoof usually

♦ Swollen coronet ruptures, discharging pus between claws
♦ Rarely penetration to deeper structures

Heel abscess (infectious bulbar necrosis)
♦ Pus under-runs horn at heel
♦ Usually medial claw of hind hoof
♦ Swelling of interdigital skin
♦ Pain on compression of heel, pus may be squeezed out of sinuses into interdigital space
♦ Whole back of foot swollen if interphalangeal joint involved

Diagnosis

Resembles:
♦ Infectious footrot
♦ Polyarthritis
♦ Shelly hoof

Treatment

♦ Surgical drainage imperative; may need only trimming of underrun horn; or amputation of claw
♦ Plus parenteral treatment with antibacterial, e.g. potentiated sulfonamide or broad spectrum antibiotic for 3 days, local dressing

FOOTROT OF PIGS [VM8 p. 877]

Etiology

Secondary infection of traumatic lesion; mixed bacterial population includes *Fusobacterium necrophorum*, *Actinomyces pyogenes*, staphylococci, and unidentified spirochetes.

Epidemiology

♦ Probably universal occurrence
♦ In all ages, with a special susceptibility in neonates
♦ Common in pigs housed on abrasive floors, e.g. woven wire, expanded metal, recently laid alkaline concrete, poorly laid concrete
♦ Wet conditions underfoot macerate horn, facilitate wear of horn
♦ Dietary deficiency, e.g. of biotin, may predispose
♦ Morbidity up to 65%
♦ Causes weight loss and reproductive inefficiency

Clinical findings

Sole abrasion injuries
♦ Sole erosion at heel or toe
♦ Sole bruising with hemorrhagic streaks in horn
♦ Separation of hard, horny wall from sole or heel to form a fissure at white line, or a crack in the lower part of the lateral claw wall
♦ Cracks, fissures, usually in lateral claw of one foot, deep enough to permit entry of infection into lamellar tissue cause severe lameness
♦ Heat, pain in claw
♦ Infection may track up to, discharge at, coronet, including formation of a granulomatous lesion at discharge site
♦ Pus discharge very small volume
♦ Recovery rate with treatment only fair

Sequels
♦ Permanent hoof deformity
♦ Secondary abscessation at other sites

Neonatal foot abscess
♦ Primary lesions at:
  • Point of toe at white line
  • Heel bulb
  • Haired skin at coronet, including interdigital coronet
♦ Minor lesions are superficial abrasions, ulcers of hoof wall, heel bulb, interphalangeal skin, with no penetration of deep tissues
♦ Major lesions have deep, diffuse suppuration, fibrosis around tendons, joints, bones causing severe swelling
♦ Hind limbs, especially medial claws, have most lesions, in fore limbs lesions in lateral claws
♦ Pus discharges from coronet
♦ Horn of claw may slough
♦ Skin necrosis over pressure points

Clinical pathology

Culture of pus to determine orientation treatment should take.

Necropsy findings

Lamellar necrosis and horn abrasion.

Diagnosis

Resembles:
♦ Foot and mouth disease
♦ Vesicular exanthema of swine
♦ Swine vesicular disease
♦ Vesicular stomatitis

Treatment

♦ Antibacterial treatment with sulfonamides
♦ Indifferent results with deep lesions involving tendons, joints; these respond reasonably to claw amputation

Control

♦ Ensure diet adequate in biotin
♦ Reduce abrasiveness of flooring
♦ Footbath containing 5–10% formalin

ORAL AND LARYNGEAL NECROBACILLOSIS (INCLUDES CALF DIPHTHERIA AND NECROTIC STOMATITIS)
[VM8 p. 879]

Etiology

Fusobacterium necrophorum.

Epidemiology

♦ Disease of cattle, mostly calves to 3 months (necrotic stomatitis), sometimes yearlings up to 18 months (calf diphtheria)
♦ Most common in groups kept in confinement in unsanitary conditions
♦ Infection transmitted by inhalation, ingestion from contaminated eating and drinking utensils
♦ Nutritionally deficient calves, or calves with intercurrent disease predisposed
♦ Calf diphtheria (larynx lesions) may be associated with laryngeal papillomatosis

Clinical findings

Necrotic stomatitis
♦ Fever, anorexia, depression
♦ Breath smells foul
♦ Stringy saliva, with feed, hangs from mouth
♦ Cheek swelling
♦ Deep, necrotic ulcers in cheek mucosa
♦ Lateral tongue ulcer, tongue swollen, protrudes
♦ Necrosis may spread to pharynx, eye sockets
♦ Similar lesions on vulva, coronets in a few cases
♦ Death due to toxemia, asphyxia, pneumonia

Calf diphtheria
♦ Moist painful cough
♦ Severe inspiratory dyspnea
♦ Salivation drools
♦ Painful swallowing
♦ Complete anorexia
♦ Profound toxemia
♦ Fever
♦ Purulent nasal discharge
♦ Nasal breath foul
♦ Throat painful on palpation, swollen
♦ Lesions seen in pharynx viewed through mouth speculum
  • Larynx, glottis mucosa edematous, inflamed
  • Necrotic lesion on arytenoid cartilage, vocal cords
♦ May be secondary pneumonia

Clinical pathology

Bacteriological examination of swab from lesion confirms diagnosis.

Necropsy findings

♦ Severe edema, inflammation, swelling around lesion
♦ Large masses cheesy, necrotic material

Diagnosis

Necrotic stomatitis resembles:
♦ Lingual actinobacillosis
♦ Grass seed abscess
♦ Oral foreign body

Calf diphtheria resembles:
♦ Traumatic pharyngitis
♦ Pharyngeal foreign body
♦ Pharynx/larynx neoplasm
♦ Retropharyngeal lymph node hyperplasia
♦ Laryngeal chondritis, inherited in Texel sheep

Treatment

♦ Parenteral potentiated sulfonamides or broad spectrum antibiotic very effective treatment in early cases

♦ Corticosteroids may reduce dyspnea more quickly than antibacterials alone
♦ Tracheotomy may be necessary in cases facing death due to asphyxia

Control

♦ Hygiene in feeding and drinking arrangements
♦ Prophylactic antibiotic feeding when outbreak looms

NECROTIC RHINITIS (BULLNOSE)
[VM8 p. 880]

Etiology

Fusobacterium necrophorum credited with being the cause.

Epidemiology

♦ Occurs in young growing pigs
♦ Often associated with poor hygiene

Clinical findings

♦ Toxemia
♦ Weight loss
♦ Facial swelling
♦ Dyspnea in some
♦ Difficult mastication in some
♦ Some deaths

Diagnosis

Resembles:
♦ Atrophic rhinitis
♦ Necrotic ulcer

Treatment

Potentiated sulfonamides or broad-spectrum antibiotics begun early halt progress of disease.

Control

Hygiene in feeding, watering arrangements.

DISEASES CAUSED BY *PSEUDOMONAS* spp.

Occasional cases of systemic invasion after pseudomonas mastitis in cows causing fibrinous pleurisy, pericarditis, and chronic pyelonephritis. Occasional cases of acute fatal pneumonia in pigs due to *Pseudomonas* spp.

MELIOIDOSIS [VM8 p. 881]

Etiology

Pseudomonas pseudomallei.

Epidemiology

- Infection in all species, most prevalent in rodents
- Commonest in swampy areas, in tropics, in summer

Source and transmission
- Feces of infected animals
- Rodents important because disease chronic
- Long survival of bacteria, up to 30 months in warm, moist soil
- Water-borne infection
- Transmission by ingestion, cutaneous abrasion, and insect transport

Importance
- Fatal zoonosis
- Death losses in animals
- Resemblance to glanders

Risk factors
- Starvation and other stress of patient

Clinical findings

Sheep
- High fever, anorexia
- Lameness
- Thick purulent ocular and nasal discharges
- May be incoordination
- Head deviation, circling
- Nystagmus, blindness
- Hyperesthesia, convulsions, death

Goats
Some acute as in sheep, more often chronic.

Pigs
- Cervical lymphadenitis, or
- Posterior paresis
- Fever, anorexia
- Cough

- Oculonasal discharge
- Some deaths

Horse
- Acute metastatic pneumonia with high fever, short course, or
- Colic
- Diarrhea
- Limb lymphangitis
- Emaciation, anasarca
- Death after several month course

Clinical pathology

- Culture of organism from discharges
- Serological tests available
- Horses may react positively to mallein

Necropsy findings

- Multiple abscesses in most organs, subcutaneous sites, lymph nodes
- Thick, green, caseous pus in abscesses in sheep
- Nasal mucosal lesions leave ragged ulcers
- Polyarthritis, meningoencephalitis in experimental cases

Diagnosis

- In sheep resembles caseous lymphadenitis
- In horses resembles:
  - glanders
  - nasal actinobacillosis

Treatment and control

- Little information available
- Oxytetracycline and chloramphenicol highly regarded
- Eliminate infected animals
- Avoid exposure of humans to infection

DISEASES CAUSED BY *CAMPYLOBACTER* spp.

Campylobacter fetus var. *venerealis* [VM8 p. 882]

Causes abortion, infertility (vibriosis) in cattle.

Campylobacter fetus subsp. *fetus* [VM8 p. 882]

Causes:
♦ Sporadic abortions in cattle
♦ Enzootic abortion in sheep

Suspected of causing:
♦ Bacteremia in humans
♦ Enteritis in cattle

Campylobacter sputorum subsp. *mucosalis* [VM8 p. 882]

Suspected of causing porcine intestinal adenomatosis.

Campylobacter intestinalis, *C. coli* and *C. jejuni* [VM8 p. 882]

♦ Found in alimentary tracts of healthy animals
♦ Strong association between milk infected with these organisms and diarrhea in humans, especially residents on farms
♦ Organisms also in meat of infected animals at slaughter

Campylobacter fecalis [VM8 p. 883]

Found in intestinal lesions, experimentally causes diarrhea in calves.

C. coli (*Vibrio coli*) [VM8 p. 883]

Thought to cause:
♦ Colitis, diarrhea in piglets and calves
♦ Abortion in sheep

C. jejuni [VM8 p. 883]

♦ Originally nominated as cause of bovine winter dysentery
♦ Found in feces of diarrheic calves
♦ Experimentally causes diarrhea in calves
♦ Found in feces in outbreaks severe gastroenteritis in lambs
♦ Suspected of causing abortion in beef cattle, sheep

C. fetus subsp. *intestinalis* [VM8 p. 883]

Thought to cause diarrhea in calves.

Unidentified *Campylobacter* spp. [VM8 p. 883]

Thought to cause:
♦ **Weaner colitis** in recently weaned sheep; morbidity rate 20–75%; case fatality rate 3%
♦ Persistent, non-responsive diarrhea in foals

DISEASES CAUSED BY *LEPTOSPIRA* spp.

Some features of the etiology, epidemiology, pathogenesis, clinical pathology, treatment and control of leptospirosis are common to all animal species and are dealt with in composite statements. There are however sufficient differences between the animal species in matters of epidemiology, pathogenesis, clinical findings, clinical pathology and necropsy findings for the diseases to be dealt with separately under the headings of:
♦ Bovine leptospirosis
♦ Ovine and caprine leptospirosis
♦ Porcine leptospirosis
♦ Equine leptospirosis

LEPTOSPIROSIS (ALL SPECIES)

Etiology

♦ *Leptospira interrogans* has over 200 serovars
♦ the common serovars and their hosts are listed in table 20.1
♦ Other notable serovars recorded in farm animals include *australis, balcanicus, ballum, canicola, copenhageni, grippotyphosa, hebdomadis, hyos (mitis), muenchen, sejroe, szwajizak*

Table 20.1 Hosts of Common Leptospira Interrogans Serovars. (Adapted from VM8, page 885.)

Serovar	Maintenance host	Accidental host
Hardjo-bovis (North America)	Cattle	Sheep and humans
Hardjo-prajitno (Europe)	Cattle	Sheep and humans
Bratislava	Pigs and horses	—
Pomona (kennewicki)	Pigs, skunks, raccoons and opossums	Sheep and cattle
Grippotyphosa	Raccoons, opossums and squirrels	Sheep and cattle
Icterohaemorrhagiae	Brown rats	Cattle and pigs

Epidemiology

Occurrence
♦ Patchy, uneven distribution worldwide
♦ Enzootic in some countries, animal losses minor, important as a zoonosis
♦ Epizootic occurrence in some countries, animal losses high, sporadic as a zoonosis
♦ Some low prevalence countries experienced original epizootics, but disease now quiescent, enzootic, under control in limited areas, sporadic zoonosis
♦ Occurs all species (Table 20.1)

Source and transmission
♦ Infection excreted in urine, aborted fetuses, uterine discharges from infected animal
♦ Contamination of pasture, feed, and drinking water
♦ Clinically recovered animals, especially pigs, may pass leptospira in urine for a year; duration of leptospiruria very variable between species, e.g. lengthy in pigs, negligible period in horses, and often intermittent in a particular patient
♦ Importance of wildlife as source demonstrated in Table 20.1
♦ Entry via mucosal or cutaneous abrasions; transmission by ingestion, skin contact
♦ Leptospira in semen of infected male (possibly for only a limited period during bacteremia), venereal, artificial insemination transmission occurs
♦ In utero transmission occurs

Risk factors
♦ pH of <6 or >8 inhibitory
♦ Temperatures <7–10°C or >34–36°C (<47–50°F or >93–96°F) are inhibitory
♦ Dryness inhibits; the organism survives for long periods in free ground water, especially stagnant water; in soil of average dampness for 6 weeks
♦ High incidence most common in:
  • Heavily irrigated pasture
  • Temperate climates with high rainfall
  • Paddocks with drinking water in ponds
  • Marshy areas, muddy fields, feedlots
  • Wet seasons

Clinical findings
♦ Differs between species
♦ Consult following descriptions

BOVINE LEPTOSPIROSIS
[VM8 p. 890]

Etiology

See Table 20.1. *Leptospira interrogans* serovar *hardjo*, *L. pomona* the important infections.

Epidemiology

Occurrence
♦ Morbidity 10–30% (infection prevalence up to 100%)
♦ Case fatality rate 5%; much higher in calves than adults
♦ Abortion rate up to 30%

Importance
Abortions, loss of milk production, calf deaths are major losses.

Clinical findings

Calves – L. pomona
♦ Incubation period 3–7 days
♦ Calves up to 1 month most susceptible
♦ High fever
♦ Anorexia, depression
♦ Mucosal petechiation
♦ Hemoglobinuria, mucosal pallor, jaundice
♦ Tachycardia, loud heart sounds, large amplitude pulse
♦ Dyspnea

♦ Most die after course of 2–3 days
♦ Survivors have long convalescence

Adults – L. pomona

♦ Mild systemic reaction
♦ Milk yield reduced severely, udder limp
♦ Milk yellow–orange color, thick, may contain blood clots in a few
♦ High cell count in milk from all 4 quarters
♦ Severe lameness, synovitis in a few
♦ Necrotic dermatitis, probably due to photosensitisation rarely
♦ Abortion at systemic episode *or* 3–4 weeks later *or* without preceding illness
♦ Rare cases of meningitis with signs of —
  • Muscular rigidity
  • Incoordination
  • Saliva drooling
  • Conjunctivitis

Adults – L. hardjo

♦ fever, anorexia, disinclination to move
♦ Agalactia, milk in all quarters yellow–orange, may contain clots
♦ Herd yield may drop significantly; morbidity up to 50%
♦ Udder flabby, no pain or heat
♦ High milk cell count in all quarters
♦ Abortion several weeks after systemic episode *or* unassociated with previous illness

Clinical pathology and necropsy findings

See composite description for all species, below.

Diagnosis

Acute leptospirosis resembles:
♦ Babesiosis
♦ Anaplasmosis
♦ Rape or kale poisoning
♦ Postparturient hemoglobinuria
♦ Bacillary hemoglobinuria

Mastitis (see Table 15.1).

Treatment and control

See composite description for all species, below.

OVINE AND CAPRINE
LEPTOSPIROSIS [VM8 p. 891]

Etiology

See Table 20.1. *L. pomona, L. hardjo* the common infections

Epidemiology

Occurrence

♦ Morbidity up to 100%, case fatality rate up to 20% (45% in goats)

Importance

♦ Main losses are deaths of neonates, feedlot lambs, loss of condition in subacute infections
♦ Potential infection source for cattle

Clinical findings

Acute – L. pomona

♦ Most found dead, presumed from septicemia
♦ Lambs most susceptible
♦ Fever, depression
♦ Dyspnea, snuffling respiration
♦ Hemoglobinuria, jaundice, pallor in a few
♦ Pregnant ewes abort
♦ Death after 12 hour course

Subacute – L. hardjo

♦ Abortion
♦ Agalactia, as in cows

Clinical pathology and necropsy findings

See composite description for all species, below.

Diagnosis

Acute disease resembles:

♦ Chronic copper poisoning
♦ Rape and kale poisoning

Treatment and control

See composite description for all species, below.

PORCINE LEPTOSPIROSIS
[VM8 p. 890]

Etiology

See Table 15.1.
♦ *L. pomona* has been the prominent infection, *L. tarassovi* less so
♦ *L. ballum, bratislava, copenhageni. muenchen, hardjo,* now more common

Epidemiology

Importance
♦ Losses due equally to abortions, neonate deaths; rearing rate may fall to 10–30%
♦ Potentially more important disease in intensive housing due to increased opportunities for transmission

Clinical findings

♦ **Abortion** storm in naive herd; 2–4 weeks before term; abortion rate declines with time
♦ Piglets at term dead or weak, die quickly
♦ **Septicemia/hemolysis** as in calves occurs rarely

Clinical pathology and necropsy findings

See composite description for all species, below.

Diagnosis

Abortion differential diagnosis (see Table 20.2).

Treatment and control

See composite description for all species, below.

EQUINE LEPTOSPIROSIS
[VM8 p. 891]

Etiology

See Table 20.1. Prevalent serovar varies widely; *L. bratislava* a common finding

Epidemiology

Occurrence
Up to 30% morbidity in infected groups.

Importance
♦ Mild disease in horses
♦ Losses negligible except for periodic ophthalmia
♦ Possible involvement in abortions

Clinical findings

Systemic infection
♦ Mild fever
♦ Anorexia, depression

♦ Dyspnea
♦ Hemoglobinuria
♦ Jaundice in some
♦ Sequels include:
  • Abortion at month 7–10
  • Periodic ophthalmia

Periodic ophthalmia
Recurrent attacks of:
♦ Photophobia
♦ Conjunctivitis, lacrimation
♦ Keratitis
♦ Pericorneal corona of blood vessels
♦ Hypopyon
♦ Iridocyclitis
♦ Terminally blindness in both eyes

Foal septicemia
A combined *L. pomona–Rhodococcus equi* septicemia in foals causes interstitial nephritis/uremia, pneumonia, enteritis

Clinical pathology and necropsy findings

See composite description for all species, below.

Diagnosis

Acute disease resembles:
♦ Alloimmune hemolytic anemia of newborn
♦ Infectious equine anemia
♦ Myoglobinuria of Azoturia
♦ Babesiosis

Abortion resembles:
♦ Equine viral rhinopneumonitis
♦ Equine viral arteritis
♦ *Salmonella abortusequi*
♦ *Streptococcus zooepidemicus*

Treatment and control

See composite description for all species, below.

LEPTOSPIROSIS

Clinical pathology (all species)

Acute infection
♦ Blood culture positive, only during early septicemic phase, *or*
♦ Transport of blood in special medium then intraperitoneal injection into guinea-pigs
♦ Hemoglobinuria
♦ Hemolytic anemia

Table 20.2 Diagnostic summary of common causes of abortion, mummification and stillbirths in swine [VM8 p. 895]

Disease	Epidemiology	Clinical features	Laboratory diagnosis		
			Isolation of agent	*Serology*	
Leptospirosis (*L. interrogans* serovar *pomona*)	Abortion last 2–3 weeks of gestation. Follows introduction of infected boar or sow or contamination of water supply	Abortion, sow systemically normal. Weak piglets sometimes	Fetal tissues and *urine of sow*	Positive or rising titers in aborting sows	
Brucellosis (*Br. suis*)	Abortion may occur any time during gestation. Spread by coitus	Embryonic death infertility, abortion. Orchitis in boars	Fetal injuries	Positive titers in herd	
Porcine parvovirus infection	Herd outbreak when introduced for first time. Subsequently herd immunity develops and problem sporadic, affecting primarily gilts. May be continual low-grade problem in piggeries where sows are stalled. Due to incomplete spread	Abortion outbreaks possible. Mainly mummification, stillbirth and infertility. Sow clinically normal	Virus detectable by hemagglutinating antibody or fluorescent antibody in fetuses less than 16 cm crown-rump (C–R) length	Antibody present in fetuses greater than 16 cm C–R length. Antibody in high titer in sow	
SMEDI virus	Poorly defined. Similar to parvovirus. Sporadic, affecting gilts primarily	Small litter size, uneven pigs and poor piglet viability, stillbirth and mummification. Infertility	Virus difficult to isolate from affected fetuses	Antibody in fetus, greater than 16 cm C–R length, and sow	
Porcine reproductive respiratory syndrome (PRRS) (LELYSTAD VIRUS)	Epidemics of reproductive failure	Abortion, mummified stillbirths, fetuses, weak piglets, increased preweaning mortality	—	Serology	

Continued overleaf

Table 20.2 (Cont'd)

Disease	Epidemiology	Clinical features	Laboratory diagnosis		Serology
			Isolation of agent		
Aujeszky's disease (pseudorabies)	Abortion usually 10–20 days after clinical illness. At any time but especially first 2 months of pregnancy. Concurrent or preceding clinical disease in young pigs in herd	Sows may show mild clinical disease at time of infection, anorexia, depression, transient pyrexia. Abortion or stillbirth or mummified fetuses at term	Difficult. CNS and lungs of fetus and vaginal swab sow		Positive titers in herdmates
Hog cholera (swine fever)	Usually signs of clinical disease within piggery. Low virulence strains may produce reproductive/ teratogenic effects only	Abortion of sows during or following acute clinical disease. Also embryonic death, small litter size, stillbirth and mummification. 'Trembling pigs' at birth may be only manifestation	Fetal pigs and affected pigs within herd. Transmission studies		Positive titers in herds and resistant to challenge

Other agents such as *Erysipelothris*, Japanese hemagglutinating virus, Japanese encephalitis virus, fungi, nutritional deficiency may produce abortion or reproductive inefficiency. Many outbreaks of abortion in sows remain undiagnosed and there must be important agents as yet unrecognized producing this syndrome.

♦ Leukopenia in cattle, leukocytosis other species

Abortion
Organism detectable in body organs.

Postfever period
♦ Leptospira disappear from blood
♦ Leptospira in urine; demonstrate by dark ground illumination, culture, guinea-pig inoculation, fluorescent staining of antibody, nucleic acid hybridization, polymerase chain reaction
♦ Leptospira in milk detected by complement fixation test for antibodies
♦ Serological tests develop positive results; rising titers in microscopic agglutination test (MAT)

Chronic disease
♦ MAT test ineffective because titer low
♦ ELISA used
♦ Leptospiral antibodies in aqueous humor more accurate than serology in diagnosis of ophthalmia

Herd test
♦ Necessary when no acute cases current at time of visit
♦ Serological test 15–25% of each age group, local wildlife if possible
♦ Paired sera collected from serologically positive animals

Necropsy (composite description for all species)

Acute disease
♦ Anemia, jaundice, hemoglobinuria
♦ Ulcers, hemorrhages in abomasal mucosa of cattle
♦ Pulmonary edema, emphysema in cattle with hemoglobinuria
♦ Interstitial nephritis, diffuse or focal

Chronic disease
♦ Interstitial nephritis causes small white foci in cortex
♦ Centrilobular hepatic necrosis
♦ Leptospirae in tissues

Aborted fetus
♦ Usually too autolyzed to be useful; fluorescent antibody test serology may give positive result
♦ Small, white foci in liver in pig fetus

Diagnosis
See individual description for each species.

Treatment and control
See composite description for all species, below.

Treatment
Leptospira pomona
♦ Control the septicemia by parenteral streptomycin (12 mg/kg body weight twice daily for 3 days) or a tetracycline; early treatment essential, before renal lesion develops
♦ To control the leptospiruria of carrier cattle, pigs a single intramuscular injection of 25 mg/kg body weight streptomycin simultaneously to all animals in group *plus* vaccination to prevent new cases
♦ Mass medication (800 g oxytetracycline/ tonne of feed for 8–11 days) recommended instead of individual injections for pigs

Leptospira hardjo
♦ Susceptible to penicillin G, ampicillin, tetracycline, erythromycin, streptomycin

Periodic ophthalmia
♦ Systemic antibiotic plus systemic corticosteroid, subconjunctival in chronic cases
♦ Atropine eye ointment three times daily

Control
There is a great deal of indecision about making recommendations for the control of leptospirosis because of:
♦ The natural tendency of the disease to be clinically self-limiting
♦ The difficulty of detecting carriers of the infection
♦ The difficulty of curing carriers of infection, assessing their status after treatment

Eradication
Cattle Not attempted because of:
♦ Inability to select carriers accurately
♦ Probability of breakdown by reinfection from wildlife, rodents
♦ Failure of medication to clear all leptospira from urine of carriers

Pigs All pigs considered carriers so *either*:
♦ Treat all pigs in the group individually with a single intramuscular injection of 25 mg/ kg body weight streptomycin *plus* vaccination to prevent new cases *or*
♦ Mass medication (800 g oxytetracycline/ tonne of feed for 8–11 days)

Containment

Limiting the prevalence to financially acceptable level in herds in enzootic area by:

♦ Hygiene – avoiding animal contact with polluted areas, e.g. swamp, damp pens; avoid contact with sources (deer, rodents)
♦ Vaccination with bacterins containing epidemiologically relevant serotypes; immunity duration 12 months; does not interfere with microscopic agglutination test
♦ After an outbreak herd immunity reduces clinical prevalence so that costs of vaccination need to be taken into account when advising a farmer whether or not to vaccinate
♦ In **dairy herds**, artificial insemination bulls to be guaranteed free; vaccination all cattle annually before breeding season commencing at 4–6 months old
♦ In **beef herds**, annual vaccination of bulls, replacement heifers, and 2–3 year old cows a few weeks before bulls turned in with cows; bulls to come from leptospira-free herds; calves commence vaccination at 4–6 months, then annually; cows failing to carry a calf to term or has a stillborn or weak calf culled
♦ In **pig herds**, annual vaccination sows, gilts at breeding time with bacterin containing *L. pomona, L. tarassovi*

SWINE DYSENTERY [VM8 p. 899]

Etiology

Treponema hyodysenteriae the primary cause but presence of one or more anaerobes necessary for pathogenicity.

Epidemiology

Occurrence

♦ Worldwide, very common, high prevalence
♦ Mostly in 7–16 week pigs, some older, rarely adults, suckers
♦ Morbidity 10–75%, case fatality 50%

Source and transmission

♦ In feces of affected pigs
♦ Ingestion, oral fecal cycling
♦ Incubation period 7–14 days usual; can be much longer
♦ Small proportion of recovered pigs, treated or not, can be carriers for 50–90 days
♦ Carrier pigs transmit infection; also become clinical cases under stress or treatment with sodium arsanilate

Risk factors

♦ Carrier pigs may carry high antibody titers against *T. hyodysenteriae* while infective
♦ Recovered untreated pigs immune to reinfection for 16–17 weeks
♦ Most outbreaks due to introduction of infected pigs
♦ Overcrowding and fecal waste build-up predispose
♦ Fecal effluent from adjoining pens spreads infection
♦ Mixing of pens of weaners, continuous supplementation of population enhance chances of infection
♦ Drying, heating, disinfection destroy organism

Importance

♦ Heavy death losses
♦ Severe reduction production efficiency
♦ Control in many herds dependent on costly prophylactic medication

Clinical findings

♦ Outbreak usually starts slowly but affects most in group in few to 14 days
♦ Rarely sudden death without preliminary diarrhea in a few pigs as first sign
♦ Moderate fever, mild depression, anorexia
♦ Feces have porridge-like consistency, passed anywhere
  • Light gray to black color
  • Contain much mucus, some blood flecks, epithelial casts
  • Much blood in some
♦ Dehydration, gaunt abdomen,
♦ Death due to dehydration, toxemia over course of some days to several weeks; rarely after several days with profuse hemorrhagic diarrhea
♦ Good response to treatment but recurrence when treatment withdrawn
♦ Rarely a chronic syndrome with persistent diarrhea, failure to grow
♦ Survivors have illness duration of 3–4 weeks

Clinical pathology

♦ Organism demonstrable:
  • As motile organisms by dark ground illumination
  • Culture after careful transfer in transport medium
  • Fluorescent antibody staining
♦ Specific identification of infection by *T. hyodysenteriae* by microscopic agglutination test or disk growth-inhibition test

Table 20.3 Suggested drugs for treatment and control of swine dysentery [VM8 p. 902]

	Treatment		Control
Drug	Water (mg/4 liters)	Feed (mg/kg)	Feed (mg/kg)
Organic arsenicals			
Sodium arsanilate	700	—	—
Arsanilic acid	—	150–250	90–150
3-Nitro–4-hydroxyphenylarsonate	540	—	—
Tiamulin (31)	240	—	40
Tylosin (37)	50–1000	—	100
3-Acetyl–4″-isovaleryltylosin (36)	—	—	55 or 110
Virginiamycin (32)	—	100	25–100
Carbadox (38)	—	50	50
Nitroimidazoles			
Dimetridazole (41)	1000	300–500	100–250
Ronidazole	240	120	60–120

NB: All water treatment should be given for 5–7 days. Feed medication for treatment should continue for at least 14 days and preferably 21 days. Drug withdrawal periods and legality should be determined to local regulation. Prophylactic levels may be permitted on a continuous basis until shortly before the pigs are sent to slaughter.

♦ Carrier pigs identified by serological tests:
  • ELISA has high sensitivity
  • Microtitration agglutination test
  • Indirect fluorescent antibody test

Necropsy findings

Typical lesions include:
♦ Colitis, typhlitis; necrosis, hemorrhage into lumen early then fibrinonecrotic, diphtheritic membrane
♦ Enlarged, congested draining lymph nodes
♦ Stomach fundus hyperemia
♦ Survivors may have chronic 'white spots' (enlarged lymphoid nodules) under serosal surface

Diagnosis

Resembles:
♦ Coliform gastroenteritis
♦ Salmonellosis
♦ Hog cholera
♦ Intestinal hemorrhage syndrome
♦ Esophogastric ulcer

Treatment

For drugs and dose rates consult Table 20.3.
♦ In **outbreak**:
  • Treat affected pigs individually
  • Treat others in pen with medication in drinking water (or feed) for several days at therapeutic levels, then continue at prophylactic level for 3–4 weeks
♦ Arsenicals most economic and effective but some risk of toxicity so surveillance at all times; 7-day medication periods alternated with 7-day no-treatment periods avoids most problems but often impractical
♦ Problems with swine dysentery medication include:
  • Failure of some outbreaks to respond
  • Relapses or new cases after treatment withdrawn, due usually to ineffective drug or inadequate dosage, or to failure to develop immunity during treatment because the pigs were treated earlier when not infected
  • Unexplained more severely affected cases in treated pigs than in untreated controls
♦ Avoidance of problems best achieved by always using highly effective drugs and using full doses for recommended periods
♦ Recurrence of disease after treatment means all carriers were not eliminated or failure to clean and disinfect pens, and rid environment of the bacteria

Control

Control depends on disinfection of the environment, elimination of carrier animals so that the environment is not reinfected, and avoiding introduction of carrier pigs. Elimination of carriers can be done by culling, but their accurate identification is a problem, or by vigorous medication. No completely satisfactory vaccine is available.

Eradication

Recommended for stud herds.

♦ Establishment of a specific-pathogen-free (SPF) herd will eliminate the disease but unexplained breakdowns occur; care needed with introduction new genetic material, only semen, SPF pigs or similar to be used
♦ **Barrier method** concentrates on the sow; feed tiamulin (20 mg/kg body weight from 10 days before farrowing to 5 days after when piglets weaned, removed to strict isolation pen
♦ Virtual eradication achieved by treatment all pigs with tiamulin 10 mg/kg body weight I/M daily for 5 days **plus** cleaning, disinfection, rodent control

Containment

Recommended for commercial herds in which frequent introductions of pigs of questionable disease history are unavoidable.

♦ Early treatment of affected pigs and in-contacts as soon as disease occurs with recommended levels of appropriate drugs for recommended periods (see Table 20.3)
♦ Prophylactic mass medication for each draft of introductions

PORCINE ULCERATIVE
GRANULOMA (NECROTIC ULCER)
[VM8 p. 905]

Etiology

Borrelia suilla.

Epidemiology

♦ Limited occurrence, uncommon disease
♦ On farms practicing poor hygiene
♦ Causes deaths of young pigs, unsightly blemish in sows

Clinical findings

♦ Initially a few small, hard, fibrous swellings
♦ On ventral abdomen of sow
♦ Face of sucking pigs; whole litter may be affected
♦ In weaned pigs along lower edge of both ears at base causing tissue loss, sloughing of ear
♦ After 2–3 weeks form persistent ulcer, raised edges, center is granulation tissue covered with sticky, gray pus
♦ Lesions expand to 20–30 cm dia. on sow belly
♦ On face erode lips, cheeks, jawbone; teeth shed

Clinical pathology

Bacteria in smears and biopsy.

Necropsy findings

Skin lesions only.

Diagnosis

Resembles:
♦ Sarcoptic mange
♦ Trauma from ear biting and snout rubbing
♦ Udder actinomycosis

Treatment

♦ Penicillin, single injection
♦ Potassium iodide orally
♦ Early cases respond to topical application of tetracycline spray, sulfonamide dust

Control

♦ Improved hygiene in pens
♦ Prompt disinfection skin wounds

BORRELIOSIS (LYME BORRELIOSIS,
LYME DISEASE) [VM8 p. 906]

Etiology

Borrelia burgdorferi.

Epidemiology

Occurrence

♦ Most countries
♦ Most species
♦ Distribution related to density of tick population; common where deer plentiful, in areas with dense vegetation, humid climate
♦ Up to 10% of horses in area, 60% on individual farms, seropositive
♦ Peaks of incidence spring and autumn
♦ May be clusters of cases in foals at weaning on enzootic farms

Source and transmission

◆ Small wild animals, e.g. field mice; white-tailed deer are reservoir
◆ Transmission by *Ixodes* spp., *Dermacentor variabilis*, *Amblyomma americanum* ticks, tabanid flies, mosquitoes
◆ Bacteria also in urine, skin contact may transmit
◆ In utero transmission causes deaths in foals and calves

Importance

◆ An important zoonosis

Clinical findings

◆ Indefinite syndromes including:

Horse

◆ Mild fever
◆ Sporadic lameness, laminitis, swollen joints
◆ Stiff gait, muscle pain
◆ Anterior uveitis
◆ Nervous system involvement in some including:
  • Depression, behavioural changes
  • Head tilt
  • Dysphagia
◆ Abortion, stillbirths
◆ Early embryonic loss or conception failure

Cattle and sheep

◆ Often groups affected
◆ Fever, mild, persistent
◆ Lameness, laminitis
◆ Stiff gait, swollen joints
◆ Erythema of udder skin or interdigital skin
◆ Decreased milk production
◆ Chronic weight loss
◆ Abortion
◆ Chronic weight loss

Clinical pathology

◆ Dark field microscopy or culture may reveal organism in blood, milk, urine
◆ Accurate indirect immunofluorescent antibody, ELISA, western blot analysis tests available

Necropsy findings

◆ Polysynovitis
◆ Lymphadenopathy
◆ Multifocal, interstitial myocarditis
◆ Interstitial pneumonia
◆ Glomerulonephritis
◆ Emaciation

Diagnosis

Resembles:
◆ Bovine ephemeral fever
◆ Mycoplasma arthritis
◆ Streptococcal arthritis
◆ Tick pyemia
◆ Laminitis
◆ Bovine, ovine erysipelas

Treatment

Horses

◆ Procaine penicillin 30 000–45 000 iu/kg body weight daily for 10 days, followed by benzathine penicillin on alternate days
◆ Oxytetracycline 6–12 mg/kg body weight I/V once daily for 21 days
◆ Phenylbutazone for the laminitis

Cattle

Penicillin or oxytetracycline daily for 21 days.

Control

Tick control.

DISEASES CAUSED BY *MYCOPLASMA* SPP.

MISCELLANEOUS MYCOPLASMOSES

Poorly defined disease states in which myco-plasmas are possibly implicated include the following.

Diseases of the genital tract
[VM8 p. 908]

Suggested relationships are:
♦ Vulvovaginitis, endometritis, salpingitis, temporary infertility in female ruminants; in ewes – *M. capricolium*
♦ Persistent infection in bull genital tract – *M. agalactia* var. *bovis*
♦ Granular vulvitis ewes – *Ureaplasma* spp.
♦ Granular vaginitis, transitory endometri-tis, salpingitis in cows – *Ureaplasma* spp.
♦ Abortion in mares – *Acholeplasma* spp.
♦ Unspecified infertility in cows – *M. bovige-nitalium*

Diseases of the respiratory tract [VM8 p. 908]

Reportings include, as secondary infections:
♦ Pneumonia in sheep – *Mycoplasma dispar, M. ovipneumoniae, M. arginini*
♦ Pneumonia in goats – *M. agalactia, M. mycoides, M. mycoides* var. *capri, M. mycoides* var *mycoides, M. ovipneumo-niae, Acholeplasma laidlawii*
♦ Pneumonia in calves – *M. agalactia* var *bovis, M. arginini, M. bovis, M. bovirhinis, M. dispar, M. ovipneumoniae, Acholep-lasma laidlawii, Ureaplasma* spp.
♦ Pleurisy in horses – *M. felis*

Diseases of the eye
[VM8 p. 909]

Keratoconjunctivitis in ruminants – *M. bovoculi (A. oculi)*

Mycoplasmal arthritides
[VM8 p. 909]

♦ Arthritis, polyarthritis in pigs – *M. hyosy-noviae, M. hyorhinis*
♦ Arthritis in goats, sheep – *M. capricolium, M. mycoides* var. *mycoides, M. putrifa-ciens* (plus mastitis)
See also Table 20.4.

CONTAGIOUS BOVINE PLEUROPNEUMONIA (CBPP)
[VM8 p. 910]

A highly infectious septicemia of cattle, one of the world's major plagues of cattle.

Etiology

Mycoplasma mycoides var. *mycoides* (small colony type).

Epidemiology

Occurrence
♦ Eradicated from most developed countries but recurring in Europe in recent years
♦ Only cattle, rare in buffalo, yak, bison, reindeer, and antelopes. Strong immunity after attack
♦ Massive outbreaks in susceptible cattle, especially in transit or housed
♦ Morbidity 90%, case fatality rate 50%; 25% remain as recovered carriers

Source and transmission
♦ Asymptomatic carriers, overt cases; car-riers infective up to 3 years
♦ Transmission by inhalation

Risk factors
♦ Organism sensitive to heat, dryness, disin-fectants; mediate contagion possible but unlikely
♦ Spreads less in arid zones

Clinical findings

♦ Incubation period 3–6 weeks
♦ Sudden onset of high fever, anorexia, milk yield fall
♦ Dyspnea; shallow, grunting respiration,
♦ Painful cough back arched, head extended
♦ Pleuritic friction sounds followed by dull-ness
♦ Edema of throat, brisket in some
♦ Ruminal atony, no exercise tolerance

Clinical pathology

Complement fixation tests, ELISA sufficient-ly accurate to make eradication practicable.

Necropsy findings

Acute

Table 20.4 Summary of systemic mycoplasmoses of sheep and goats [VM8 p. 910]

Bacterial species	Animals affected	Disease caused	Pathogenicity
M. agalactiae	Sheep/goats	Contagious agalactia, arthritis, pneumonia, granular vaginitis, pinkeye	High
M. arginini	Sheep/goats	Pneumonia, arthritis, vaginitis, pinkeye, mastitis	Low
M. capricolum	Sheep/goats	Arthritis, mastitis, pneumonia	High
M. mycoides subsp. capri	Goats	Contagious caprine pleuropneumonia, pneumonia, arthritis	Moderate
M. mycoides subsp. mycoides (large colony type)	Sheep/goats	Contagious caprine pleuropneumonia, mastitis, arthritis, high mortality in young kids	Moderate
M. ovipneumoniae	Sheep/goats	Pneumonia	Commonly precursor to pneumonic pasteurellosis
M. putrefaciens	Goats	Mastitis and arthritis	High
Acholeplasma laidlawii	Sheep/goats	Bacteria found in lungs	Non-pathogenic
Ureaplasma sp.	Sheep/goats	Vaginitis	
Mycoplasma strain F38	Goats	Contagious caprine pleuropneumonia	Low
	Sheep/goats		High pathogenicity

♦ Fibrinous pleurisy
♦ Extensive pleural effusion
♦ 'Marbled' consolidation of much of lungs
♦ Greatly distended interlobular septa

Chronic
♦ Encapsulated chronic foci (sequestra)
♦ Fibrous adhesions
♦ Organism in impression smears or culture

Diagnosis

Resembles:
♦ Pneumonic pasteurellosis
♦ Acute pulmonary emphysema, edema and interstitial pneumonia
♦ Viral pneumonia of calves
♦ Lungworm infestation

Treatment

♦ Only where disease endemic
♦ Sulfadimidine widely used; tylosin, spiramycin effective

Control

For herds:
♦ Avoid collecting herd together
♦ Remove clinical cases
♦ Remove positive reactors to CF test or ELISA
♦ Retest at 2 months intervals till 2 successive tests clean
♦ Culled animals slaughtered on farm or to abattoir and slaughter under close supervision
♦ Vaccination with live vaccine made from strain of organism suited to country and type of cattle

To maintain a free area:
♦ Restrict entry to animals not in contact with infected animals or in infected area for 6 months
♦ Animals vaccinated at least 2 months and not in contact with infection

Nomadic herds – restrain occurrence by annual vaccination all cattle.

CONTAGIOUS CAPRINE
PLEUROPNEUMONIA (CCPP)
[VM8 p. 914]

Etiology

Mycoplasma (strain F38).

Epidemiology

♦ Similar to the bovine disease
♦ Prevalent in North Africa and the Mediterranean countries

Clinical findings

♦ Cough, dyspnea
♦ Lagging, lying down a lot
♦ Fever
♦ Death in as short a period as 2 days

Clinical pathology

Complement fixation, ELISA, latex agglutination tests available.

Necropsy findings

Marbled consolidation as in cattle disease, but no sequestra, less interlobular septal reaction.

Diagnosis

Resembles pneumonias caused by:
♦ *M. mycoides* subsp. *capri*
♦ *M. mycoides* subsp. *mycoides*
♦ *M. capriolum*

Treatment

Tylosin or oxytetracycline both very effective.

Control

Vaccination twice yearly practiced in endemic areas.

CONTAGIOUS AGALACTIA OF
GOATS AND SHEEP [VM8 p. 914]

Etiology

M. agalactiae most favored to be cause.

Epidemiology

♦ Occurrence same as caprine pleuropneumonia
♦ Case fatality rate high, survivors culled for blind quarters

Clinical findings

- Sudden onset severe mastitis, arthritis, ophthalmitis
- Abortion
- Course up to several months

Clinical pathology

- Culture of organism from milk
- Complement fixation, ELISA satisfactory serological tests

Diagnosis

Resembles pneumonia caused by:
- M. mycoides var. mycoides
- M. arginini
- M. capricolium
- M. putrefaciens

Treatment

Early treatment with tylosin, erythromycin, chlortetracycline effective.

Control

Vaccination effective in control and aid to eradication.

MYCOPLASMAL ARTHRITIS OF CATTLE [VM8 p. 915]

Etiology

- Mycoplasma agalactia var. bovis, principal cause of the disease in feedlot cattle
- M. bovis, M. alkalescens cause calf polyarthritis

Epidemiology

Occurrence
- 6–8 month old feedlot cattle several weeks after introduction
- Morbidity 18–85%; case fatality 3–50%
- Occurs in calves sucking cows in which mycoplasma mastitis is occurring
- Occurs in calves with enzootic pneumonia due to M. bovis

Risk factors
- Long transport
- Mixing groups of cattle

Clinical findings

- Lameness, stiff gait
- Moderate fever, anorexia, weight loss
- Limb joints, tendon sheaths swollen
- Recumbent, decubitus ulcers
- Pneumonia in some
- Spontaneous recovery in 10–14 days or
- Euthanasia due to continued recumbency

Clinical pathology

- Inflammatory synovial aspirates
- Culture of organism from aspirate

Necropsy findings

- Fibrinous synovitis, severe thickening, edema of synovial membrane
- Fibrinous taeniosynovitis
- Pneumonia, pleurisy, pericarditis in some
- Culture of organism often difficult

Diagnosis

Resembles:
- Bovine ephemeral fever
- Streptococcal arthritis
- Laminitis
- Bovine erysipelas

Treatment

- Mycoplasma spp. sensitive to tylosin, oxytetracycline, lincomycin, oleandomycin but response poor in clinical cases
- Intra-articular antibiotic plus corticosteroid advised

Control

- Disease usually disappears from group spontaneously
- Long-term feeding with tiamulin hydrogen fumarate, or formalinized M. bovis vaccine used

ENZOOTIC PNEUMONIA OF PIGS [VM8 p. 916]

Etiology

Mycoplasma hyopneumoniae (syn. M. suipneumoniae). Pasteurella multocida a common secondary invader.

Epidemiology

Occurrence

♦ Worldwide
♦ High incidence in intensive pig-raising enterprises
♦ 40–80% morbidity; case fatality rate low without potent secondary invader
♦ Peak incidence in 16–20 week old pigs; all ages affected during first outbreak in herd

Source and transmission
♦ Source is respiratory tract of infected pig
♦ Transmission direct by pig to pig inhalation; number of organisms to effect infection small so that wind a possible mechanism for long distance transmission
♦ Sow to piglet the usual cycle
♦ Spread enhanced by stress and group mingling at weaning

Risk factors
♦ Concurrent infection with lungworms, migrating ascarids, adenovirus, transmissible gastroenteritis
♦ Secondary invasion of lesions by pasteurellae, streptococci, mycoplasmas, *Bordetella bronchiseptica*, *Klebsiella pneumoniae*
♦ Proximity to infected herds
♦ Intensive management in finishing period including management errors such as:
 • Continuous input of pigs instead of all-in, all-out operations
 • Fattening units buying pigs at open sales
 • Fluctuating temperatures, humidity
 • Irregular ventilation rates
 • Semisolid pen partitions
 • Large numbers of pigs in common air space
 • Dusty atmosphere

Importance
Growth rate of affected pigs subnormal, *or if* growth rate maintained by good management, feed conversion efficiency reduced.

Clinical findings

Incubation period 10–16 days.

Initial outbreak in a naive herd (Epizootic disease)
♦ 100% morbidity in all age pigs
♦ Severe dyspnea
♦ Fever in some
♦ Some deaths
♦ Subsides to chronic disease in herd after 3 month course

Chronic (enzootic disease)
♦ Mostly in feeder pigs; may be in suckers
♦ Insidious onset

♦ Persistent, dry, hacking cough; worst at feeding time, and getting up in the morning; can be elicited by forced exercise; usually disappears in 2–3 weeks
♦ Rare to find dyspnea, fever, anorexia
♦ Some pigs slow in weight gain; others unaffected

Sequel
Acute bacterial pneumonia.

Clinical pathology

♦ Serological tests adequate for herd diagnosis include:
 • Complement fixation
 • Indirect hemagglutination
 • ELISA
♦ Test adequate for accurate definition of *M. hyosynoviae*, without reacting with other *Mycoplasma* spp. awaited

Necropsy findings

♦ Clearly demarcated lesions along ventral borders of all lobes but especially right anterior lobes
♦ Lesions plum-colored, grayish, resemble lymphoid tissue
♦ Mycoplasmas cultured or diagnosed on basis of immunofluorescent staining of lung sections

Diagnosis

Resembles:
♦ Swine influenza
♦ *Actinobacillus pleuropneumoniae* pneumonia
♦ Lungworm
♦ Ascariasis

Treatment

♦ No effective treatment including tiamulin, tylosin
♦ Fluoroquinolones, e.g. ciprofloxacin active in vitro
♦ For severely affected pigs, possibly with secondary bacterial infection, vigorous individual treatment with broad spectrum antibiotic, tetracycline usually used
♦ For in-contact pens tetracyclines, tylosin, spiramycin fed at 200 mg/kg body weight for 5–10 days

Control

Eradication
♦ Because of the mode of transmission eradi-

cation by breaking the chain of infection achieves eradication relatively easily; the problems are the high cost, and the ease with which the pneumonia-free herd is reinfected

♦ The only really satisfactory procedure for breeding units is by repopulation with specific-pathogen-free (SPF) pigs alternative, risky, but much cheaper procedures are:
  • **Snatching** neonates at birth; rearing in isolation
  • **Isolated farrowing** of sows, usually in individual pens erected outside
♦ All procedures need to maintain constant surveillance by necropsy examination of a sample of young pigs from each litter for lesions of enzootic pneumonia

Containment at low infection level

Important practices which reduce infection incidence or disease severity include:

♦ Low intensity of management
♦ Small herds
♦ Sows can be farrowed in isolation
♦ Litters reared separately
♦ Less than 25 weaner pigs per pen
♦ Less than 100 pigs in any airspace
♦ Optimal temperature, humidity, and ventilation in housing
♦ Dust, ammonia, and hydrogen sulfide content of air kept low
♦ Efficient cleaning and disinfection program
♦ Purchase fattening pigs direct from breeder or pneumonia-free source
♦ When purchasing pigs avoid coughing, uneven litters
♦ Purchased high-risk feeder pigs fed antibiotic supplemented feed for 2 weeks after introduction (tetracycline, tylosin, spiramycin at 100–200 mg/kg feed); more intensive medication for higher-risk operations
♦ Introduced pigs best kept in isolation and finished as separate batch
♦ An efficient vaccine is not as yet available
♦ All-in, all-out management system

MYCOPLASMAL ARTHRITIS IN
PIGS [VM8 p. 923]

Etiology

♦ *Mycoplasma hyorhinis* in young pigs
♦ *Mycoplasma hyosynoviae* in growing pigs

Epidemiology

Occurrence

♦ Widespread in young pigs

♦ *M. hyorhinis* arthritis commonest in 3–10 week old pigs; sporadic cases, occasional outbreaks; causes runting; up to 10% case fatality
♦ *M. hyosynoviae* arthritis commonest in pigs over 3 months old; morbidity usually 5–15%, up to 50%; up to 15% affected chronically; a major problem in some herds

Source and transmission

♦ *M. hyorhinis* a common inhabitant of respiratory tract, conjunctiva of normal pigs
♦ *M. hyosynoviae* a common inhabitants of pharyngeal and tonsillar mucosae of normal pigs
♦ Transmission by aerosol inhalation, direct contact, possibly indirect because survival in environment up to 4 weeks (*M. hyosynoviae*)

Clinical findings

M. hyorhinis infection
♦ Transient fever, depression, anorexia
♦ Dyspnea, abdominal breathing
♦ Pleural friction rub in some
♦ Joints swollen, painful
♦ Recumbent, reluctant to rise
♦ Many recover spontaneously in 1–2 weeks, others remain illthrifty
♦ Many pigs affected insidiously without dramatic clinical signs, just unthrifty runts after weaning

M. hyosynoviae infection
♦ Sudden onset acute lameness in one or more, usually major, joints
♦ Joint swelling minimal
♦ Most recover in 3–10 days; some permanently recumbent

Clinical pathology

♦ Synovial aspirate inflammatory fluid
♦ Organisms identified by immunofluorescent techniques
♦ Complement fixation test positive after acute phase

Necropsy findings

♦ Serofibrinous pleuritis, pericarditis, peritonitis in *M. hyorhinis* infection; fibrinous adhesions in serous cavities in chronic cases
♦ In both infections synovial hypertrophy, serosanguineous synovial fluid in affected joints; thickened joint capsules, articular erosion in chronic cases
♦ Organisms more readily detected in acute cases

Diagnosis

Resembles:
♦ Streptococcal arthritis
♦ Glasser's disease

Treatment

♦ Tylosin 1–2 mg/kg (or lincomycin 2.5 mg/kg, or tiamulin 10–15 mg/kg) body weight for 3 days effective

♦ Early treatment of *M. hyosynoviae* with parenteral corticosteroid reduces occurrence chronic laminitis

Control

♦ Minimization of stress
♦ Tylosin or tetracycline in feed or drinking water during stress
♦ Early weaning recommended to reduce infection rate of *M. hyosynoviae*

21 DISEASES CAUSED BY VIRUSES AND CHLAMYDIA – I

VIRAL DISEASES WITH MANIFESTATIONS ATTRIBUTABLE TO INVOLVEMENT OF THE BODY AS A WHOLE

HOG CHOLERA (CLASSIC SWINE FEVER) [VM8 p. 927]

Etiology

Hog cholera virus is:
♦ A pestivirus of the family Togaviridae
♦ One antigenic type; multiple strains of varying virulence
♦ Antigenically related to bovine virus diarrhea virus

Epidemiology

Occurrence
♦ Worldwide but now eradicated from many countries; in some of which it has recurred
♦ Pigs only
♦ At one time identified only as catastrophic outbreaks with morbidity and case fatality rates approximating 100%; now a mild form of the disease which spreads slowly is also recognized

Source and transmission
♦ The source of the virus is always an infected pig; in all secretions of subclinical carriers or incubating, sick or convalescent cases
♦ Subclinical carriers may excrete virus in urine for very long periods
♦ Ingestion the usual route, possibly inhalation

Risk factors
♦ The **virulent** virus is very infectious, only small doses are needed to infect
♦ The **less virulent** virus is less infectious, spreading slowly, and causing clinical disease only in fetuses, neonates
♦ The virus is susceptible to heat and dryness,

surviving only 1–2 days in outdoor pens but it persists in raw meat for up to 84 days, in frozen meat for over 4 years; spread by feeding raw offal, garbage the principal method of transmission
♦ Spread also common by mechanical dissemination on clothing, motor vehicles, vaccinating equipment

Importance
♦ Enormous wastage due to pig deaths, costs of vaccination, eradication
♦ Occurrence in a country restricts its opportunities to sell pig products overseas

Clinical findings

Acute disease
♦ Incubation period 5–10 days
♦ Early in outbreak young pigs may die without prior signs
♦ Anorexia, depression, drooping posture, tail limp
♦ Disinclined to move, staggering gait, recumbency piled on top of each other
♦ High fever
♦ Constipation, then diarrhea, vomiting
♦ Diffuse purple discoloration of belly skin
♦ Conjunctivitis with mucopurulent eye discharge in most
♦ Nervous signs, tremor, circling, ataxia, convulsions in early stages in some
♦ Death after 5–7 day course

Chronic hog cholera
♦ Longer incubation period
♦ Weight loss to emaciation
♦ Dermatitis, alopecia, purple blotching of belly skin
♦ High liability to secondary infection

Nervous syndrome

♦ Short incubation, short course
♦ Lateral recumbency
♦ Tetanic/clonic convulsions, some continuous, some intermittent
♦ Squealing during convulsion in some
♦ Terminal coma for several hours
♦ Milder disease in a few cases of:
  • Tremor
  • Stumbling gait
  • Blindness
  • Pica

Reproductive inefficiency

♦ Abortion
♦ Small litter size
♦ Mummification, stillbirths

Congenital defects

For example:
♦ Cerebellar hypoplasia
♦ Myoclonia congenita
♦ Microcephaly
♦ Pulmonary hypogenesis
♦ Joint deformity

Clinical pathology

♦ In acute disease, marked leukopenia early, leukocytosis in late stages
♦ Animal inoculation in immune, non-immune pigs the ultimate test for diagnosis of disease in a country
♦ Serological tests used but limited value in acute disease; commonly cross-react with bovine virus diarrhea virus, give positive reactions with vaccinates; tests used include
  • ELISA excellent for herd diagnosis
  • Neutralizing peroxidase-linked antibody assay

Necropsy findings

No changes in peracute cases.

Acute cases

♦ Generalized petechiation common but not constant; most visible under kidney capsule, in bladder, larynx, lymph nodes, at ileocecal valve
♦ Lymph node enlargement
♦ Infarcts in spleen, gall bladder mucosa
♦ Non-suppurative encephalomyelitis
♦ Detection of virus antigen in tissue or tissue culture by:
  • Fluorescent antibody staining
  • Agar gel precipitation test

Diagnosis

Acute hog cholera resembles:
♦ African swine fever
♦ Salmonellosis
♦ Acute erysipelas
♦ Acute pasteurellosis
Nervous form resembles:
♦ Viral encephalomyelitis
♦ Salmonellosis

Treatment

Hyperimmune serum has been used.

Control

Outbreak control in hog-cholera-free areas

♦ Eradication by slaughter of infected, in-contact pigs
♦ Quarantine all piggeries; no movement unless to immediate slaughter
♦ All pig transports, premises, utensils disinfected with 5% cresylic acid
♦ Footwear, clothing, and vehicle tires disinfected before leaving infected premises
♦ Garbage feeding forbidden, or thoroughly boiled

Outbreak control in enzootic area

♦ Isolate infected animals; hygiene to contain infection
♦ Burn dead animals
♦ Scrape, clean disinfect premises with 5% cresylic acid
♦ Hyperimmune serum to pigs in infected pens, vaccination later
♦ Vaccination in-contact pens, all other pigs on the property
♦ Intelligent use of the best vaccine:
  • Killed and chemically inactivated vaccines, e.g. crystal violet vaccine, are insufficiently immunogenic
  • Living attenuated virus vaccine preferred
  • Virulent virus, combined with serum, gives more solid immunity but risk of causing disease
♦ Educate farmers to:
  • Stop garbage feeding, or boil it properly
  • Avoid buying suspect pigs and selling sick, suspect pigs

Eradication

♦ Reduce infection rate by:
  • Eliminating garbage feeding
  • Widespread vaccination program
Final program to include:
♦ Cessation of vaccination to prevent crea-

tion of carrier pigs, and mild and chronic forms of the disease
♦ Complete prohibition of community feeder pig sales
♦ Elimination of carriers from infected herds; difficulty is identifying them; simpler but more costly to slaughter out all the infected herds, burning all carcases to prevent recycling through swill cycle

AFRICAN SWINE FEVER (AFRICAN PIG DISEASE, WARTHOG DISEASE)
[VM8 p. 935]

Etiology

An arbovirus tentatively classified as belonging to the family Iridoviridae.

Epidemiology

Occurrence
♦ Originated in Africa as disease of warthogs, wild pigs with cycles recurring every 10–12 years
♦ Now a serious threat to pig production in the Mediterranean countries, West Indies; eradicated from Spain, France, Italy, Belgium in recent years
♦ Originally appeared as an epidemic with morbidity, case fatality rates approximating 100%; now subsided ta a case fatality rate of <2%

Source and transmission
♦ Clinically normal, viremic warthogs, wild pigs, sick and clinically normal, long-time carriers amongst domestic pigs are source
♦ Transmission in Africa by tick *Ornithodorus moubata*; virus persists in tick for long periods; in Europe by *Ornithodorus erraticus*. Other *Ornithodorus* spp. ticks in North America and *Haematopinus suis* are potential vectors
♦ Transmission between domestic pigs in close contact with each other is by ingestion of feed contaminated by feces, or other excretions of infected pig
♦ Spread between pens probably by infected fomites including uncooked garbage

Risk factors
♦ A number of strains of varying virulence exists
♦ Virus resists most environmental insults

Importance
♦ Has caused massive death losses
♦ Presence in a country invites disbarment of its pork industry from international trade

Clinical findings

Acute disease
♦ Early outbreaks when disease introduced to naive herd
♦ 5–15 day incubation
♦ High fever for 4 days
♦ Purplish blotching belly, snout, limbs, ears skin
♦ Anorexia, depression, huddling together
♦ Disinclination to move, stumbling gait,, especially hind limbs
♦ Nasal, ocular mucopurulent discharge
♦ Dyspnea, cough in some
♦ Diarrhea, dysentery, vomiting in some
♦ Abortion
♦ Death in all cases after 2–4 days, preceded in some by convulsions

Subacute and chronic disease
♦ Depression, fever for 2–3 weeks, some continue eating
♦ Subacute cases recover
♦ Chronic cases emaciated, soft, edematous swellings over joints, under mandible
♦ Case fatality about 5%

Clinical pathology

♦ Severe leukopenia by day 4; pronounced lymphopenia, immature neutrophils; hypergammaglobulinemia in chronic cases
♦ Antigen detected by fluorescent antibody technique in tonsil, lymph node
♦ Serological tests recommended include:
  • ELISA
  • Immunoblotting assay
  • Monoclonal antibody immunoperoxidase test

Necropsy findings

♦ As for hog cholera but more severe
♦ Generalized petechiation common but not constant; most visible under kidney capsule, in bladder, larynx, lymph nodes, at the ileocecal valve
♦ Lymph node enlargement due to lymphadenitis
♦ Infarcts in spleen and gall bladder mucosa
♦ Pericarditis
♦ Interstitial pneumonia
♦ Button ulcers in cecum/colon
♦ Non-suppurative encephalomyelitis
♦ Marked lymphocyte karyorrhexis
♦ For detection of virus in tissue use:
  • ELISA
  • Radioimmunoassay tests
  • Growth in swine monocyte culture

Diagnosis

Resembles hog cholera.

Treatment

Nil.

Control

♦ Prohibition of imports and introductions
♦ Tick control
♦ No vaccine available
♦ In outbreak
  • Quarantine
  • Slaughter infected and in contact pigs
  • Hygiene of pens and utensils using strong caustic soda solution .

EQUINE INFECTIOUS ANEMIA
(SWAMP FEVER) [VM8 p. 940]

Etiology

Retrovirus (subfamily Lentivirinae) with many serotypes and a lot of antigenic drift between them.

Epidemiology

♦ Worldwide
♦ Horses only, all ages and classes
♦ Highest incidence in wooded, wet, warm environments
♦ With large insect populations, especially biting flies (e.g. *Stomoxys* spp) and mosquitoes (*Psorophora columbiae*)
♦ Slow spread in a community
♦ Sporadic cases only
♦ Morbidity very low,; mortality rate exceeds 50%

Source

♦ Infected animals, mostly subclinical carriers can remain infective for years
♦ Non-sterile animal products of equine origin, administered by injection

Transmission

♦ Insect bite
♦ Passive by hypodermic needle or surgical instrument
♦ Milk of infected dam
♦ Semen of infected stallion
♦ Via intact mucosa by swabbing in dope testing

Risk factors

♦ Summer–autumn
♦ Bush-covered terrain
♦ Heavy insect populations

Clinical findings

♦ Slow spread in a community
♦ Recurrent attacks

First attack

♦ Incubation period 2–4 weeks
♦ Anorexia, depression, weight loss
♦ Tremor
♦ Staggering walk, recumbency
♦ Intermittent fever
♦ Jaundice
♦ Ventral, preputial edema
♦ Mucosal, conjunctival petechiation
♦ Tachycardia, cardiac arrhythmia constant signs
♦ Serosanguineous nasal discharge
♦ Profuse diarrhea in some
♦ Splenic enlargement palpable rectally
♦ Abortion
♦ Course of few days to 3 weeks
♦ Most cases show temporary improvement then repeat attack
♦ Others recumbent, die gradually in 10–14 days

Relapse attacks

♦ Milder signs for 2 weeks
♦ Poor work performance
♦ Mucosal pallor
♦ Attacks cease after a year

Clinical pathology

♦ Marked thrombocytopenia in some
♦ Erythrocyte count falls after first attack
♦ Leukopenia, neutropenia, lymphopenia
♦ Blood changes severe in initial attack, subdued subsequently
♦ Episodes of hemolytic disease, blood loss anemia
♦ Agar gel immunodiffusion test (AGID) used widely for identification of disease, suitable for eradication program
♦ ELISA, indirect hemagglutination, complement fixation tests also available

Necropsy findings

Acute stage

♦ Jaundice
♦ General petechiation
♦ Subcutis edema
♦ Spleen and liver enlargement

Chronic stage
- Pallor
- Emaciation
- Proliferation of reticuloendothelial tissue, vascular intima, round cell infiltrations in liver, glomerulitis, hemosiderosis.

Diagnosis

Resembles:
- Purpura hemorrhagica
- Babesiosis
- Ehrlichiosis
- Leptospirosis
- Strongylosis
- Fascioliasis

Treatment

Supportive blood transfusions, haematinics.

Control

- Eradication by AGID test, slaughter of reactors, compensation
- Probability of reinfection by insect vectors discourages draconian measures
- Prevention of introduction requires two negative AGID tests 6 months apart in quarantine or under close surveillance
- Vaccines available but not in general use
- Hygiene needed in sterilizing surgical equipment
- Single-use hypodermic needles
- Insect repellents and control reduce spread.

BOVINE EPHEMERAL FEVER (BEF)
[VM8 p. 944]

Etiology

Unnamed, insect-borne rhabdovirus.

Epidemiology

Occurrence
- African continent, Asia, Australia
- Only cattle affected; serological evidence of infection in African wildlife
- Mostly in 6 months to 2 years old
- In enzootic areas morbidity 5–10%
- In naive area outbreaks morbidity 35–100%, case fatality rate <1%

Source and transmission
- Source is cattle with clinical disease
- Possibly unknown other silent hosts
- Transmitted by mosquitoes (*Aedes*, *Ano-*

pheles, Culex spp.), sandflies (*Culicoides brevitarsis*)

Risk factors
- Summer disease
- Spread on prevailing wind
- Cyclical diminution, then resurgence as population loses immunity

Importance
- Loss of production on a large scale in outbreak
- Temporary infertility, likelihood of mastitis

Clinical findings

- Acute onset
- A number affected at same time
- Fever, anorexia, drop in milk yield
- Diarrhea or constipation
- Stringy nasal, watery ocular discharges
- Head-shaking, tremor
- Stiffness, muscle spasms, arched back, feet placed under the body
- Hind limb paresis, then recumbency for about 48 hours
- Recumbent posture like milk fever
- Some have subcutaneous emphysema
- Spontaneous recovery after 3–5 days
- Few develop aspiration pneumonia or myopathy and permanent recumbency

Clinical pathology

- Leukocytosis, left shift, lymphopenia early
- Plasma fibrinogen levels elevated
- Many well-regarded serological tests, including AGID and a blocking ELISA

Necropsy findings

- Moderate serofibrinous polyserositis in all cavities plus aggregations of neutrophils in surrounding tissues
- Lymph nodes enlarged

Diagnosis

Resembles:
- Traumatic reticuloperitonitis
- Laminitis
- Parturient paresis

Treatment

Phenylbutazone, flunixin meglumine cause complete remission of signs.

Control

Vaccination is the only prospect, but no widely accepted and tested vaccine available commercially.

AFRICAN HORSE SICKNESS (AHS)
[VM8 p. 946]

Etiology

An orbivirus with nine known, probably many more, antigenic strains.

Epidemiology

Occurrence
♦ African continent, spread in recent times to Spain and Portugal
♦ Horses, mules, donkeys, zebras with decreasing frequency
♦ Dogs by eating infected meat
♦ Goats, ferrets, mice, guinea-pigs, rats by experimental infection
♦ Elephants seroconvert on exposure
♦ Infection prevalence, morbidity, varies with insect population; case fatality rate 90%

Source and transmission
♦ Infected Equidae
♦ Possibly also a silent host, e.g. dogs, elephants
♦ Transmission only by insect vector, e.g. *Hyalomma dromedarii* (tick), *Culicoides* spp. (biting midge), *Aedes aegypti, Anopheles stephensi, Culex pipiens* (mosquitoes)

Risk factors
♦ Low, swampy areas with high insect populations
♦ Warm weather
♦ Cyclic outbreaks at 10–20 year intervals
♦ Strong immunity in survivors

Importance
♦ Heavy death losses
♦ Continued cost of control because eradication impossible

Clinical findings

Pulmonary horse sickness
♦ The common form in naive horses
♦ Incubation period 5–7 days
♦ Anorexia
♦ Intermittent fever
♦ Dyspnea, paroxysmal cough

♦ Profuse, yellow, serous to frothy, nasal discharge
♦ Profuse sweating
♦ Staggery gait, recumbency
♦ Death at day 4–5

Cardiac horse sickness
♦ Common in enzootic areas
♦ Incubation period up to 3 weeks
♦ Restless, mild abdominal pain in some
♦ Intermittent fever
♦ Late edema of temporal fossae, eyelids, lips, chest in some
♦ Bluish oral mucosa
♦ Sublingual petechiae in some
♦ Muffled heart sounds due to hydropericardium
♦ Crackling and absent breath sounds due to pulmonary edema
♦ Dysphagia, nasal regurgitation
♦ Most die after course up to 2 weeks

Horse sickness fever
♦ In enzootic areas, in partially immune horses
♦ Intermittent, mild fever for 1–3 days
♦ Anorexia
♦ Conjunctivitis
♦ Moderate dyspnea

Clinical pathology

Effective tests include:
♦ Agar gel immunodiffusion test (AGID)
♦ Indirect fluorescent antibody (IFA)
♦ Complement fixation test (CF)
♦ Virus neutralization
♦ ELISA tests

Necropsy findings

Pulmonary horse sickness
♦ Hydrothorax, pulmonary edema, ascites
♦ Bowel wall edema
♦ Liver congestion

Cardiac horse sickness
♦ Hydropericardium, anasarca, especially the head
♦ Endocardial hemorrhage, myocardial degeneration

Diagnosis

♦ Outbreaks of disease resembling pulmonary horse sickness do not occur
♦ **Cardiac horse sickness** resembles:
  • Purpura hemorrhagica
  • Equine infectious anemia

Treatment and Control

◆ No treatment
◆ Introduction to a country may be airborne insects, infected horses by aircraft
◆ Importation may be permitted into 30-day, insect-proof quarantine, from free areas, vaccination of all horses in 16 km radius of quarantine point
◆ In enzootic area, vaccinate all equidae in area or in buffer to limit spread
◆ Vaccine must contain multiple relevant strains
◆ Commonest is a killed, whole virus vaccine, two injections, one month apart, repeated every 6 months

ENCEPHALOMYOCARDITIS VIRUS
DISEASE OF PIGS [VM8 p. 949]

Etiology

A cardiovirus of the family Picornaviridae.

Epidemiology

Occurrence
◆ Reported from many countries
◆ A virus infection of rodents transmitted to pigs, humans
◆ High incidence of subclinical infections
◆ Myocarditis common in young pigs, sporadic cases or outbreaks, case fatality rate 50%
◆ Also causes significant reproductive failure especially stillbirths, fetal mummification in gilts, sows
◆ Disease in pigs may be related to plague of rats and mice

Clinical findings

Myocarditis in young pigs
◆ Found dead or drop dead during feeding or excitement
◆ Inappetence, depression
◆ Tremor, incoordination
◆ Dyspnea
◆ Death after course of few days

Reproductive disease
◆ Inappetence, fever in dam
◆ Farrowing at about 110 days
◆ Mummified fetuses, stillbirths, weak piglets dying of crush injury

Clinical pathology

◆ Neutralizing antibodies 5–7 days after infection in sows, healthy in-contact pigs; persist several months
◆ Serological tests used include:
  • Hemagglutination inhibition
  • Agar gel immunodiffusion
  • Microtiter serum neutralization test

Necropsy findings

◆ Skin reddening
◆ Excess fibrinous fluid in serosal cavities
◆ Myocardial necrosis appearing as focal, diffuse myocardial pallor
◆ Virus in heart muscle, brain, and other tissues

Diagnosis

Resembles:
◆ Peracute septicemias of sucking pigs, e.g. colibacillosis
◆ Gut edema
◆ Mulberry heart disease
◆ Nutritional deficiency vitamin E and selenium

Treatment

Nil.

Control

Rodent control.

RIFT VALLEY FEVER (RVF)
[VM8 p. 950]

Etiology

A phlebovirus, of the family Bunyaviridae; 3 strains.

Epidemiology

Occurrence
◆ African continent only; large potential for spread
◆ Susceptible hosts include all ruminants, monkeys, humans, rodents, possibly horses; resistant species – pigs, poultry, rabbits, guinea-pigs
◆ Outbreaks outside an enzootic area kill many young ruminants and cause abortions in adults

Source and transmission

♦ Viremic animals; up to 20% cattle in enzootic areas seroconvert each year
♦ Transmission by mosquitoes, other blood-sucking insects

Risk factors

♦ Forested areas with heavy insect populations worst
♦ Cyclical outbreaks at 5 year intervals; large outbreaks in humans

Importance

♦ Death losses in animals
♦ Serious zoonosis

Clinical findings

Young ruminants

♦ 12 hour incubation period
♦ Fever
♦ Staggery gait, recumbency
♦ Death within 36 hours

Adults

Some deaths. Abortion the common finding.

Clinical pathology

♦ Severe leukopenia
♦ Efficient serological tests include ELISA, serum neutralization, hemagglutination, agar gel immunodiffusion, complement fixation tests

Necropsy findings

♦ Severe hepatic necrosis, especially lambs and calves
♦ Specific diagnosis by immunohistochemical localization of viral antigen

Diagnosis

Resembles:
♦ Wesselbrons disease
♦ Bluetongue in sheep
♦ Bovine ephemeral fever
♦ Enterotoxemia

Treatment

Nil.

Control

♦ Prevention of introduction requires prohibited importation animals, products, insects from infected countries

♦ Human carriers may be the vehicle
♦ Insect control and vaccination in infected areas
♦ Annual vaccination with killed or mutagenic attenuated vaccine recommended; simple attenuated vaccines abortigenic, teratogenic

AKABANE VIRUS DISEASE OF CATTLE (ENZOOTIC BOVINE ARTHROGRYPOSIS AND HYDRANENCEPHALY) [VM8 p. 951]

Etiology

A bunyavirus.

Epidemiology

Occurrence

Cyclic (5–10 years) epizootics Australia, Israel, Kenya, Japan, and Korea

Source and transmission

♦ From infected domestic ruminants
♦ Seroconversion also in camels and horses
♦ Transmission by *Culicoides brevitarsis, C. nebeculosis* (biting midges), possibly others

Risk factors

♦ Wet season, large insect population
♦ Large population of early pregnant cows, ewes and does in a seasonal breeding program

Clinical findings

♦ Abortions, premature births in autumn, in some countries only
♦ Deformed young in midwinter
♦ First affected young have arthrogryposis:
  • Dystokia
  • dully formed but underweight
  • Unable to rise, stand, or walk
  • Congenital articular rigidity in 1 to 4 limbs; limb fixed usually in flexion, few in extension
  • Limb muscles severe atrophy
  • Vertebral column deformity
♦ In mid-outbreak some calves with arthrogryposis and hydranencephaly
♦ **Hydranencephaly** in second half of outbreak:
  • Calf can stand, walk

- Blind, lack normal instincts; no dam-seeking but can suck
- Very late cases ataxic, weak and fall easily.

Clinical pathology

LISA test shows high antibody titer in dam and surviving neonates.

Necropsy findings

Arthrogryposis

Joint fixation, joint surfaces normal, tendon contracture, joints freed by severing tendons, muscle atrophy. Ventral horn cells deficient in spinal cord.

Hydranencephaly

Cerebral hemispheres absent, replaced by fluid-filled meninges; porencephaly only in some, others have small brain stem and cerebellum.

Diagnosis

Resembles:
♦ Inherited congenital articular rigidity
♦ Inherited arthrogryposis
♦ Nutritional deficiency of manganese
♦ Poisoning by *Nicotiana, Datura, Lupinus* spp.
♦ Other viruses known or suspected of causing similar deformities to Akabane virus include:
  • Cache Valley virus
  • Chuzan virus
  • Aino virus

Treatment

Calves not viable because lesion irreversible.

Control

♦ Only feasible control is vaccination
♦ An effective killed vaccine available but use unlikely because of infrequence of disease.

ENZOOTIC BOVINE LEUKOSIS (BOVINE LYMPHOSARCOMA)
[VM8 p. 954]

Etiology

The bovine leukemia virus, a C type retrovirus.

Epidemiology

Occurrence
♦ Many countries especially Europe, North and South America
♦ Natural infection only in cattle, experimental transmission to sheep is easy
♦ Does not spread quickly; herd infection rate small; within herd infection prevalence up to 100%, within herd mortality 2–5%
♦ Prevalence higher in dairy than in beef herds
♦ No breed susceptibility
♦ Rarely in animals younger than 2 years

Source and transmission
♦ Infected cattle the source; infected animals permanently infected and act as source of infection in spite of development of specific antibodies
♦ Close physical contact and exchange of infective biological material required for transmission
♦ Virus contained in lymphocytes in blood, milk, tumor masses
♦ Transmission by biting insects, bats or human interventions such as dehorning shears, emasculator; not by artificial insemination or embryo transfer unless the material contains lymphocytes; transmission by rectal examination is possible but judged to occur very rarely
♦ Transmission by drinking infected milk may occur in the very young but appears to occur very rarely
♦ Transplacental transmission occurs in a small proportion, probably less than 10%, of cows at risk

Risk factors
♦ Most patients infected by the virus do not develop the neoplastic disease. Those that do are predisposed by their genetic makeup
♦ Similarly, patients with the persistent lymphocytosis form of the disease are so because of their genetic constitution
♦ Distinct familial tendency to develop the full-blown disease or the persistent lymphocytosis; but genetic resistance can be overcome by large dose of virus, period of stress

♦ Increased prevalence after 24 months old
♦ New herd infections usually caused by introduction of an infected animal

Importance

♦ Serious cause of wastage by death, culling on individual farms; loss to the industry minor because of low prevalence
♦ Stud herds likely to suffer decreased demand for their cattle
♦ All the evidence points to enzootic bovine leukosis **not** being a zoonosis

Clinical findings

Adult multicentric lymphosarcoma

♦ Incubation period 4–5 years, i.e. signs appear in the 4–8 year age group
♦ Many have had lymphocytosis without clinical signs for years
♦ 5–10% die suddenly without prior signs; death due to:
  • Adrenal gland involvement
  • Abomasal ulcer rupture
  • Splenic rupture
♦ Most have course 1 week to several months with signs:
  • Weight loss
  • Anorexia
  • Anemia, pallor
  • Weakness, stumbling gait, difficulty rising
  • Some have fever (when tumor growth rapid)
  • Tachycardia, arrhythmia (myocardial involvement)
  • Any one of the following syndromes, or multiple combinations of them
  • When diagnostic clinical signs present death only 2–3 weeks away

Superficial lymphadenectasia

♦ Superficial lymph node enlargement an early sign in most cases
♦ Multiple enlarged haemolymph nodes on perineum and flanks
♦ Enlarged nodes palpable rectally, often with spread to peritoneum and pelvic viscera
♦ In many all the nodes are enlarged, in others only a few, e.g. the nodes of the head plus the mandibular symphysis
♦ Lesions firm, resilient
♦ Occasionally body surface covered with multiple 5–10 cm dia. subcutaneous masses

Abomasal lymphosarcoma

Abomasal wall involvement causes:
♦ Capricious appetite
♦ Persistent, sloppy diarrhea
♦ Melena from a bleeding ulcer
♦ Chronic bloat due to mediastinal lymph node enlargement

Cardiac lymphosarcoma

Right ventricular wall involvement cause right heart congestive failure:
♦ Muffled heart sounds due to hydropericardium
♦ Dyspnea due to hydrothorax
♦ Jugular vein engorgement
♦ Brisket, intermandibular space edema
♦ Tachycardia, arrhythmia
♦ Systolic murmur with an associated jugula pulse exaggeration
♦ Liver enlargement
♦ Diarrhea due to portal hypertension

Peripheral nerve root, spinal cord tumor

♦ Gradual onset of paralysis in hind limbs over several weeks, sometimes one limb more than the other
♦ Begins as knuckling at fetlock
♦ Stumbling gait
♦ Difficulty rising
♦ Recumbency

Cutaneous lymphosarcoma

♦ Very rare; seen only in cattle less than 3 years old
♦ Cutaneous plaques 1–5 cm dia. on neck back, croup, and sides
♦ Scab develops, hair lost, scab shed, plaque shrinks, disappears, recurs several years later with general involvement of interna organs

Bone leukosis

In calf form of disease: lameness, posterior ataxia, dyspnea, lymphadenectasia; multiple bone infarcts, bone marrow necrosis.

Juvenile lymphosarcoma

♦ In calves 2 weeks to 6 months; may be present at birth or as late as 2 years
♦ Gradual weight loss
♦ Sudden enlargement all lymph nodes
♦ Depression, fever, weakness, tachycardia
♦ Posterior paresis
♦ Bloat in some cases
♦ Congestive heart failure in some

Miscellaneous lesions

Include:
♦ Cranial meningeal lesions causing signs of

space-occupying lesion with localizing signs (see brain tumor)

- Retropharyngeal lymph node enlargement causing dyspnea, snoring (see pharyngeal obstruction)
- Periorbital lesions causing uni- or bilateral eye protrusion
- Periureteral lesion causing uni- or bilateral hydronephrosis
- Uterine wall with lesions palpable like irregularly shaped cotyledons
- Kidney tumors causing irregularly shaped kidney, possibly uremia
- Thymic tumor, chiefly in young beef cattle causing dyspnea, jugular vein engorgement, brisket edema

Clinical pathology

Diagnostic tests to be used vary with the stage of the disease.

Diagnosis of viral infection

- used in very early stages or when seeking a definitive, etiological diagnosis
- Serological test acceptable for diagnosis because of cost of virus identification
- Preferred serological tests:
  - Agar gel diffusion test (AGID) – the official screening test to identify presence of infection in herd
  - Radioimmunoassay (RIA); for identification of individual cases
  - ELISA for herd diagnosis – more sensitive than AGID
  - A protein immunoblot test – comparable to ELISA
- Virological tests include:
  - Patient leukocytes inoculated onto lamb spleen cell tissue culture
  - Transmission of infection from patient to seronegative sheep
  - Virus identified by:
  - Electron microscopy
  - Fluorescent antibody technique (FAT)
  - Enzyme-linked immunoabsorbent assay (ELISA)
  - Radioimmunoassay (RIA)
  - Syncytial infectivity assay

Diagnosis of persistent lymphocytosis

- An elevation of absolute lymphocyte count to more than 3 times the standard deviation above the normal mean for the breed, age group, persisting for more than 3 months
- More than 25% of the cells being abnormal, immature also considered to be diagnostic

Diagnosis of lymphosarcoma

Histological examination of needle biopsy aspirate is adequate.

Necropsy findings

- Firm, white tumor masses in any organ
- in neonates and young patients, common sites in kidney, thymus, liver, spleen, lymph nodes
- In adults, heart, abomasum, and spinal cord are common sites
- Cardiac lesions most commonly in right atrium
- Abomasum lesion is gross, uneven thickening in submucosa, especially close to pylorus; similar lesions also in intestine wall; some lesions ulcerated
- Nervous system lesions include thickening of nerve roots close to cord at lumbosacral, rarely cervical, level
- Swollen lymph nodes may contain yellow necrotic center
- Tumors are masses of lymphocytic cells

Diagnosis

Differential diagnosis of each of the common syndromes of enzootic bovine leukosis includes the following.

Lymphadenectasia

- Tuberculosis
- Fat necrosis for internal lymph node involvement

Abomasal lymphosarcoma

- Abomasal ulcer
- Johne's disease

Cardiac lymphosarcoma

- Traumatic pericarditis
- Valvular disease, endocarditis

Spinal cord nerve roots lymphosarcoma

- Rabies
- Spinal cord abscess
- Spondylosis

Treatment

- Has been undertaken to prolong life of patient for purpose of obtaining semen or ova for multiplication
- Drugs used include nitrogen mustard, triethylenemelamine, L-asparaginase

Control

Eradication

♦ Severest policy is eradication in herds, reduction of prevalence to virtual eradication
level in an area
♦ Compulsory cull and slaughter programs
based on AGID test used but very expensive in terms of cows destroyed due to
positive persistent lymphocytosis test
♦ Any eradication program runs the risks of
reinfection of herd by importation of
infected animal, and introduction of infection by insect vectors

Limitation of incidence

♦ Embryo transfer from infected dams to
negative recipients plus immediate isolation of neonates
♦ Alternative is a two-herd scheme based on
need for close contact for spread to occur –
test-and-segregate method: herd divided
on basis of AGID test; herds maintained at
least 200 meters apart, with another location for quarantine of imported animals
which need to be tested twice at 30-day
intervals
♦ Herd retested every 3 then 6 months until
herd free
♦ Avoidance of procedures likely to transmit
infection, e.g. dehorning, castration without disinfection
♦ Calves reared on milk from seronegative
cows
♦ Insect control

PORCINE EPIZOOTIC LYMPHOSARCOMA [VM8 p. 960]

♦ Rare pig disease of unidentified cause in
young animals
♦ Signs include:
• Emaciation, stunted growth
• Anorexia
• Pot belly
• Peripheral lymph node enlargement
• Lymphocytosis, immature cells

EQUINE SPORADIC LYMPHOSARCOMA [VM8 p. 960]

♦ In horses older than 6 years
♦ Subcutaneous enlargements, may ulcerate
♦ Lymphadenectasia, internal, external
♦ Jugular vein engorgement
♦ Cardiac irregularity
♦ Exophthalmia
♦ Anasarca
♦ Eyelid swelling, bilateral
♦ Most patients die within a month
Also recorded in horses are:
♦ Malignant lymphoma with ulcerative
pharyngitis
♦ Diffuse small intestinal lymphoma in adult
horses characterized by:
• Malabsorption syndrome, with or with-
out diarrhea
• Hypoalbuminemia
• Serum gamma globulin levels elevated
• Anemia

VIRAL DISEASES CHARACTERIZED BY ALIMENTARY TRACT SIGNS

FOOT AND MOUTH DISEASE (FMD, APHTHOUS FEVER) [VM8 p. 965]

Etiology

♦ An aphthovirus of the Picornaviridiae fam-
ily
♦ Seven major serotypes A, O, C, SAT
(Southern African Territories) 1, SAT 2,
SAT 3, Asia 1
♦ A large number of antigenically different
subtypes of varying virulence; strains with
animal host specificity
♦ Mutation within serotypes common

Epidemiology

Occurrence

♦ All cloven-hoofed domestic and wild animals
♦ Notable eradications, freedom in some
countries but enzootic in Africa, South
America, Asia, much of Europe
♦ Main serotypes have limited geographical
prevalence
♦ Occurs as outbreaks, mostly when infection introduced into a naive country, or
introduction of a new serotype into an
enzootic country
♦ Morbidity approximates 100%; case fatality rate low, e.g. 2% in adults, up to 20% in
calves

Source and transmission

- Source is excretions of infected animals, clinical cases or inert carriers
- Transmission by ingestion or inhalation of virus on fomites, in meat, other products, in all excretions and secretions or by direct contact
- Common source introducing virus to naive country is meat scraps fed in swill to pigs

Risk factors

- Virus very resistant to environmental influence, surviving a year in premises, 10–12 weeks in clothing, 4 weeks on hair, long periods on pasture in cool weather but susceptible to sunlight, dryness, heat, pH changes away from neutral, insensitive to freezing, most disinfectants except caustic soda and formalin
- Virus survives long periods in aerosol form in temperate, tropical climates, travels long distances (e.g. 250 km) in direction of prevailing wind
- After an attack, cattle are immune 4 years, pigs 5 months; new outbreaks during immune period usually due to infection by new serotype

Importance

The most important bovine disease because of the savage restriction on importation of animals and their products from countries where FMD occurs.

Clinical findings

Cattle

- Incubation 3–6 days
- High fever
- Dramatic fall in milk yield
- Severe depression, anorexia
- Acute, painful stomatitis
- Stringy saliva drools from mouth
- Lip smacking
- Careful chewing
- Vesicles, bullae, containing clear, serous fluid, on buccal mucosa, tongue, dental pad, on coronets and skin of interdigital cleft
- Vesicles rupture easily, leaving raw circular area
- Severe lameness, often recumbency, due to coronet lesions
- Acute weight loss, reduced milk production
- Lesions heal quickly, course of a week
- **Complications** include:
  - Heavy mortality in calves due to myocarditis

- Sudden death with heart irregularity due to myocarditis
- Dysentery, diarrhea
- Ascending posterior paralysis
- **Sequels** include:
- Abortion
- Mastitis
- 'Panting' with dyspnea, hair overgrowth, poor heat tolerance
- Diabetes mellitus

Sheep, goats, pigs

- Mild form of cattle disease
- The only severe lesions are on the feet causing lameness
- Some pigs have dramatic lesions on snout
- High lamb mortality due to myocarditis

Clinical pathology

- Tests used on fresh fluid from vesicles, sera used for identification of FMD virus, its serotype, and differentiation from the other vesicular diseases include:
  - Tissue culture, neutralization by specific sera
  - Complement fixation test
  - Virus infection associated antigen test (VIA)
  - ELISA, indirect ELISA
  - Propagation of virus in unweaned white mice
  - Intradermal injection into guinea pig plantar pads
  - Large animal inoculation helps separate the vesicular diseases (see Table 21.1)

Necropsy findings

- Vesicles and erosions on buccal mucosa, coronets, and udder
- Secondary bacterial infection causes ulceration of vesicular lesions
- Vesicles may extend down alimentary and respiratory tracts
- Hemorrhages, pale streaking in myocardium in neonates, rarely adults

Diagnosis

Resembles:

- Vesicular stomatitis, and other vesiculoviruses
- Vesicular exanthema of swine
- Swine vesicular disease
- Mycotoxins from fungal infections of celery and, parsnips
- Bluetongue in sheep

Table 21.1 Differentiation of acute vesicular diseases [VM8 p. 970]

Animal species	Route of inoculation	Foot-and-mouth disease	Vesicular stomatitis	Vesicular exanthema of swine	Swine vesicular disease	Bluetongue
NATURAL INFECTION						
Cattle		+	+	−	−	(rarely occurs)
Pig*		+	+	+	+	−
Sheep and goat		+	±|+	−	−	+
Horse		−	+	−	−	−
EXPERIMENTAL TRANSMISSION						
Cattle	Intradermal in tongue, gums, lips	+	+	−	−	+
	Intramuscular	+	−	−	−	
Pig*	Intradermal in snout, lips	+	+	+	+	
	Intravenous	+	+	+	+	+
	Intramuscular	+	−	−	+	
Sheep and goat	Various	+	+	−	(+) (no lesions)	+
Horse	Intradermal in tongue	−	+	+ (some strains)	−	
	Intramuscular			(some strains)	−	−
Guinea-pig	Intradermal in footpad	+	+	−	−	−
UWW mice		+	+	−	+	+ (hamster also)
Adult chicken	Intradermal in tongue	+	+	−	−	−

*White-skinned pigs fed on parsnips or celery and exposed to sunlight develop vesicles.

Treatment

Flunixin meglumide provides good symptomatic response.

Control

The choice is between:
 Eradication, suited to countries with sea boundaries or FMD-free neighbours
 Vaccination when threat of reinvasion constant
 Combination of vaccination until incidence low then eradication

Eradication
♦ Clinical cases, in-contacts slaughtered, buried or burned
♦ No reclamation of meat
♦ Milk destroyed
♦ Disinfection or destruction of all inert material, including vehicles and housing
♦ Disinfection by 2% sodium hydroxide or formalin or 5% sodium carbonate *after* complete cleaning
♦ Farm left unstocked 6 months
♦ Trial restocking with sentinel herd first
♦ Clothing chemically disinfected or boiled
♦ All movement off and on to farm supervised
♦ Quarantine all farms within 16–24 km radius; no animal movement, only supervised human movements

Entry prevention
For protection of a clean population includes:
♦ Complete embargo on importation of animals, products, contact materials from hazardous environments; exceptions must be tested by lengthy quarantine period and adequate negative tests
♦ Embargo on meats or refuse from transport vehicles
♦ Clothing, effects of humans from high risk origins disinfected
♦ Semen, fertilized ova, except those with intact zona pellucida, banned from hazardous origins

Vaccination
♦ Mass vaccination of all ruminants annually used in high risk countries
♦ Ring or frontier vaccination used to contain an outbreak or protect a boundary
♦ Killed, trivalent (O, A, C strains) vaccines grown on tissue culture the standard; protection for 6–8 months
♦ Preparation of vaccines containing other, locally more relevant serotypes now common
♦ Progam continues as annual plus calves every 6 months to ensure first vaccination at 4–10 months
♦ Attenuated, lapinized vaccines used extensively in countries where prevalence high and killed vaccines inadequate

SWINE VESICULAR DISEASE
[VM8 p. 974]

Etiology

An enterovirus of family Picornaviridae.

Epidemiology

Occurrence
♦ Comparatively new disease, since 1966
♦ Patchy occurrence in Europe and Asia
♦ Only in pigs; high morbidity but a mild disease with no fatalities

Source and transmission
♦ In vesicle fluid, oral, nasal secretions, feces
♦ Infection mostly short lives (3 weeks); some chronic for 3 months
♦ Rapid spread in group, transmission by direct contact or infected environment, through damaged skin or mucosae

Risk factors
♦ Virus extremely resistant to environmental conditions; survives long periods (6 months) on fomites, in meat, uncooked garbage
♦ Disinfection requires 2% sodium hydroxide, 8% formaldehyde or sodium hypochlorite 0.04% in sites free of organic matter; heating must exceed 68°C (154°F)
♦ Several strains of varying virulence suspected

Importance
Similarity to FMD necessitates prompt eradication causing serious losses.

Pathogenesis

♦ Invasion leads to viremia, localization in vesicles at buccal mucosa, snout skin, coronets, myocardium
♦ Massive discharge of virus from vesicle

Clinical findings

♦ Incubation period 2–14 days
♦ So mild that sick pigs may be missed
♦ Most pigs in pen will be affected
♦ Transient fever, anorexia
♦ Mild lameness, arched back; may not be evident in soft bedding
♦ Vesicles commonest at coronary band at heel, belly, tongue, lips, snout; commence as swollen, blanched skin, then vesicles, rupture, ulcers in some; may be very few in number in some outbreaks
♦ Rarely ataxia, circling, head pressing, convulsions
♦ Production loss minor
♦ Herd course 2–3 weeks

Clinical pathology

♦ Antigen demonstrated in vesicle tissue by fluorescent antibody, direct complement fixation test, grown on tissue culture
♦ Antibodies produced in 4–6 days, detected by serological tests including:
  • Virus neutralization
  • Double immunodiffusion
  • Counterimmunoelectrophoresis
  • ELISA

Necropsy findings

♦ No gross lesions to differentiate disease from other vesicular diseases
♦ Skin lesions plus necrotic foci in tonsils, renal pelvis, bladder, salivary glands, pancreas, myocardium
♦ Non-purulent meningoencephalitis

Diagnosis

For differentiation from other vesicular disease see Table 21.1.

Other causes of foot lameness in pigs include porcine foot rot.

Treatment

Nil.

Control

♦ Eradication by slaughter of clinical cases and in-contact pigs mandatory in most situations
♦ Depopulation, rigorous disinfection of site, complete disposal of carcases; no meat salvage

♦ Problem is mild nature of disease, prospect that infected pigs go unnoticed
♦ Complete prohibition of garbage feeding
♦ Closing of markets except for pigs going direct to slaughter
♦ No vaccination accredited for use
♦ Trial repopulation at 2–3 months

VESICULAR STOMATITIS
[VM8 p. 976]

Etiology

♦ A vesiculovirus, family Rhabdoviridae, in two antigenically distinct types – New Jersey (most common and virulent) and Indiana – and a number of subtypes

Epidemiology

Occurrence

♦ Western hemisphere
♦ Only in enzootics; cyclical outbreaks every 10–20 years.
♦ In cattle, deer, horses, donkeys, pigs; humans susceptible; not goats, sheep
♦ Seroconversion occurs in some rodent, ungulate, carnivoral wildlife
♦ No mortality, morbidity usually 5–10%, rarely 80% in dairy herds

Source and transmission

♦ Infected animals, especially deer, possibly wildlife reservoir
♦ Spread within herds by ingestion food infected by virus from ruptured oral vesicles, by milking procedures and embryo transfer
♦ Between herds spread by insect vector Simulium vittatum (biting fly), Aedes spp.(mosquitoes), Lutzomyia trapidoi (sand fly)

Risk factors

Heavy rainfall, low-lying, tropical areas.

Importance

♦ Interrupts milk supply
♦ Close resemblance to foot-and-mouth disease causes international consternation
♦ Causes a mild disease in humans

Clinical findings

♦ Incubation period a few days

Cattle

Fever
- Vesicles on lips, tongue dorsum, dental pad, buccal mucosa generally
- Ruptured vesicles cause ropy salivation
- Anorexia in most cases
- Some outbreaks lack vesicles, only erosive, necrotic lesions
- Teat lesions in milking cows can cause mastitis; rarely lesions on feet
- Recovery in 3–4 days

Horses
- Similar to cattle but lesions may be limited to tongue dorsum, lips
- Rarely lesions on udder or prepuce

Pigs

Lesions on or behind snout, or on feet, causing lameness.

Clinical pathology

Serological tests include complement fixation, serum neutralization, immunoelectroosmophoresis.

Necropsy findings

Necropsy not usually undertaken; no gross lesions other than vesicles.

Diagnosis

Resembles:
- Foot-and-mouth disease
- Necrotic glossitis in cattle
- Swine vesicular disease

Treatment and control

- Non-steroidal anti-inflammatories hasten recovery, reduce illness severity
- Hygiene to reduce spread within a milking herd
- Vaccination a possible technique, but mildness and infrequency of disease and low incidence do not encourage development

VESICULAR EXANTHEMA OF
SWINE [VM8 p. 978]

Etiology

A calicivirus of the family Caliciviridae; a number of antigenically different strains.

Epidemiology

Occurrence
- Has occurred only in continental USA, Hawaii, and Iceland
- Eradicated in 1959, after 27 years of existence
- Only in pigs, all ages and breeds
- Mild disease, low case fatality rate, less than 5%, higher in unweaned pigs

Source and transmission
- Live pigs, infected pork
- Virus in feces, saliva for up to 5 days after signs commence
- Infected pork scraps in raw garbage cause spread between farms
- On farm spread mostly by direct contact
- Virus resistant but indirect transmission uncommon
- Many subclinical cases
- Possibly a marine virus originated in marine animal garbage fed to pigs

Risk factors
- Readily destroyed by disinfectants
- Survives well in environment and meat
- Immunity for 20 months after attack

Importance
- Causes severe weight loss
- Abortion loss, sows go dry, piglet deaths
- Causes confusion with FMD diagnosis

Clinical findings

- Incubation period 1–3 days
- Severe depression, anorexia
- High fever
- Vesicles in mouth, on snout, teats, udder, coronet skin, sole, heel bulbs, between claws; commence as bleached area, fills with clear fluid, rupture leaving raw surface at 24–48 hours
- May be second crop of vesicles with face, tongue swelling
- In some outbreaks feet lesions predominate; cause severe lameness
- Recovery in 1–2 weeks
- Abortion, agalactia common

Clinical pathology

- Vesicle fluid checked for virus by tissue culture, animal transmission (see Table 21.1)
- Serological tests include complement fixation, virus neutralization in cell culture, gel diffusion precipitin tests

Necropsy findings

No diagnostic lesions other than superficial oral and skin lesions.

Diagnosis

For differential diagnosis vesicular diseases see Table 21.1.
Resembles lameness caused by:
◆ Porcine footrot
◆ Polyarthritis

Treatment

Nil.

Control

Eradication should be attempted:
◆ Slaughter all clinical cases, in contact pigs
◆ Destruction of carcases
◆ Clean and disinfect premises with 2% sodium hydroxide
◆ Ban garbage feeding

RINDERPEST (CATTLE PLAGUE)
[VM8 p. 980]

Etiology

A morbillivirus of the family Paramyxoviridae, with many strains of varying virulence but all antigenically identical.

Epidemiology

Occurrence
◆ An ancient European and Asiatic cattle plague
◆ Causes devastating epizootics in Asia, Africa, and the Middle East
◆ All ruminants and pigs susceptible but natural infection occurs commonly only in all ages and breeds of cattle and buffalo
◆ Susceptibility of goats and sheep varies between types of sheep; may play a part in epidemiology, pigs and camels do not
◆ Many ruminant wildlife become affected when cattle epizootics occurring
◆ Morbidity varies widely with history of disease; naive herds likely to be 100%; in enzootic areas usually 30%; case fatality rates likely to be 25–90%

Source and transmission
◆ In all secretions, excretions of clinical cases; uncommon for recovered animals to be source of virus for more than a few days
◆ Pigs, sheep, goats, camels, wild ruminant may be source; disease spreads readily t cattle from pigs, not from sheep and goats
◆ Ingestion, inhalation of aerosol; close contact needed because virus does not surviv more than a few hours outside the body; u to 30 minutes as aerosol in humid atmos phere

Risk factors
◆ Susceptible to most disinfectants, heat, dry ness, relatively resistant to cold
◆ Immunity after natural infection is long probably for life
◆ Infection causes extensive lymphocyte des truction and immunosuppression

Importance
◆ Massive death losses in nomadic popu lations or in enzootic countries where annual vaccination allowed to lapse
◆ Losses may be due to dehydration or secondary infections in immunosuppressed patients
◆ Introduction to a country would require a slaughter-out policy and loss of export markets

Clinical findings

Syndromes similar in all species except European pig breeds, clinically inapparent disease; Asian pig breeds develop full syndrome.

Acute rinderpest – in naive cattle
◆ Incubation period 6–9 days
◆ High fever without localizing signs for several days
◆ Anorexia, milk yield decline
◆ Lacrimation
◆ Dry, staring coat
◆ Mucosal phase of erosions on buccal, nasal mucosae, conjunctivae
◆ Mucopurulent discharge, blepharospasm
◆ Drooling of bubbly, clear, blood-stained saliva, becoming mucopurulent
◆ Serous nasal discharge, becomes purulent
◆ Mouth erosions are discrete, gray, raised, necrotic lesions, 1–5 mm dia., inside lower lip, cheek mucosa at commissures, then tongue underside, dorsum
◆ Similar lesions on nasal, vulvar, vaginal mucosae
◆ Vulvar enlargement, mucosal hyperemia
◆ Lesions slough leaving raw, red, clear-edged areas, coalesce to form ulcers
◆ Severe diarrhea, sometimes dysentery, tenesmus
◆ Skin at perineum, scrotum, flanks, inner

aspects of thighs becomes moist, erythematous, covered with scabs
♦ Course of 3–5 days, temperature falls suddenly, mucosal lesions worsen, *plus*
♦ Dyspnea, cough
♦ Severe dehydration
♦ Abdominal pain in some
♦ Recumbency, death at day 6–12
♦ Survivors abort, have 2 week convalescence

Subacute form – in previously exposed cattle in enzootic area
♦ Mild fever, anorexia, depression
♦ Mucosal lesion catarrhal only
♦ Diarrhea without dysentery
♦ Secondary protozoan disease may overshadow rinderpest
♦ A skin form also occurs with no systemic reaction; only multiple pustules on neck, withers, inside thighs, scrotum

Clinical pathology

♦ Early severe leukopenia, lymphopenia
♦ Fatal dehydration
♦ Clinical diagnosis confirmed by detection of virus antigen in:
  • Needle biopsy of lymph node by agar gel diffusion technique
  • Mucosal scraping, nasal, ocular discharges by complement fixation, counterimmunoelectrophoresis, DNA probes, polymerase chain reaction, and other tests
  • In lymphocyte cultures
♦ Serological tests include virus neutralization tests, ELISA, rapid dot–enzyme immunoassay
♦ Confirmation by transmission to susceptible animals practiced but dangerous, expensive

Necropsy findings

♦ Dehydration, emaciation, soiled with feces
♦ Necrotic erosions, with ulceration in mouth, pharynx, upper esophagus, *not* forestomachs, severe in abomasum, few only in small intestine, severe in large intestine causing zebra stripes of erythema running transversely across colonic mucosa
♦ Necrotic erosions also on upper respiratory mucosa, lower reproductive tract of females
♦ Characteristic histopathological lesions include the mucosal erosions, massive lymphocyte destruction in lymph nodes

Diagnosis

In cattle resembles:
♦ Foot-and-mouth disease
♦ Hemorrhagic septicemia
♦ Bovine malignant catarrh
♦ Mucosal disease
♦ Jembrana disease
In sheep and goats resembles:
♦ Peste des petits ruminants
♦ Bluetongue
♦ Sheep and goat pox
♦ Nairobi sheep disease

Treatment

Not undertaken.

Control

Rinderpest-free countries
♦ Prevention of introduction of animals from high-risk counties, especially wild ruminants to zoos and game parks
♦ Barrier zone of vaccinated animals at high-risk land borders
♦ If outbreak occurs:
  • Complete prohibition all livestock (ruminants and pigs) movement
  • Slaughter of cases and in-contacts
  • Disposal of cadavers on the farm
  • Cleaning and disinfection of premises, utensils, gear
  • Vaccination if outbreak likely to get out of control

Enzootic countries
♦ Vaccination all susceptible animal species annually until 90% immune status achieved
♦ Thereafter calves vaccinated, and again the next year until no outbreaks for 5 years
♦ Outbreaks dealt with by preventing animal movement and ring vaccination around area

Vaccination
♦ Choice of the correct vaccination for each situation is critical
♦ Vaccines capable of causing severe adverse reactions; British breeds, young animals most susceptible; vaccines to be used in adult cattle of native breeds must be much more potent if the immunity produced is to be sufficient
♦ Vaccination causes lymphopenia and reduction of immunity in vaccinates, leading to activation of infection, especially of protozoa

- Calves from immune cows will be immune for 4–8 months, vaccination of them is not recommended until 9 months of age
- All strains of rinderpest virus have same antigenicity so no difficulties with strains included in vaccine
- All vaccines now use attenuated strains of the virus; goat-adapted, rabbit-adapted, chicken embryo-adapted viruses used
- Cell culture vaccines now used almost universally; duration of immunity may be 10 years; vaccine capable of variable degrees of attenuation
- A recombinant vaccine offers many advantages

PESTE DES PETITS RUMINANTS
(PPR, GOAT PLAGUE, OR KATA)
[VM8 p. 986]

Etiology

A morbillivirus of the Paramyxoviridae family closely related to rinderpest virus.

Epidemiology

Occurrence
- Africa and Asia
- Goats, sheep, some wild ruminants
- Morbidity rates im enzootic areas, herds are 50–90%; case fatality rates in goats (55–85%) much higher than in sheep

Source and transmission
- Infection derives from a clinical case, or inapparent carrier
- Transmission by inhalation, conjunctiva or ingestion

Risk factors
- Goats more susceptible than sheep
- Kids less than 4 months old likely to have passive maternal immunity
- Kids 4–12 months old are most susceptible
- Sahelian (Sub-Saharan) breeds of sheep, goats more resistant than dwarf breeds
- Introduced animals, or animals returned unsold from a market are at great risk
- Solid immunity after an attack

Importance
- Heavy death losses in goats, less in sheep
- Most important disease of small ruminants in West Africa

Clinical findings

Acute
- The common disease in goats
- Incubation period 3–6 days
- Similar to rinderpest plus dyspnea
- High fever
- Severe depression
- Sneezing, serous nasal, ocular discharge
- Focal necrotic lesions in mouth, coalesce forming diphtheritic plaques
- Severe halitosis
- Sore mouth, swollen lips, anorexia,
- Nasal, ocular discharges become mucopurulent, mats eyelids, blocks nares
- Profuse, mucoid, blood-stained diarrhea
- Dyspnea, cough, lung sounds crackling, loud
- Vulvar, preputial superficial erosions
- Death after course of 1 week

Subacute
- The common disease in sheep
- Same syndrome only milder
- Most recover after 2 week course
- Ecthyma a common complication

Clinical pathology

- Leukopenia/lymphopenia as in rinderpest but not as severe
- Severe dehydration
- Virus antigen demonstrable in ocular, nasal discharges, pharynx, feces using following tests:
  - Counterimmunoelectrophoresis
  - Agar gel immunodiffusion
- Serological tests available include:
  - ELISA
  - Immune electrophoresis
  - Complement fixation

Necropsy findings

- Dehydration, emaciation
- Hindquarters soiled with feces
- Eyelids matted, nostrils blocked by exudate
- Discrete erosions oral mucosa, pharynx, upper esophagus, abomasum, distal small intestine
- Hemorrhagic ulceration at ileocecal area, creating zebra stripes across colon
- Mucopurulent exudate nasal cavities to larynx, trachea contains froth, pulmonary edema
- Interstitial pneumonia
- Identification of virus antigen in lymphoid tissue using:
  - Immunohistochemical techniques

- DOT-ELISA
♦ For differentiation of PPR and rinderpest viruses use:
  - Serum neutralization test on tissue culture, or
  - DNA probe

Diagnosis

Resembles:
♦ Rinderpest
♦ Heartwater
♦ Pneumonic pasteurellosis
♦ Contagious caprine pleuropneumonia
♦ Contagious ovine pleuropneumonia
♦ Coccidiosis
♦ Ecthyma
♦ Nairobi sheep disease

Treatment

♦ Isolate patients
♦ Hyperimmune serum produced in cattle hyperimmunised against rinderpest
♦ Parenteral broad spectrum antibiotic against secondary bacterial infection
♦ Fluid therapy

Control

♦ Avoid introduction of high-risk animals, especially market purchases
♦ Tissue culture rinderpest vaccine first at 3–4 months old
♦ Other vaccines likely to be effective include recombinant vaccine, a PPR homologous attenuated tissue culture vaccine

NAIROBI SHEEP DISEASE (NSD)
[VM8 p. 988]

Etiology

A nairovirus of the family Bunyaviridae.

Epidemiology

Occurrence
♦ East Africa
♦ Sheep and goats
♦ Animals reared in enzootic areas usually immune
♦ Disease occurs when naive animals introduced to area
♦ Case mortality up to 90%

Source and transmission
♦ Transmitted transstadially, transovarially by tick *Rhipicephalus appendiculatus*
♦ Virus persists in ticks for long periods

Importance
Causes a mild febrile disease in humans.

Clinical findings

♦ Fever
♦ Anorexia
♦ Nasal discharge
♦ Dyspnea
♦ Severe diarrhea, some with dysentery
♦ Abortion
♦ Death after course of 3–9 days

Clinical pathology

Available serological tests include:
♦ Hemagglutination test
♦ Indirect immunofluorescence
♦ ELISA

Necropsy findings

♦ Serositis
♦ Lymphadenopathy
♦ Abomasal, intestinal mucosal hyperemia
♦ Virus can be isolated from tissues in tissue culture or in infant mice

Diagnosis

Resembles:
♦ Peste des petits ruminants
♦ Parasitic gastroenteritis
♦ Salmonellosis

Treatment

Nil.

Control

♦ Animals to be moved to enzootic areas vaccinated before shipment
♦ Inactivated vaccine used but not field tested

BOVINE MALIGNANT CATARRH
(BMC, MALIGNANT HEAD
CATARRH, MALIGNANT
CATARRHAL FEVER) [VM8 p. 989]

Etiology

♦ Two antigenically distinct viruses cause identical clinical diseases:

- Alcelaphine BMC virus (wildebeeste-associated)
- Unspecified but probably a herpesvirus (sheep-associated)
♦ Neither virus causes disease in its principal host
♦ The alcelaphine virus readily cultivated and transmitted; the sheep-associated agent is neither

Epidemiology

Occurrence
♦ Most countries
♦ Only cattle, buffalo, some ruminant wild-life, e.g. deer, bison
♦ Outbreaks in cattle commingled with wil-debeeste, hartebeeste
♦ Rare, sporadic cases in cattle
♦ Devastating outbreaks very rarely in cattle commingled with lambing ewes carrying the agent

Source and transmission
♦ Healthy, primary young (e.g. 3–4 month wildebeeste) host
♦ Virus does not survive outside the host
♦ Transmission by inhalation or ingestion of alcelaphine virus
♦ Sheep-associated virus probably by inges-tion feed contaminated by placental fluids

Importance
Case fatality rate 100%. Sporadic losses ex-cept rare outbreaks in cattle run with sheep.

Clinical findings

♦ Incubation period 3–8 weeks

Head-and-eye form
♦ Sudden onset dejection, anorexia, agalac-tia, high fever
♦ Tachycardia
♦ Profuse mucopurulent nasal discharge
♦ Stertorous dyspnea
♦ Ocular discharge, eyelid edema, blepharos-pasm, scleral vessel congestion
♦ Oral lesions commence as discrete patches, then diffuse areas superficial necrosis an-terior nasal, buccal mucosae and muzzle
♦ Sore mouth, ropy strings of saliva, smac-king of lips, mucosa slimy to touch
♦ Scabby lesions at back of pastern, teats, vulva, scrotum
♦ Corneal opacity commencing at corneos-cleral junction
♦ Hypopyon in some
♦ Incoordination, paresis in one limb

♦ Demented appearance
♦ Tremor
♦ Nystagmus
♦ Head-pushing
♦ Paralysis, convulsions before death at about 7 days

Peracute (alimentary) form
♦ Outbreak with 80–90% morbidity, 100% mortality
♦ High fever
♦ Dyspnea
♦ Profuse diarrhea
♦ Corneal opacity, hypopyon common
♦ Erosive oral, cutaneous lesions diffuse, very severe
♦ Terminal convulsions after course 3–4 days.

Clinical pathology

♦ Leukopenia in some cases
♦ Transmission attempted to susceptible calves using donor large volume, whole blood taken at fever peak, immediate trans-fusion
♦ Serological tests available for wildebeeste-associated virus
♦ Sheep-associated agent undetectable

Necropsy findings

♦ Oral mucosal erosions
♦ Similar lesions esophagus, abomasum, in-testines, trachea
♦ Lymph nodes swollen
♦ Affected epithelium erodes leaving raw surface
♦ Perivascular, mononuclear cuffing most organs with intense inflammatory reaction
♦ Diagnosis in cattle depends on histopatho-logical findings

Diagnosis

Resembles:
♦ Mucosal disease
♦ Rinderpest
♦ Papular stomatitis
♦ Foot-and-mouth disease
♦ Vesicular stomatitis
♦ Photosensitive dermatitis

Treatment and control

♦ Non-steroidal anti-inflammatories may ease discomfort but death inexorable

Avoid cohabitation with lambing ewes, wildebeeste

Vaccination not a likely prospect

BOVINE VIRUS DIARRHEA (BVD),
MUCOSAL DISEASE (MD)
[VM8 p. 993]

Etiology

A pestivirus of the family Flaviviridae.

Epidemiology

Occurrence
♦ Worldwide
♦ Cattle
♦ Infection prevalence very high , 60–80%; mucosal disease morbidity rate very low (e.g. <5% of animals in herd less than 2 years of age); case fatality rate approximately 100%

Source and transmission
♦ Main source is persistently infected, clinically normal, animal; these are usually a very small proportion of the herd but a maternal family of them can develop in a herd as all of the dam's offspring become permanently viremic
♦ Direct contact between animals via all secretions, excretions, including semen
♦ Transplacentally to fetus from permanently or transiently infected dam
♦ Via insect bites

Risk factors
♦ Virus has great antigenic diversity amongst strains so that vaccination or natural infection cannot be guaranteed to provide protection against all strains
♦ **Mucosal disease** occurs usually at 6–24 months of age, precipitated by a superinfection with a cytopathic strain of the BVD virus in a patient which has been rendered immunotolerant and permanently viremic by a non-cytopathic strain of the virus acquired during early fetal life

Economic importance
♦ Losses due to introduction of **bovine virus diarrhea virus (BVDV)** into a susceptible herd containing pregnant females include:
♦ Abortions
♦ Congenital defects
♦ Stillbirths
♦ Neonatal deaths
♦ Growth retardation, pre- and postnatal
♦ Reproductive inefficiency
♦ Yearling deaths due to **mucosal disease**
♦ Culling of permanently infected animals
♦ After the initial experience of the herd with the infection, and the disease is enzootic in the herd, losses are greatly reduced unless heifers are allowed to reach breeding age without being exposed to natural infection or vaccinated

Clinical findings

Bovine virus diarrhea
♦ In animals any age never previously exposed to BVD virus
♦ Often subclinical
♦ Mild fever
♦ Anorexia
♦ Mild diarrhea
♦ Leukopenia
♦ Many of group affected
♦ All recover after course of 2–3 days
♦ All group seroconvert at this time; same happens in fetuses infected in utero after 150–180 days of pregnancy

Acute mucosal disease
♦ Sudden onset in animals older than 6–24 months infected in utero before 150 days of pregnancy
♦ Mostly sporadic cases only over several months; rarely a small group affected
♦ Fever, depression, anorexia
♦ Drool saliva, wetting hair around mouth
♦ Profuse, foul-smelling diarrhea, contains mucus, blood in some; occasionally fibrin tags, casts; rarely no diarrhea in cases with short history
♦ Tenesmus common
♦ Discrete, shallow erosions on buccal mucosa; coalesce leaving large areas of mucosa without epithelium
♦ Lesions inside lips, on gums, dental pad, tongue, mouth commissures, posterior hard palate
♦ Lesions on muzzle covering it with scabs, debris
♦ Lesion may be scarce in 20% of cases near end of outbreak; few small lesions usually detectable on posterior hard palate
♦ Tachycardia
♦ Polypnea
♦ Ruminal movements absent
♦ Dehydration, weakness, recumbency
♦ Over 90% die after a course of 5–7 days

Chronic mucosal disease
♦ Some acute cases persist with intermittent bouts of diarrhea

♦ Anorexia
♦ Emaciation
♦ Rough, dry hair coat
♦ Chronic bloat
♦ Hoof deformity
♦ Chronic oral erosions
♦ Chronic, scabby skin lesions at perineum, scrotum, preputial orifice, vulva, between thighs, skin/horn junction around dew claws, heels, interdigital clefts
♦ Heavy dandruff deposits
♦ Death from inanition after course of up to 18 months

Unthrifty, persistently viremic calves
♦ May be small at birth
♦ May fail to grow normally
♦ May survive for months, develop fatal mucosal disease, pneumonia
♦ No mucosal, skin lesions
♦ Seronegative to BVD virus

Congenital defects
♦ Cerebellar, cerebellar/ocular agenesis
♦ Ocular defects including
  • Retinal atrophy
  • Optic neuritis
  • Cataract
  • Microphthalmia
♦ Brachygnathism
♦ Musculoskeletal deformities
♦ Alopecia, curly hair coat
♦ Intrauterine growth retardation

Reproductive inefficiency
Significant wastage due to abortion, still-births, early neonatal deaths and failure to conceive reported but not established as cause–effect relationship; much of the wastage can be eliminated by maximizing immunity to the BVDV before breeding.

Clinical pathology
♦ Severe leukopenia in acute mucosal disease.

Virus identification
♦ Difficult; techniques used include:
  • Polymerase chain reaction
  • Indirect, immunoperoxidase staining
♦ Serological tests used to identify animals carrying the virus include:
  • Direct or indirect immunofluorescent or enzyme-linked antibody staining
  • Immunodiffusion
  • Antigen-capture ELISA

• Monoclonal antibody techniques
• Viral RNA oligonucleotide fingerprinting
• Dot blot assay

Serology
Techniques used to detect presence of antibody include:
♦ Virus neutralization teat
♦ Complement fixation
♦ Immunofluorescent staining
♦ A range of ELISAs

Necropsy findings
♦ Similar findings in most forms of the disease
♦ Shallow erosions, lacking surrounding inflammation, with raw, red base on muzzle, in mouth, pharynx, larynx, posterior nares, esophagus, pillars of rumen, folds of omasum, sides of abomasal folds
♦ In chronic mucosal disease necrotic epithelium not eroded, creating elevated, friable plaques in mouth, rumen
♦ Coagulated blood, fibrin overlaying eroded Peyer's patches in small intestine
♦ Mucosa in large intestine congested in tiger stripe pattern
♦ Congenital defects include cerebellar hypoplasia, cataracts, retinal degeneration, hypoplasia, neuritis of optic nerves

Diagnosis
Resembles:
♦ Rinderpest
♦ Bovine malignant catarrh
♦ Foot-and-mouth disease
♦ Vesicular stomatitis
♦ Bluetongue
♦ Papular stomatitis
♦ Infectious bovine rhinotracheitis (alimentary form in neonates)
♦ Necrotic stomatitis

Treatment
Nil.

Control
Eradication
♦ Eradication of the disease from herds has been achieved but is very complicated and expensive because of the overpowering need to detect and eliminate permanently viremic, serologically negative animals that represent the continuing source of infection

♦ The permanently infected, viremic animals have a short life expectancy and, provided no additional ones are added because the herd is close, it can be anticipated that some herds will automatically clear themselves of the infection

Vaccination

♦ Vaccination of all animals before puberty, effectively 3–6 weeks before breeding, is a standard recommendation but is not effective in persistently viremic calves which may or may not respond to the vaccine depending on whether the vaccine strains are antigenically identical to the infecting one. Therefore the vaccinated calf may subsequently succumb to mucosal disease, either as a result of infection with the vaccine strain or by another, different strain

♦ Vaccination of cattle destined for feedlots serves no useful purpose

♦ An important vaccination strategy in breeding females, to ensure maximum reproductive is maintained, is vaccination at least several 3–6 weeks before breeding commences

♦ Vaccinating pregnant cows lacking any neutralizing antibody with modified live virus vaccines between 50 and 190 days of pregnancy exposes the fetus to infection and the possible development of congenital defects

Introduced animals

♦ These can reasonably be considered free of the infection if they are strongly seropositive or are negative but from a known free herd

BOVINE PAPULAR STOMATITIS
[VM8 p. 1009]

Etiology

A parapoxvirus of the family Poxviridae; several strains; probably identical with pseudocowpox virus.

Epidemiology

Occurrence
♦ Most countries
♦ Cattle only
♦ Young animals 2 weeks to 2 years
♦ Morbidity often 100%

Importance
♦ Mild disease causing no wastage
♦ Confuses diagnosis of cattle diseases characterized by oral mucosal lesions

Clinical findings

♦ Transient fever, anorexia, increased salivation, weight loss in some
♦ Mostly disease unnoticed unless oral mucosae examined for other reason
♦ Round, papules, 0.5–1.0 cm dia. on muzzle, inside oral cavity, nostrils
♦ Lesions expand peripherally, may coalesce, periphery reddened, centre sunken, rough, external lesions may be covered by scab
♦ Lesions heal quickly but epithelium discolored so lesion sites visible several weeks
♦ Quick recurrence common so disease may persist several months

Clinical pathology

♦ Virus detectable by electron microscopy of saliva
♦ Cytoplasmic inclusions in mucosal cells
♦ Virus neutralization test available
♦ Indirect immunofluorescence test used also

Necropsy findings

Not applicable.

Diagnosis

♦ When it accompanies ostertagiasis or other cause of parasitic gastroenteritis in calves this disease resembles:
• Mucosal disease
• Bovine virus diarrhea
• Bovine malignant catarrh
• Foot-and-mouth disease
• Rinderpest
♦ Bovine papular stomatitis virus may contribute to the development of 'rat-tail syndrome' in sarcocystosis

Treatment

No treatment necessary.

Control

No control practiced.

TRANSMISSIBLE
GASTROENTERITIS (TGE) OF PIGS
[VM8 p. 1009]

Etiology

♦ A coronavirus of the family Coronaviridae; one antigenic type
♦ The virus is not related to most other por-

cine coronaviruses but is related antigenically to the porcine respiratory coronavirus

Epidemiology

Occurrence

⧫ Most countries, especially northern hemisphere
⧫ Pigs only
⧫ In outbreaks in naive herds infection prevalence explosive, close to 100%, but clinical disease mild except in unweaned piglets, lactating sows; case fatality rate very low except in unweaned piglets (up to 100%); outbreak terminates in 3–5 weeks; herd immunity prevents further attacks for 3–6 years
⧫ Nature of outbreak different in herds practicing intensive husbandry, continuous farrowing, continuous introduction of susceptible pigs into infective environment; outbreaks greatly prolonged, recrudescence more likely, for longer periods, and at shorter intervals; also atypical forms of disease with low morbidity, mortality, no clinical signs until 2–4 weeks old

Source and transmission

⧫ Introduced, infected pigs
⧫ Virus shed in large quantities in feces of infected pigs for some weeks, in respiratory aerosol, in sow's milk
⧫ Clinically normal feeder pigs can be carriers
⧫ In meat scraps, virus resists freezing
⧫ Transmission by birds, on inert objects such as footwear and vehicle tires
⧫ Transmission by oral and respiratory routes
⧫ Spread within herd very rapid

Risk factors

⧫ Lack of previous exposure to infection
⧫ Spread, severity enhanced by cold or draughty environment
⧫ Virus survives poorly outside host, easily destroyed by disinfectants, boiling, drying, sunlight

Importance

⧫ Major enzootic disease in most countries
⧫ Wastage due to piglet deaths, no production from a large part of the investment for a long period, lost productivity of surviving pigs

Clinical findings

Acute piglet disease

⧫ Incubation period 24–48 hours
⧫ Vomiting, yellow, foamy, slimy
⧫ Profuse diarrhea, watery, yellow–green, offensive odor, contains milk clots
⧫ Transient fever in some
⧫ Depression, dehydration
⧫ Hair coat ruffled,
⧫ Weakness, emaciation, death on day 2–5
⧫ Survivors emaciated, gain weight slowly
⧫ Disease becomes less severe as outbreak proceeds

Acute in older pigs

⧫ Many infections subclinical
⧫ Signs similar but milder
⧫ Fever, anorexia
⧫ Diarrhea in some
⧫ Agalactia in lactating sows
⧫ Course up to 10 days

Subacute in young pigs

⧫ In enzootic herds
⧫ Mild diarrhea only
⧫ Subsequent slow weight gain

Clinical pathology

⧫ Severe dehydration, metabolic acidosis, marked hypoglycemia
⧫ Virus detected in feces and fresh tissue by:
  • ELISA
  • Immune electron microscopy
  • Fluorescent antibody staining
  • Immunoperoxidase test
  • Capture-enzyme immune assay
  • Reversed passive hemagglutination test
  • Solid-phase immune electron microscopic technique
⧫ Serological tests for antibody include:
  • Serum neutralization test
  • ELISA
  • Competitive ELISA

Necropsy findings

⧫ Lesions confined to intestines and stomach; may be minor
⧫ Intestinal wall thin, translucent
⧫ Intestine distended with fluid ingesta
⧫ Villous atrophy detectable microscopically, but recovers over a 7-day period
⧫ Intestinal wall thickening in chronic cases, similar to that in regional ileitis
⧫ Cardiac, skeletal muscle deterioration in some cases

Diagnosis

Resembles:
⧫ Rotavirus infection

* **Porcine epidemic diarrhea**, in UK, cause unknown, no villous atrophy, affects pigs of all ages
* Hog cholera
* Vomiting and wasting disease
* Colibacillosis

Treatment

* No specific treatment
* Supportive oral fluid, electrolyte therapy

Control

* Of an outbreak impossible because of explosive nature
* Plan 1 – isolate farrowing sows individually with strict hygiene to avoid virus contact with piglets; needs exceptional facilities
* Plan 2 – maximize contact of pregnant sows with virus by mixing them with infected pigs, *or* oral dosing or feeding with feces or ground up intestine from affected piglets
* Vaccines do not provide adequate immunity; natural infection does

VOMITING AND WASTING
DISEASE OF PIGS
(HEMAGGLUTINATING
ENCEPHALOMYELITIS VIRUS
DISEASE OF PIGS) [VM8 p. 1015]

Etiology

A hemagglutinating coronavirus, family Coronaviridae.

Epidemiology

Occurrence

* Canada, USA, Europe, UK, Australia
* Infection very widespread, clinical disease rare
* In naive herds occurs as outbreaks; also area outbreaks
* After initial outbreak further litters unaffected
* Morbidity 100%, case fatality high
* Pigs 2 days to 3 weeks old; encephalitic disease in younger pigs in this age group

Source and transmission

* Infected pigs transfer disease between herds
* Transmission oral or respiratory

Risk factors

Strain virulence and litter susceptibility affect which of the syndromes appears.

Importance

Massive losses of baby pigs in initial outbreaks.

Clinical findings

* Sows and young litters
* Sows may show mild fever, anorexia for several days for 1–2 days
* Piglets show one of the following syndromes

Encephalomyelitis

* Depression, then anorexia
* Rapid emaciation
* Hyperesthesia, incoordination, muscle tremor, occasional vomiting
* After 48–72 hours paddling convulsions, death after course of 2–3 days

Vomiting and wasting

* Yellow–green vomitus, for several days
* Anorexia
* Thirst, with ineffective attempts to drink
* Transient fever in some
* Feces dry, hard
* Mild diarrhea in some older pigs
* Severe, rapid dehydration, emaciation
* Die or euthanised after course of 2 days to 3 weeks

Clinical pathology

* Virus in tissues demonstrated by:
  * Hemagglutination
  * Fluorescent antibody
  * Electron microscopy
* Serological tests include:
  * Virus neutralization
  * Hemagglutination inhibition
  * Agar gel immunodiffusion

Necropsy findings

* No gross lesions
* Non-suppurative encephalomyelitis in pigs affected by the nervous syndrome

Diagnosis

The vomiting and wasting syndrome is distinctive.

The encephalomyelitis disease resembles:
* Porcine viral encephalomyelitis

♦ Porcine encephalomyocarditis virus infection

Treatment

Nil.

Control

Prior exposure of sow to infection at least 10 days prior to farrowing, by purposeful exposure.

VIRAL DIARRHEA OF YOUNG
ANIMALS [VM8 p. 1016]

Etiology

♦ **Rotaviruses**, several serotypes, in calves, lambs, piglets, and foals, with no cross-protection between serotypes
♦ **Pararotaviruses** in piglets, calves, and lambs
♦ **Coronaviruses** in calves and piglets
♦ **Adenovirus in calves**
♦ **Parvovirus in calves**
♦ The **Breda** virus in calves
♦ Multiple virus infections, combinations of a virus with *Escherichia coli* occur

Epidemiology

Calf – rotavirus
Occurrence:
♦ Infection ubiquitous in all countries, all ages, all species; diarrhea outbreaks in young only
♦ Interspecies infections with a virus an unknown quantity in field cases; some cross-infections by experimental transmission
♦ Infection prevalence in young adults up to 100%, of clinical disease up to 60%; case fatality rates vary 5–60% depending on adequacy of colostral protection, coexistence of colibacillosis, general care of the calves

Source and transmission:
♦ Only feces of infected animals; adults the source for the young
♦ Virus resistant to common disinfectants; infection via fomites important
♦ Transmission by ingestion

Risk factors:
♦ Mortality 100% at birth, mild disease at 3–4 weeks
♦ Inadequate colostrum intake; colostrum of low antibody content; colostral antibodies protect against diarrhea only for the first 5–7 days of life

Calf – coronavirus
Occurrence:
♦ Worldwide
♦ Important cause of diarrhea in calves 3–21 days old
♦ Infection prevalence in adults up to 60%; estimated diarrhea prevalence in young 10–80%

Source and transmission:
♦ In feces, especially adults in winter, at parturition
♦ Fecal and oral transmission assumed; aerosol transmission possible

Calf – parvovirus
♦ In outbreaks of postweaning diarrhea in beef calves
♦ May be associated with subclinical coccidiosis

Calf – Breda virus
♦ Common infection, sometimes associated with diarrhea outbreaks
♦ Not considered a major pathogen

Lambs – rotavirus
♦ Rotavirus in sporadic diarrhea of lambs younger than 3 weeks
♦ Mild diarrheic disease experimentally; recovery in a few days
♦ Mortality high in mixed infection with *Escherichia coli*

Piglets – rotavirus
♦ Ubiquitous
♦ In 1–4 week piglets depending on decline of passive maternal immunity
♦ Commonest in piglets weaned early at 3 weeks in intensive management systems
♦ Morbidity up to 80%; case fatality 5–20%; many subclinical infections
♦ Direct transmission, plus virus surviving in dirty pens, perpetuates infection between groups in piggery
♦ Gilts, sows transmit virus before farrowing through lactation
♦ Combined rotavirus – *Escherichia coli* or *Isospora suis* infections associated with diarrhea in piglets

Piglets – pararotaviruses and enteroviruses
♦ Potential enteric pathogens; found in many pre- and postweaning diarrhea outbreaks

Piglets – corona-like virus (porcine epidemic diarrhea virus)
♦ Causes diarrhea outbreaks in any age pigs except sucking pigs (type 1) or all ages (type 2)

Foals – rotavirus
♦ Major cause of diarrhea in foals up to 3 months old especially on horse farms with high population density
♦ Combines with *Salmonella* spp.

Clinical findings

Calves – rotavirus
♦ In calves over 4 days old
♦ Sudden onset profuse, pale yellow, mucoid diarrhea containing blood flecks
♦ No toxemia
♦ Recovery in a few days
♦ Explosive outbreaks, up to 50% of 5–14 day old calves affected
♦ Mixed infections with:
  • *Escherichia coli* cause severe dehydration, some deaths
  • Coronavirus

Calves – coronavirus
♦ In 1–7 day old calves
♦ Mucoid, slimy, dark green to light brown, voluminous diarrhea for several days
♦ Severe dehydration, some deaths

Lambs – rotavirus
♦ Dullness, profuse diarrhea
♦ Some deaths

Pigs – rotavirus
♦ In nursing piglets 1–4 weeks old, or may be a major problem in pigs after weaning
♦ Most of litter have profuse liquid diarrhea
♦ Dehydration
♦ Recover in few days unless complicated by *E. coli*

Pigs – epidemic diarrhea type 2
♦ All age pigs
♦ Profuse fluid diarrhea
♦ Explosive outbreaks, 100% morbidity; case fatality rate high in piglets under 3 weeks old

Foals – virus diarrhea
♦ Depression, failure to suck, recumbent
♦ Fever
♦ Rapid, shallow respiration
♦ Profuse, non-fetid, watery diarrhea
♦ Severe dehydration, electrolyte imbalance

♦ Recovery with treatment after 2–4 day course; fatal cases die within 24 hours

Clinical pathology

♦ Feces (or loops of gut) checked for virus by tests including:
  • Electron microscopy
  • Immunofluorescent staining
  • Immunodiffusion test
  • ELISA
  • Cell culture
  • Counterimmunoelectrophoresis
  • And many others, some of them specially created tests for use in field situations, e.g. Rotazyme test
♦ Serological tests available include ELISA, radioimmunoassay, agar gel immunodiffusion

Necropsy findings

♦ Dehydration
♦ Fluid-filled, atonic intestine, abomasum distension
♦ Microscopically villous atrophy, villous fusion

Diagnosis

Resembles:

Calves
♦ Enteric colibacillosis
♦ Cryptosporidiosis
♦ Bovine virus diarrhea possibly

Piglets
♦ Transmissible gastroenteritis
♦ Enteric colibacillosis
♦ Coccidiosis
♦ Hemorrhagic enterotoxemia due to *Clostridium perfringens* type C

Lambs
♦ Coliform septicemia
♦ Lamb dysentery

Foals
♦ Salmonellosis
♦ *Clostridium perfringens* type B
♦ foal heat diarrhea due to excess milk supply

Treatment

♦ Broad-spectrum antibiotic therapy usual to control possible secondary invaders

♦ Fluid, electrolyte therapy as for undifferentiated calf diarrhea (p. 296) for up to 72 hours
♦ Withhold milk for 24–48 hours beneficial; often impracticable
♦ Isolate affected animals where possible

Control

See under undifferentiated calf diarrhea (p. 296) for basic recommendations.

Vaccination of neonate
♦ Modified live, orally-administered rotavirus, or rotavirus and coronavirus combination, vaccine used extensively with little advantage gained
♦ Parenteral vaccination of the pregnant dam to enhance passive transfer of immuno-globulins from dam to calf intestinal lumen
♦ One of the problems is the rapid decline in antibody content of the colostrum after parturition and the need to maintain the intestinal antibody content for longer periods
♦ In handfed neonates collection, storage and feeding of the colostrum over an extended period reduces the prevalence of diarrhea in the calves, but the use of multiple, adjuvanted vaccines, in calves nursing their dams increases and extends the colostral antibody content of the dam's milk but has not been shown to significantly reduce the prevalence of diarrhea

WINTER DYSENTERY OF CATTLE
[VM8 p. 1026]

Etiology

A coronavirus; *Campylobacter fetus* var *jejuni* was thought to be the cause.

Epidemiology

Occurrence
♦ In many countries in cattle, possibly sheep
♦ Outbreaks in adult milking cows, especially recently calved
♦ Young animals only mildly affected
♦ Commonest in housed cattle in winter
♦ Morbidity 50% within a few days, 100% within a week; case fatality rate <1%

Source and transmission
♦ Feces from clinical cases, silent carriers carry virus
♦ Disease highly contagious, brought onto farm by infected carrier, on boots and vehicle tires
♦ Contamination via feed and drinking water, infection by ingestion

Risk factors
♦ Immunity for 6 months after attack
♦ Recurrence in herd after 2–3 years (varies from few months to 10 years); in frequent recurrences attacks mild, in widely separated outbreaks disease more severe

Importance
Serious loss of body weight, milk production for up to 2 weeks, sometimes to 1 month; cows in late lactation may go dry.

Clinical findings

Cattle
♦ Incubation 3–7 days
♦ Explosive outbreak of explosive diarrhea; most of herd affected in 4–7 days
♦ Transient fever early, subsides with diarrhea onset
♦ Precipitate milk yield fall for 1 week
♦ Transient anorexia
♦ Slight weight loss
♦ Feces thin, watery, homogeneous, little odor, no mucus, epithelial shreds, dark green to black; passed with no warning, with great velocity, especially with cough
♦ Nasolacrimal discharge
♦ Herd-wide cough in some outbreaks
♦ Rarely severe dehydration, weakness, blood flecks or clots in feces
♦ Feces normal in 2–3 days; herd normal in 2 weeks

Sheep
♦ Diarrhea
♦ Emaciation

Clinical pathology

♦ ELISA used to demonstrate coronavirus; alternative is gold electron microscopy
♦ Significant rise in sera antibodies in serial samples 8 weeks apart

Necropsy findings

♦ Examination not usually available without secondary invaders
♦ Abomasal hyperemia, mild catarrhal enteritis in small intestine

Diagnosis

Resembles:
- Salmonellosis
- Acute arsenic poisoning
- Coccidiosis

Treatment

- Probably unnecessary because of spontaneous recovery
- Sulfonamides, nitrofurazone, copper sulphate (30 ml of 5% solution) are favorite remedies

Control

- Control efforts helpless in face of high infectivity
- Hygiene with boots, clothing, instruments advised

BLUETONGUE [VM8 p. 1028]

Etiology

An arthropod-borne orbivirus of the family Reoviridae; at least 24 serotypes with a great deal of variability in virulence and genetic composition within the serotypes.

Epidemiology

Occurrence
- In countries between latitudes 40°N and 35°S where vector survives
- Enzootic areas, where disease occurs in introduced animals, bordered by areas where occasional epizootics occur
- Spread can occur over large distances when vector carried by strong wind
- Serotypes of varying virulence have geographical localizations causing a patchy distribution of the clinical disease, often unrelated to serological findings
- In naive herd morbidity up to 75%; case fatality up to 50%, but both usually much lower
- Seasonal depending on insect life cycle

Source and transmission
- Transmitted by *Culicoides* spp., replicates in the insect, released through salivary glands
- Mechanical transmission by other biting insects possible; ticks, mosquitoes, ked suspected
- Infection persists in carrier ruminants, probably cattle
- Over-wintering in the insect also probable
- Transmitted in semen, not in transplanted embryos

Risk factors
- Virus resistant to decomposition and some virucidal agents but sensitive to acid, 3% sodium hydroxide, Wescodyne
- Sheep breeds vary in susceptibility, e.g. Merinos and British breeds more susceptible than native African breeds
- Exposure to solar radiation increases severity of signs
- Immunity is strain-specific; a new strain in an area means new outbreaks, possibly a series of varying virulence

Importance
- Heavy death rate, recovered animals lose fleece or develop break in staple
- Abortions

Clinical findings

Sheep – naturally occurring, florid bluetongue
- Incubation period less than 1 week
- High fever
- 48 hours later mucopurulent, often blood-stained nasal discharge
- Frothy, blood-stained, malodorous salivation
- Buccal, nasal mucosal hyperemia, edema causing swelling of lips, tongue
- Involuntary lip twitches
- Lenticular, necrotic ulcers on sides of swollen, sometimes blue-hued, tongue
- Similar lesions at mouth commissures, tips of buccal papillae, around anus and vulva
- Prehension, mastication, swallowing difficult and painful
- Vomiting, aspiration pneumonia in a few
- Facial swelling
- Swelling, drooping of ears
- Haired skin hyperemic
- Severe conjunctivitis, lacrimation in some
- Respiration obstructed, stertorous, rapid
- Diarrhea and dysentery in some
- Laminitis and coronitis accompanied in some by:
  - Lameness
  - Recumbency
  - Dark red to purple band in skin just above coronet a diagnostic sign
- Wryneck, with head, neck twisted to one side in a few cases
- Gait stiff, stumbling
- Rapid weight loss
- Death after 6-day course

♦ Several months convalescence in survivors
♦ Sequels include:
  • Fleece falls out
  • Hooves crack, slough
  • Skin wrinkling, cracking around lips, muzzle
  • Congenital defects, porencephaly, cerebral necrosis, in a few

Sheep – subacute syndromes in enzootic areas

♦ Abortion without prior fever
♦ Emaciation, weakness, long convalescence without local lesions

Cattle

♦ Most infections subclinical
♦ Fever
♦ Stiff, lame gait
♦ Laminitis all feet
♦ Lip edema, inappetence, excess salivation, fetid breath
♦ Ulcerative lesions on tongue, lips, dental pad, muzzle
♦ Nasal discharge
♦ Severe coronitis, hoof sloughing in a few
♦ Photodermatitis in a few
♦ Abortion
♦ Congenital defects including:
  • Hydranencephaly
  • Microcephaly
  • Blindness
  • Limb curvature
  • Jaw deformity

Goats

♦ Mild to moderate fever
♦ Mucosal and conjunctival hyperemia

Deer

Disease identical with epizootic hemorrhagic disease.

Clinical pathology

♦ Serum creatinine kinase levels elevated
♦ Severe leukopenia and lymphopenia
♦ Isolation of virus from blood by:
  • Tissue culture
  • Transmission to experimental animals
  • In situ nucleic acid hybridization
  • Polymerase chain reaction
♦ Serological tests have problems including viremic animals with no antibodies; tests in use include:
  • Agar gel immunodiffusion
  • Competitive and blocking ELISAs
  • Serum virus neutralization

Necropsy findings

♦ Skin, mucosal lesions as above
♦ Generalized edema
♦ Hyperemia, hemorrhage, necrosis of skeletal and cardiac muscle
♦ Aspiration pneumonia
♦ Distinctive hemorrhage at base of pulmonary artery
♦ Abomasal mucosa hyperemic, edematous, hemorrhagic, ulcerated
♦ Hemorrhages, hyaline degeneration of skeletal muscle

Diagnosis

Resembles:
♦ Foot-and-mouth disease
♦ Contagious ecthyma
♦ Ulcerative dermatosis
♦ Ibaraki disease
♦ Enzootic hemorrhagic disease in deer

Treatment

Affected animals confined away from sun, treated to control secondary infection.

Control

♦ Prevention of entry by:
  • Prevention of importation of possible carrier animals, or testing in quarantine
  • Similar precautions with semen
  • Spraying of aircraft to prevent insect introductions
♦ Control of insect vectors impractical

Vaccination

♦ Serotypes in vaccine need to be constantly reviewed as important ones in environment change frequently
♦ Attempts to vaccinate wild ruminants, the important carriers, via feed unsuccessful; vaccination has to be parenteral
♦ Egg-attenuated living polyvalent virus vaccine the standard
♦ Annual revaccination prior to expected vector proliferation
♦ Lambing deferred until after insect season, then vaccinated more than 2 weeks after weaning, when maternal immunity has declined
♦ Cattle should also be vaccinated
♦ Vaccination of pregnant ewes (4–8 weeks pregnant) may lead to congenital defects:
  • Retinal dysplasia
  • Limb edema, spasticity

• Dummy syndrome with brain hypo-plasia, hydranencephaly

EPIZOOTIC HEMORRHAGIC
DISEASE [VM8 p. 1032]

Etiology

A serogroup of Orbivirus closely related to bluetongue virus.

Epidemiology

♦ An acute, infectious, hemorrhagic disease of deer
♦ Cattle are infected but develop no lesions or signs
♦ Same geographical distribution as bluetongue virus

22 DISEASES CAUSED BY VIRUSES AND CHLAMYDIA – II

VIRAL DISEASES CHARACTERIZED BY RESPIRATORY SIGNS

The following viral diseases cause similar diseases to those caused by equine herpesviruses 1 and 2, and to strangles. They confuse the diagnosis of these diseases and, on their own account, cause disruption of racing and breeding programs. All of the virus diseases of the equine respiratory tract reduce the resistance of the tract to other diseases, and affected horses should be withdrawn from active training for at least 30 days.

EQUINE RHINOVIRUS INFECTION
[VM8 p. 1034]

Etiology

♦ Equine rhinoviruses 1, 2, 3
♦ Only no. 1 known to cause illness

Epidemiology

♦ Occur in most horse populations
♦ Transmitted by inhalation
♦ 100% morbidity, strong immunity

Clinical findings

♦ 3–8 day incubation
♦ Fever
♦ Pharyngitis, pharyngeal lymphadenitis
♦ Nasal discharge
♦ Persistent cough
♦ Spontaneous recovery after 3 weeks course

EQUINE ADENOVIRUS INFECTION
[VM8 p. 1035]

Epidemiology

♦ The common infection in foals with combined immunodeficiency disease
♦ Also occurs independently in all ages

Clinical findings

Adults and foals
♦ Mild respiratory disease
♦ Fever
♦ Conjunctivitis
♦ Cough
♦ Nasal discharge
♦ Transient diarrhea

Foals
Dyspnea due to severe non-fatal pneumonia.

Clinical pathology

♦ Inclusion bodies in smears of nasal mucosa or conjunctiva
♦ Wide range of serological tests

EQUINE PARAINFLUENZA VIRUS
AND REOVIRUS INFECTIONS [VM8
p. 1034]

Parainfluenza 2 (PI-3), and a range of reovirus serotypes cause rare, mild disease similar to rhinovirus and adenovirus infection

EQUINE COITAL EXANTHEMA
[VM8 p. 1034]

Etiology

Equine herpesvirus-3.

Epidemiology

Sexually transmitted.

Clinical findings

- 2–10 day incubation period
- Papular, then pustular, then necrotic lesions in vagina, extending in some to vulva and perineum; also prepuce, penis
- Lesions in some on muzzle, around nostrils, on conjunctiva
- Spontaneous recovery in 14 days

Diagnosis

Resembles:
- Dourine
- Vesicular stomatitis
- Mouth lesions caused by hairy caterpillar invasion of pasture, or grasses with bristly seed heads

EQUINE VIRAL
RHINOPNEUMONITIS (EVR)
[VM8 p. 1036]

Etiology

- Any of 3 herpesviruses
  - EHV-1 (subtype 1 causes abortion, subtype 2 abortion or respiratory disease)
  - EHV-2 causes **equine cytomegalovirus syndrome**, a fever, nasal discharge and lymphadenopathy disease of 1 week duration in foals
  - (EHV-3 causes equine coital exanthema)
  - EHV-4 causes the respiratory tract syndrome **equine viral rhinopneumonitis**

Epidemiology

Occurrence
- High prevalence in most countries
- Mostly young horses

Source and transmission
- Other infected horses; infection rate probably maintained by prolonged infectivity

- Transmission by inhalation principally; also ingestion contaminated materials
- Virus survives up to 45 days in environment

Risk factors
- Possible carrier state in other species, e.g. llama, rodents
- Immunity after infection or vaccination short

Importance
- Reduction of immunity to bacterial disease
- Interference with training, performance contests
- Abortion outbreaks cause great financial loss

Clinical findings

Respiratory disease
- Incubation period 2–20 days
- Fever
- Conjunctivitis
- Cough
- Slight lymph node enlargement
- Diarrhea rarely
- Limb edema rarely
- Recovery after 5 day course, 3 weeks in some

Complications
- Streptococcal secondary invaders common
- Foals may develop primary viral pneumonia

Abortion
- Outbreak, up to 90% mares in group
- Up to 4 months after mild (easily unobserved) respiratory disease
- As early as 5th month, commonest at 8–10th month
- Easy abortion, placenta passed, no mammary development in some

Neonatal viremia and septicemia
- Infected foals, normal at birth; weaken, die about day 3
- Severe depression
- Dyspnea in some
- Secondary infection with *Escherichia coli, Actinobacillus equuli*

Paralytic syndrome
- Occurs separate from or included in outbreak of respiratory and abortion disease
- Commonest in reinfections, possibly after vaccinations

♦ Mostly in mares; foals, stallions also affected
♦ Incubation period 7 days
♦ Incoordination, paresis
♦ Urinary incontinence in some
♦ Recumbency
♦ Euthanasia at up to 1 month

Clinical pathology

♦ Severe leucopenia
♦ Serological tests used include CF, ELISA, polymerase chain reaction in increasing order of sensitivity
♦ Virus neutralizing antibodies not good indicator of patient's resistance; lymphocyte transformation test a better indicator of the cell-mediated immunity, the critical feature of immunity to this disease

Necropsy findings

Respiratory disease Rhinitis, pneumonitis.
Paralytic syndrome Acute disseminated encephalopathy
Aborted fetuses Focal hepatic necrosis with acidophilic antibodies in hepatic parenchyma, bronchial, and alveolar epithelium. Clear serous fluid in pleural and peritoneal cavities.

Diagnosis

Respiratory disease resembles:
♦ Equine influenza
♦ Equine viral arteritis
♦ Rhinovirus
♦ Adenovirus
♦ Reovirus
♦ Parainfluenza

Other causes of abortion include:
♦ Equine viral arteritis
♦ *Salmonella abortivoequina*
♦ *Streptococcus zooepidemicus*

Paralytic syndrome resembles:
♦ Botulism
♦ Equine encephalomyelitis
♦ Borna disease and others

Treatment and control

♦ Customary to administer antibiotics to counter secondary invaders
♦ Vaccination widely practiced; has some constraints
♦ Living attenuated vaccines, e.g. a cell-culture adapted live virus vaccine, are market leaders because they neither spread from vaccinates nor cause disease
♦ Problem is short duration of vaccine protection
♦ Many other vaccines on trial
♦ Present recommendation is use vaccine only if disease a serious problem
♦ Isolation of infected mares and the avoidance of movement of stud mares are critical to control on stud farms

EQUINE VIRAL ARTERITIS [EVA]
[VM8 p. 1040]

Etiology

An arterivirus of the family Togaviridae with some antigenic heterogeneity.

Epidemiology

♦ Infrequent outbreaks in most countries
♦ Horses only, all age groups

Source and transmission

♦ Infected horses, including long-term carriers
♦ Transmission by inhalation thought to be main mechanism
♦ Possibly also ingestion, venereal transmission

Importance

♦ Severe disease, with low case fatality rate
♦ Also causes abortion

Clinical findings

Most outbreaks at present time are of inapparent illness plus epidemic abortion; classic disease in naive herd is:
♦ Incubation period 1–6 days
♦ Fever
♦ Nasal discharge
♦ Mucosal petechiation
♦ Conjunctivitis with severe ocular discharge, keratitis, eyelid edema, blepharospasm, aqueous humor opacity
♦ Dyspnea
♦ Cough only in some and severe only in bad cases
♦ Anorexia
♦ Colic in some
♦ Rarely diarrhea, jaundice
♦ Edema of lower limbs, belly wall, prepuce, scrotum in stallions

- Fatal cases dehydrated, recumbent, die after course of 3–8 days

Abortion At time of systemic illness; placenta passed with fetus.

Clinical pathology

- Serological tests available; used to illustrate rising antibody titer level, include:
  - Complement fixation
  - Virus neutralisation
  - ELISA
- Pronounced leukopenia, especially lymphocytes, at height of fever

Necropsy findings

- Congestion, petechiation upper respiratory tract
- Edema lung, mediastinum
- Pleural, peritoneal effusion
- Subserosal petechiation
- Catarrhal, hemorrhagic enteritis
- General vascular endothelial lesion with necrosis vascular wall musculature

Diagnosis

Respiratory syndrome resembles:
- Equine viral rhinopneumonitis
- Equine influenza
- **Getah** virus disease

Local edema syndrome resembles:
- Purpura hemorrhagica
- African horse sickness
- Urticaria

Other causes of abortion include:
- Equine viral pneumonitis
- *Salmonella abortivoequina*
- *Streptococcus zooepidemicus*

Treatment and control

- No specific treatment
- Vaccines undergoing trial; killed vaccines preferred
- Attenuated vaccines in use but include risk of starting disease in vaccinated herds

EQUINE INFLUENZA [VM8 p. 1042]

Etiology

- IA/E1, IA/E2 serotypes of the influenza virus
- Especially the H3N8 subtype of the IA/E2

virus; causes the most virulent form of the disease
- Chinese virus IA/E1/Jilin has low cross-reactivity with western viruses

Epidemiology

Occurrence
- Most countries in recent times
- Individual serotypes have limited geographical prevalence
- Horses only, all ages but especially up to 2 years
- Explosive outbreaks at long intervals, due usually to advent of a new virus subtype

Source and transmission
- Inhalation, possibly ingestion, of exhaled infection from infected clinical case, infective for about a week
- Virus viable on fomites 1–2 days

Risk factors
- Antigenic drift, especially in IA/E2, means new cohorts of horses continually develop susceptibility horses
- Most outbreaks in busy racing season when horses are moved about
- Immunity after infection lasts 1–2 years

Importance
- Major cause of disruption of racing calendar and performance horse programs
- Affected horses out of work for at least 30 days

Clinical findings

- Incubation period 2–3 days
- Fever
- Dry, hacking cough
- Minor nasal discharge
- Head lymph nodes swollen
- Depression, anorexia, stiff gait, difficulty rising, in some cases
- Spontaneous recovery after course of 1–3 weeks

Complications
- Pneumonia in foals
- Severe, persistent cough
- Limb edema
- Pneumonia
- Guttural pouch empyema
- Chronic pharyngitis

Herd history
- Characteristic is speed of spread, most animals clinically affected within a few days
- In vaccinated herds signs much less visible, sometimes limited to hind limb edema.

Clinical pathology

- Serological tests used to follow titers over time include:
  - Complement fixation
  - Hemagglutination inhibition
  - Serum neutralisation
  - ELISA used routinely

For speed during outbreak indirect immuno-fluorescence used on pharyngeal smears

Necropsy findings

- Largely irrelevant because disease rarely fatal
- Lesions restricted to bronchiolitis

Diagnosis

Resembles:
- Equine viral rhinopneumonitis
- Equine viral arteritis
- Infections with Getah virus
- Parainfluenza, reovirus, adenovirus, rhinovirus infections

Treatment and control

- Recommended treatment, prophylactic hygiene procedures are non-specific
- Water-soluble vaccines widely used but resistance brief and incomplete; also some adverse reactions
- Vaccinations commence with 2 injections at 6 months, repeated annually, with supplementary vaccinations at 6 month intervals if outbreak looms

Area vaccination program includes:
- Vaccinate all horses entering racing stable, sale ring, horse show
- No racing for 10 days after vaccination
- International travel horses vaccinated before departure
- Vaccine to contain both viruses

GETAH VIRUS DISEASE OF
HORSES [VM8 p. 1041]

In horses and pigs in Japan. Probably transmitted by *Aedes vexans* mosquitoes. Causes fever, mucosal exanthema, limb edema

CAPRINE ENZOOTIC NASAL
GRANULOMA [VM8 p. 1044]

Etiology

Retrovirus.

Epidemiology

- Goats and sheep
- History of similar cases in flock
- Purebred, cross-bred goats 7 months to 8 years

Clinical findings

- Serous–mucoid nasal discharge
- Cough
- Stertor, dyspnea
- Skull deformity, eye protrusion in some
- Weight loss, emaciation, death after long course

Necropsy findings

- Low grade neoplasms of nasal glands as adenopapilloma, adenocarcinoma, plus inflammatory nodules, on ethmoid mucosa; may be uni-, usually bilateral
- Tumors may cause skull deformity

CAPRINE HERPESVIRUS-1
[VM8 p. 1045]

Etiology

Caprine herpesvirus-1.

Epidemiology

- Widespread in some countries
- Commonest in young kids
- High morbidity, case fatality rate
- Systemic disease transmitted by ingestion or inhalation
- Sexually transmitted disease in adults

Clinical findings

Newborn kids
- Anorexia
- Dyspnea, cyanosis
- Abdominal pain
- In some cases —
  - Diarrhea, dysentery
  - Vesicles, ulcers at coronets
  - Conjunctivitis
  - Nasal discharge

- Oral mucosal erosions
- Cutaneous petechial hemorrhages

Adults

♦ Abortion, stillbirths, neonatal deaths
♦ Vulvar edema, erythema
♦ Vaginal mucosal erosions, discharge
♦ Hyperemia, ulceration of penis, prepuce; preputial discharge

Clinical pathology

♦ Serum neutralization, ELISA and radio-immunoassay tests used in diagnosis
♦ Lymphopenia a consistent finding
♦ Intranuclear inclusion bodies in some

Necropsy findings

Neonates

♦ Vesicles, ulcers on coronets
♦ Necrosis, ulceration forestomachs and intestines

Adults

♦ Vulvar, vaginal erosions, ulceration
♦ Placentitis in does
♦ Similar lesions in prepuce, on penis

Diagnosis

Resembles:
♦ Caprine mycoplasmoses
♦ Venereal ulcerative dermatosis

SWINE INFLUENZA [VM8 p. 1045]

Etiology

Type A influenza virus of family Orthomyxoviridae.

Epidemiology

Occurrence

♦ Widespread infection in many countries
♦ Explosive outbreaks; high morbidity; case fatality less than 5%
♦ Mostly in young pigs; all ages in a naive herd susceptible

Source and transmission

♦ Inapparent carriers thought to be source
♦ Transmission by aerosol inhalation

Risk factors

♦ Most common during cold weather, late fall to spring
♦ Many pigs may be affected at once, suggesting prior infections being activated by external factor such as inclement weather

Importance

A mild disease with few death losses except in neonates; some weight gain wastage, risk of secondary bacterial infection especially *Haemophilus*, *Pasteurella* spp.

Clinical findings

♦ Incubation period 2–7 days
♦ High fever depression, anorexia
♦ Disinclined to rise, move
♦ Stiff gait
♦ Labored dyspnea
♦ Sneezing, paroxysms of painful coughing
♦ Conjunctival congestion, watery ocular, nasal discharge
♦ Rapid recovery in most after course of 4–6 days
♦ Weight loss rapidly regained
♦ Clonic convulsions terminally in few fatal cases

Clinical pathology

♦ Tissue culture isolation of virus; indirect immunofluorescence staining, using monoclonal antibodies, of nasal epithelial smear quicker, simpler
♦ Virus neutralization test, hemagglutination inhibition tests used to identify infected animals

Necropsy findings

♦ Enlarged throat, cervical, mediastinal lymph nodes
♦ Congestion upper respiratory tract mucosa
♦ Much tenacious exudate in bronchi
♦ Atelectasis ventral lung borders
♦ Necrotising bronchitis, bronchiolitis

Diagnosis

Resembles:
♦ Enzootic pneumonia
♦ Inclusion body rhinitis
♦ Atrophic rhinitis
♦ Hog cholera

Treatment

♦ Broad-spectrum antibacterial treatment, administered in feed to counteract secondary invaders is a common strategy
♦ Dust-free, well ventilated, warm housing

Control

♦ Avoidance of importations of high risk animals, stress to precipitate disease
♦ Vaccines not used routinely because of variability in antigenicity, infrequent occurrence of disease

PORCINE EPIDEMIC ABORTION
AND RESPIRATORY SYNDROME
(PEARS; BLUE-EARED PIG DISEASE,
SWINE INFERTILITY AND
RESPIRATORY SYNDROME (SIRS);
PORCINE REPRODUCTIVE AND
RESPIRATORY SYNDROME)
[VM8 p. 1048]

Etiology

The **Lelystad virus** of the Togaviridae family

Epidemiology

♦ First reported in USA in 1988; in Canada, UK, Europe since then; rapid spread indicates wind-borne transmission. Spread between farms can be by infected pigs
♦ High herd morbidity in infected countries
♦ Disease affects pregnant gilts, sows, unweaned, weaned young pigs and feeder pigs
♦ Losses due to abortions, stillbirths, small litter sizes, deaths of neonates, respiratory illness of feeder pigs, costs of eradication
♦ Presence of disease in a country may result in restrictions on the importation of its pork products

Clinical findings

Gilts, sows of any parity
♦ Fever, anorexia for several days
♦ Severe dyspnea, diarrhea common
♦ Mid- to later-term abortions
♦ Many autolyzed or mummified fetuses
♦ Stillbirths, weak neonates

Nearby nursing or weaned pigs
♦ Morbidity up to 30%; case fatality rate 5–10%
♦ Dyspnea, polypnea

♦ Subnormal growth rates
♦ Bluish discoloration of ears, abdomen, vulva in some

Herd history
Course in herd 6–12 weeks.

Clinical pathology

An ELISA, an indirect fluorescent antibody assay available.

Necropsy findings

No characteristic lesions in adults, feeder pigs or fetuses.

Diagnosis

The reproductive disease resembles:
♦ Leptospirosis
♦ Encephalomyocarditis virus infection
♦ Parvovirus infection
♦ Hog cholera
♦ Fumonisin poisoning

The respiratory syndrome resembles:
♦ Enzootic swine pneumonia
♦ *Actinobacillus pleuropneumoniae* infection
♦ Swine influenza complicated by *Haemophilus*, *Pasteurella* spp.
♦ *Metastrongylus* spp. infestation
♦ *Ascaris lumbricoides* infestation
♦ A severe necrotizing pneumonia in pigs characterized by fever, dyspnea, slow growth rates associated with a new influenza-A virus reported in Canada

Treatment

None recommended.

Control

Too little known to recommend other than basic rules for containment of a highly infectious disease.

INCLUSION BODY RHINITIS
(GENERALIZED CYTOMEGALIC
INCLUSION BODY DISEASE OF
SWINE) [VM8 p. 1050]

Etiology

A beta herpesvirus of the family Herpesviridae.

Epidemiology

Occurrence
♦ Worldwide, very common minor disease of young pigs
♦ Even occurs in reputable SPF herds
♦ Outbreaks, affecting a number of litters
♦ Morbidity 100%; case fatality nil

Source and transmission
♦ From upper respiratory tract of infected pigs for 2–4 weeks after infection
♦ Direct transmission
♦ Inhalation of aerosol also
♦ Transplacental occurs

Importance
♦ Inclusion body rhinitis may be precursor to atrophic rhinitis
♦ Generalized cytomegalic virus disease causes death losses

Clinical findings

♦ Pigs up to 10 weeks old; older pigs in naive herd

Inclusion body rhinitis
♦ Paroxysms of sneezing
♦ Minor serous nasal discharge, rarely blood stained
♦ Black, brown exudate around eyes
♦ Recovery after 2–4 week course

Generalized cytomegalic disease
♦ Scouring during first week of life
♦ Skin pallor, anemia
♦ Edema creates appearance of plumpness in neck, forequarters
♦ Sudden death in 2–4 week old pigs; mortality rate in litter up to 50%; several litters affected

Clinical pathology

♦ Diagnostic intranuclear inclusion bodies in exfoliated nasal mucosal cells obtained in nasal swab
♦ Serological tests include:
  • Indirect immunofluorescence
  • ELISA

Necropsy findings

♦ Intranuclear inclusion bodies in nasal epithelium
♦ Generalized petechiation at necropsy in some cases of generalized cytomegalic virus disease

Diagnosis

Resembles swine influenza.
The anemia of generalized cytomegalic disease resembles:
♦ Nutritional deficiency of iron
♦ eperythrozoonosis
♦ blood loss anemias due to hemorrhagic disease

Treatment

Nil.

Control

♦ Avoidance of stressful management procedures
♦ See also atrophic rhinitis

ENZOOTIC PNEUMONIA OF CALVES (VIRAL PNEUMONIA OF CALVES) [VM8 p. 1051]

Etiology

♦ A series of viruses, sometimes in association with *Mycoplasma* spp., other bacteria
♦ Viruses include:
  • Parainfluenza-3 (PI-3) paramyxovirus
  • Bovine respiratory syncytial virus (BRSV)
  • Bovine virus diarrhea virus (BVDV)
  • Other viruses, not considered to be important include rhinoviruses, adenoviruses, reoviruses, enteroviruses
♦ Common mycoplasmas are *M. bovis*, *M. dispar*, *M. bovirhinis*, *Ureaplasma diversum*
♦ Other associated bacteria include *Pasteurella hemolytica*, *P. multocida*, *Chlamydia* spp.

Epidemiology

Occurrence
♦ Worldwide
♦ Primarily a disease of housed dairy calves 2–5 months old
♦ Less commonly in dairy calves as young as 1 week, growing cattle up to 12 months
♦ Common, important disease of beef calves in housed veal-producing units
♦ Also rarely in beef herds at pasture
♦ Morbidity up to 100%; very variable depending on housing, identity of the virus;

case fatality rate usually less than 5%, up to 30% with BRSV

Source and transmission
Direct or aerosol transmission from infected animal discharging virus from respiratory, nasal mucosa.

Risk factors
♦ Environmental factors including ambient temperature, overcrowding, ventilation, critical to spread
♦ Parainfluenza-3 virus ubiquitous, may be activated to pathogenic status by presence of other agents or adverse environmental conditions
♦ Spread between herds by introduced animals
♦ Calves have passive immunity to most of the pathogens until 2–4 weeks of age and develop infections between then and 2–4 months of age
♦ Herd immunity may restrict disease to appearance in introduced animals
♦ Continual throughput of calves predisposes; all-in, all-out policy with cleaning/disinfection break of 6–7 days reduces prevalence

Importance
♦ Many death losses
♦ High costs of treatment
♦ Prolongation of stay in veal calf-rearing unit
♦ Reduction of future vigor, disease resistance of survivors

Clinical findings

Parainfluenza-3 virus
♦ Incubation period 5–7 days
♦ Fever
♦ Nasal discharge, small amount, mucopurulent
♦ Harsh, dry cough, easily stimulated by trachea pinch
♦ Polypnea, dyspnea
♦ Loud breath sounds anterior, ventral parts of lung
♦ Recovery in most cases after course of 4–7 days; rare sudden deaths

Bovine respiratory syncytial virus (BRSV)
♦ Generally similar to PI-3 infection but commonly much more severe e.g.:
♦ Longer course of several weeks
♦ Mouth breathing, frothy salivation
♦ Expiratory grunt
♦ Crackling sounds on auscultation caused by bronchiolitis, emphysema
♦ Subcutaneous emphysema along the back in some

Secondary bacterial pneumonia
♦ Fever, dyspnea more severe
♦ Severe toxemia, with depression, anorexia
♦ Crackling breath sounds due to bronchopneumonia
♦ Pleuritic friction rub in some
♦ Some response to antibiotic treatment, does not occur in pure virus pneumonia

Clinical pathology

♦ Fluorescent antibody technique for virus identification in transtracheal aspirate, lung lavage or nasopharyngeal swabs
♦ BRSV isolation difficult; serological test used:
  • Modified indirect fluorescent antibody test
  • Indirect hemagglutination
  • ELISA

Necropsy findings

PI-3 infection
♦ Atelectasis, consolidation of ventral, anterior margins of lungs without a bronchiolar reaction; little diaphragmatic lobe involvement
♦ Lesion is interstitial pneumonia
♦ Intracytoplasmic inclusion bodies in lung tissue in PI-3 infection

BRSV infection
♦ Similar lesions, more severe, plus emphysema
♦ Multinucleated syncytia containing intracytoplasmic inclusion bodies

Bacterial secondary pneumonia
♦ Bronchopneumonia, mottled red and gray lobular hepatization, serofibrinous pleurisy, suppuration in some.

Diagnosis

Resembles pneumonia due to:
♦ *Pasteurella* spp.
♦ *Klebsiella* spp.
♦ *Streptococcus* spp.
♦ *Mycoplasma* spp.
♦ Lungworms
♦ Aspiration pneumonia

- Acute bovine pulmonary edema, emphysema

Treatment

- Viral pneumonia will not respond to antibacterial therapy but broad-spectrum agent usually administered to ensure no secondary bacterial invasion (see undifferentiated bovine respiratory disease)
- Bronchodilators, non-steroidal inflammatory agents currently being used; flunixin meglumine appears to have modest beneficial effects

Control

- Depends on effective animal, environmental management, isolation of introduced animals
- Major problem is protection of calves housed indoors through winter months; farmer tendency is to pack the animals in, conserve heat by reducing ventilation to minimum, minimal bedding; better result achieved by keeping in small groups in movable igloos or similar light-framed buildings, with access to open, below-freezing air
- Vaccines against PI-3 are used but have no proven value
- An inactivated, adjuvanted vaccine against BRSV reduces the incidence of that disease

VIRAL PNEUMONIA IN OLDER
CALVES, YEARLINGS, AND ADULT
CATTLE [VM8 p. 1059]

The same general description as the one given for enzootic calf pneumonia (above) also fits the pneumonia usually encountered in older calves up to 8 months of age except that the bovine respiratory syncytial virus is the more common infection, the disease is commoner in beef herds at range, and the disease is more severe.

INFECTIOUS BOVINE
RHINOTRACHEITIS (IBR:
REDNOSE) (VM8 p. 1061)

Etiology

- Bovid herpesvirus-1, an alphaherpesvirus of the family Herpesviridae causes IVM8

and infectious bovine pustular vulvovaginitis and balanoposthitis
- Several different genotypes identifiable by DNA restriction endonuclease fingerprinting techniques:
  - Bovine herpesvirus-1.1 (BHV-1.1) are the respiratory viruses; they are abortigenic and can cause infertility
  - BHV-1.2 are the pustular vulvovaginitis viruses; of these BHV-1.2a strains are abortigenic, BHV-1.2b strains are not
- BEHV (bovine encephalitis herpesvirus) cause of encephalitis in cattle; a BHV-1.3 virus also isolated from a non-suppurative meningoencephalitis of calves.

Epidemiology

Occurrence

- In all forms of cattle enterprise in most countries
- Infection very widespread in domestic cattle, deer, buffalo and many wild ruminants
- Morbidity greatest in feedlots (up to 35%) least in range herds, up to 8% in dairy herds; the case fatality rate is very low in the uncomplicated respiratory disease, e.g. 1%

Source and transmission

- Inhalation of aerosol-borne infection from infected animals in respiratory disease
- Venereal transmission of venereal disease (virus survives in frozen semen)
- Introduction of infected animals often precedes outbreak
- All animals from infected herds must be considered carriers

Risk factors

- Respiratory, genital diseases rarely occur together in the same herd
- Non-immune naive or unvaccinated herds, neonates with no passive maternal immunity very susceptible to infection; systemic disease more likely to occur in them
- After infection the virus often becomes latent, to be reactivated by later stress, making the patient a clinical case or a subclinical carrier
- Placenta may harbour latent virus for periods up to 90 days

Importance

Losses due to epidemics of abortion, infertility, production loss due to respiratory disease, deaths from the systemic disease in neonates.

Clinical findings

Respiratory disease
- Incubation period 10–20 days
- Mild syndrome in enzootic herds, severe in naive herds
- Sudden onset of fever
- Anorexia
- Marked nasal mucosal hyperemia
- Small areas of grayish necrosis on anterior nasal mucosa
- Serous nasal and ocular discharge
- Salivation excessive
- Drastic milk yield decline
- Rapid, shallow respiration
- Normal lung sounds
- Low exercise tolerance
- Conjunctivitis in some outbreaks
  - One or both eyes
  - Conjunctiva red, swollen
  - No corneal involvement other than minor edema
  - Profuse, serous ocular discharge
- Short explosive cough, only in some outbreaks
- Rarely sudden death due to obstructive bronchiolitis
- Temperature declines after 3–4 days, recovery complete after 10–14 day course in most cases

Complications
- Longer illness with severe tracheitis/bronchitis in feeder cattle; mucopurulent nasal discharge
- Death due to bronchopneumonia after illness lasting up to 4 months
- Partial nasal obstruction, due to thickened mucosa, causing stertorous respiration

Neonatal viremia
- Within first week of life
- May be outbreaks in herds where herd immunity has declined
- Sudden fever, anorexia
- Salivation, rhinitis, conjunctivitis, often unilateral
- Oral mucosa hyperemic, soft palate erosions, covered with tenacious exudate
- Acute pharyngitis, esophagitis, dysphagia, aspiration pneumonia
- Laryngitis causing dyspnea
- Bronchopneumonia with crackles, wheezes, loud breath sounds
- Diarrhea, dehydration in some
- Necropsy lesions include larynx edema, bronchopneumonia, pulmonary edema, aspiration pneumonia

Encephalitic disease
- In calves younger than 6 months
- Incoordination
- Alternating excitement, depression
- Blindness
- Salivation
- Bellowing
- Convulsions
- Usually fatal

Abortion
- Occurs some weeks up to 90 days after the respiratory disease or vaccination of non-immune pregnant cows with modified live virus vaccine derived from bovine tissue culture
- Commonest in cows 6–8 months pregnant
- Placental retention common
- No residual infertility

Clinical pathology

- For diagnosis, tissue culture of virus from cotton-polyester nasal swabs, plus rising antibody titers
- Available serological tests include:
  - ELISA
  - Indirect or passive hemagglutination
  - Immunoperoxidase test
  - Virus neutralization
  - Indirect immunofluorescence
- Virus identification also possible by:
  - Dot-blot hybridisation assay
  - Restriction endonuclease analysis

Necropsy findings

Respiratory disease
- Gross lesions on muzzle, nasal cavities, pharynx, larynx, trachea, terminating in large bronchi
- Lesions are swelling, congestion, some petechiation, catarrhal exudate, small numbers of necrotic foci in trachea
- Necrotic, fibrinopurulent lesions in secondary bacterial infection
- Virus isolated by cell culture

Neonatal viremia
- Severe epithelial necrosis in esophagus, rumen
- Multiple focal lesions in edematous larynx epithelium
- Bronchopneumonia

Aborted fetus
Focal necrotic hepatitis.

Encephalitis
* Lesions in cerebral cortex, internal capsule
* Immunoperoxidase test using monoclonal antibodies specific for diagnosis of BHV-1 encephalitis

Diagnosis

Respiratory disease resembles:
* Pneumonic pasteurellosis
* Bovine virus diarrhea
* Bovine malignant catarrh
* Calf diphtheria
* Enzootic calf pneumonia
* Viral calf pneumonia
* Allergic rhinitis
* Nasal granuloma

Treatment

* Broad-spectrum antibacterials are standard to avoid secondary bacterial invasion
* Tracheitis with bronchopneumonia resistant to treatment

Control

Eradication
* Difficult but necessary in stud herds wishing to export seronegative cattle; eradicated from Switzerland in the 1980s
* Two herd scheme with calves moved to free herd at weaning
* Seropositive animals culled
* All introductions must be seronegative
* Vaccination prohibited

Containment by vaccination or natural exposure
* Modified live virus, either intramuscular or intranasal, and inactivated vaccines are used
* Inactivated vaccines not fully proven as protective
* Intranasal vaccination safe for pregnant cows, and valuable for the prevention of abortion, and gives rapid protection against the respiratory disease; significant protection in the face of an outbreak
* Intramuscular vaccination is abortigenic
* Bulls in artificial insemination centers should be seronegative and negative to regular checks of semen for presence of virus

CHRONIC ENZOOTIC PNEUMONIA OF SHEEP (CHRONIC NON-PROGRESSIVE PNEUMONIA, ATYPICAL PNEUMONIA, PROLIFERATIVE, EXUDATIVE PNEUMONIA) [VM8 p. 1070]

Etiology

* Not identified; suspect pathogens include:
  * *Mycoplasma ovipneumoniae*
  * *Bordetella parapertussis*
  * Chlamydia
  * Parainfluenza-3 virus
  * Adenovirus
  * A respiratory syncytial virus
  * Reovirus
* *Pasteurella hemolytica* a common secondary invader

Epidemiology

* Chronic, low pathogenicity pneumonia of young sheep common to all countries
* Up to 85% lambs in a flock may have lesions
* Seasonal occurrence in cooler months
* Commoner when exposed to chilling rain for long periods

Importance
* Causes significant growth retardation, weight gain
* Some carcase rejection because of pleurisy
* Death losses when enzootic bacterial pneumonia (e.g. *Actinomyces pyogenes*) also present

Clinical findings

* Insidious onset
* Persists in a flock for 4–7 months
* Poor weight gains, growth retardation

Clinical pathology

Undefined.

Necropsy findings

Proliferative, exudative pneumonia.

Diagnosis

Resembles:
* *Pasteurella haemolytica* pneumonia
* Maedi

- Jaagsiekte
- Lungworm infestation

Treatment

Nil.

Control

Not specified

OVINE PROGRESSIVE PNEUMONIA
(MAEDI, MAEDI–VISNA)
[VM8 p. 1071]

Etiology

- Ovine retrovirus of the family Lentivirinae; many genetic variants in isolates
- Closely related viruses cause visna, caprine arthritis encephalitis

Epidemiology

Occurrence
- Most major sheep-raising countries
- Only in sheep and goats; all breeds, all ages
- No identified wild ruminants infected

Source and transmission
- In infected milk from carrier ewe
- Lateral transmission in adults
- Spread rapid; all flock infected within 2 years
- Very rapid spread when flock also infected with pulmonary adenomatosis
- Morbidity up to 70%; case fatality rate 100%

Clinical findings

- Incubation period 2 years
- Most clinical cases older than 3 years
- Insidious onset, slow progress
- Listless
- Body weight loss, emaciation
- Exercise intolerance
- Dyspnea later
- Cough
- Nasal discharge
- Temperature high normal
- Udder enlarged, firm, teats limp, little milk, milk normal; may be the only clinical abnormality
- Arthritis only seen in USA; carpal joints swollen, lame
- Always fatal after course of 3–10 months

- Respiratory signs may be minimal relative to emaciation

Clinical pathology

- Moderate hypochromic anemia
- Leukocytosis in preclinical stage
- Hypergammaglobulinemia
- Virus isolated in cell culture
- Serological tests include:
  - Complement fixation
  - Virus neutralization test
  - ELISA
- Agar gel immunodiffusion test
- Indirect immunofluorescence test

Necropsy findings

- Lungs large, heavy, do not collapse, gray–blue to gray–yellow color; chronic interstitial pneumonia with lymphoid tissue proliferation
- Bronchial, mediastinal lymph nodes enlarged
- Similar lesions in udder

Diagnosis

The respiratory disease resembles:
- jaagsiekte
- Parasitic pneumonia
- Melioidosis

Udder disease resembles:
- Mastitis
- Caprine arthritis encephalitis

Emaciation disease resembles:
- Johne's disease
- Caseous lymphadenitis

Treatment

Nil.

Control

Complete depopulation of sheep in a country has been the control program used; alternatives are:

Separation at birth Lambs taken at birth, reared separately, artificially; no colostrum

Test and segregate:
- All positive reactors to serological test, and their progeny, culled
- Annual retest until two consecutive negative tests

♦ Introductions to either system must be seronegatives
♦ Shed lambing very conducive to spread and should be discontinued

PULMONARY ADENOMATOSIS (JAAGSIEKTE, OVINE PULMONARY CARCINOMA) [VM8 p. 1075]

Etiology

♦ Uncertain; probably a retrovirus
♦ A herpesvirus also isolated from the lungs of animals sick with the disease

Epidemiology

Occurrence
♦ In most sheep-raising countries
♦ Clinical disease very patchy in distribution
♦ Almost entirely in mature sheep; very rarely in 3–6 months lambs; goats infected experimentally
♦ Morbidity usually 5% per year, up to 20%
♦ Case fatality 100%
♦ Occurs in restricted areas, e.g. certain parts of UK

Source and transmission
♦ Retrovirus identified in lung tissue
♦ Aerosol transmission of infectious agent from copious nasal discharge suspected
♦ Genetic susceptibility suspected

Clinical findings

♦ Incubation period usually 1–3 years
♦ First illness at 2, usually 3–4 years
♦ Occasional cough
♦ Exercise intolerance; panting after exercise
♦ Emaciation
♦ Appetite, temperature normal
♦ Dyspnea
♦ Lacrimation
♦ Profuse, watery, nasal discharge
♦ Up to 200 ml watery mucus runs from nostrils if sheep held up by hind limbs

♦ Moist crackles audible over lungs; audible at a distance from a group of affected sheep resembling the sound of boiling porridge
♦ Always fatal after prolonged course 6 weeks to 4 months

Complications
♦ Cor pulmonale
♦ Pneumonic pasteurellosis

Clinical pathology

No tests available.

Necropsy findings

♦ Lungs grossly increased in size, weight up to 3 times normal
♦ Extensive areas neoplastic tissue, especially at ventral borders of apical lobes
♦ Excess frothy fluid in bronchi
♦ Bronchial, mediastinal lymph nodes enlarged, contain small metastases in some
♦ Lesions are adenomatous ingrowths of alveolar epithelium
♦ Pneumonic pasteurellosis, with abscesses, pleurisy common complication

Diagnosis

Resembles:
♦ Jaagsiekte
♦ Parasitic pneumonia
♦ Melioidosis

Treatment

Nil.

Control

♦ Eradicated from Iceland by complete depopulation of sheep from country
♦ Because of lack of diagnostic test recommendation for herd eradication is culling of clinical cases, and all their progeny at the earliest sign of disease

VIRAL DISEASES CHARACTERIZED BY NERVOUS SIGNS

VIRAL ENCEPHALOMYELITIS OF
HORSES [VM8 p. 1077]

Etiology

♦ An alphavirus of the family Togaviridae
♦ Three immunologically distinct strains
with differing virulences: Eastern (EEE),
Western (WEE), Venezuelan (VEE), and
antigenic variants within these strains

Epidemiology

Occurrence
♦ Only in Canada, USA, Central and South
America
♦ WEE in the west of North America extending eastward to Appalachians; EEE in the
east and south extending west to mid-west,
plus Caribbean islands, Central and South
America; VEE in many South, Central
American countries, also in West Indies,
southern USA
♦ Infection prevalence much higher than
clinical disease morbidity; variable depending on insect population, and terrain,
influencing exposure to insect bite; in outbreaks morbidity up to 20%
♦ Case fatality rate 20–30% with WEE, 40–
90% with VEE, WEE. Mortality rate in
young foals from unvaccinated mares
100%

Source and transmission
♦ WEE and EEE are bird diseases, accidental
infections in horses, mules, donkeys, humans, possibly monkeys; disease in birds
may be fatal or innocuous
♦ Pigs and wild ruminants may be seropositive but no clinical disease; many animal
species susceptible to experimental infection
♦ Spread by bites of mosquitoes, ticks, blood-
sucking bugs, chicken mites, lice
♦ Virus life cycle passed in *Aedes, Culex,
Mansonia* spp. mosquitoes
♦ Major route of spread is from birds to
horses
♦ Wild birds, small vertebrates including
snakes, turtles form infection reservoir
♦ Long-distance transmission probably by
wind transport of infective mosquitoes
♦ The VEE virus produces a high level of
viremia in horses which act as amplifiers;
the infection cycle with small rodents and
birds is at a low level

Risk factors
♦ strain virulence; WEE least virulent, EEE,
VEE equally virulent
♦ Season; most prevalent when mosquitoes
active; thus summer, but also year-round in
tropical areas
♦ Swamps favor occurrence
♦ Young horses most susceptible
♦ Immunity after natural infection lasts 2
years

Importance
A serious zoonosis with all 3 strains.

Clinical findings

♦ Diseases caused by all viruses clinically
indistinguishable
♦ Incubation period 1–3 weeks
♦ Fever, anorexia, depression for 24 hours;
may be mild and pass unnoticed
♦ Hypersensitivity to sound and touch
♦ Transient excitement, restlessness, blind-
ness in some
♦ Walk into objects, circling
♦ Shoulder, facial muscle tremor; penis erec-
tion
♦ Severe mental depression phase follows:
  • Stand with head hung low
  • Appear to be asleep with feed hanging
    from mouth
  • May eat or drink if feed placed in mouth
  • Pupillary light reflex persists
  • Can be roused but soon lapses
♦ Paralysis phase follows:
  • Patient unable to hold up head
  • Lower lip pendulous
  • Tongue may hang out
  • Head-pressing or leaning back on halter
  • Incoordination, especially hind limbs
  • Unable to swallow
  • Defecation, urination suppressed
  • Recumbency
♦ Death after course of 2–4 days in most
cases
♦ Survivors deficient mentally, do not re-
spond to signals

Clinical pathology

♦ A four-fold increase in antibodies in acute,
convalescent sera 10–14 days apart pro-
vides positive diagnosis using as the test:
  • Complement fixation
  • Hemagglutination inhibition
  • Virus neutralization

- Single negative sera may mislead because of 5–10 day lead time between infection and antibody appearance
- Single positive may mislead because titers stay high for years
- Culture of virus from blood may be achieved with VEE because of high viremia, but unlikely with other two viruses

Necropsy findings

- No gross changes
- Liquefactive necrosis, hemorrhages in cerebral cortex; most severe in EEE, medium in VEE, least in WEE.
- Transmission using brain as source by:
  - Injection into sucking mouse brain or duck embryo tissue culture
  - Fluorescent antibody test

Diagnosis

Resembles:

- Hepatic encephalopathy
- Borna disease
- Japanese encephalitis
- Snowshoe hare virus encephalitis of horses
- West Nile virus encephalitis
- Equine degenerative myeloencephalopathy
- Botulism
- Poisoning by fumonisin, sesquiterpene lactones
- Sporadic cases of:
  - Brain tumor
  - cholesteatoma
  - Hydrocephalus

Treatment

- Supportive treatment may enable animal to survive, but may be mentally deficient
- Nurse recumbent patients on good bedding
- Support standing patients in sling, feed via nasal tube

Control

A five point program:

- Accurate clinical/laboratory test available
- Sentinel animals to monitor presence of virus in area
- Quarantine laws to control movement of infected animals
- Insect abatement policy; indoor housing at night

Vaccination – WEE, EEE

- Highly effective formalin-inactivated vaccines available for WEE, EEE; combined vaccine if both viruses possible in area
- Vaccinations begun before insect season starts
- Course of 2 vaccinations, 10 days apart, then annual revaccination
- Foals from vaccinated dams vaccinated at 6–8 months
- Foals from unvaccinated dams at 2–3 months, again at 1 year
- Rare complication is post-vaccinal hepatitis

Vaccination – VEE

- Objective, besides preventing infection, is to reduce number of viremic horses to act as donors
- Tissue-culture attenuated vaccine used; antibody titre higher in horses not previously vaccinated with WEE, VEE vaccines
- Combination vaccine including WEE, EEE, VEE available, effective

JAPANESE ENCEPHALITIS
[VM8 p. 1085]

Etiology

A flavivirus of the family Flaviviridae

Epidemiology

- A disease of humans, transmissible to all animal species
- Sporadic clinical cases in racehorses in Malaysia, also in pigs; symptomless in cattle, sheep, goats
- Mosquito-transmitted; commonest in summer; overwinters in mosquito
- Maintained in population by human–mosquito–pig cycle with pigs the major source of virus
- Can cause heavy death losses in swine

Clinical findings

Mild cases

- Fever, anorexia
- Sluggish movements
- Jaundice in some
- Recovery after course of 2–3 days

Moderate cases

- Mild fever
- Somnolence, pronounced lethargy
- Mucosae jaundiced, petechiated
- Labial paralysis
- Difficult swallowing
- Radial paralysis
- Staggery gait, incoordination, easy falling
- Neck rigidity
- Blindness
- Recovery in most after course of 4–9 days

Severe cases

- Uncommon; 5% of cases
- High fever
- Hyperexcitability
- Tremor
- Profuse sweating
- Violent uncontrolled activity
- Fatal termination in some

Abortion

Sows abort or produce dead pigs at term.

Clinical pathology

ELISA available

Necropsy findings

Non-suppurative encephalitis.

Diagnosis

Resembles:

- Hepatic encephalopathy
- Borna disease
- Japanese encephalitis
- Snowshoe hare virus encephalitis of horses
- West Nile virus encephalitis
- Equine degenerative myeloencephalopathy
- Botulism
- Poisoning by fumonisin, sesquiterpene lactones

Treatment

Nil.

Control

- Excellent protection against encephalitis but no protection against stillbirths with formalin-killed vaccine
- Live, attenuated vaccine protects against stillbirths, encephalitis

BORNA DISEASE [VM8 p. 1086]

Etiology

An unclassified virus indistinguishable from the virus of Near Eastern equine encephalomyelitis; it is possible they are the same disease.

Epidemiology

- Affects horses, rarely as outbreaks in sheep; possibly humans
- Transmission method unknown; presumed ingestion or inhalation
- Virus resistant to environmental influences
- Low morbidity, most die

Clinical findings

- Many subclinical cases
- Incubation period 4 weeks to 6 months
- Fever
- Pharyngeal paralysis, no feed taken
- Hyperesthesia
- Tremor
- Lethargy, somnolence
- Flaccid paralysis
- Death after 1–3 week course

Clinical pathology

Infection identified by tests including:

- Complement fixation
- Fluorescent antibody

Necropsy findings

- No gross findings
- Typical viral encephalitis in brain stem and spinal cord
- Diagnostic intracellular inclusion bodies in brain nerve cells

Diagnosis

Resembles:

- hepatic encephalopathy
- Borna disease
- Japanese encephalitis
- Snowshoe hare virus encephalitis of horses West Nile virus encephalitis
- Equine degenerative myeloencephalopathy
- Botulism
- Poisoning by fumonisin, sesquiterpene lactones

Treatment

Nil.

Control

Lapinized vaccine effective.

OTHER EQUINE
ENCEPHALOMYELITIDES
[VM8 p. 1086]

West Nile virus meningoencephalitis
[VM8 p. 1086]

♦ In horses, humans in French Mediterranean littoral
♦ Insect transmitted
♦ Fever, incoordination, paresis, paralysis, 2–3 weeks course

Murray Valley encephalitis
[VM8 p. 1086]

Serological evidence of infection in horses of this human disease in Australia; histological evidence of encephalitis

Powassan virus [VM8 p. 1086]

♦ The infection, primarily of wildlife, has occurred in horses in Canada, associated with a non-suppurative, focal, necrotizing meningoencephalitis
♦ Tick-transmitted
♦ Clinical tremor, staggering, recumbency and non-suppurative encephalomyelitis produced experimentally

California serogroup of viruses
[VM8 p. 1087]

♦ Cause acute encephalitis in horses
♦ Includes snowshoe hare virus, Jamestown canyon virus, occur in Canada, maintained in a horse–mosquito–small wild mammal cycle
♦ Main Drain virus isolated from a horse with encephalitis in California, in a rodent–*Culicoides* spp.–horse cycle

RABIES [VM8 p. 1087]

Etiology

A lyssavirus of the family Rhabdoviridae

Epidemiology

Occurrence
♦ All warm-blooded animals except, possibly, the opossum
♦ In most countries except those with sea boundaries, e.g. UK, Australia, New Zealand

Source and transmission
♦ Variable sources including wolves, foxes, mongoose, raccoons, skunks, fruit and vampire bats, with domestic dogs and cats often forming the last link from the wild animal reservoir to humans and domestic livestock
♦ Transmission is via the saliva of infected patient, during a bite, or manipulation such as drenching
♦ Rabid dogs cause more deaths than foxes because they bite many animals, foxes tend to bite only a few
♦ Inhalation of aerosolized urine from infected, symptomless fruit bats in caves also a route of transmission
♦ Transmission is also possible by ingestion if the dose is large enough; knowledge put to use in vaccinating wildlife by baiting

Risk factors
♦ Fragile virus; dies in dried saliva in few hours; susceptible to most disinfectants
♦ Variation in susceptibility: fox, coyote extremely susceptible; cattle, cats highly susceptible; dogs, sheep, cattle moderately susceptible

Importance
♦ Deaths losses in livestock rarely great
♦ Most importance relates to rabies as a zoonosis with a 100% case fatality rate

Clinical findings

Incubation period 3 weeks to 3 months

Paralytic rabies – cattle
♦ Knuckling at fetlocks in hind limb
♦ Swaying, sagging of hindquarters while walking
♦ Deviation of tail to one side, tail flaccidity
♦ Decreased sensation tail head, perineum
♦ Anus paralysis, straining with sucking, blowing of air
♦ Staggery gait, recumbency
♦ Drooling of saliva, jaw sags; inability to close jaw, unable to swallow, constant chewing movements

- Some patients unable to eat, others eat until a few hours before death
- Course up to 7 days

Furious rabies – cattle

- Tense, alert appearance
- Hypersensitive to sound or movement
- Some patients attack another animal or object
- Ineffectual attempts to bite
- Gait incoordinated
- Continuous, hoarse bellowing
- Sexual activity exaggerated, e.g. bulls will mount trucks
- After course of 24–48 hours, flaccid paralysis, death

Sheep

- Often a number affected at one time
- Similar syndrome to cattle
- Most cases paralytic
- A few patients attempt to bite, pull their wool, show sexual excitement

Goat

- Most cases aggressive
- Continuous bleating common

Horses

- Ataxia, paresis of hindquarters
- Loss of tail, anal sphincter tone
- Staggery gait, sudden onset of lameness in one hind limb, recumbency
- Pharyngeal paralysis, drooling saliva, teeth not closed
- Colic
- Furious rabies in a few include signs of:
  - Hyperesthesia, excitement
  - Aggressiveness with biting, kicking
  - Chewing foreign materials, own skin
  - Blind charges, circling
  - Sudden falling, rolling
  - Tremor of hind limbs, crouching
  - Frequent whinnying with abnormal voice
- Course 1–7 days

Pigs

- Very variable syndrome; signs seen include:
- Excitement, tendency to attack or dullness, incoordination
- Nose twitch, rapid chewing movements, excess salivation
- Clonic convulsions, walking backwards
- Terminal paralysis
- Death after a course of 12–48 hours

Clinical pathology

- A diagnosis usually made on clinical, confirmed on necropsy, grounds
- Serological tests used to determine immunological status include:
  - Virus neutralisation
  - Passive hemagglutination
  - Complement fixation
  - Radioimmunoassay
  - Indirect fluorescent antibody staining
  - ELISA

Necropsy findings

- Rabies suspect kept in isolation; if alive at 10 days rabies eliminated as diagnosis
- Brain removed after euthanasia during clinical stage checked for rabies virus by:
  - Fluorescent antibody test (FAT) on impression smear
  - In cases where FAT negative, and human exposure involved, intracerebral injection in unweaned white mice; nervous signs in mice at 4–18 days; brain in some harvested and FAT applied; other mice allowed to die, brain checked for Negri bodies or tissue culture infection test
  - Histological check for Negri bodies

Diagnosis

In cattle resembles:

- Acute or subacute lead poisoning
- Lactation tetany
- Hypovitaminosis A
- Polioencephalomalacia
- Listeriosis

In sheep resembles:

- Enterotoxemia
- Pregnancy toxemia
- Louping-ill

In pigs resembles:

- Pseudorabies
- Porcine viral encephalomyelitis
- Hog cholera
- African swine fever
- Streptococcal meningitis

In horses resembles:

- Viral encephalomyelitis
- Brain cholesteomata
- hepatic encephalopathy

Treatment

- None attempted after clinical signs evident
- Prophylaxis after bite by rabies suspect:

- Thorough washing of wounds with soap and water
- Ensure patient maintained in isolation for 10 days

Control

Control introduction of dogs with prohibition of entry from country where disease occurs, plus strict quarantine for 6 months; 12 months safer; vaccination, twice, with an inactivated vaccine while in quarantine recommended
- Where disease enzootic:
  - Control of wildlife, possibly oral vaccination distributed by aircraft
  - Control of dogs by registration, muzzling, allowing them out only on leash
  - Vaccinate dogs, cats; mostly live vaccine strains, e.g. FLURY, ERA, Kelev strains used annually

PSEUDORABIES (AUJESZKY'S DISEASE) [VM8 p. 1094]

Etiology

Porcine herpesvirus-1 of the family Herpesviridae; a number of genomically different strains, identifiable by restriction endonuclease analysis, DNA hybridisation

Epidemiology

Occurrence
- A major disease of pig industry worldwide
- Primarily a pig disease; occurs incidentally, rarely in most other species, e.g. in goats, cattle comingled with pigs
- Outbreaks in naive herds, very rapid spread, lasts 1–2 months
- Infection prevalence usually 100%; morbidity rate very low in adults; case fatality rate varies, up to 100% in piglets, 5% in growing pigs

Source and transmission
- Pigs, possibly rodents, the source
- Clinically normal carriers; also animals with latent infection capable of being activated
- Vaccination minimizes clinical disease but not infection; virus can continue replicating in vaccinated or recovered pig or piglets with maternal antibodies
- Spreads to other species also, but not spread between those species
- Spread by direct contact via nasal mucosa, abraded skin, plus ingestion of contaminated water, feed, possibly by inhalation, possibly by aerosol transport over long distances; in utero transmission, via milk also occurs

Risk factors
- Large breeding units
- Gilts in same shed as sows
- Clinical cases
- Keeping growing pigs in confined quarters
- Concurrent infection with *Actinobacillus pleuropneumonia*
- Virus survives 2–7 weeks in environment, up to 5 weeks in meat, only hours in an aerosol
- Susceptible to most disinfectants; 5.25% sodium hypochlorite best

Importance
- Losses include direct wastage due to deaths, abortions, stillbirths plus indirect costs of laboratory diagnosis, culling, vaccination
- Transmissible to humans

Clinical findings

Pigs
- Variable depending on strain of virus
- Nervous, reproduction or respiratory syndromes

Piglets up to 1 month old
- Fever
- Hind limb incoordination, sideways progression
- Tremor
- Recumbency, paddling movements
- Lateral head deviation
- Mouth frothing
- Nystagmus
- Blindness in some outbreaks
- Convulsive episodes in some
- Snoring respiration, abdominal dyspnea, vomiting diarrhea in some
- Deaths after 12 hour course

Growing pigs
- Much less severe than in piglets; much variation depending on strain of virus
- Fever, depression, vomiting, sneezing, nasal discharge, cough, dyspnea, tremor, incoordination, recumbency, convulsions, *or*
- Incoordination, leg weakness

Adult pigs

♦ Anorexia, dullness, agalactia, constipation, *or*
♦ Fever, sneezing, nasal pruritus, vomiting, incoordination, convulsions, death

Early pregnant sows

Embryonic death, abortion, mummified fetus of all or part of litter

Adult cattle

♦ Sudden death without prior illness, *or*
♦ Intense local pruritus, violent licking, rubbing or chewing of part
♦ Most common about head, flanks, feet
♦ Intense excitement, convulsions, bellowing
♦ Mania
♦ Circling
♦ Diaphragm spasm
♦ Opisthotonus
♦ Ataxia
♦ Salivation
♦ Dyspnea
♦ Fever
♦ Paralysis, death after course of 6–48 hours

Young calves

♦ Encephalitis, without pruritus
♦ Erosions in mouth, esophagus
♦ Most cases die

Goats

♦ Restless
♦ Pruritus in some
♦ Getting up, lying down frequently
♦ Profuse sweating
♦ Convulsions
♦ Terminal paralysis

Dogs, cats

♦ Syndrome as in cattle
♦ Death in 24 hours

Clinical pathology

♦ Serological tests suitable for herd diagnosis:
  • Virus neutralisation
  • ELISA
  • Latex agglutination
  • Radial immunodiffusion enzyme assay
  • Dot enzyme immunoassay
♦ Antibody titer rise necessary for diagnosis of active infection
♦ None of the tests is capable of differentiating between infection and vaccination titers; the Gi-ELISA can differentiate in herds specifically vaccinated with G negative vaccines
♦ Virus identified by immunofluorescen staining in smears made from swabs, usin special materials, of nasal, vaginal mucosa

Necropsy findings

♦ No specific gross lesions
♦ In histological specimens severe, extensiv neuronal damage, perivascular cuffing foal necrosis in spinal cord and brain
♦ Intranuclear inclusions in necrotizin lesions in upper respiratory tract, lungs
♦ Placentitis, intranuclear inclusions in abor tion cases
♦ Virus in tissues identified by:
  • Direct immunofluorescence of im pression smear
  • Immunoperoxidase test
♦ DNA hybridization dot blot assay

Diagnosis

Resembles:
♦ Viral encephalomyelitis
♦ Rabies
♦ Streptococcal meningitis
♦ Hypoglycemia in baby pigs
♦ Louping ill
♦ Japanese encephalitis
♦ Salmonellosis
♦ Glasser's disease
♦ Septicemic colibacillosis
♦ Erysipelas
♦ Gut edema
♦ Salt poisoning
♦ Organophosphate poisoning

Treatment

♦ No effective remedy
♦ Hyperimmune serum at time of infection will reduce mortality rate

Control

♦ Difficult, unreliable because healthy pigs may shed virus for several months
♦ Eradication in breeding herds can be attempted by:
  • Depopulation when infection prevalence >50%
  • Program of intensive serological testing, culling of reactors possible in herds with infection prevalence <50%
  • Progeny segregation with segregation after weaning, vaccination of dams, frequent serotesting of free herd

◆ Vaccination used in commercial piggeries to:
  • Reduce clinical disease in an outbreak
  • Reduce prevalence in an enzootic herd
◆ Vaccines include modified live virus, inactivated virus administered intranasally or parenterally; intranasal preferred; attenuated vaccines may not be safe for piglets or pregnant sows
◆ Genetically engineered vaccines also in use; combined with special serological test to differentiate between serum titers due to natural infection and vaccination has been used in effective eradication program

VIRAL ENCEPHALOMYELITIS OF PIGS (TESCHEN DISEASE, TALFAN DISEASE, POLIOMYELITIS SUUM)
[VM8 p. 1103]

Etiology

A number of antigenically related enteroviruses of the family Picornaviridae, including Teschen, Talfan, Konratice, Reporyje, with varying virulence.

Epidemiology

Occurrence
◆ Worldwide; most virulent strains still in Central Europe, where disease originated
◆ Mostly a disease of young pigs, rarely adults
◆ In enzootic herds herd immunity develops and disease limited to weaned, early grower pigs, suckers protected by maternal antibodies

Source and transmission
◆ Virus in feces
◆ Spread from infected pigs by ingestion and inhalation
◆ Spread in herd very rapid

Risk factors
Resistant to environmental conditions, especially drying.

Importance
◆ Wastage due to deaths, some cripples
◆ Infection prevalence very high in enzootic area; morbidity variable, usually low (5–50%), sporadic cases or few in each litter; case fatality rate 70–90% in Teschen disease, much lower in Talfan

Clinical findings

Acute disease – Teschen disease
◆ Incubation period 10–12 days
◆ Fever, anorexia, vomiting
◆ Voice abnormality or loss (laryngeal paralysis)
◆ Hyperesthesia, easily startled, loud squealing response to noise
◆ Facial paralysis in some
◆ Limb stiffness
◆ Opisthotonus
◆ Falling to one side
◆ Tremor
◆ Nystagmus
◆ Violent clonic convulsions
◆ Death after course of 3–4 days, *or*
◆ Survival with flaccid paralysis, especially hind limbs
◆ Some cases pass direct to flaccidity without convulsions

Subacute disease – Talfan disease (UK), viral encephalomyelitis (USA, Australia), poliomyelitis suum (Europe) in piglets up to 2 weeks old
◆ Sudden onset, short-lived outbreaks
◆ Most common, severe in pigs less than 2 weeks old (morbidity, case fatality rates near 100%)
◆ Younger piglets affected, many recover
◆ Sows may be mildly, transiently ill
◆ Anorexia,
◆ Constipation
◆ Weight loss
◆ Vomiting
◆ Diarrhea in some
◆ Hyperesthesia
◆ Tremor
◆ Knuckled fetlocks
◆ Ataxia
◆ Walking backwards
◆ Dog-sitting posture
◆ Lateral recumbency terminally
◆ Paddling convulsions
◆ Nystagmus, blindness
◆ Dyspnea

Subacute disease in piglets 4–6 weeks old
◆ Rarely also in sows, gilts
◆ Transient anorexia
◆ Transient swaying drunken gait

Clinical pathology

Serological tests include:
  • Virus neutralisation
  • Complement fixation

Necropsy findings

+ Diffuse non-suppurative encephalomyelitis in brain stem and spinal cord
+ Virus present in tissue in small amounts, difficult to identify

Diagnosis

Resembles:
+ Pseudorabies
+ Hemagglutinating encephalomyelitis virus disease
+ Rabies
+ Streptococcal meningitis
+ Hypoglycemia in baby pigs
+ Louping ill
+ Japanese encephalitis
+ Salmonellosis
+ Glasser's disease
+ Septicemic colibacillosis
+ Erysipelas
+ Gut edema
+ Salt poisoning
+ Organophosphate poisoning

Treatment

None recommended

Control

+ A closed herd policy to limit entry.
+ Sporadic occurrence has not warranted a specific control policy
+ A formalin-killed and a modified live virus are current in Europe
+ Eradication has been achieved by slaughter of infected herds plus ring vaccination around them

SPORADIC BOVINE ENCEPHALOMYELITIS (SBE, BUSS DISEASE, TRANSMISSIBLE SEROSITIS) [VM8 p. 1105]

Etiology

Chlamydia psittaci

Epidemiology

Occurrence
+ Reported at low prevalence only in a few countries
+ Cattle and buffalo only
+ Calves younger than 6 months most susceptible

+ Sporadic small outbreaks, single cases, enzootic some herds
+ May be high infection prevalence
+ Morbidity rate 5 (adults)–50% (calves); case fatality 30%

Source and transmission
+ Infected animals the source; transmission mode unknown
+ infectious agent appears to be in feces for several weeks after infection

Risk factors
Chlamydia susceptible to disinfectants, resistant to freezing.

Clinical findings

+ Incubation period 4 days to 4 weeks
+ Depression, inactivity, fever for several days then
+ Nasal discharge, salivation
+ Dyspnea, cough in some
+ Diarrhea in some
+ Stiff gait, fetlock knuckling
+ Staggery gait, circling, easy falling
+ Opisthotonus in some
+ Death or recovery after course of 3 days to 3 weeks
+ Survivors slow to regain serious weight loss

Clinical pathology

+ Infectious agent isolatable from blood
+ Complement fixation test

Necropsy findings

+ Fibrinous peritonitis, pleurisy, pericarditis
+ Diffuse encephalomyelitis, meningitis, especially cerebellar, medullary area
+ Elementary bodies in tissues

Diagnosis

Resembles:
+ Pneumonic pasteurellosis
+ Bovine malignant catarrh
+ Listeriosis
+ Rabies
+ Lead poisoning

Treatment

Irregular results of field treatment with a tetracycline, but generally good if administered early in course.

Control

olation of clinical cases recommended.

VINE ENCEPHALOMYELITIS (LOUPING-ILL) [VM8 p. 1106]

Etiology

A flavivirus of the family Flaviviridae; concurrent infection with tick-borne fever agent (*Cytoecetes phagocytophila*) enhances pathogenicity of louping-ill virus.

Epidemiology

Occurrence
‣ Patchy distribution in UK, Scandinavia, Europe, Middle East related to distribution of tick vector
‣ Predominantly in sheep but can infect many species, including cattle, humans
‣ Infection prevalence high in enzootic areas, herds; passive immunity spares neonates; morbidity 5–60%, highest in lambs, yearlings; most infections subclinical

Source and transmission
‣ Only sheep, red grouse, possibly horse, red deer, elk sufficiently viremic to be donors
‣ Reservoir, transmitter tick *Ixodes ricinus*; not transmitted transovarially; inhalation transmission to humans, ingestion in pigs, via milk in goats

Risk factors
‣ Spring and fall when tick active
‣ Immunosuppression increases chances of infection

Importance
A zoonosis to pathologists

Clinical findings

Sheep
‣ Incubation period 2–4 days
‣ Transient high fever with regression followed by
‣ Secondary fever plus:
  • Standing apart, opisthotonus
  • Lip, nostril-twitching
  • Tremor of neck and limbs
  • Bounding gait due to stiff, jerky movements – louping
  • Hind limb incoordination
  • Walks into objects, head-pressing
  • Hypersensitivity to touch, sound in some
‣ Recumbency, convulsions, paralysis, death after course of 2 days plus
‣ Survivors miss the recumbent–convulsive stage, persist, some with persistent torticollis, posterior paresis

Cattle
As for sheep plus:
‣ Eeyelid blinking, eye rolling
‣ Convulsions common

Goats
Usually subclinical in adults but kids drinking infected milk may develop acute disease

Horse
Similar to sheep

Clinical pathology

Virus isolatable from blood in viremic stage
‣ Serological tests include —
  • Hemagglutination inhibition
  • complement fixation
‣ Virus neutralisation

Necropsy findings

‣ No gross findings
‣ Perivascular cell accumulations in meninges, and brain spinal cord
‣ Virus detectable in tissue by fluorescent antibody

Diagnosis

In lambs resembles:
‣ Swayback
‣ Tick pyemia
‣ Spinal abscess

In yearlings resembles:
‣ Spinal trauma
‣ Coenurosis
‣ Polioencephalomalacia

In adults resembles:
‣ Scrapie
‣ Many poisonous plants
‣ Tetanus
‣ Hypocalcemia
‣ Pregnancy toxemia
‣ Hypomagnesemia
‣ Ovine radial polyneuropathy

Treatment

♦ Antiserum helpful if given within 48 hours of first signs
♦ Sedate, isolate clinical cases

Control

Vaccination

♦ The favoured option
♦ Formalinized brain tissue vaccine effective; has transmitted scrapie
♦ In oil the vaccine gives immunity for up to 3 years
♦ Vaccination late in pregnancy protects lambs

Other measures

♦ Tick control
♦ Eradication of reservoir in sheep, red grouse

CAPRIDE ARTHRITIS
ENCEPHALITIS (CAE) [VM8 p. 1110]

Etiology

A series of genetically distinct, non-oncogenic retroviruses of the family Lentivirinae, with varying virulences

Epidemiology

Occurrence

♦ Worldwide
♦ Highest prevalence in developed countries which have imported dairy goats from Europe and North America

Source and transmission

♦ Infection at birth persists for life; only few develop clinical disease
♦ Mostly doe-to-kid via colostrum and milk
♦ Intra-uterine possible but insignificant in control program
♦ Some spread by direct contact between goats especially via shared milking facilities

Risk factors

♦ Patchy distribution with most in exotic dairy breeds, and in family-owned herds as distinct from institutional herds, due possibly to more importations in family herds
♦ Higher prevalence in Angora than dairy goats

Importance

♦ Serious production and death losses
♦ Known infection in herd severely limi value of sale goats

Clinical findings

Arthritic disease

♦ Visible mostly in carpal joint (big knee some tarsal joints
♦ Sudden or insidious
♦ Uni- or bilateral
♦ Often no lameness; mild if present
♦ Some goats live normal life span; othe emaciate, develop poor hair coat, recumbent with decubitus ulcers
♦ Course several months
♦ Atlantal, supraspinous bursae enlarge i some
♦ Some may also have indurative mastit (see below)
♦ Pneumonic disease in some

Pneumonic disease

Increasing dyspnea

Indurative mastitis (hard udder)

♦ Develops a few days after kidding
♦ Udder firm, hard
♦ No milk can be expressed
♦ No toxemia, abnormal milk
♦ May improve a little with time

Leukoencephalitis

♦ Principally in kids 1–5 months old
♦ Uni- or bilateral weakness posterior pare sis, ataxia
♦ Eventually all 4 limbs paretic, recumbency
♦ May be one limb affected with propriocep tive deficit
♦ Head tilt, torticollis, circling
♦ Bright, alert, drink well
♦ Most kids euthanised after course of abou 10 days

Clinical pathology

♦ Synovia brown, red-tinged with very high cell count, mostly mononuclears
♦ May be high cell count, protein content ir cerebrospinal fluid
♦ Agar gel immunodiffusion test used to detect experience of infection
♦ Virus identified by culture from explant o tissue
♦ Delay between infection and positive AGID test may be over 1 year

Necropsy findings

- Emaciation
- Chronic polysynovitis with degenerative joint disease in most joints
- Gross lymph node enlargement
- Interstitial pneumonia
- Nervous system lesions in white matter especially of spinal cord, sometimes cerebellum, brain stem

Diagnosis

Arthritic disease resembles arthritis caused by:

- *Mycoplasma* spp.
- *Chlamydia* spp.
- *Corynebacterium* spp.

Encephalomyelitis resembles:

- Swayback
- Spinal abscess
- Spinal nematodiasis
- Listeriosis
- Polioencephalomalacia

Treatment

Nil.

Control

- Identify infected animals, cull them or manage in separate herd
- Separate kids from infected dams before they suck; rear on pasteurized milk; test by AGID regularly, cull positive reactors
- Hygiene at milking
- Voluntary control programs for area control; accredited herds must pass negative herd test twice at 6 month interval
- Quarantine, test introduced animals

IMMUNE DEFICIENCY DISEASE OF LLAMAS [VM8 p. 1111]

- Retrovirus infection detected by reverse transcriptase activity suspected of causing immunodeficiency in llamas
- Characterised by ill-thrift, anemia, leukopenia, recurrent infection

SCRAPIE [VM8 p. 1112]

Etiology

- The largely unidentified but acknowledged infectious **scrapie agent**, a small unconventional virus, a virion, is the cause but the

susceptibility of the host, and the incubation period for the clinical signs of the disease, are determined by the host's genetic makeup
- The prototype disease for the transmissible subacute spongiform encephalopathies including as well:
  - Chronic wasting disease of deer and elk
  - Transmissible mink encephalopathy
  - Kuru of humans
  - Creutzfeldt-Jakob disease of humans
  - Bovine spongiform encephalopathy (BSE)

Epidemiology

Occurrence

- No identifying test so exact details unknown
- UK principally, also enzootic in North America, Europe; reports of occurrence in a few other countries
- Called **rida** in Iceland
- Disease of mature sheep; transmissible to goats, rare natural occurrence in them; can persist in a goat herd, separated from sheep
- In infected flocks morbidity averages 1% annually (0.1–10%), rarely reaches 40%; can cause collapse of flock; case fatality rate 100%

Source and transmission

- Transmitted from an infected sheep laterally by contagion or from dam to lamb, subject to the recipient having a suitable, susceptible, inherited tendency; vertical transmission appears unlikely
- Means of transmission uncertain but probably from placenta, fetal fluids to newborn lamb
- Lateral transmission probably by ingestion of contaminated pasture
- Scrapie agent not in semen, rarely in fetus

Risk factors

- Scrapie agent very resistant to chemical, physical influences; survives boiling, freezing, survives long periods in dead, formalinised tissues; on pasture duration probably exceeds 3 years
- Scrapie agent fails to provoke any protective response in the host
- Susceptibility to development of clinical disease inherited, probably via an inherited long or short incubation period gene (the SIP – Scrapie incubation period gene)
- Age of appearance of clinical disease in

sheep 2.5–4.5 years, rarely younger than 1.5 years; in goats range is 2–7 years
♦ Most susceptible age is young sheep

Importance
♦ Wastage due to death plus heavy culling of related sheep
♦ Presence in a stud flock a serious impediment to sale of sheep

Clinical findings

♦ Incubation period several months to 3 years
♦ Transient episodes of collapse or behavior change, e.g. aggression such as charging dogs and gates
♦ Rubbing, biting of fleece (pruritus) begins; may be unobserved but causes bilateral ragged appearance, loss of fleece, chiefly over rump, thighs, tail base, neck dorsum, poll; less common sites side of neck, ribs behind shoulders
♦ Stilted gait
♦ Weight loss but appetite seems good
♦ Fine tremor, intermittent head nodding, jerking at rest
♦ Hyperexcitability
♦ Pruritus becomes intense, scratching with hind feet, biting evident, causing face swelling, ear hematoma
♦ Application of light pressure to fleece causes characteristic **nibbling/licking** reaction
♦ Serious gait problems appear:
  • Incomplete hock flexion
  • Shortened step
  • Weakness
  • Lack of balance
♦ When chased, sheep grossly incoordinated, falls easily, has transient convulsions
♦ Swallowing difficult, prehension normal, vomiting
♦ Voice tremble or complete loss
♦ Blindness
♦ Terminally anorexia, emaciation, recumbency, limb hyperextension
♦ Always fatal after a course of 2–12 months

Clinical pathology

No antemortem tests available.

Necropsy findings

♦ Trauma due to rubbing
♦ Essential lesion is vacuolation of neurones in spinal cord, medulla, pons, midbrain, consequential Wallerian degeneration in dorsal, ventral, ventrolateral columns o spinal cord, nerve fibers in cerebellar peduncles, optic nerves, plus degeneration o cerebellar, hypothalamoneurohypophy seal systems
♦ Conclusive lesion is amyloid scrapie associated fibrils in brain; these can be used to transmit the disease

Diagnosis

Resembles:
♦ Louping ill
♦ Pseudorabies
♦ Photosensitisation
♦ Pregnancy toxemia
♦ Lice, ked, itchmite infestation

Treatment

Nil.

Control

♦ No effective control
♦ Newly imported disease eradicated by slaughter of all infected flock plus in-contact sheep
♦ In enzootic flocks, countries control by slaughter elimination of clinical cases, susceptible families, avoidance of contact with placenta of diseased ewes
♦ Depopulation program requires infected farms to be left unstocked for 2 years, plus extensive cleaning, disinfection of farm area

BOVINE SPONGIFORM
ENCEPHALOPATHY (BSE, MAD
COW DISEASE) [VM8 p. 1116]

Etiology

Suspected cause is sheep-derived scrapie agent

Epidemiology

Occurrence
♦ Cattle, especially dairy herds, are the important subjects; rare cases in exotic zoo ruminants, cats fed BSE-infected meat
♦ Significant occurrence only in UK or cattle imported from UK
♦ Sporadic cases in native cattle in number of countries; disease may have been unrecognized for many years

♦ Disease appeared for first time in 1985, related to change in meat-meal producing procedure several years before
♦ Since then has developed into major epizootic involving more than 90 000 cattle by 1992
♦ Incidence in individual herds less than 2%; case fatality 100%
♦ Mature animals, average age 4–5 years (22 months–15 years)

Source and transmission

♦ Brain tissue of latent scrapie-infected sheep, used in feed supplement fed to cattle after inappropriate sterilization procedure
♦ Use of brain tissue from latent infected cattle may have amplified occurrence
♦ Ingestion; a poor means of transmission, accounting for the low in-herd incidence
♦ No evidence indicating direct horizontal transmission between cattle but cases occur in animals not fed infected meat products
♦ Apparent vertical transmission may occur due to contact of calf with placenta, fetal fluids, as in scrapie in sheep

Importance

♦ Significant death losses overall but single farm losses small
♦ Potentially a serious zoonosis for veterinarians, animal handlers; press reports of occurrence of fatal Creutzfeldt-Jakob disease in farmers associated with infected herds
♦ Concern about transmission to humans detracts from popularity of meat

Clinical findings

♦ Incubation period 1–2 years
♦ Signs progressive over time but variable from day to day
♦ Apprehensive behavior, reluctance to pass through gate, milking shed; appear disoriented, staring at imaginary objects, presumably for long periods
♦ Hyperesthesia to sound, touch
♦ Excessive grooming, licking, show nibbling response to scratch reflex
♦ Kicking during milking, resistant to handling
♦ Hind limb ataxia early; swaying gait, difficulty turning, knuckling, stumbling, falling, difficulty rising
♦ Weight loss, milk yield decline in most cases
♦ Euthanasia usually because of recumbency or difficulty in handling after course 1–6 months

Clinical pathology

No antemortem tests available

Necropsy findings

♦ No gross lesions
♦ Critical lesion is bilaterally symmetrical intracytoplasmic vacuolation of neurones and gray matter neuropil
♦ Scrapie associated fibrils visualisable in brain by electron microscopy

Diagnosis

Resembles:
♦ Hypomagnesemia
♦ Nervous acetonemia
♦ Rabies
♦ Lead poisoning
♦ Polioencephalomalacia
♦ Brain abscess
♦ Spinal abscess
♦ Hepatic encephalopathy
♦ Tremorgenic toxins, e.g. swainsonine, ergotamine

Treatment

Nil.

Control

♦ Elimination of feeds containing animal protein derived from animals capable of containing scrapie agent
♦ Compulsory slaughter of clinical cases
♦ Meat or milk from infected animals not allowed to enter human food chain

VISNA (MAEDI–VISNA)
[VM8 p. 1120]

Etiology

The maedi–visna virus; visna is the neurological manifestation of the virus.

Epidemiology

♦ Rare disease of sheep, more common and severe in Icelandic sheep than other breeds
♦ Eradicated from Iceland, rarely seen elsewhere
♦ Occasionally in goats
♦ Always occurs in association with maedi
♦ Case fatality rate 100%

Clinical findings – sheep and goats

♦ Incubation period 2 years
♦ Insidious onset
♦ Lagging behind flock
♦ Weight loss
♦ Ataxia due to hypermetria, fall easily
♦ Severe facial muscle tremor
♦ Fetlock knuckling, standing on hoof dorsum
♦ Head tilt in some
♦ Periods of normality but disease progressive
♦ Death or euthanasia after course of several months

Clinical pathology

♦ Increased monocytes, some gammaglobulin, in cerebrospinal fluid
♦ Serological tests include —
  • Complement fixation
  • Virus neutralization test
  • ELISA
  • Agar gel immunodiffusion test
  • Indirect immunofluorescence test

Necropsy findings

♦ Muscle wasting
♦ Chronic interstitial pneumonia with lymphoid tissue proliferation in some.

Diagnosis

Resembles:
♦ Scrapie
♦ Segmental axonopathy

BORDER DISEASE (HAIRY SHAKER DISEASE OF LAMBS, HAIRY SHAKERS, HYPOMYELINOGENESIS CONGENITAL] [VM8 p. 1121]

Etiology

♦ A pestivirus of the family Togaviridae; serologically related to:
  • Bovine diarrhea virus
  • Hog cholera virus
♦ Several strains with varying pathogenicities

Epidemiology

Occurrence
♦ Most sheep-producing countries
♦ Principally in sheep, rarely goats

♦ Infection prevalence very variable between countries, regions; much higher than morbidity
♦ Abortion, neonatal lamb deaths 25–75% in naive flock
♦ After initial outbreak of abortions, flock immunity leads to high incidence of congenitally defective lambs

Source and transmission
♦ In utero transmission, effect varies: lambs infected prior to immune competence may die, or survive in persistently viremic state; provide major source of infection in flock
♦ Introduction to flock by purchased sheep
♦ Contact transmission between sheep by oral, conjunctival routes from virus in all excretions
♦ Some transmission possible via fetal fluids, placenta of infected abortus
♦ Possible virus reservoirs in cattle and deer

Risk factors
♦ Varying severity of interactions between virus and different host genotypes
♦ Disease, as distinct from infection, occurs only in pregnant animals
♦ Morbidity low in flocks with high level of flock immunity

Importance
♦ Heavy wastage due to lamb losses in initial outbreak
♦ Subsequently losses due to congenital defects in lambs

Clinical findings

Congenital defects in lambs include:
♦ Low birth weight
♦ Decreased crown–rump length
♦ Short tibia–radius length
♦ Shortened longitudinal axis of head, cranium slightly domed
♦ Rhythmic tremors of pelvic, upper hind limb muscles, and head and neck causing head-bobbing; tremors absent during sleep, worst during motion; fade as lamb gets older
♦ Difficulty rising
♦ Erratic hindquarter gait
♦ Lambs may be unable to suck teats
♦ Fleece hairy, rough in smooth-coated breeds, not visible in breeds with kempy fleece; may be total or patchy abnormal pigmentation of fleece
♦ Lamb unthrifty, most die around weaning

of intercurrent disease or mucosal disease-like syndrome

Lambs with hydranencephaly, cerebellar dysplasia display circling, head-pressing, nystagmus, gross incoordination

Clinical pathology

Diagnosis made on basis of combination of serology and virus isolation

Newborn lambs with persistent viremia infected early in pregnancy:
- Serologically negative in precolostral sera; lambs that have taken colostrum will be seropositive until maternal antibodies disappear
- Virus in blood buffy coat

Newborn lambs infected late in pregnancy:
- Seropositive in precolostral sera
- Free of virus in blood

Persistently infected older sheep detectable by culturing blood of seronegatives

Aborting ewes – serological tests unhelpful because of time lapse between infection and abortion

Necropsy findings

- Congenital defects includ:
  - Small brain and spinal cord
  - Arthrogryposis
  - Hydranencephaly
  - Porencephaly
- Demyelination, myelin dysmorphogenesis
- Brain size, demyelination repair with time
- Best diagnostic aid is immunofluorescent staining

Diagnosis

The **abortion** form resembles:
- Rift Valley fever
- Wesselbrons disease
- Tick-borne fever
- Chlamydiosis
- Listeriosis
- Toxoplasmosis
- Leptospirosis

The **nervous syndrome** may be confused with:
- Enzootic ataxia
- Caprine encephalomyelitis

Treatment

- With careful nursing many will survive but will be unthrifty and susceptible to intercurrent disease.

Control

- Cull persistently infected sheep; many show no clinical abnormality; lambs abnormal at birth may be normal at 2 months old
- Identification of permanently infected ewe lambs destined for breeding possible (see above in clinical pathology) but expensive
- Permanently infected sheep may be run with breeding flock, provided they are not pregnant to maintain high immunity level
- Avoid introduction of untested sheep into clean flock
- Seriousness of disease fades after first abortion outbreak

VIRAL DISEASES CHARACTERIZED BY SKIN LESIONS

CONTAGIOUS ECTHYMA
(CONTAGIOUS PUSTULAR
DERMATITIS, ORF, SCABBY
MOUTH, SORE MOUTH)
[VM8 p. 1125]

Etiology

A parapox virus of the family Poxviridae

Epidemiology

Occurrence
- Worldwide in sheep and goats
- In enzootic areas mostly in 3–6 months lambs; in naive flocks in lambs a few days old, adult sheep

- Morbidity rate 70–80%; case fatality rate small, may reach 15% in lambs with complicating secondary bacterial infection, blowfly strike; up to 75% in septicemic form in neonates

Source and transmission
- Contact with infected animals, or
- Infected inanimate objects, e.g. pasture plants, stubble, spiky plants

Risk factors
- Outbreaks at any time; mostly on dry pasture in summer
- In many wild small ruminants including musk ox, wild thar, and buffalo and camel

- Transmission by use of surgical appliance, e.g. ear tag pliers, emasculators
- No maternal antibodies in colostrum, neonates susceptible
- Immunity after natural infection up to 3 years
- Virus resistant, can survive for years in dry scabs

Importance
- Interference with feeding causes some weight loss
- A minor zoonosis

Clinical findings

- Thick, tenacious, discrete, 0.5 cm dia. scabs covering a raised, ulcerated area of inflammation and granulation
- Lesions at mucocutaneous junction, first usually at oral commissures
- Spread to muzzle, lips, nostrils, surrounding haired skin, sometimes onto buccal mucosa; these may form painful proliferative lesions generally in mouth and at gingival margins of incisor teeth
- Often so numerous they coalesce
- Fissures cause soreness
- Scabs crumble easily but difficult to remove
- Lambs restricted in sucking, grazing, lose weight
- Rarely systemic invasion with lesions at coronets, ears, around anus, vulva, preputial orifice, on teats, udder skin, or extensively on nasal, buccal mucosae; systemic reaction; lesions may spread to trachea, lungs, causing pneumonia or to esophagus to abomasum, small intestine, causing gastroenteritis
- Spontaneous recovery in 2–3 weeks

Complications
- Secondary infection with Fusobacterium necrophorum
- Extensive, large lesions over head, neck, sides, flanks, not on face or around orifices recorded in goats
- Profuse, verrucose lesions at edge of burn injury
- Malignant form, oral lesions extending down alimentary tract, then hoof-shedding, lesions on scrotum with scrotum filled with fluid
- Malignant form especially in housed, colostrum-free lambs

Clinical pathology

- Tests not usually needed for diagnosis
- Serological tests available include:

- Complement fixation
- Gel diffusion test
- Virus neutralization
- Virus identification by
- Electron microscopy
- Tissue culture

Necropsy findings

- Ulcerative lesions in nasal cavities, trachea esophagus, abomasum, small intestine i malignant cases.

Diagnosis

Resembles:
- Bluetongue
- Ulcerative dermatosis
- Mycotic dermatitis
- Facial eczema
- Strawberry foot rot
- Sheeppox

Treatment

- Debridement delays healing
- Diathermy debridement, cryosurgery may be needed for removal of granulomatous oral lesions
- Soft, palatable feed useful in severe cases

Control

- In outbreak isolate early cases, vaccinate remainder; not useful if incidence already high
- In flocks with persistent problem annual vaccination of 6–8 week lambs; prelambing ewe vaccination ineffective
- Lambs inspected 2 weeks after vaccination to ensure lesions at skin vaccination site
- Local autogenous, live-virus vaccine most effective
- Commercial vaccine of attenuated virus available

PAPILLOMATOSIS [VM8 p. 1127]

Etiology

- Six bovine papillomaviruses (BVP1–6) cause cutaneous warts in cattle and horses
- BVP1,5,6 cause warts on the udder and teats
- BVP2,3 cause general skin warts
- BVP4 causes papillomata of esophagus to intestine
- Other regional bovine papillomas with probable viral specificity are those of:

- Mouth
- Larynx
- Interdigital fibropapillomata
- Ocular squamous cell carcinoma

Ear cancer of sheep, equine sarcoid may also have specific papillomavirus etiology

Epidemiology

Occurrence

Universal

Common only in cattle and horses, rarely pigs and sheep

Young animals most susceptible

Sometimes congenital in horses

Source and transmission

- Contact infection with infected animals through cutaneous abrasions, from virus lodged on barbed wire, grass seeds, etc.
- Crops of warts along path of wire scratches, tattoo marks, etc.
- Perianal warts spread by rectal examinations

Importance

- Esthetic effect limits sales of stud stock
- On teats interfere with milking
- At anus interfere with breeding

Clinical findings

Cattle

- Incubation period 3–8 weeks
- Solid outgrowths of skin and connective tissue
- Sessile or pedunculated, smooth or ulcerated surface, cauliflower appearance in many cases
- On any part of body
- Disappear spontaneously most cases, course up to one year

Teat warts may be elongated rice grain form, flat round types, or frond-like; may obstruct milking machine cups.

Perianal warts around anus and vulva, on prepuce and penis, make mating impracticable.

Oral warts seen only at necropsy, common in some localities.

Interdigital fibropapillomas, round, circumscribed lesions on heel pads of cows are probably spirochetal in origin.

Reticular papillomas can cause chronic ruminal tympany.

Goats

- Commonest on unpigmented skin, often on udder
- Spontaneous regression; some may recur

Horses

- Very small, multiple lesions on lower face, lips, muzzle, nose
- Rarely in mouth, on conjunctiva, penis and vulva
- Mostly in young, including congenital
- Prolonged course may be due to immunodeficiency

Clinical pathology

ELISA and restriction endonuclease analysis available for diagnosis.

Necropsy findings

- Applicable only to internal occurrences
- Usually non-clinical occurrences of typical wart-like papillomas in cattle, observed at autopsy and abattoir including urinary bladder, all levels of alimentary tract; often associated with parallel occurrence of carcinoma suggesting etiological relationship

Diagnosis

Resemble:

- Atypical, long-duration, true papillomas in cattle, without the usual dermal fibroplasia, caused by a non-transmissible, papilloma-like virus; characteristically, low, flat, circular, sessile lesions may coalesce to form large masses
- Sarcoids in horses
- Squamous cell carcinoma

Treatment

- Spontaneous recovery the best treatment
- Surgical removal used for lesions that are untimely, badly located, subject to frequent trauma
- Removal by excision, or by vaccination with an autogenous, intradermal vaccine from patient's lesion
- Commercial vaccine may be tissue cultured virus or homogenized wart tissue, live or formalin-killed
- 2 injections 2 weeks apart
- Recovery in 3–6 weeks in most, except teats which respond poorly
- Many local or parenteral treatments used by farmers; most have no beneficial effect; many not tested

Control

♦ Prophylactic vaccination not usually practiced because of low prevalence.

SARCOID [VM8 p. 1130]

Etiology

Multifactorial cause probably including papillomavirus (BVP1 and 2), possibly retrovirus.

Epidemiology

♦ Horses (mostly Appaloosa, Arabian, Quarterhorse), donkeys, mules
♦ Genetic susceptibility probable, via major histocompatibility complex
♦ More common in geldings than stallions
♦ Incidence increases with age.

Clinical findings

♦ Single or multiple, hairless, sometimes ulcerated, solid skin structures resembling large warts
♦ Mostly on lower limbs
♦ Some on lips, eyelids, eyes, penile sheath, base of ears
♦ Four types:
  • Verrucose, wart-like, dry, flat, horny, sessile or pedunculated
  • Proud flesh, spreading ulcer type
♦ Combination of the above
♦ Slow-growing, slight thickening skin thickening with rough surface

Clinical pathology

Identification by histological examination of biopsy sample.

Necropsy findings

Skin lesions only.

Diagnosis

Resembles:
♦ Papillomas
♦ Other skin tumors
♦ Cutaneous habronemiasis
♦ Phycomycosis

Treatment

♦ Surgery, especially cryosurgery, effective if all tissue removed

♦ Recurrences common
♦ Other well-regarded treatments include:
  • Radiotherapy
  • Local hyperthermia
  • Intralesional injection of BCG vaccine preferably a mycobacterial cell-wall fraction vaccine to avoid hypersensitivity reactions
♦ Very large or multiple lesions respond poorly to all treatments

LUMPY SKIN DISEASE (LSD, KNOPVELSIEKTE) [VM8 p. 1131]

Etiology

♦ Neethling poxvirus, a capripoxvirus
♦ Identical with another capripoxvirus, the Kenya sheep and goat pox virus (SGPV) but different from Middle East SGPV, also a capripoxvirus

Epidemiology

♦ Enzootic in Africa, Egypt, Israel
♦ Morbidity 20%, case fatality 2% in enzootic area
♦ 80% morbidity in susceptible population
♦ Only cattle affected, all ages and types

Source and transmission

♦ Source is infected cattle
♦ Transmission by bites of unspecified insects, probably *Stomoxys, Biomyia, Culicoides, Glossinia, Musca* spp. bites
♦ Transmission by ingestion possible

Risk factors

♦ European breeds more susceptible than Brahman types
♦ Most prevalent in season with heavy insect population

Importance

♦ Loss of milk, hide damage, weight loss
♦ High risk disease for other countries

Clinical findings

♦ Incubation period 2–4 weeks
♦ Fever
♦ Initial lacrimation, nasal discharge, salivation, lameness in some
♦ Skin lesions about 1 week later
♦ Multiple, round, firm, 1–4 cm diameter intradermal nodules
♦ In severe cases nodules also in:

- Nasal cavities, causing nasal discharge, respiratory obstruction, stertor, dyspnea
- Mouth, causing salivation, or
- On conjunctiva, prepuce, vulva
♦ Most lesions regress spontaneously
♦ Some persist as hard lumps or ulcers
♦ Local lymph nodes swollen
♦ Lymphatic obstruction causes limb edema
♦ Recovery after course 2–4 weeks

Clinical pathology

♦ Granulomatous lesion in biopsy
♦ Intracellular, eosinophilic inclusions in early lesions
♦ Fluorescent antibody, virus neutralization tests available

Necropsy findings

♦ Animals dead of spread to internal organs have typical granulomatous lesions in alimentary and respiratory tracts
♦ Pneumonia in a few

Diagnosis

Resembles:
♦ **Generalised bovine herpesvirus-2** (the bovine ulcerative mammillitis virus) infection (USA); probably identical with 'Allerton type lumpy skin disease' (UK); lesions are not granulomas but superficial, ring-like lesions with an intact central skin area with raised edges
♦ Urticaria

Treatment and control

♦ Control of infected cattle movements
♦ Insect control
♦ Vaccination with tissue-culture, living virus vaccine effective
♦ Vaccination with attenuated sheep pox virus

VIRAL PAPULAR DERMATITIS
[VM8 p. 1133]

Etiology

Unidentified virus.

Epidemiology

♦ Recorded in USA and Australia
♦ Outbreaks in introduced horses
♦ Sudden outbreaks suggest insect vector

Clinical findings

♦ Fever
♦ Then firm papules, 0.5–2 cm dia.
♦ After 5 days top scab sloughs, leaving alopecic area
♦ No itchiness, no systemic reaction
♦ Lesions subside spontaneously 10 days to 6 weeks

COWPOX AND BUFFALOPOX
[VM8 p. 1133]

Etiology

♦ Cowpox virus an orthopoxvirus closely related to the antigenically identical buffalopox, and to smallpox viruses.

Epidemiology

Cowpox very rare; now seen only in circus animals and cats.

Source and transmission
♦ From infected animals
♦ Transmitted by milking machine liners, milkers' hands
♦ Entry through teat abrasions, possibly insect bites
♦ Immunity after infection several years plus

Clinical findings

♦ Incubation period 3–6 days
♦ Lesions (see above) usually not seen until scab stage in dry cows; in cows being milked scabs replaced by ulcers
♦ Lesions on teats and udder floor
♦ Soreness interferes with milk letdown
♦ Mastitis a common sequel
♦ Uncommon spread of lesions to thighs, perineum, vulva, mouth; scrotal lesions

Clinical pathology

Virus cultivable, identified by electron microscopy

Diagnosis

Resembles:
♦ Udder impetigo
♦ Bovine ulcerative mammillitis
♦ Lumpy cow disease
♦ Generalized herpesvirus-2 infection
♦ Pseudocowpox
♦ Mycotic dermatitis

♦ Photosensitive dermatitis
♦ Black spot

Treatment and control

♦ Topical ointment before milking, astringent mixture after each milking
♦ Intensive teat-dipping program with standard mastitis control preparations
♦ Tinctures preferred if clinical cases occurring

PSEUDOCOWPOX (MILKERS'
NODULE) [VM8 p. 1135]

Etiology

A parapoxvirus, similar to those of infectious papular stomatitis, contagious ecthyma.

Epidemiology

♦ Worldwide occurrence
♦ Slow-spreading disease with morbidity at any one time about 10%, but almost all cows will eventually succumb

Source and transmission
♦ From infected cows, via teat cup liners, hands, cloths, insects
♦ Entry via skin lesions

Risk factors
♦ Introduced or freshly calved cows most susceptible
♦ All cows over 2 years affected

Importance
♦ Benign disease but interferes with easy milking
♦ Secondary mastitis a sequel

Clinical findings

♦ Lesions may be on all teats
♦ Erythema first, then painful vesicle, then pustule briefly, then scab
♦ Scab separates leaving central, raised granuloma, surrounded by ring or horseshoe-shaped crescent of small scabs
♦ Lesions regress spontaneously in about 3 weeks
♦ Disease disappears from herd but may recur quickly

Clinical pathology

Tissue culture and electron microscopy useful for laboratory identification.

Diagnosis

Resembles:
♦ Cowpox
♦ Bovine ulcerative mammillitis
♦ Udder impetigo
♦ Mycotic dermatitis
♦ Teat papilloma

Treatment and control

♦ Emollient ointment before milking
♦ Triple dye, or other astringent mixture, after milking
♦ Iodophor teat dip as udder disinfectant
♦ Teat cup sterilization between cows

BOVINE ULCERATIVE
MAMMILLITIS [VM8 p. 1136]

Etiology

Bovine herpesvirus-2 (BHV2).

Epidemiology

Occurrence
♦ Massive outbreaks in milking herds
♦ Young cows more susceptible than older ones
♦ Morbidity averages 30%, nil mortality
♦ Outbreak subsides, disease disappears at about 4 months
♦ After first outbreak only heifers affected

Source and transmission
♦ Brought in by introduced cows or unknown, probably biting insects
♦ Rapidity of spread in herd suggests physical contact via milking machine cups, hands, with some other factor causing penetration into teat tissue

Importance
♦ Mastitis a common sequel
♦ Severe interference with milking, yield down

Clinical findings

♦ Incubation period 5–10 days
♦ Lesions usually begin in freshly calved cows, then spread to rest of herd

- Teat, udder lesions
- Most severe in fresh cows
- Vesicles coalesce causing extensive weeping and sloughing of udder skin
- Lesions on teats in mid-lactation cows are large skin areas which slough leaving chronic ulcers that heal in 3–4 months
- Minor lesions are circles of erythema enclosing dry skin or elevated papules; heal in 10 days
- Rarely ulcers in mouth and vagina

Clinical pathology

- Virus cultivable
- High serum antibody levels persist several years

Diagnosis

Resembles:
- Peracute staphylococcal mastitis
- Photosensitive dermatitis
- Another herpesvirus (strain DN599) also causes mammary pustular dermatitis

Treatment and control

- Crystal violet or triple dye lotions after milking
- Emollient ointment before milking to soften scabs, relieve discomfort
- Iodophor teat disinfectant, udder wash to reduce spread in milking shed

SHEEPPOX AND GOATPOX
[VM8 p. 1138]

Etiology

Three viruses affect the small ruminants —
- **Sheeppox virus** (SPV), a capripoxvirus affecting only sheep
- **Sheep and goatpox virus** (SGPV), a capripoxvirus affecting sheep and goats
- **Kenya sheep and goatpox virus** (KSGPV), related to lumpy skin disease virus, affects sheep and goats

Epidemiology

- Occur in most developing countries
- Serious disease, causing many losses
- Case fatality rate nearly 50% lambs in susceptible groups
- Highly contagious by direct contact or inhalation
- An important threat to countries with large sheep populations

Clinical findings

Sheeppox in sheep
- Incubation period 2–14 days

Lambs
- Severe depression, recumbency, high fever
- Nasal, ocular discharges
- May die before pox lesions develop
- Lesions on unwoolled skin, buccal, respiratory, vaginal mucosae
- Typical lesion progression from nodule to vesicle to pustule, to scab

Adults
- Skin lesions only, under tail, skin generally.

Goatpox in sheep
- More severe than sheeppox
- Lesions on udder and teats, buccal mucosa, lips

Goatpox in goats
- Mild disease in adults, severe fatal disease in kids
- Lesions same as sheeppox in sheep.

Clinical pathology

Indirect fluorescent antibody (FAT) test or immunodiffusion techniques suited to identification of virus.

Necropsy findings

Malignant form in lambs, kids have lesions in respiratory tract with a secondary pneumonia in some, lesions in alimentary tract accompany a bloody diarrhea

Diagnosis

Resembles:
- Bluetongue
- Contagious ecthyma

Treatment and control

- In free countries prohibition of importation of sheep and goats from infected countries
- If disease introduced then destruction of flock
- Excellent commercial, single virus or mixed virus vaccines, providing long-term immunity, available

CAMELPOX [VM8 p. 1139]

Etiology and epidemiology

♦ Several strains of an orthopoxvirus
♦ Case fatality rate may be 5%.

Clinical findings

♦ Incubation period 3 – 15 days
♦ Typical pox lesions on hairless parts of body in young camels
♦ Benign course for 2–3 weeks

Clinical pathology

ELISA available

Diagnosis

Resembles contagious ecthyma.

Control

Tissue culture vaccine.

SWINEPOX [VM8 p. 1139]

Etiology

Suipoxvirus of family Poxviridae

Epidemiology

Occurrence
♦ Occurs in all swine-raising countries
♦ High morbidity in infected herds; case fatality rate in suckers can be high
♦ In enzootic herds cases only in introduced or young animals

Source and transmission
♦ From infected pigs
♦ Transmission by contact; udder lesions on sows to facial skin if suckers
♦ Transmitted also by bites of *Haematopinus suis*
♦ Possibly intra-uterine; some cases appear to be congenital

Clinical findings

♦ Typical pox lesions (see cowpox) anywhere on body
♦ In adults common on belly, inside thighs
♦ In sucking pigs many lesions on face, con-junctivitis, keratitis; also systemic infection, fever, some deaths
♦ Congenital infection – striking pox lesions at birth in stillborn or weak piglets

Diagnosis

Resembles:
♦ Tyroglyphid mite infestation
♦ Sarcoptic mange
♦ Ringworm
♦ Pityriasis rosea

Treatment and control

♦ No treatment applicable
♦ Louse control
♦ No vaccine available

HORSEPOX [VM8 p. 1140]

Etiology

Poxvirus antigenically identical with cowpox

Epidemiology

♦ Very rare, sporadic cases in Europe
♦ Benign disease, occasional deaths in young
♦ Spread by contact
♦ Solid immunity after an attack

Clinical findings

♦ Typical pox lesions on lower limbs causing lameness, *or*
♦ On buccal mucosa spreading to pharynx causing salivation, anorexia
♦ Rarely lesions on vulva, conjunctiva or generally

Diagnosis

Resembles:
♦ Greasy heel
♦ Vesicular stomatitis
♦ Viral papular dermatitis
♦ Molluscum contagiosum
♦ Uasin gishu

Treatment

Astringent lotions.

Control

Strict hygiene in stabling and care of grooming kits and the like.

ULCERATIVE DERMATOSIS OF
SHEEP [VM8 p. 1140]

Etiology

Virus antigenically identical to ecthyma
virus.

Epidemiology

Sporadic cases, not highly contagious
Morbidity rate 15–20% usual; may be up
to 60%; case fatality rate low if sheep in
good condition, disease not neglected
Transmission probably by physical contact
at mating

Clinical findings

♦ Raw, granulating ulcers on skin of lips,
  nostrils, feet, legs, external genitalia
♦ Lesions may be restricted to genitalia or
  lower limbs
♦ Facial lesions rare

Diagnosis

Resembles:
♦ Ecthyma
♦ Infectious balanoposthitis
♦ Strawberry foot rot
♦ foot rot
♦ Interdigital abscess

DISEASES CAUSED BY *CHLAMYDIA PSITTACI*

Chlamydia psittaci cause:
♦ Sporadic bovine encephalomyelitis
♦ Ovine contagious ophthalmia

Occasional cases of:
♦ **Pneumonia** in most species
♦ **Abortion** in cows
♦ **Orchitis/epididymitis** in male ruminants
♦ **Enteritis** in calves

Confirmation of infection is by:
♦ Complement fixation test
♦ ELISA

Preferred treatment is tetracyclines

CHLAMYDIAL POLYARTHRITIS
[VM8 p. 1143]

Epidemiology

♦ In calves, foals lambs
♦ Uncommon but fatal in calves
♦ Common feedlot disease of lambs
♦ High morbidity; low case fatality rate in
  ewes

Clinical findings

♦ Depression, fever
♦ Joint-swelling
♦ Lame, stiff gait
♦ Unwilling to move
♦ Recumbency
♦ Conjunctivitis

Necropsy findings

♦ Lung and renal abscess
♦ Encephalomyelitis

Diagnosis

Resembles:
♦ *Mycoplasma* spp. infection
♦ *Hemophilus* spp. infections

CHLAMYDIAL ABORTION
[VM8 p. 1143]

Epidemiology

♦ Common goat and sheep abortion
♦ Sporadic occurrence in cattle
♦ Transmission by inhalation, ingestion of
  pasture contaminated by uterine discharge,
  placenta

Clinical findings

♦ Abortion in late pregnancy
♦ Retained placenta, metritis common
  sequels
♦ Stillbirths, neonatal mortalities

Clinical pathology

♦ ELISA and complement fixation tests
  available.

Necropsy findings

♦ Areas of necrosis, thickening of placenta
♦ Focal hepatic necrosis in some fetuses

Control

♦ Adjuvanted, killed vaccine effective.

23 DISEASES CAUSED BY RICKETTSIA

OVINE AND CAPRINE
CONTAGIOUS OPHTHALMIA
(OVINE AND CAPRINE
INFECTIOUS
KERATOCONJUNCTIVITIS,
CONTAGIOUS
CONJUNCTIVOKERATITIS, PINK
EYE) [VM8 p. 1144]

Etiology

♦ This disease is till classified as being caused by *Rickettsia conjunctivae* in sheep, goats, *R. rupricaprae* in chamois
♦ Bulk of evidence incriminates *Mycoplasma conjunctivae*

Epidemiology

Occurrence

♦ Common in most countries
♦ All breeds
♦ Recently weaned lambs worst affected
♦ Spread through flock rapid
♦ Morbidity 10–15%, up to 80%; case fatality rate nil

Source and transmission

♦ Tears of infected sheep
♦ Direct transmission by immediate contact, exhaled droplets
♦ Indirect transmission by dust, flies, long grass

Risk factors

♦ Warm, summer months with plenty of dust, long grass, flies
♦ Frequent mustering, e.g. to treat cases
♦ Recent previous infection leads to premunity due to persistence of infection in eye
♦ Possibly some flock immunity; disease not inclined to recur for several years

Importance

♦ Minor inconvenience by interfering with grazing
♦ Some interference with weight gain

Clinical findings – Sheep

♦ One or both eyes
♦ Lacrimation, blepharospasm
♦ Brown discoloration below eye due to dust accumulation in tears
♦ Cornea cloudiness, vascularisation in some; most commonly at dorsal corneoscleral junction
♦ Corneal ulcer in some
♦ Severe signs commence to improve by day 3; complete recovery by day 10

Complications

♦ Corneal cloudiness may persist longer or permanently, causing blindness
♦ Ulceration may lead to collapse of eye

Goats

♦ Milder disease with little keratitis
♦ Granular lesions on palpebral conjunctiva, third eyelid

Clinical pathology

Swabs, scrapings of conjunctiva stained with fluorescent antibody identify *Rickettsia*, *Mycoplasma*, *Chlamydia* spp.

Diagnosis

In goats resembles:
Idiopathic caprine keratoconjunctivitis characterized by:
♦ 20–50% morbidity
♦ Conjunctivitis, opacity, vascularisation, ulceration
♦ Severe corneal edema forming vesicles
♦ Healing period 2–4 weeks

In sheep resembles *Chlamydia psittaci*, *Branhamella ovis* also isolated from cases

Treatment

♦ Often left untreated because of practical difficulty in pastured sheep, plus
♦ Will mean repeated close contact between sheep, possibly enhancing spread

♦ Effective treatment leads to quicker rein-fection
♦ Local treatment with:
  • 2.5% zinc sulfate solution
  • 0.5% ointment or 1.0% solution ethidium bromide
♦ Oxytetracycline powder or lotion
♦ Cloxacillin ophthalmic ointment
♦ Parenteral treatment with long-acting tetracycline or tiamulin recommended for specific *Mycoplasma* spp. infection

Control

Move to less dusty, traumatic, fly-infested environment

EPERYTHROZOONOSIS

is listed in Chapter 25.

ANAPLASMOSIS [VM8 p. 1146]

Etiology

♦ Cattle, wild ruminants *Anaplasma marginale*, possibly *A. caudatum*. *A. centrale* causes mild disease in cattle
♦ Sheep and goats *A. ovina*

Epidemiology

Occurrence
♦ All continents
♦ Enzootic in tropical areas where vectors persist
♦ Sporadic in temperate regions
♦ Infection prevalence 60–90% in enzootic areas; 3.6–37% in temperate climate; case fatality rate in outbreak 30–50%

Source and transmission
♦ Infected domestic, wild ruminants with rickettsia in blood stream
♦ Long-term survivors persist as subclinical carriers
♦ Insect vectors include:
  • Ticks *Dermacentor*, *Boophilus*, *Rhipicephalus*, *Argas* spp.; life cycle in tick
  • Biting flies *Tabanid* spp.; eye gnats (*Hippelates* spp.) mechanical transmission only
♦ Mechanical transmission on needles, scalpels, castrating, spaying, dehorning instruments
♦ Transmission in fluids, tissues, blood trans-fusion, embryo transplants, whole blood vaccines
♦ Intrauterine infection occurs

Risk factors
♦ Age; young cattle infected, stay infected for life but no clinical illness; 94% clinical cases in cattle over 3 years old
♦ Clinical disease rare in enzootic area; occurs when seronegative animals introduced
♦ Clinical disease outbreak in normally free area recently invaded by vector
♦ Stress, especially nutritional as in entry to feedlot, likely to stimulate clinical disease in subclinical carriers

Importance
♦ Limits productivity in enzootic area
♦ Significant death losses in outbreaks

Clinical findings

Cattle
♦ Incubation period 3–4 weeks for tick-borne infection, 2–5 weeks for mechanical transmission
♦ Peracute cases die in 24 hours after high fever, pallor, jaundice, dyspnea – usually adult dairy cattle
♦ Acute cases show moderate fluctuating fever for up to 2 weeks
♦ Moderate anorexia
♦ Severe weight loss
♦ Mucosae pale, jaundiced
♦ Hyperexcitability, including aggression, in some
♦ No hemoglobinuria
♦ Patient may die at this stage
♦ Complications:
  • Abortion
  • Testicular hypofunction for several months

Sheep, goats
♦ Mostly subclinical
♦ Same syndrome of severe anemia as in cattle in some goats

Clinical pathology

♦ Clinical disease only if >15% erythrocytes parasitized; may reach 90% in acute disease
♦ Severe erythrocyte depletion
♦ Immature erythrocytes in blood
♦ Small, dot-like protozoa at periphery of

10–50% red cells stained with Giemsa or Diff-Quik stain
♦ Transmission experiments to splenectomised animals
♦ Detecting carrier animals:
  • Complement fixation test
  • Capillary agglutination, or card test
  • Indirect fluorescent antibody
  • Dot-ELISA, antigen capture ELISA
  • Nucleic acid probe analysis
♦ Vaccinated animals also react

Necropsy findings

♦ Pallor, jaundice, emaciation
♦ Thin, watery blood
♦ Liver enlarged, deep orange color
♦ Spleen enlarged with soft pulp
♦ Protozoa in stained peripheral blood smears

Diagnosis

Resembles:
Other causes of anemia including:
♦ Babesiosis
♦ *Borrelia theileri* infections

Treatment

Clinical cases
♦ Tetracycline 6–10 mg/kg body weight, either as single dose or repeated twice more; clinical signs relieved but patient stays a carrier
♦ Long-acting tetracycline 20 mg/kg body weight I/M every 7 days for 2–4 injections sterilizes patient; one such injection cures patient but does not sterilize patient
♦ Imidocarb (3 mg/kg body weight) and amicarbalide (20 mg/kg divided into 2 daily doses, cure illness but do not sterilize
♦ Supportive blood transfusions

Carriers
♦ Parenteral tetracycline 10–30 mg/kg body weight daily for 10–16 days, *or* 23 mg/kg intravenously for 5 days
♦ Oral tetracycline 10 mg/kg for 30–60 days, *or* 1 mg/kg for 120 days also recommended

Control

Enzootic area
♦ Eradication not a practical solution because so many insect vectors, wild reservoirs, inaccuracy of testing for carriers, long term of carrier state
♦ Insect control

♦ Hygiene at surgery, injections
♦ **Vaccination**
  • Living *A. marginale*
  • Attenuated *A. marginale*
  • Killed *A. marginale*
  • Live *A. centrale*
♦ Choice of a vaccine depends on susceptibility of the vaccinees, the level of resistance required, prevalence of anaplasmosis in local cattle, the problems that arise from use of whole-blood vaccines

Prevention of introduction
♦ Only seronegative animals admitted
♦ Use of killed vaccine if risk high

In an outbreak
♦ Treat clinical cases
♦ Prophylactic daily dosing in feed of in-contacts (see above), *or*
♦ Treat all cattle once with therapeutic dose of tetracycline, repeat 4–6 weeks later
♦ When outbreak over test and treat or cull seropositives; vaccinates will be seropositive for up to 15 months

TICK-BORNE FEVER [VM8 p. 1151]

Etiology

Cytoecetes phagocytophila; strains vary in antigenicity, pathogenicity

Epidemiology

Occurrence
♦ Some parts of Europe and Scandinavia
♦ Enzootic in areas inhabited by ticks
♦ Sheep, cattle, goats, deer, possibly horses
♦ All ages
♦ Infection morbidity high; disease morbidity, case fatality rates low

Source and transmission
♦ Infected animals remain carriers for life
♦ Transmitted by tick (*Ixodes ricinus*) bites; organism does not pass to next generation of ticks

Risk factors
♦ Disease more severe in young
♦ Seasonal occurrence in spring and fall coinciding with tick activity

Importance
♦ Disease benign but some abortions, weight loss in young
♦ Increases susceptibility of patient to other

disease, e.g. staphylococcal pyemia, pneumonia, louping-ill.

Clinical findings

Cattle
- Incubation period 6–7 days
- Moderate fever 2–8 days
- Recurrent febrile episodes with:
  - Milk yield loss
  - Lethargy
  - Polypnea, cough
- Abortion
- Some sudden deaths

Sheep
- Same disease but milder
- Rams temporarily sterile

Goats and horses
- High fever
- Dullness
- Tachycardia

Clinical pathology

- Transient, severe thrombocytopenia
- Prolonged neutropenia, lymphocytopenia
- Rickettsiae in neutrophils, monocytes in blood smears during febrile periods
- Serological tests used include:
  - Counterimmunoelectrophoresis
  - Indirect immunofluorescence

Necropsy findings

- Splenomegaly in sheep
- Depletion of lymphocyte reserves

Diagnosis

In cattle resembles bovine petechial fever.

Treatment

- Tetracycline 10 mg/kg body weight I/V, one injection
- Potentiated sulfonamide
- Patient not sterilized, clinical disease may recur

Control

- Tick control by dipping program
- Keep animals off tick-ridden terrain during active tick period, especially lambs less than 6 weeks old, naive late pregnants
- Some protection provided before going onto tick-infested land, or before commencement of tick season by:
- Single injection therapeutic dose of long-acting tetracycline
- Dipping of flock

HEARTWATER (COWDRIOSIS)
[VM8 p. 1153]

Etiology

Cowdria ruminantium

Epidemiology

Occurrence
- Only in Africa, Madagascar, West Indies
- In imported cattle, sheep, goats south of Sahara; Angora goats very susceptible
- Morbidity sheep, goats 10%; case fatality 50%; less in cattle

Source and transmission
- Infected animals, including symptomless carriers
- Transmission transstadially, but not transovarially, by many *Amblyomma* spp. ticks

Risk factors
- Less severe in indigenous breeds, game animals, reared in enzootic area
- Recovered animals immune up to 4 years

Importance
- Very important in Africa
- Most losses in exotic ruminants introduced to enzootic area, during active tick season

Clinical findings

Incubation period 1–3 weeks

Peracute disease
- Fever
- Prostration
- Terminal convulsions
- Death in all cases after 1–2 day course

Acute disease
- Fever
- Anorexia
- Listlessness
- Polypnea
- Ataxia
- Chewing movements
- Eyelid-twitching
- Circling

♦ Aggressiveness
♦ Blindness
♦ Recumbency
♦ Convulsions
♦ Profuse, fetid diarrhea in many cases
♦ Death after 6 day course in 50–90% cases (5–10% in calves below 4 weeks old)

Subacute disease
♦ Similar, less severe disease
♦ Death after course of 2 weeks, *or*
♦ Spontaneous, gradual recovery

Mild disease
♦ Mostly subclinical
♦ Mainly in indigenous, wild ruminants

Clinical pathology

♦ May be neutropenia, eosinopenia, lymphocytosis
♦ Transmission by injection of blood into sheep
♦ Serological tests include
  • Indirect fluorescent antibody test
♦ ELISA

Necropsy findings

♦ Ascites, hydrothorax, hydropericardium
♦ Pulmonary edema
♦ Generalized subserosal hemorrhages
♦ Lymph nodes, spleen markedly enlarged
♦ Microscopic perivascular edema in brain
♦ Rickettsiae identifiable in Giemsa stain of brain impression smear

Diagnosis

Peracute cases resemble anthrax.
  Acute disease resemble:
♦ Rabies
♦ Sporadic bovine encephalomyelitis
♦ Tetanus
♦ Cerebral theileriasis
♦ Babesiasis
♦ Trypanosomiasis
♦ Hypomagnesemia
♦ Strychnine poisoning
♦ Lead poisoning
♦ Organophosphate poisoning

Treatment

Tetracyclines effective in early stages.

Control

♦ Contrived infection by injection of heartwater-infected blood followed by treatment with tetracycline used as a hazardous but effective vaccination procedure
♦ Immunity after such vaccination wanes unless continual reinfection maintained
♦ Tick control keeps disease in check

EQUINE EHRLICHIOSIS
[VM8 p. 1155]

Etiology

Ehrlichia equi

Epidemiology

♦ Occurs in horses in USA during fall to spring
♦ Minor disease in young; severe in horses over 3 years old

Clinical findings

♦ High fever
♦ Pallor, jaundice
♦ Anorexia, depression
♦ Hyperpnea
♦ Reluctant to move, incoordination
♦ Edema, heat of extremities
♦ Spontaneous recovery within 2–3 weeks

Clinical pathology

♦ Diagnosis based on detection of inclusion bodies in neutrophils, eosinophils
♦ Marked, transient leukopenia, thrombocytopenia
♦ Indirect fluorescent antibody test positive for over 300 days after infection

Necropsy findings

♦ Petechiation
♦ Limb edema
♦ Vasculitis on microscopic examination

Diagnosis

Resembles:
♦ Equine infectious anemia
♦ Equine monocytic ehrlichiosis
♦ Potomac horse fever

Treatment

Rapid cure with intravenous oxytetracycline

EQUINE MONOCYTIC
EHRLICHIOSIS (EQUINE
ERHLICHIAL COLITIS, POTOMAC
HORSE FEVER) [VM8 p. 1155]

Etiology

Ehrlichia risticii

Epidemiology

Occurrence
♦ Occurs in North America and Europe
♦ Only in horses but transmissible experimentally to other species, including dogs and cats
♦ Infection prevalence close to 30%; many subclinicals; case fatality rate 10%

Source and transmission
♦ Infected horses unlikely as source; they develop sterile immunity
♦ Transmission mode unknown; possibly tick vector
♦ Is transmissible orally
♦ Dogs, rabbits, red fox could be reservoir hosts

Risk factors
♦ Sporadic, seasonal (summer, fall)
♦ Commonest near large rivers
♦ Clinical disease uncommon in horses younger than one year; some peracute cases in foals
♦ Solid immunity for 20 months after infection

Clinical findings

Incubation period (experimental) 7 days

Acute
♦ Acute onset
♦ Depression, anorexia
♦ Congested mucosae
♦ High fever
♦ Decreased intestinal sounds early then tinkling sounds accompanying:
  • Profuse, projectile diarrhea at 24–72 hours, lasting 10 days
  • Rapid onset dehydration, hypovolemic shock
  • Acute or subacute colic

  • Laminitis at day 3
  • Subcutaneous edema, belly, lower limbs

Subacute
♦ Fever plus anorexia only, *or*
♦ Mild colic only, *or*
♦ Belly, limb edema only

Clinical pathology

♦ Organism cultivable
♦ Demonstration of organism on blood smear if very early in course, before clinical signs
♦ Serological tests include:
♦ Indirect immunofluorescence
♦ ELISA
♦ Rising titers indicate infection but interpretation difficult because of persistence of high titers
♦ Significant leukopenia early, leukocytosis later
♦ Hemoconcentration during dehydration

Necropsy findings

♦ Intestinal mucosal congestion, hemorrhage, erosions or ulcers, concentrated in cecum and colon
♦ Mesenteric lymph nodes swollen, edematous
♦ Subcutaneous edema belly wall
♦ Laminitis in some

Diagnosis

Resembles:
♦ Salmonellosis
♦ Antibiotic-induced enterocolitis
♦ Phenylbutazone poisoning
♦ Colitis-X

Treatment

♦ Oxytetracycline 6.6 mg/kg body weight I/V for 5 days, early in disease; hazardous because it may cause enterocolitis
♦ Intensive intravenous fluid therapy

Control

♦ Tick control recommended but disease still occurs
♦ Inactivated, whole cell, adjuvanted vaccine provides resistance but horses not fully protected after 6 months; needs 2 initial

injections with revaccination at 4 month intervals

JEMBRANA DISEASE [VM8 p. 1157]

Etiology

Cause not identified; intracellular, rickettsia-like bodies in lymph node lymphocytes, monocytes; thought to be an ehrlichiosis.

Epidemiology

♦ Occurred in Bali, Indonesia during 1964–1967
♦ Subsequently less severe disease
♦ Bali cattle, buffaloes; transmissible experimentally to other species
♦ Bacteremia, persists 2 years
♦ Possible insect transmission, or mechanically by needles
♦ Heavy mortalities

Clinical findings

♦ Fever, anorexia
♦ Generalized lymph node enlargement
♦ Nasal discharge
♦ Saliva drools
♦ Anemia
♦ Diarrhea, dysentery
♦ Rarely oral mucosal erosions
♦ Hemorrhages in oral, vaginal mucosa, rarely in anterior chamber of eye

Clinical pathology

♦ Rickettsia-like bodies in blood during febrile phase
♦ Moderate anemia
♦ Leukopenia, lymphopenia, eosinopenia, thrombocytopenia

Necropsy findings

♦ Generalized lymph node massive enlargement
♦ Generalised hemorrhages
♦ Spleen enlargement
♦ Rare intestinal mucosal erosions

Diagnosis

Resembles:
♦ Rinderpest
♦ Mucosal disease
♦ Salmonellosis

♦ Arsenic poisoning
♦ Ostertagiasis

Treatment and control

None specified.

'Q' FEVER [VM8 p. 1158]

Etiology

Coxiella burnetti, a rickettsia

Epidemiology

♦ Organism has worldwide distribution with cycles in wildlife and their ectoparasites
♦ Infection in ruminants main source of infection for humans
♦ Clinical disease rare in animals; a serious infection in humans, especially farm families drinking raw milk
♦ Organism in feces, urine, placenta, fetal fluids, milk; occurrence in humans often associated with contact with parturient animals
♦ Transmission mode uncertain
♦ Infection morbidity very variable
♦ Infection can persist several months in environment; resistant to most disinfectants, destroyed by pasteurization

Clinical findings

Very heavy infections can cause late abortion in sheep and goats; probably not in cattle.

Clinical pathology

♦ Seropositivity common in enzootic area
♦ Isolation of organism critical for diagnosis of disease in animals

Necropsy findings

No lesions.

Control

♦ Herds, flocks providing raw milk in enzootic areas should be free of infection
♦ Vaccination of humans at risk is practiced

BOVINE PETECHIAL FEVER (ONDIRI DISEASE) [VM8 p. 1159]

Etiology

Ehrlichia ondiri

Epidemiology

- Occurs in cattle in Kenya grazing high altitude scrub pasture
- Indigenous cattle appear to be resistant; only introduced animals affected
- Bushbuck thought to be natural reservoir
- Transmission thought to be by insect vector
- Recovered cattle immune 2 years; latently infected

Clinical findings

- High fever
- Mucosal petechiae
- Epistaxis
- Melena
- Hyphaema in some

Clinical pathology

- Organisms in granulocytes, monocytes during febrile period

24 DISEASES CAUSED BY ALGAE AND FUNGI

ALGAL INFECTIONS

Asymptomatic systemic *Prototheca* spp. infections, some with lymphadenitis, in cattle, sheep. See also protothecal mastitis, algal poisoning.

SYSTEMIC AND MISCELLANEOUS MYCOSES

Systemic fungal infections [VM8 p. 1160]
These are environmental infections originating from environmental sources, especially dust by inhalation. Some, mostly *Aspergillus, Mucor, Candida* spp., are from alimentary tract beginning as rumenitis, abomasitis, pharyngitis.

Mycotic abortion [VM8 p. 1160] Secondary to pulmonary and systemic infection in housed cattle, mycotic abortion has assumed small but notable prevalence, especially when haymaking is affected by rain. Common infections *Aspergillus, Mucor* spp., occasionally *Mortierella wolfii, Petriellidium boydii*. Treatment of systemic fungal infections is not widely documented. Nystatin is reported on most favorably as treatment

COCCIDIOIDOMYCOSIS
[VM8 p. 1161]

Epidemiology

♦ Cattle, sheep, horses, humans in southwestern United States
♦ Related to environment in dusty feed lots
♦ Rarely clinical illness

Clinical
♦ Horses and sheep show weight loss, fever
♦ Persistent cough
♦ Recurring, subcutaneous, pectoral abscesses
♦ Wheezing breath sounds

♦ Leg edema
♦ Intermittent colic

Necropsy findings

♦ Pus in pulmonary, mesenteric lymph node granulomas
♦ Sometimes calcified
♦ Some resemblance to tuberculosis, caseous lymphadenitis

Treatment and control

♦ No effective treatment or control other than dust prevention.

MUCORMYCOSIS (ZYGOMYCOSIS)
[VM8 p. 1161]

♦ Placental infection with *Rhizopus, Absidia, Mucor* spp., cause necrosis of maternal cotyledons and abortion in cattle
♦ *Absidia* spp. in bovine preputial catarrh
♦ Asymptomatic mesenteric lymph node, intestinal mural granulomas in pigs
♦ Ulcerative esophagitis, gastritis or abomasitis, enteritis associated with prolonged antibiotic therapy causes vomiting, diarrhea in young calves, pigs
♦ Primary **rumenitis**, due to lactic acid production in heavily grain fed cattle, infected by *Rhizopus* spp. Often terminates as fatal peritonitis
♦ Sporadic outbreaks *Candida* spp. porcine dermatitis

446

ASPERGILLOSIS [VM8 p. 1162]

◆ Systemic infection with *Aspergillus* spp. in all species, after prolonged antibiotic therapy; primary lesion in intestinal wall, secondaries liver, mesenteric lymph nodes, lungs, placenta causing abortion (6–8 months in cows), and congenital cutaneous and systemic infections in calves
◆ Gastroenteritis with chronic diarrhea in calves
◆ Chronic, subacute or acute pneumonia in calves, lambs, foals in dusty, poorly ventilated housing
◆ Systemic infections with pulmonary and lymph node localizations in racing camels
◆ Keratitis in eyes after prolonged antibiotic treatment of traumatic lesions

HISTOPLASMOSIS [VM8 p. 1162]

◆ The systemic form of *H. capsulatum* infection in epizootic lymphangitis.
◆ *Histoplasma capsulatum* in pulmonary infections by inhalation from contaminated dust
◆ Necropsy lesions – macrophages packed with fungal cells, in any organ causing fever, weight loss, localizing signs related to location of lesions, and sensitivity to histplasmin

RHINOSPORIDIOSIS [VM8 p. 1162]

◆ *Rhinosporidium seeberi* causes large nasal polyps, respiratory stertor, dyspnea, blood-stained nasal discharge in cattle, horses
◆ Suspected also in etiology of some cases of nasal granuloma.

CRYPTOCOCCOSIS (EUROPEAN BLASTOMYCOSIS, TORULOSIS) [VM8 p. 1163]

◆ *Cryptococcus neoformans* occurs rarely in systemic infections, nasal myxomatous polyps, mastitis, placentitis or granulomatous meningoencephalitis

MONILIASIS (CANDIDIASIS) [VM8 p. 1163]

◆ Oral pharyngeal infection by *Candida albicans* in malnourished piglets causing vomiting, emaciation, white pseudomembrane in fauces
◆ Chronic, slowly progressive, fatal pneumonia in feedlot cattle
◆ *C. parapsilosis* can cause bovine abortion with congenital, systemic infection

NORTH AMERICAN BLASTOMYCOSIS [VM8 p. 1164]

◆ Rare infection (*Blastomyces dermatiditis*) in humans; responds poorly to treatment
◆ Perineal abscesses in one horse.

DERMATOMYCOSES

RINGWORM [VM8 p. 1164]

Etiology

All species Alternaria spp., *Trichophyton mentagrophytes, T. verrucosum*

Horse Keratinomyces allejoi, *Microsporum equinum, M. gypseum, Trichophyton equinum, T. mentagrophytes, T. quinckeanum, T. verrucosum,*

Donkey T. mentagrophytes, T. verrucosum

Cattle Scopulariopsis brevicaulis, T. megnini, T. mentagrophytes, T. verrucosum, T. verrucosum var album, T. verrucosum var discoides

Pig M. canis, M. nanum, T. mentagrophytes, T. rubrum, T. verrucosum

Sheep M. canis, T. gypseum, T, mentagrophytes, T. quinckeanum, T. verrucosum var. ochraceum

Goat T. verrucosum

Epidemiology

Occurrence
Common only in horses and cattle

Risk factors
◆ Housed groups of animals
◆ Close physical contact
◆ Grooming
◆ Interchangeable harness and rugs
◆ Introduced carrier animals

- Infected housing
- High humidity
- Young animals

Clinical findings

Cattle
- Thick, gray, rounded, 3 cm dia. crusts, coalesce in bad cases
- Moist skin under at first, later dry
- Hairs lost, dandruff accumulates
- General distribution, but most lesions on head, neck, perineum

Horse
- Patches of bald, shining skin
- May be fine, scabs, lesions; coalesce readily forming extensive bald patches due to *T. equinum*
- Smaller, thick scabs due to *M. gypseum*
- Commonly widespread over body
- May begin at girth, neck, head limbs

Pigs
- Spreading ring of inflammation around single, scabby, alopecic centre
- One lesion may cover whole side of large pig
- Scabs thin, dry flakes

Sheep
- Lesions on head, not woolled area
- Disappear spontaneously at 4–5 weeks but persist in flock
- Round bald lesions with gray crust

Goat
Lesions like sheep but general spread over body

Clinical pathology

Skin scrapings for
- Spores, hyphae in smears
- Fungi in cultures causing color change in special medium
- Selection of scraping site by detection green fluorescence infected hairs under Wood's lamp; not all fungi fluoresce.

Diagnosis

Resembles:
- Mycotic dermatitis in cattle and horses
- Queensland Itch in horses
- Tinea versicolor (*Melazzesia furfur*) on goats' teats, with small, scaly, circular lesions
- Pityriasis rosea, tyrogliphosis in pigs.

Treatment

Spontaneous recovery usual, especially in young but treatment recommended to prevent environmental contamination.

Individual animals
Local treatment Brush off, dispose of scabs, apply:
- Weak iodine solution, tincture
- Whitfield ointment
- 10% ammoniated mercury ointment
- 1:200 to 1:1000 solution quaternary ammonium compounds
- Proprietary ointments and lotions containing organic fungistatic agents, e.g. captan, thiabendazole

Systemic treatment:
- Sodium iodide 10% solution, 1 g/14 kg body weight I/V widely used
- Griseofulvin used but too expensive for most cases

Groups of animals
- A spray preparation, e.g. 0.1 to 0.01% natamycin, nanamycin A, 2 sprayings 4 days apart; captan, 1:300, twice 2 weeks apart, also effective
- Vaccine as used in control also widely used

Control

- Isolate, treat infected animals
- Destroy bedding
- Disinfect accommodation and harnesses with commercial agricultural fungistat eg. iodophors solution, quaternary ammonium compound solution, Bordeaux mixture
- Vaccinate with commercial vaccine

EPIZOOTIC LYMPHANGITIS
(PSEUDOGLANDERS, EQUINE
BLASTOMYCOSIS, EQUINE
HISTOPLASMOSIS) [VM8 p. 1167]

Etiology

Gram-positive fungus *Histoplasma farciminosum*.

Epidemiology

♦ Horses only
♦ Still occurs as outbreaks in Africa, Asia, Mediterranean littoral
♦ Spread by direct contact, gear, equipment
♦ Entry by cutaneous abrasions lower limbs
♦ Wastage due to loss of function

Clinical findings

♦ Indolent ulcer at primary lesion
♦ Draining lymphatics thicken, develop nodules
♦ Nodules, lymph nodes enlarge, may rupture discharging thick, creamy pus
♦ No pain, no itching
♦ Lesions mostly on limbs; can be general
♦ Occasionally on nasal septum, in eye or sinuses or lungs
♦ Disease persists 9–12 months

Clinical pathology

♦ Gram-positive, double-walled yeast-like cells in discharges
♦ Fluorescent antibody test

Necropsy findings

Granulomas in lymphatics, lymph nodes, rarely lungs.

Diagnosis

Resembles:
♦ Glanders but pus creamy, characteristic yeast cells, rare pulmonary involvement
♦ Sporotrichosis

Treatment and control

♦ Parenteral iodides possibly effective
♦ In early cases excision of lesions
♦ Slaughter clinical cases, strict hygiene, quarantine infected groups
♦ Killed vaccines widely used

SPOROTRICHOSIS [VM8 p. 1169]

Etiology

Sporotrichum schencki, gram-positive fungus.

Epidemiology

♦ Mostly horses, rare cases other species
♦ Spread by contact with infected cases, or contaminated environment
♦ Entry through skin wounds
♦ Slow spread in group
♦ Low mortality rate

Clinical findings

♦ Small, painless, cutaneous nodules on lower limbs
♦ Discharge a little pus, heal 3–4 weeks
♦ Lymphangitis in some
♦ New lesions may continue to appear for months

Clinical pathology

♦ Small number of gram-positive, single-walled, fungal spores
♦ Can be cultured, passaged to rats, hamsters

Diagnosis

Resembles:
♦ Glanders
♦ Epizootic lymphangitis, differentiated by recognition of spores
♦ Maduromycotic mycetoma

Treatment and control

♦ Systemic iodides, sodium parenterally or potassium orally
♦ Griseofulvin effective systemically
♦ Iodine tincture on discharging sites
♦ Strict hygiene, isolation

SWAMP CANCER (EQUINE PHYCOMYCOSIS, CUTANEOUS PITHYOSIS, HYPHOMYCOSIS, DESTRUENS, FLORIDA HORSE LEECH, BURSATTEE) [VM8 p. 1169]

Etiology

♦ Principally *Pythium insidiosum* (= *Hyphomyces destruens*)
♦ *Basidiobolus haptosporus, Conodobolus coronatus* also implicated

Epidemiology

♦ Common in tropics
♦ In horses; rarely in cattle, dogs, humans
♦ Summer disease with high prevalence in animals standing in water for long periods

Clinical findings

♦ Lesions on lower limbs, ventral abdomen, below medial eye canthus, alae nasi, lips

- Initial lesion a rapidly enlarging, itchy nodule
- Large cutaneous granulomas with ulcer center raised edges

Clinical pathology

- Culture of fungus difficult
- Agar gel, double diffusion, complement fixation, intradermal hypersensitivity tests available
- Fungus, 'grains' in biopsy material

Diagnosis

Resembles:
- Cutaneous habronemiasis
- Maduromycotic mycetoma

Treatment and control

- Surgical excision of small lesions
- Parenteral iodine injection
- Long course of amphotericin parenterally, plus local infiltration and excision
- Good prophylactic, therapeutic effect from a vaccine, but severe systemic and local reactions common

MADUROMYCOTIC MYCETOMA (MADUROMYCOSIS) [VM8 p. 1170]

Etiology

Brachycladium spiciferum (Helminthosporium spiciferum, Curvularia geniculata, Monosporium apiospermum).

Epidemiology

In horses.

Clinical findings

- 1–2.5 cm dia. cutaneous nodules over most of body, most common at fetlock, coronet
- Some discharge exudate
- Biopsy shows mottled appearance of brown specks in pink tissue

Clinical pathology

Fungus in pus

Diagnosis

Resembles equine cutaneous pythiosis

25 DISEASES CAUSED BY PROTOZOA

BABESIOSIS (TEXAS FEVER, REDWATER FEVER, CATTLE TICK FEVER) [VM8 p. 1171]

Etiology

Cattle
♦ *Babesia bovis* (includes *B. argentina, B. berbera*)
♦ *B. bigemina*
♦ *B. major*
♦ *B. divergens*

Water buffalo (*Bubalis bubalis*)
♦ *B. bovis*
♦ *B. bigemina*
♦ Sheep and goats
♦ *B. motasi*
♦ *B. ovis*

Pigs
♦ *B. trautmanni*
♦ *B. perroncitoi*

Horses
♦ *B. equi*
♦ *B. caballi*

Epidemiology

Occurrence
♦ Limited to distribution of insect vectors
♦ Cattle – *B. bigemina, B. bovis* in the tropics and subtropics; *B. major, B. divergens* in temperate regions
♦ Sheep – south-east Europe, UK, Africa, South America
♦ Pig – south-east Europe, Africa
♦ Horse, donkey, mule, zebra – southern Europe, Asia, North and South Americas
♦ Morbidity variable with tick prevalence; case fatality rate close to 100% in adults, near to nil in yearlings

Source and transmission
♦ Only in blood stream of hosts in active phase of disease

♦ Transmitted by ticks, pass part of life cycle in tick, some protozoa persist through several generations of ticks:
  • Cattle – *Boophilus, Rhipicephalus, Haemaphysalis, Ixodes* spp.
  • Sheep – *Rhipicephalus, Haemaphysalis* spp.
  • Pigs – *Rhipicephalus, Boophilus* spp.
  • Horses – *Dermacentor. Rhipicephalus, Hyalomma* spp.
♦ Infection persists in adult animals for up to 2 years
♦ In an enzootic area with constant reinfection, carrier state persists for life
♦ Infection can be passed between animals on needles, instruments

Risk factors
♦ Infection, and premunity persists for about 6 months in the absence of reinfection, then sterile immunity for 6 months; a total immune period of 1 year
♦ Afrikander, zebu cattle breeds resistant to tick infestation, and some *Babesia* spp. infections
♦ Calves, foals from immune dams immune till 6 months
♦ Disease much milder in young animals
♦ Introduced, naive cattle most susceptible
♦ Existing immunity may be overcome by nutritional or other stress
♦ Heaviest losses in marginal areas where ticks may be absent, animals lose immunity, for some years
♦ Seasonal variation in tick population can cause summer prevalence of disease

Importance
♦ Heavy losses by death, reduced productivity
♦ Heavy costs of tick control
♦ Limitation of livestock movement

Clinical findings

Cattle
♦ Incubation period 2–3 weeks
♦ Many inapparent infections in young animals

- Acute onset high fever, depression
- Tachycardia, tachypnea
- Anorexia, milk yield depression, weight loss
- Rumination ceases
- Mucosae congested, then pale, then jaundice
- Urine dark red, brown, frothy
- **Pipestem** feces (thin stream of liquid feces ejected forcibly)
- Death in many after course of 24 hours
- Survivors ill for 3 weeks

Complications
- Abortion
- Cerebral babesiosis:
  - Incoordination, posterior paralysis, or
  - Mania, convulsions, coma

Horses
- Incubation period 8–10 days
- Reluctant to move, some recumbent
- Intermittent fever
- Edema head, belly wall, fetlocks
- Hemoglobinuria unusual
- Jaundice slight
- Red urine, pallor, jaundice, mucosal petechiation, weakness in young horses
- Constipation, colic in some
- Some deaths as early as 24 hours, most at 8–10 days
- Long convalescence in survivors
- Survivors are carriers for up to 4 years

Other species
As for cattle.

Clinical pathology

- Existing infection identified by:
  - Demonstration of protozoa in peripheral blood smear
  - Transmission of infection by blood infusion into susceptible, usually splenectomised, subject
- Infection experienced during past year established by serological tests including, for cattle:
  - Complement fixation
  - Indirect fluorescent antibody
  - Indirect hemagglutination
  - ELISA, microplate ELISA
  - Latex agglutination
  - DNA probes
  - And many others
- Some of these tests available for other species; most used are ELISAs
- Hematology examination marked by low erythrocyte count, hemoglobin content,

peak at 9–16 days after infection; thrombocytopenia, low fibrinogen content

Necropsy findings

- Jaundice
- Splenomegaly, soft, pulpy contents
- Liver, kidneys enlarged, dark
- Red–brown urine
- Marked intravascular clotting
- Protozoa in impression smears from heart muscle, brain, other tissues for 8 hours after death

Diagnosis

Cattle
Resembles:
- Eperythrozoonosis
- leptospirosis
- *Theileria annulata* infection
- Postparturient hemoglobinuria
- Bacillary hemoglobinuria
- S-methyl-L-cysteine sulfoxide poisoning

Horses
Resembles azoturia

Treatment

- To be effective treatment must be urgent
- No effect on protozoa in ticks so tick elimination also necessary

Cattle
- Effective drugs include:
  - Diminazene aceturate
  - Imidocarb dipropionate
  - Amicarbalide diisethionate
- Many other drugs, especially acaprin, piroparv are safe, moderately efficient drugs in extensive use in enzootic countries and have the advantage of not completely sterilising the patient, permitting a state of premunity

Horses
- Many drugs used; imidocarb most favored
- Severe local reactions to some babesicides

Sheep
- Diminazene aceturate recommended

Control

- Eradication from large areas achieved by tick control

♦ Control short of eradication depends on:
  • Limitation without elimination of tick population plus
  • Vaccination of susceptible introduced animals, or animals in high risk, border zones with:
    • Living protozoa, or
    • Living protozoa plus chemosterilant (chemoimmunization), or
    • Killed, adjuvanted vaccines, or
    • Attenuated vaccines, especially irradiated ones, or
    • Long-acting chemosterilant, e.g. imidocarb (chemoprophylaxis)
♦ Animals vaccinated with live protozoa must be kept under observation and treated with babesicides if their reaction is excessive, but not to the point of chemosterilization
♦ Vaccination breakdowns may be due to failure to include all relevant protozoa and their local strains in the vaccine
♦ Whole-blood vaccines have transmitted other pathogens, e.g. enzootic bovine leukosis virus

EPERYTHROZOONOSIS
[VM8 p. 1180]

Etiology

The species-specific rickettsiae *Eperythrozoon ovis, E. suis* etc., *E. wenyoni* in cattle.

Epidemiology

Occurrence
♦ Widespread, in most countries but a minor disease
♦ Sheep, goats, pigs, cattle, llamas, wildlife
♦ Subclinical infection common
♦ Occurs as outbreaks in stressed groups
♦ Source is permanently infected animals
♦ Transmission by any means of transmitting infected blood, especially biting insect, e.g. pig lice, mosquitoes; also vaccination, castration
♦ Transplacental infection likely
♦ Patients infected probably for life

Clinical findings

Incubation period about 1–3 weeks.

Pigs
♦ Fever, tachycardia
♦ Mucosal pallor
♦ Jaundice in some
♦ Weight loss

♦ Reproductive failure due to delayed estrus cycles, embryonic death
♦ Hind limb weakness

Cattle
♦ Rare disease
♦ Fever, stiff gait lassitude
♦ Milk yield depression
♦ Diarrhea
♦ Lymph node enlargement
♦ Swelling of teats, hind limbs

Sheep
♦ Rarely sudden death with hemoglobinuria, jaundice
♦ Common syndrome is mild with:
  • Fever, depression
  • Anemia, low exercise tolerance
  • Weight loss, wool yield reduced

Clinical pathology

♦ Epicellular parasites on erythrocytes in stained blood smear
♦ Profound hypoglycemia
♦ Significant anemia
♦ Leukopenia
♦ Serological tests used include:
  • Complement fixation
  • Indirect fluorescent antibody
  • ELISA
  • Indirect hemagglutination
♦ Transmission to splenectomized animal used for identification

Necropsy findings

A generally non-fatal disease

Diagnosis

Resembles:
♦ Blood loss anemia
♦ Poor production performance

Treatment

♦ Organic arsenicals widely used
♦ Babesicides e.g. imidocarb also recommended
♦ Tetracycline effective in pigs
♦ Reinfection occurs quickly

Control

No effective programs listed.

COCCIDIOSIS [VM8 p. 1181]

Etiology

♦ Cattle – *Eimeria zuernii, E. bovis, E. ellipsoidalis*
♦ Sheep – *E. arloingi A, E. weybridgenis, E. crandallis, E. ahsata, E. ovinoidalis, E. gilruthi*
♦ Goats – *E. arloingi, E. faurei, E. gilruthi, E. caprovina, E. ninakohlyakimovae, E. christensi*
♦ Pigs – *Isospora suis, Eimeria debliecki, E. scabra, E. perminuta*
♦ Horses – *Eimeria leuckarti*

Epidemiology

Occurrence
♦ Worldwide
♦ All domestic animals
♦ Outbreaks in cattle, sheep, goats, piglets; sporadic cases only in foals
♦ Infection prevalence very high; morbidity 10–15%, rarely up to 80%; case fatality low

Source and transmission
♦ Feces of infected, often subclinical, cases
♦ Transmission by ingestion of contaminated water, feed; licking hair coat
♦ Large numbers of oocysts need to be ingested for clinical signs to develop
♦ Oocysts in feces may survive 2 years; need warmth, moisture to sporulate; inactivated by hot, dry or below-freezing temperatures

Risk factors
♦ Close confinement permitting maximum contamination of feed, water by feces; frequent recycling leads to build-up of massive levels of oocyst intake
♦ Species-specific; no passage between host species
♦ Young animals most susceptible
♦ Seasonal when animals penned, e.g. beef calves put into feedlots after weaning
♦ In lambs when ewes penned for lambing supervision
♦ Exposure to severe cold or other stress may precipitate clinical disease
♦ Concentration of grazing around water supplies
♦ Infections with more than one coccidia species exacerbates disease
♦ Immunity develops after infection; naive animals most susceptible; degree of immunity varies with coccidial species

Importance
Death, productivity losses common in calves, occasionally in pigs.

Clinical findings

Cattle
♦ Incubation period 14–30 days
♦ Sudden onset severe diarrhea
♦ Foul-smelling, fluid feces containing mucus, blood (dark, tarry staining, to streaks or clots to passage of whole blood)
♦ Perineum, tail smeared with blood-stained feces
♦ Severe straining in most cases; rectal prolapse in some
♦ Rare cases of hemorrhagic anemia
♦ Reduced feed intake
♦ Recovery in most after 5–6 day course
♦ Long convalescence to regain lost weight

Nervous coccidiosis
♦ Up to 50% calves with clinical coccidiosis in the outbreak may develop the nervous disease
♦ Tremor
♦ Hyperesthesia
♦ Paddling convulsions with head ventroflexion
♦ Nystagmus
♦ Death in 80–90% after course of 24 hours

Lambs
♦ Similar syndrome to calves but much less dysentery
♦ Anorexia, low weight gain, emaciation
♦ Soft feces, smudged perineum
♦ Weakness, recumbency
♦ Recovery or high death rate in feedlot lambs after 1–3 weeks
♦ Doubts about the clinical disease and mortalities being due to coccidiosis

Foals
♦ Diarrhea for several days
♦ Fatal intestinal hemorrhage in some

Piglets
♦ Severe outbreaks in entire litters of 5–15 day old pigs
♦ Anorexia, depression
♦ Profuse, yellow, apparently foamy, watery diarrhea for several days
♦ Dehydration
♦ Vomiting in some
♦ Case fatality rate up to 20%

Clinical pathology

♦ Heavy oocyst population in feces develops 2–4 days after diarrhea onset; period of oocyst discharge varies but count may be low a few days after peak of illness
♦ Oocyst count >5000/g feces indicates diagnosis of coccidiosis; may be as high as 100 000/g in normal animals

Necropsy findings

♦ Hemorrhagic enteritis; ulceration, mucosal necrosis in some
♦ Mucosal thickening in cecum, colon, rectum, ileum
♦ Small white cyst-like bodies in tips of villi in terminal ileum in some
♦ Blood-stained feces in intestine
♦ Anemia
♦ More small intestine involvement in lambs than in calves; includes villous atrophy

Diagnosis

Resembles:
♦ Colibacillosis
♦ Salmonellosis
♦ Clostridiosis (*Clostridium perfringens* type C)
♦ Intestinal helminthiasis
♦ Mixed infections with the above or with viral enteritides present diagnostic problems

Treatment

♦ Coccidiosis a self-limiting disease; late treatment of clinical cases unlikely to exert any effect on outcome
♦ Isolate clinical cases (see Table 25.1 for recommended treatments); sulfadimidine, amprolium most widely used
♦ Reduce stocking rate
♦ Clean pens
♦ Provide water, feed troughs not able to be contaminated by infected feces
♦ Supportive treatment with fluids, electrolytes; blood transfusions in some

Control

♦ Control difficult to achieve consistently
♦ Well-drained, frequently cleaned pens for young stock in confined accommodation
♦ Minimize fouling of feed and water with feces, hair coats, fleece
♦ Frequent field rotation for stock at pasture
♦ Use of coccidiostats in feed to keep oocyst level low but permit development of immunity. See Table 25.1 for details of drugs used
♦ Variable results with effective drugs because their use may commence at insusceptible stage of the life-cycle; situation further complicated by common infections with a number of coccidial species with different life cycles
♦ Feeding coccidiostats for very young pigs difficult; avoided by feeding drug to sow before and after farrowing but results unsatisfactory

SARCOCYSTOSIS (SARCOSPORIDIOSIS) [VM8 p. 1191]

Etiology

Sarcocystis spp. (see Table 25.2), coccidian parasites in phylum Apicomplexa.

Epidemiology

Occurrence
In infected countries morbidity close to 100% in cattle, sheep and horses, lower in pigs; mostly asymptomatic; clinical disease rare.

Source and transmission
♦ Prey–predator life cycle; definitive host a carnivorous predator
♦ Farm dogs and cats fed uncooked offal from farm butchered animals, cohabit with livestock, fecal contamination of their feed
♦ Oocysts, then sporocysts formed in predator gut, passed in feces, contaminate feed, consumed by intermediate host, e.g. ruminant, pass through gut mucosa into blood stream, then localization in striated muscle, nervous tissue developing into sarcocysts found at meat inspection

Risk factors
♦ All ages
♦ Some sarcocyst species more pathogenic than others
♦ Disease worse when heavy sporocyst ingestion
♦ Monensin may potentiate

Importance
♦ Cause meat condemnation at abattoir, e.g. the cat–sheep parasite
♦ Rare clinical disease in livestock

Table 25.1 Chemotherapeutics which have been recommended for the treatment and control of coccidiosis in calves and lambs [VM8 p. 1189]

Chemotherapeutic agent	Treatment	Prevention
Sulfamidine (sulfamethazine)	*Calves and lambs*: 140 mg/kg body weight orally daily for 3 days individually	*Calves*: in feed 35 mg/kg body weight for 15 days *Lambs*: daily dose 25 mg/kg body weight for 1 week
Nitrofurazone	*Calves and lambs*: 15 mg/kg body weight daily for 7 days or 0.04% in feed for 7 days. In water at 0.0133% for 7 days	*Calves*: In feed at 33 mg/kg body weight for 2 weeks *Lambs*: in feed at 0.04% for 21 days
Amprolium	*Calves*: individual dose at 10 mg/kg body weight daily for 5 days (50) or 65 mg/kg body weight one dose (51)	*Calves*: in feed at 5 mg/kg body weight for 21 days *Lambs*: in feed, 50 mg/kg body weight for 21 days
Monensin	*Lambs*: 3 mg/kg body weight daily for 20 days beginning on 13th day following experimental inoculation (41)	*Calves*: 20 mg/kg feed fed continuously *Calves*: 16.5 0r 33 g/tonne for 31 days
Lasalocid		*Lambs*: 25–100 mg/kg feed from weaning until market. Also, in ewe's diet from 2 weeks before and until 60 days after lambing

Table 25.2 Sarcocystic species in agricultural animals [VM8 p. 1191]

Intermediate host	Sarcocystis spp.	Synonyms	Definitive host
Cattle	S. cruzi	S. bovicanis	Dog, wolf, coyote, fox, raccoon
	S. hirsuta	S. bovifelis	Cat
	S. hominis	S. bovihominis	Humans
Sheep	S. tenella	S. ovicanis	Dog, coyote, fox
	S. arieticanis	—	Dog
	S. gigantea	S. ovifelis	Cat
	S. medusiformis	—	Cat
Goats	S. capracanis	—	Dog, coyote, fox
	S. hericanis	—	Dog
	S. moulei	—	Cat
Pigs	S. miescheriana	S. suicanis	Dog, raccoon, wolf
	S. suihominis	—	Human
	S. porcifelis	—	Cat
Horses	S. bertrami	S. equicanis	Dog
	—	S. fayeri	
	S. neurona	—	not determined

Clinical findings

Cattle – acute
♦ Incubation period 23–26 days
♦ Anorexia, fever, weight loss, reduced milk yield
♦ Nervousness, tremor
♦ Excessive salivation
♦ Lameness
♦ Tail switch loss (rat-tail)
♦ Anemia
♦ Abortion

Cattle – chronic
♦ Poor weight gain
♦ Loss of hair on neck, rump, tail switch

Sheep – non-suppurative encephalomyelitis
Ataxia, flaccid paralysis.

Sheep – chronic
♦ Reduced growth rate
♦ Possibly esophageal dysfunction, regurgitation

Horses
Probably cause of **protozoal myeloencephalitis.**

Clinical pathology

♦ Incidental findings include:
  • Anemia
  • High serum levels creatine phosphokinase, lactic dehydrogenase, aspartate aminotransferase
♦ Serological evidence of infection in –
  • ELISA
  • Indirect hemagglutination test

Necropsy findings

♦ Emaciation, lymphadenopathy, laminitis, anemia, ascites
♦ Vasculitis, widespread hemorrhages
♦ Erosions, ulcers oral, esophageal mucosae
♦ Necrotizing myocarditis
♦ Necrotizing encephalomyelitis
♦ Schizonts in tissues

Diagnosis

Resembles:
♦ Septicemia
♦ Hemorrhagic disease
♦ Bracken poisoning

Treatment

Amprolium, salinomycin may relieve signs; monensin has exacerbated muscle lesions.

Control

♦ Separation of farm livestock and dogs, cats
♦ No uncooked meat offal fed to dogs, cats

EQUINE PROTOZOAL MYELOENCEPHALITIS
[VM8 p. 1193]

Etiology

Sarcocystis neurona.

Epidemiology

♦ Horses, ponies in USA
♦ All ages, breeds, reported mostly in 1–7 year old thoroughbreds, standardbreds
♦ Individual cases

Clinical findings

♦ Insidious onset ataxia, progressing to paresis, muscle atrophy, sensory deficits in one limb, or
♦ Cranial nerve involvement, e.g. blindness, facial paralysis, dysphagia
♦ Signs may deteriorate to euthanasia level in weeks or remain static for long periods

Clinical pathology

♦ No laboratory test available
♦ Elevated protein, leukocytes in cerebrospinal fluid

Necropsy findings

♦ Necrotizing, non-suppurative encephalitis, myelitis
♦ Protozoan organisms in tissues

Diagnosis

Resembles diseases caused by myeloencephalitis.

Treatment

♦ Long-term (at least 6 weeks) treatment with potentiated sulfonamide and pyrimethamine; residual nervous deficit probable
♦ Corticosteroid administration hastens progress of disease

BOVINE PROTOZOAL ABORTION
[VM8 p. 1194]

Etiology

Protozoan parasite resembling *Neospora caninum*, possibly *Sarcosporidia* spp.

Epidemiology

♦ Recorded in Australia, New Zealand, USA
♦ Probably a disease in an intermediate host with the definitive host a carnivore
♦ Occurs as epizootics during a 1–2 month period, in large, dry-lot dairies; also sporadic cases in chronic pattern

Clinical findings

♦ Autolyzed fetuses at 3–8.5 months fetal age, or
♦ Live-born, premature calves
♦ Some neonatal calves with sporozoan encephalomyelitis
♦ No sickness, milk drop or future conception problem in dam
♦ Repeat abortions possible in same cow

Clinical pathology

♦ No tests available

Necropsy findings

♦ Fetal non-suppurative encephalomyelitis, myocarditis
♦ Protozoa in tissues identified by immunohistochemical test utilizing *Neosporum caninum* antiserum

Diagnosis

Resembles:
♦ Brucellosis
♦ Vibriosis
♦ Leptospirosis
♦ Infectious bovine rhinotracheitis
♦ Mycotic abortion
♦ Epizootic abortion
♦ Trichomoniasis
♦ Listeriosis
♦ Salmonellosis

Treatment

No treatment identified.

Control

Depends on identification of protozoan and its life-cycle.

CRYPTOSPORIDIOSIS [VM8 p. 1195]

Etiology

Cryptosporidium parvum.

Epidemiology

Occurrence
♦ Worldwide distribution
♦ In neonates of all species, especially calves, lambs, kids; not considered a significant enteric pathogen in pigs, foals
♦ Infection prevalence 70%; case fatality may be high in severe outbreaks

Source and transmission
♦ Infected animals of any species, including humans
♦ A typical enteric protozoan life cycle of 6 stages includes excystation, asexual merogony, gametogony, fertilization, oocyst formation, sporozoite formation; oocysts sporulate, and are infective, in host cells, not after passage to the exterior
♦ Infective oocysts in feces of infected animals; large numbers in brief patent period cause rapid build-up and danger period
♦ Maximum discharge from 9–14 day old calves, rare in adults
♦ Transmission direct or via infected fomites, surviving several months in cool, moist conditions; most disinfectants, drying, low or high temperatures destroy the oocysts

Risk factors
♦ *C. parvum* a common infection in healthy animals; disease due to concurrent:
  • Infection with other pathogens e.g. rotavirus, coronavirus
  • Immunodeficiency
  • Managemental, environmental stress
♦ Recovered animals immune but are not carriers
♦ Greatest disease incidence in 5–15 day old calves, lambs 4–10 days, kids 5–21 days, foals 5 days–6 weeks; wider age group, up to market age in affected in pigs

Importance
An important zoonosis in immunologically compromised human patients.

Clinical findings

In 5–15 day old calves:
♦ Self-limiting, mild to moderate diarrhea, with yellow, watery feces containing mucus
♦ Unresponsive to standard scour treatments
♦ Severe weight loss
♦ Apathy, anorexia, dehydration
♦ Rarely weakness, recumbency
♦ Spontaneous recovery after course of 6–10 days

♦ Deaths usually related to under-nutrition, cold stress during diarrhea period

Clinical pathology

Diagnosis based on detection of otherwise difficult to find oocysts in feces by one of:
  • Special staining
  • Flotation
  • ELISA
♦ Immunofluorescence technique

Necropsy findings

♦ Villous atrophy in ileum, cecum, colon
♦ Dehydration, emaciation, serous atrophy
♦ Cryptosporidia visible microscopically in small intestinal microvilli

Diagnosis

Resembles:
♦ Colibacillosis
♦ Rotavirus infection
♦ Coronavirus
♦ Salmonellosis
♦ Possible disease caused by *Cryptosporidium muris* infection

Treatment

♦ Standard antiprotozoal, antimicrobial drugs have no apparent therapeutic effect
♦ Anticoccidial prophylactics ineffective; preliminary trials suggest effectiveness of halofuginone (60–125 μg/kg body weight orally per day for 7 days)
♦ Supportive treatment with fluids, electrolytes, continue full milk intake

Control

♦ Reduce fecal–oral cycle by clean environment
♦ Ensure adequate colostrum intake
♦ Individual pens for calves for first 2 weeks
♦ Disinfection of oocytes by application of 5% ammonia, 10% formol saline, ammonium hydroxide, hydrogen peroxide, chlorine-dioxide based disinfectants
♦ Isolation of sick calves
♦ All-in, all-out management of calf houses

GIARDIASIS (LAMBLIASIS)
[VM8 p. 1199]

Etiology

♦ *Giardia duodenalis* (*G. intestinalis*, *G. lamblia*, *Lamblia intestinalis*)

♦ The one species thought to infect all animal species

Epidemiology

♦ Most continents
♦ All species except possibly pigs
♦ Infection prevalence up to 18–36% in sheep, 10–28% in cattle
♦ Greater susceptibility in young; possible occurrence in chronic diarrhea in adult horses
♦ Many infections asymptomatic
♦ Animals appear to act as infection reservoir for humans
♦ Infectious period several months
♦ Infection by ingestion of infective cysts from fecal contamination
♦ Transmission by direct contact, infected fomites or water

Clinical findings

Calves
♦ Semifluid, pasty diarrhea with mucus for 2 days to 6 weeks
♦ Slow growth rate

Clinical pathology

Cysts demonstrated in feces by flotation on zinc sulfate or graded glucose solution.

Necropsy findings

Cysts in smears of small intestinal mucosa.

Diagnosis

Resembles:
♦ Colibacillosis
♦ Rotavirus infection
♦ Coronavirus infection
♦ Cryptosporidiosis
♦ Coccidiosis
♦ Salmonellosis

Treatment

♦ Dimetridazole (50 mg/kg daily for 5 days), quinacrine (1 mg/kg twice daily for 7 days) appear very effective
♦ Parasite also susceptible to furazolidone, albendazole

Control

Procedures designed to break the fecal–oral cycle (see cryptosporidiosis).

BESNOITIOSIS [VM8 p. 1200]

Etiology

Besnoitia besnoiti.

Epidemiology

♦ Occurs in tropical and subtropical countries
♦ Morbidity variable; many subclinical cases, case fatality 10%
♦ Primary host probably cats
♦ Intermediate host infection in cattle, goats, horses, many wildlife
♦ Transmission mode undefined, possibly ingestion infected cat feces
♦ Can be mechanically transmitted by syringe, biting flies
♦ Both stages of life-cycle contagious:
  • Endozoites cause acute disease
  • Cystozoite causes chronic disease
♦ Can cause severe production loss in cattle

Clinical findings

Cattle – acute disease
♦ High fever, increased heart and respiratory rate
♦ Warm, painful swellings on belly wall, sternal area
♦ Stiff movements
♦ Superficial lymph nodes swollen
♦ Diarrhea in some
♦ Abortion
♦ Nasal discharge
♦ Lacrimation, then mucopurulent, some blood-stained
♦ Small, white, elevated macules on nasal mucosa, scleral conjunctivae
♦ With time, skin grossly thickened, alopecia
♦ Severe dermatitis over most of body
♦ Bulls temporarily sterile
♦ Course of disease several months

Cattle – chronic disease
♦ In enzootic area
♦ Alopecia
♦ Thickened wrinkled skin in folds at neck, shoulder, rump
♦ Small, subcutaneous lumps
♦ Lesions on teats and lips of suckling calves

Goats
♦ As for cattle with worst lesions at fetlock
♦ White, gritty, subcutaneous granules over hindquarters

Horses
♦ Similar to cattle, neither as severe nor as prolonged.

Clinical pathology

♦ Cysts containing spindle-shaped spores in skin, scleral scrapings, sections
♦ Serological tests include:
  • Indirect immunofluorescence technique
  • ELISA

Necropsy findings

Cattle
♦ In severe form, widespread lesions in skeletal, heart muscle, lungs
♦ Schizonts in lesions

Diagnosis

Resembles:
♦ Sarcoptic mange
♦ Demodectic mange
♦ Mycotic dermatitis
♦ Highly chlorinated naphthalene poisoning

Treatment

No specific treatment recorded.

Control

♦ Tissue culture vaccine has moderate restraining effect.

TOXOPLASMOSIS [VM8 p. 1201]

Etiology

Toxoplasma gondii. Several strains of varying virulence.

Epidemiology

Occurrence
♦ Worldwide distribution of infection
♦ Variable infection prevalence, e.g. in pigs seropositives average 22% (0–97%); most other species average 15–25% seropositives
♦ Disease morbidity nil in farm animals except for abortion, neonatal disease in sheep, goats; abortion rate up to 50% in many countries

Source and transmission
♦ A disease of cats as the definitive host; acquire infection by ingesting uncooked, infected meat from intermediate host
♦ Cats shed oocysts in feces, ingested on contaminated feed or in drinking water by other cats or intermediate hosts
♦ All other species, including humans, intermediate hosts
♦ Oocysts can survive in environment for over 1 year

Risk factors
♦ Prevalence high in high rainfall zones, prolongs oocyst survival
♦ Cats in a sheep environment, especially where stored feed fed

Importance
♦ Important cause of abortion, neonatal mortality in sheep
♦ Serious zoonosis; large risk from cat feces but possible transmission by ingestion of infected, uncooked meat

Clinical findings

Systemic disease
♦ Rarely in cattle, sheep, goats pigs, not in horses
♦ In adults or neonates
♦ Fever
♦ Dyspnea, cough
♦ Tremor
♦ Hyperexcitability, then lethargy

Abortion and neonatal deaths
♦ Ewes and does
♦ Fetal absorption
♦ Mummified or stillborn lambs
♦ Abortion in last month, up to 50%
♦ Neonatal deaths
♦ Viable full-term lambs with ataxia, sucking disorders

Clinical pathology

Serological tests, with equivocal results, include:
♦ Complement fixation
♦ Sabin–Feldman dye test
♦ Indirect fluorescent antibody test
♦ Indirect hemagglutination test
♦ ELISA
♦ Modified direct agglutination test

Necropsy findings

- Pneumonitis, hydrothorax, ascites, lymphadenitis, intestinal ulcer, necrotic foci in liver, spleen, kidney in some
- Multiple, proliferative, necrotic granulomata, some calcified characteristic
- Lesions in nervous system, lung, myocardium
- In pregnant ewes, lesions in uterine wall, placental cotyledons, fetus – focal necrotic lesions in brain, liver, lungs
- Toxoplasma in most organs
- Confirmatory diagnosis depends on transmission to mice

Diagnosis

Resembles:
- Brucellosis
- *Campylobacter fetus* infection
- Enzootic ewe abortion
- Listeriosis
- *Salmonella abortusovis* infection
- *Salmonella dublin* infection
- Rift Valley fever
- *Coxiella burnetti* infection
- Border disease

Treatment

Sulfonamides (especially sulfadimidine, sulfamerazine, sulfadiazine) combined with pyrimethamine have some efficiency against proliferating toxoplasma in the acute stage but limited activity against tissue cysts.

Control

- Eliminate cats from farm environment
- Exposure of ewes to infection during non-pregnant stage will encourage development of immunity
- Feeding monensin, decoquinate during early pregnancy protects against infection of fetus
- Vaccination with tachyzoites from an incomplete strain (S48) of *T. gondii* causes satisfactory protection
- For protection of humans vaccination of animals against toxoplasmosis should not be permitted, infected groups of animals should be disposed of, all meat should be thoroughly cooked

THERILERIOSES [VM8 p. 1206]

Tick-borne protozoan diseases caused by *Theileria* spp. in cattle, sheep, goats, wild ungulates, and characterized by lymphoproliferative disorders. The important infections in cattle are:
- East coast fever – *Theileria parva*
- Mediterranean coast fever – *T. annulata*
- Oriental theileriosis – *T. orientalis*
- Benign theileriosis – *T. orientalis, T. mutans, T. sergenti, T. velifera, T. buffeli*
Theilerioses in sheep, goats include *T. hirci*

EAST COAST FEVER (ECF)
[VM8 p. 1207]

Etiology

Theileria parva in several variants with differing virulence:
- *T. parva parva* causing **classical ECF** transmitted from cattle to cattle by *Rhipicephalus appendiculatus*
- *T. parva lawrencei* causing **Corridor disease** transmitted from buffalo to cattle by *Rhipicephalus appendiculatus, R. zambesiensis*
- *T. parva bovis* causing **January disease** transmitted by *R. appendiculatus*

Epidemiology

Occurrence
- Africa
- Cattle, buffalo
- Morbidity, case fatality rates near 100% in naive cattle; indigenous *Bos indicus* resistant; Asiatic water buffalo fully susceptible, African buffalo immune
- In enzootic areas cattle infected as calves, develop immunity

Source and transmission
- Blood from infected cattle to *Rhipicephalus appendiculatus*
- Life cycle in tick, passage through all tick stages, transmitted via salivary gland, not via ovary to next tick generation
- Sporozoites from feeding, infected tick injected in saliva into beast after 2–4 days feeding
- Ticks remain infected for about a year

Risk factors
- Level of tick burden
- Clinical cases of the disease; subclinical carriers unusual
- Young animals less susceptible, calves develop immunity without clinical disease
- *Bos indicus* cattle less susceptible
- Ticks more plentiful in open savannah than wooded areas

- Most cases in rainy season when ticks active
- Previous infection confers lifelong immunity provided reinfection continues

Importance
- Heavy death, production losses in naive cattle
- Costs of control very heavy

Clinical findings

Classical ECF – T. parva infection
- Incubation period 1–3 weeks
- Lymph node enlargement local to infecting ticks
- Then fever, anorexia, depression, milk yield decline
- Nasal, ocular discharge
- Dyspnea
- Generalized lymphadenectasia
- Diarrhea, dysentery in some, only in late stages
- Emaciation
- Recumbency
- Terminal frothy nasal discharge
- Death after course of 7–10 days

Complication
- Turning sickness
- Corridor disease – *T. parva lawrencei* as for classical ECF plus keratitis, blepharospasm
- January disease – *T. parva bovis* mild form of classical ECF

Clinical pathology

- Schizonts sometimes seen in circulating lymphocytes
- More obvious in stained biopsy material from lymph node biopsy
- Piroplasms in erythrocytes
- Panleukopenia, thrombocytopenia, little anemia
- Serological tests include:
  - Immunofluorescence
  - Complement fixation
  - Indirect hemagglutination
  - ELISA

Necropsy findings

- Massive pulmonary edema, hyperemia, emphysema
- Hydrothorax, hydropericardium
- Emaciation
- Generalized hemorrhages
- Enlarged lymph nodes, liver, spleen

- Abomasum, intestine ulceration
- Small, lymphoid nodules in liver, kidney, alimentary tract
- Proliferating lymphoblastoid cells, with necrosis in lymphoid organs, lungs, liver, kidneys; resemble multicentric lymphoid tumor
- Schizonts in Giemsa-stained smears from tissues

Diagnosis

Resembles:
- *Theileria annulata* infection
- Trypanosomiasis
- Bovine malignant catarrh

Treatment

- To be effective must be in early stages
- Tetracyclines moderately effective
- Superseded by:
  - Halofuginone lactate, 2 oral doses 1.2 mg/kg body weight, or
  - Parvaquone I/M 2 doses 10 mg/kg 48 hours apart, or
  - Buparvaquone I/M 2 doses 2.5 mg/kg 48 hours apart

Control

- Tick control
- Avoidance of nutritional stress
- Introduction of resistant breeds
- Vaccination by immunotherapy (infection-treatment); *T. parva* sporozoites in ground up ticks injected, infection controlled by long-acting oxytetracycline (20 mg/kg body weight), or parvaquone, given at same time

TURNING SICKNESS [VM8 p. 1209]

Etiology

In southern Africa *Theileria tauratragi*. See also *T. parva lawrencei* infection.

Epidemiology

- Disease of cattle
- Infection of eland antelope, commonly non-pathogenic for cattle

Clinical findings

- Tremor
- Head-pressing

♦ Profuse salivation
♦ Convulsions

Clinical pathology

Parasitized lymphocytes may be in stained blood smears.

Necropsy findings

♦ Thrombosis, infarcts in brain, spinal cord, meninges
♦ Parasitized lymphoblasts in impression smears of brain, spinal cord

Diagnosis

Resembles other diseases characterized by encephalitis.

Treatment and control

As for classical ECF.

MEDITERRANEAN COAST FEVER
(TROPICAL THEILERIOSIS)
[VM8 p. 1210]

Etiology

Theileria annulata (syn. *T. dispar*).

Epidemiology

Occurrence
♦ Cattle; buffalo act as carriers
♦ North-east Africa, central-west Asia, Portugal, China
♦ Infection prevalence in enzootic area 100%; case fatality rate 10–20%, mainly in calves; 40–80% in introducees

Source and transmission
♦ Blood of animal with parasitemia
♦ Recovered animals act as carriers
♦ Transmitted by *Hyalomma* spp. ticks

Risk factors
♦ Highly virulent in British dairy breeds; indigenous zebu breeds resistant
♦ Calves subject to fatal disease
♦ Tends to be seasonal in summer

Importance
Major constraint on livestock improvement in enzootic areas.

Clinical findings

♦ Generally as for East Coast fever
♦ Mucosal pallor, jaundice
♦ Anorexia, fever
♦ Dyspnea
♦ Diarrhea
♦ Weight loss
♦ Rarely small cutaneous nodules containing schizonts
♦ Long course, several weeks

Clinical pathology

♦ Piroplasms in erythrocytes in blood smears, schizonts in lymphocytes
♦ Anemia
♦ Hemoglobinuria
♦ Leukopenia, lymphocytopenia, thrombocytopenia
♦ Indirect fluorescent antibody test used for serological diagnosis

Necropsy findings

As for East Coast fever plus pallor, jaundice of tissues.

Diagnosis

Resembles:
♦ East Coast fever
♦ Oriental theileriosis
♦ Babesiosis
♦ Anaplasmosis
♦ Trypanosomiasis
♦ Bovine malignant catarrh

Treatment

None recorded but buparvaquone (see under East Coast fever) should be effective.

Control

♦ Vaccination as described under East Coast fever
♦ Vaccines prepared by growing schizonts in lymphoid cell culture and attenuated also used

ORIENTAL THEILERIOSIS
[VM8 p. 1206]

Etiology

Theileria orientalis.

Epidemiology

♦ In imported cattle in Far East, Malaysia, New Zealand
♦ British breeds more susceptible than zebu breeds
♦ Transmitted by *Haemaphysalis* spp. ticks

Clinical findings

♦ Severe anemia in heavily parasitized cattle
♦ Most infestations benign

Clinical pathology

Piroplasms in erythrocytes in blood smears.

Diagnosis

♦ Resembles other diseases characterized by anemia

Control

Tick control.

BENIGN THEILERIOSIS
[VM8 p. 1207]

Etiology

T. orientalis, T. mutans, T. velifera, T. sergenti, T. buffeli.

Epidemiology

♦ Individual species located at various locations in Africa, Australia
♦ All transmitted by *Amblyomma* or *Haemaphysalis* spp. ticks

Clinical findings

♦ Generally benign infections but may cause a syndrome of fever, anorexia, anemia; may also undermine premunity against anaplasmosis, babesiosis, heartwater and vaccines against these diseases must be free of these pathogens

Treatment

Concurrent treatment with primaquone, halofuginone clears the infection with *T. buffeli.*

OVINE AND CAPRINE
THEILERIOSIS [VM8 p. 1207]

Etiology

Theileria hirci

Epidemiology

♦ North Africa, Middle East, India
♦ Morbidity rate 20%; case fatality 100%
♦ Transmitted by ticks *Rhipicephalus, Hyalomma* spp.

Clinical findings

♦ Anemia
♦ Jaundice
♦ Lymph node enlargement

Clinical pathology

♦ Piroplasms in blood smears
♦ Indirect fluorescent antibody tests

Diagnosis

Resembles benign theileriosis caused by *T. ovis, T. separata.*

Treatment

Parvaquone, buparvaquone recommended for early cases.

Control

Tick control.

DISEASES CAUSED BY TRYPANOSOMES [VM8 p. 1212]

These include:
♦ Nagana
♦ Surra
♦ Dourine
♦ Chaga's disease of humans, dogs, rarely in pigs; caused by *Trypanosoma cruzi*, transmitted by blood-sucking bugs *Rhodnius, Triatoma* spp. Occurs in the Americas
♦ *T. theileri* trypanosomiasis of cattle transmitted mechanically by many biting flies,

ticks, and transplacentally. In many countries, with very low parasitemia, low virulence, causing disease only in neonates and severely stressed animals
♦ *T. melophagium* trypanosomiasis of sheep transmitted by the ked *Melophagus ovinus*

NAGANA (SAMORE, AFRICAN TRYPANOSOMIASIS, TSETSE FLY DISEASE) [VM8 p. 1212]

Etiology

♦ *Trypanosoma vivax*
♦ *T. congolense*
♦ *T. brucei*
♦ *T. simiae*

Epidemiology

Occurrence
♦ All animal species affected, mostly in cattle
♦ Mixed infections common
♦ All occur in Africa; *T. vivax* also in Central and South America
♦ Infection prevalence very variable; present day rate about 10% in cattle
♦ Morbidity rate in outbreaks up to 70% in cattle with *T. vivax*, 100% in pigs with *T. simiae*
♦ Case fatality rate about 100% with *T. vivax*, *T. simiae*

Source and transmission
♦ From blood of an animal with parasitemia, including domestic animals with acute or chronic disease, wild animal species
♦ Transmission by *Glossina* spp. tsetse fly; *T. vivax* also mechanically by biting flies
♦ Part of life cycle of trypanosome passed in fly
♦ Infection transmitted to next host in fly's saliva
♦ Transmission also mechanically by —
  • Biting flies *Tabanus, Stomoxys, Hippobosca* spp.
  • Needles, surgical equipment
♦ Intra-uterine transmission occasionally

Risk factors
♦ Some cattle and goat breeds trypanotolerant, support limited populations of trypanosomes
♦ Density of the tsetse population
♦ Some trypanosomes, e.g. *T. vivax* maintain higher level of parasitemia, spread more readily
♦ Immunity specific to each strain, species of trypanosome

Importance
♦ Most important disease of livestock in Africa
♦ Wastage due to death, production losses, costs of control
♦ *T. brucei* possibly also infects humans

Clinical findings

♦ No pathognomonic signs or syndromes
♦ Many variations around a central clinical pattern
♦ Initial syndrome may be acute, from which the patient may die acutely or survive as chronic, or chronic from the beginning

Basic disease
♦ Incubation period 8–20 days
♦ Fever, usually intermittent
♦ Dull, anorexic
♦ Ocular discharge
♦ Lose weight
♦ Swollen lymph nodes
♦ Mucosal pallor
♦ Some have belly and throat edema
♦ Rarely diarrhea
♦ Semen quality poor
♦ Emaciation
♦ Dies after 2–4 month course

Peracute disease — *T. vivax* or multiple infection
♦ Mucosal petechiation
♦ Rhinorrhagia
♦ Dysentery
♦ Death after several weeks

Cerebral disease — *T. brucei* in horses, pigs, small ruminants
♦ Circling
♦ Head-pressing
♦ Paralysis

Species-specific syndromes
♦ *T. vivax* causes acute or chronic, severe disease in cattle, sheep goats; anemia marked
♦ *T. congolense* severe, acute or chronic disease with severe anemia in all species
♦ *T. brucei* causes subacute, chronic disease in all species characterized by anasarca, keratoconjunctivitis, cerebral disease in some
♦ *T. simiae* causes peracute, highly fatal disease in pigs

Clinical pathology

Trypanosomes visible in early stages via wet or dry stained smears

Serious variability in trypanosome concentration overcome by concentrating parasites in blood buffy layer

◆ Transmission tests cumbersome, inaccurate

◆ Serological tests to provide evidence of exposure to trypanosomes include:
  • Indirect immunofluorescence
  • Capillary agglutination
  • ELISA

Necropsy findings

◆ Non-specific lesions

◆ Anemia, emaciation, anasarca

◆ Enlargement liver, spleen, lymph nodes

◆ Generalized hemorrhages in severe cases

◆ Commonly evidence of a secondary bacterial infection

◆ Clumps of trypanosomes in blood vessels of acute cases

◆ Hyperplastic lymphoid organs

Diagnosis

Resembles other diseases characterized by septicemia

Treatment

◆ Standard treatments are likely to cause severe adverse reactions

◆ Development of resistance to each drug is common

◆ Recommended drugs include:
  • Diminazene aceturate for *T. vivax, T. congolense*
  • Homidium bromide, homidium chloride for *T. vivax, T. congolense*
  • Isometamidium for *T. vivax, T. congolense*
  • Pyrithidium bromide for *T. vivax, T. congolense*
  • Quinapyramine sulfate for *T. brucei* in horses
  • Suramin for *T. brucei* in horses, camels
  • Antrycide-Suramin for *T. simiae* in pigs

Control

◆ Tsetse fly control by use of insecticides, trapping, liberation of sterilised males

◆ Use of trypanotolerant animals

◆ Prophylactic treatment with suramin, pro-thidium, isometamidium given 4 or 5 times annually

◆ No vaccines available because of frequent variations in antigenicity

SURRA (MAL DE CADERAS, MURRINA) [VM8 p. 1218]

Etiology

Trypanosoma evansi.

Epidemiology

Occurrence

◆ Africa, Middle East, Asia, Central and South America

◆ Horses, camels mainly, buffalo, cattle also

◆ Infection prevalence 20% up to 70% in camels; case fatality rates 100% in camels, horses, much less in cattle, buffalo

Source and transmission

◆ Infected animals with parasitemia; clinical cases, recovered patients, cattle, buffalo

◆ Transmitted by biting flies, e.g. *Tabanus* spp., not tsetses, vampire bats in South America

Risk factors

◆ Wet seasons when flies plentiful

Importance

◆ Deaths, loss of productivity, costs of control make surra an important disease of camels.

Clinical findings

◆ Intermittent fever

◆ Progressive anemia

◆ Dependent edema

◆ Listlessness

◆ Weight loss

◆ Nasal, ocular discharge

◆ Terminal paresis, paralysis, convulsions

◆ Invariably fatal after course of few days up to several months in horses, course of years in camels

◆ Chronic disease includes abortion, poor milk production, work capacity reduced, irregular estrus, in cows, poor semen quality in bulls

Clinical pathology

◆ Parasites in blood films taken during acute phase

◆ In acute phase examination of buffy layer in centrifuged sample necessary

♦ Attempts at transmission with injections of blood into rodents, dogs
  • Serological tests include:
  • Complement fixation
  • Passive hemagglutination
  • Indirect fluorescent antibody
  • ELISA

Necropsy findings

♦ Emaciation
♦ Pallor, icterus in some
♦ Inflammatory changes, lymphoplasmacytic infiltrates in brain, spinal cord
♦ Trypanosomes in body fluids

Diagnosis

Resembles:
♦ *Trypanosoma brucei* infection
♦ Diseases characterized by encephalitis

Treatment

♦ Drugs recommended for nagana may be used but less effective against *T. evansi*, and toxic for horses, camels
♦ For camels quinapyramine sulphate recommended
♦ For horses diminazene aceturate recommended

Control

♦ Vector control impossible
♦ Prophylactic treatment of hosts with quinapyramine prosalt, suramin or isometamidium chloride

DOURINE [VM8 p. 1220]

Etiology

Trypanosoma equiperdum.

Epidemiology

Occurrence
♦ Africa, Asia, south-eastern Europe, South America, USA
♦ Horses, donkeys
♦ Sporadic outbreaks; case fatality rate variable from negligible to 50–75%

Source and transmission
♦ Infected, often clinically normal male or acting as passive carrier between infected mares
♦ Venereal transmission

♦ Trypanosome inhabits urethra, vagin intermittently, so not all matings infectiou
♦ Invasion through intact skin, mucosa

Risk factors
♦ Use of common stallion
♦ International movement of stallions
♦ Many subclinical cases acting as carrier for years

Importance
An uncommon, easily controlled disease.

Clinical findings

Acute venereal disease
Stallions
♦ Incubation period 1–4 weeks up to 3 months
♦ Penis, prepuce, scrotum swelling, edema
♦ Edema spreads anteriorly to chest
♦ Paraphimosis
♦ Inguinal lymph nodes swollen
♦ Moderate mucopurulent urethral dis charge

Mares
♦ Vulva swelling, edema, profuse discharge
♦ Vaginal mucosa hyperemic, ulcers in some
♦ Edema spreads to perineum, udder, belly wall

Second, skin stage
♦ 2–5 cm diameter cutaneous plaques on body, neck for hours to several days, disappear spontaneously but succeeding crops may continue for weeks

Third, nervous disease stage
♦ Anemia
♦ Emaciation
♦ Stiff, stumbling gait
♦ Paresis, paralysis
♦ Hindquarter atrophy
♦ Death or euthanasia after course of several weeks to years of intermittent attacks

Clinical pathology

♦ Trypanosomes in edema fluid, vaginal, urethral washings; in blood during week 2–5 after infection
♦ Serological tests include:
  • Complement fixation
  • Indirect fluorescent antibody
  • Capillary agglutination
  • ELISA

Necropsy findings

♦ Emaciation, subcutaneous edema, anemia
♦ Edema of external genitalia in acute case; depigmented scars, leukodermic patches, on genitalia in chronic stages
♦ Lymph node enlargement
♦ Lymphoblastic infiltration, degeneration of spinal cord, nerve trunks of hind limbs
♦ Trypanosomes in skin, mucosa in acute lesions

Diagnosis

Resembles:
♦ Equine infectious anemia
♦ Coital exanthema

Treatment

♦ Not attempted if eradication pending
♦ Variable results; poor in chronic cases
♦ Drugs used include diminazene, suramin, quinapyramine

Control

♦ Ban on importation from countries where disease occurs
♦ Eradication by identifying infected horses with complement fixation test, slaughter of positive reactors
♦ Strict control of breeding and movement of horses

26 DISEASES CAUSED BY HELMINTH PARASITES

HEPATIC FASCIOLIASIS (LIVER
FLUKE DISEASE) [VM8 p. 1230]

Etiology

Fasciola hepatica.

Epidemiology

Occurrence
♦ Worldwide
♦ Enzootic and as outbreaks in sheep, goats, cattle, occasionally horses
♦ Outbreaks of acute disease last 2–3 weeks; occur mostly in summer-autumn

Life cycle, source and transmission
♦ Flukes mature in donor host's bile ducts
♦ Eggs pass down bile duct to intestine and out with feces
♦ Eggs hatch miracidia which invade intermediate host snails, or eggs eaten by snails, hatch in snail's gut
♦ Miracidia produce cercariae in snail, emerge into pasture
♦ Cercariae encyst on grass, eaten by ruminant
♦ Metacercariae hatch from cyst, invade ruminant tissues, migrate through peritoneum to liver, through liver tissue into bile ducts
♦ Intermediate host – fresh water snails including *Lymnaea truncatula, L. columella, L. tomentosa, L. viridis, Galba bulimoides*

Risk factors
♦ Heavy fluke burden in donor host increases pasture contamination
♦ Number of eggs laid per fluke varies with season of year
♦ Pasture depth, moisture, temperature; warm, moisture needed for hatching, migration of miracidia, heavy snail population, cercariae, survival of cysts
♦ Heavy stocking increases chances of ingestion of cercariae

♦ Flukes stay years in host; many inapparent carriers
♦ Migration of immature flukes through tissue containing quiescent spores of *Clostridium* spp. may stimulate development of infectious necrotic hepatitis, bacillary hemoglobinuria

Clinical findings

Acute hepatic fascioliasis in sheep
♦ Many die without apparent illness
♦ Mostly in young sheep in summer and fall
♦ Dullness, weakness, anorexia
♦ Mucosal, conjunctival pallor, edema
♦ Pain on pressure over liver
♦ Short course, most die; outbreak lasts 2–3 weeks

Subacute hepatic fascioliasis in sheep
♦ Longer course
♦ Mucosal pallor
♦ Submandibular edema in a few
♦ Pain on pressure over liver

Chronic hepatic fascioliasis in cattle and sheep
♦ Weight loss
♦ Submandibular edema
♦ Mucosal pallor
♦ Wool-shedding
♦ Course of weeks up to 3 months in fatal cases
♦ Cattle milk yield declines, chronic diarrhea

Clinical pathology

Acute hepatic fascioliasis
♦ Severe, normochromic anemia, eosinophilia
♦ Severe hypoalbuminemia
♦ Elevated serum liver enzymes (plasma glutamate dehydrogenase, gammaglutamyl transpeptidase, sorbitol dehydrogenase)
♦ No eggs in feces

subacute, chronic hepatic
fascioliasis
  Severe hypochromic, macrocytic anemia
  Severe hypoalbuminemia
  Serum aspartase aminotransferase levels
  elevated
  Large numbers of fluke eggs in feces

Necropsy findings

Acute hepatic fascioliasis
  ◆ Swollen liver
  ◆ Many perforations in, hemorrhages under,
    capsule
  ◆ Tracts of damaged tissue in parenchyma

Chronic hepatic fascioliasis
  ◆ Large flukes in thickened, often calcified in
    cattle, enlarged bile ducts
  ◆ Fibrosed parenchyma
  ◆ Anemia, edema, emaciation

Diagnosis

Liver lesions resemble infestations with:
  ◆ Fascioloides magna; common in wild rumi-
    nants in North America; isolated out-
    breaks in sheep, goats, cattle comingling
    with deer
  ◆ Fasciola gigantica in goats, buffalo in
    Africa, Asia, USA
  ◆ Dicrocoelium dendriticum in North Amer-
    ica, Europe, Asia playing a causative role in
    infectious necrotic hepatitis

Acute hepatic fascioliasis in sheep resembles:
  ◆ Infectious necrotic hepatitis
  ◆ Acute haemonchosis
  ◆ Eperythrozoonosis
  ◆ Anthrax
  ◆ Enterotoxemia

Chronic hepatic fascioliasis resembles:
  ◆ Nutritional deficiencies of copper, cobalt
  ◆ Other internal parasitisms, especially
    ostertagiasis
  ◆ Johne's disease

Treatment

  ◆ Triclabendazole (10 mg/kg body weight in
    sheep, 12 mg/kg in cattle) very effective
    against all stages of fluke in sheep, cattle,
    horses; clorsulon (20 mg/kg) also effective
    against all ages of fluke
  ◆ Rafoxanide, closantel, brotianide all effec-
    tive but not against such young flukes as
    triclabendazole

  ◆ Many other fascioliocides in use; many not
    effective against all ages of fluke
  ◆ Most taint milk and create difficulties in
    sale of milk the day after treatment; fascio-
    licides which do not taint milk include
    oxyclozanide, bromsalans

Control

  ◆ Snail control by use of molluscicides a
    reduced activity now that effective drugs
    available; best procedure is to fence off
    swampy pieces of land
  ◆ Clearing of foliage overhanging water still
    advised
  ◆ Strategic treatments with fasciolicides, at
    times so as to:
    • Remove egg-laying flukes and reduce
      pasture contamination
    • To catch the immature flukes in the liver
      when they are susceptible to the medi-
      cation but before they commence egg
      laying
  ◆ No fixed program will suit all circum-
    stances; program must be tailored to fit
    local conditions in that particular year
  ◆ 4 treatments at 8–11 week intervals per
    year to ewes with triclabendazole very cost
    effective
  ◆ After initial heavy dosing infection rate
    much lower, lighter treatment program
    possible
  ◆ To avoid loss of milk due to tainting dairy
    cows treated at drying off

PARAMPHISTOMIASIS (STOMACH
FLUKE DISEASE) [VM8 p. 1236]

Etiology

  ◆ Paramphistomum cervi, P. microboth-
    rioides, P. licoides, P. ichikawai, P. micro-
    bothrium
  ◆ Calicophoron calicophorum, C. ijimai
  ◆ Cotylophoron cotylophorum
  ◆ Ceylonocotyle streptocoelium

Epidemiology

Occurrence
  ◆ Serious disease in cattle, sheep, goats in
    many countries
  ◆ Case fatality in cattle may be as high as
    96%, in sheep 90%
  ◆ In late summer to early winter when pas-
    ture contamination heaviest; worst after
    flooding
  ◆ All ages but most outbreaks in yearling
    class

Life cycle, source, and transmission

♦ Intermediate host is aquatic planorbid snails
♦ Immature flukes excyst in duodenum, migrate orally to rumen, reticulum; prepatent period, until egg-laying 6 weeks to 4 months

Clinical findings

Acute disease

♦ Persistent, fetid diarrhea
♦ Weakness, depression, dehydration, anorexia
♦ Some show submandibular edema, mucosal pallor
♦ Death after a course of 2–3 weeks

Chronic disease

♦ Weight loss
♦ Anemia
♦ Dry coat
♦ Milk yield reduced

Clinical pathology

♦ Usually no eggs in feces; will be in adults in herd
♦ Search for immature flukes in feces in adults in herd

Necropsy findings

♦ Emaciation, muscle atrophy, anasarca, gelatinous fat depots
♦ Mucosa of upper duodenum thickened, patchy hemorrhages under serosa, bloodstained mucus on mucosa
♦ Large numbers small, immature flukes in duodenum, some buried in mucosa

Diagnosis

Resembles:
♦ Intestinal parasitism
♦ Nutritional deficiency of copper
♦ Hepatic fascioliasis
♦ Johne's disease
♦ Infectious enteritis
♦ Poisoning with arsenic, many poisonous plants

Treatment

♦ Effective treatments against all ages of the flukes include oxyclozanide (2 doses 18.7 mg/kg 3 days apart), niclosamide (160 mg/

kg as 2 doses 3 days apart), resorantel (6 mg/kg)
♦ remove calves from infested pasture

Control

♦ On problem farms annual dosing with on of the above fasciolicides to remove adu flukes before they contaminate pasture
♦ Snail control

TAPEWORM INFESTATION
[VM8 p. 1237]

Etiology

Ruminants

♦ Moniezia benedini, M. expansa
♦ Helictometra giardi
♦ Avitellina spp.
♦ Stilesia hepatica
♦ Thyanosoma actinioides

Horses

♦ Anoplocephala magna, A. perfoliata
♦ Paranoplocephala mamillana

Epidemiology

♦ Widely distributed
♦ Only heavy infestations in young patients cause illness

Life cycle

♦ Eggs containing live embryos passed in feces
♦ Embryos eaten by intermediate host mostly oribatid mites
♦ Infection of primary host when it eats the intermediate

Clinical findings

Ruminants

♦ Heavy infestations may cause:
♦ Unthriftiness, poor coat
♦ Mild constipation or diarrhea with dysentery
♦ Anemia
♦ Stunting
♦ Pot-bellied

Horses

♦ Mild, intermittent colic
♦ Diarrhea or feces covered with bloody mucus
♦ Rarely fatal cecal rupture

Clinical pathology

- Tapeworm segments visible in feces
- Eggs singly or in capsules on flotation

Necropsy findings

- May be ulcer at attachment site in small intestine
- Thickening bile, pancreatic duct in *Thyanosoma*, *Stilesia* spp. infestations

Diagnosis

Resembles:
- Heavy nematode infestations
- Malnutrition

Treatment

Ruminants
- Niclosamide (100 mg/kg)
- Cambendazole (20 mg/kg)
- Oxfendazole, fenbendazole, albendazole (5 mg/kg)

Horses
- Niclosamide 200 mg/kg
- Pyrantel pamoate 13.2 mg/kg

Control

In enzootic area periodic dosing with a taeniacide (above), particularly in summer–fall, may benefit lamb growth

ASCARIASIS [VM8 p. 1239]

Etiology

Pigs – *Ascaris suum*
Horses – *Parascaris equorum*
Cattle and buffalo – *Toxocara vitulorum*
Sheep – rarely infected with *Ascaris lumbricoides*, the ascarid of humans

Epidemiology

Occurrence
- Worldwide
- Ascariasis limited to:
  - Pig and horse farms with dense populations
  - On same pasture year after year
  - Pigs fed on floor in pens that are never cleaned out

Life cycle – all ascarids except *T. vitulorum*

- Adults in small intestine lay very large numbers of eggs
- Passed in feces; capable of surviving up to 5 years in cool, moist surroundings
- In high humidity eggs hatch through several larval stages to become infective
- Ingested by host, hatch, pass through intestinal wall, reach liver via portal vein
- Invade blood vessels, pass to lungs
- Up trachea, swallowed, final attachment to intestine wall
- Period between infestation and commencement of worms laying eggs (prepatent period) varies (8–9 weeks for *A. suum*, 14–15 weeks for *P. equorum*). Foals can be passing eggs at 12–13 weeks old
- *T. vitulorum* larvae acquired by calf in colostrum on days 2–5 days after calving; eggs passed by calf at 3 weeks old

Clinical findings

Disease only in young.

Pigs – up to 5 months
- Poor growth
- Enzootic pneumonia, swine influenza attacks more serious
- May be cough in a few
- Dyspnea rarely
- Adult worms vomited
- Rarely obstructive jaundice with worms in bile duct
- Rarely intestine obstruction, rupture

Foals, calves
- Poor growth
- Poor coat
- Diarrhea
- Steatorrhea, anemia in calves
- Occasional colic, intestinal obstruction, perforation, convulsions in foals

A. suum infestations in atypical species
- Anorexia, fever
- Dyspnea, cough about day 8 after infection

Clinical pathology

- Massive egg numbers in clinical patients
- Eosinophilia in early stages

Necropsy findings

- Large liver, hemorrhages under capsule
- Subpleural hemorrhages, lung edema

- Blood-stained pleural fluid
- White spots, fibrosis in liver in chronic cases
- Large numbers mature worms in intestine
- *A. suum* in aberrant hosts causes lung emphysema and hemorrhages, alveolar wall thickening with fibrin

Diagnosis

In pigs resembles:
- Enzootic pneumonia
- Enteritis due to *Salmonella, Treponema*spp.

In foals resembles pneumonia caused by *Rhodoccocus* spp.

In calves resembles enteritis due to other causes

Treatment

- Ivermectin 0.3 mg/kg in pigs; 0.2 mg/kg in calves, orally to foals
- Pyrantel tartrate, levamisole and others effective also

Control

- Aimed at keeping young animals away from heavily contaminated environment; concrete pig housing, kept clean, bedding removed monthly in warm season, achieves this
- Sows treated before going into thoroughly cleaned farrowing pen, or pre-farrowing plus piglet treatment at 3–4 weeks old, followed by periodic treatment until adult or sold
- Foals a problem because mares infect them, pasture usually contaminated from previous year; clean foaling pen, exercise pens kept clean of manure, rested periodically, treat foals at 10–12 weeks old, repeat bimonthly

STRONGYLOSIS OF HORSES
(REDWORM INFESTATION)
[VM8 p. 1241]

Etiology

- Large strongyles – *Strongylus vulgaris, S. edentatus, S. equinus, Triodontophorus* spp.
- Small strongyles – *Cylicostephanus* spp., *Cylicocyclus* spp., *Cyathostomum* spp.
- Other much less common species

Epidemiology

Occurrence
- Worldwide
- Horses
- Small burdens in adult horses are source of infection for young; mares infect foals

Life cycle
- Direct; eggs in feces produce larvae in 7 days in suitable climatic conditions
- Large strongyle larvae have a migratory cycle, *S. vulgaris* migrates via small arteries to cranial mesenteric artery, thence back to large intestine wall and into lumen, with a prepatent period of 6 months; *S. edentatus* migrates via portal vessels to liver, to hemorrhagic retroperitoneal nodules and large bowel wall to be discharged into the large intestine with a prepatent period of 10 months
- Small strongyle larvae enter wall of cecum, colon; stay in subserous nodules, commence egg-laying after average 12–18 weeks; may accumulate in gut wall in hypobiotic state; synchronous emergence in winter causes severe diarrhea

Risk factors
- Survival of eggs and larvae favored by moisture, warmth, shade; desiccation destroys; larvae overwinter in Europe
- Optimum chances for infection in morning dew or after rain
- Seasonal infection peak in late summer and fall
- Continual reinfestation by increasingly burdened young horses

Importance
Wastage due to death losses, failure of young horses to grow, poor racing performance; heavy costs of treatment and control.

Clinical findings

Classical syndrome
- Poor coat
- Exercise intolerance
- Anorexia, depression, dullness, weight loss
- Emaciation, recumbency in severe cases
- Anemia, mucosal pallor in some
- Intermittent hypermotility spasmodic colic
- Thromboembolic colic
- Diarrhea or constipation

Winter cyathostomosis
♦ Caused by simultaneous maturation of large numbers of hypobiotic small strongyle larvae in stress conditions of cold, feed shortage
♦ Profuse diarrhea in adults, especially pregnant mares
♦ Rapid emaciation

Secondary diseases
♦ Migratory life cycle of large strongyles causes:
♦ Colic due to hypermotility (spasmodic colic)
♦ Intussusception, volvulus due to disordered motility
♦ Thromboembolic colic
♦ Myocardial lesion causing cardiac arrhythmia, poor racing performance
♦ Focal lesion in brain, spinal cord causing cerebrospinal nematodiasis
♦ Aortic, iliac thrombosis causing ischemia, lameness

Clinical pathology

♦ Fecal egg count to determine severity of infection, subject to variability due to immune status, worm species, relation to treatment, stage of life cycle
♦ Larval culture to determine identity of worms; commonly mixed infections
♦ Erythrocyte count, hemoglobin percentage, packed cell volume estimates of anemia status may be indicator of severity of infestation

Necropsy findings

♦ One or more of the following lesions
♦ Large numbers of adult strongyles in cecum, colon
♦ Catarrhal, hemorrhagic or fibrinous inflammation of cecum, ventral colon; excessive mucus, numerous punctate hemorrhages
♦ Many *Triodontophorus tenuicollis* larvae, small circular hemorrhages, deep mucosal ulcers in right dorsal colon
♦ Multiple subserous larvae including —
  • Nodules in intestinal wall
  • Arteritis at root of cranial mesenteric artery; may contain lamellated thrombus, cause artery occlusion with gangrene of local intestine wall
  • Arteritis at root of aorta, may rupture
♦ Focal ischemic lesions in myocardium associated with aortic arteritis

Diagnosis

Resembles other causes of poor growth in foals and yearlings:
♦ Ascariasis
♦ Mare agalactia
♦ Nutritional deficiency

Anemia in horses may also be caused by:
♦ Babesiosis
♦ Equine infectious anemia

  Equine colic has many causes (Table 5.3). Diarrhea in horses commonly caused by:
♦ Salmonellosis
♦ Colitis-X
♦ Monocytic ehrlichiosis (Potomac horse fever)
♦ Sand colic
♦ Idiopathic diarrhea

Treatment

♦ Ivermectin (0.2 mg/kg as paste) effective against all stages, all strongyle species; moxidectin has similar early reputation
♦ Phenothiazine, piperazine mixture has wide spectrum
♦ Mebendazole, cambendazole, fenbendazole, many other benzimidazoles also highly effective; often combined with piperazine because of increasing resistance of small strongyles to benzimidazoles
♦ Cases of verminous arteritis, hypobiotic larvae can be cleared with ivermectin, but structural lesions unaffected
♦ Rapid response in horses usually encouraged by treatment for anemia

Control

♦ Not possible by pasture management alone
♦ Use of anthelmintics obligatory
♦ Problem is foals run at pasture with dams who can carry heavy worm burdens without sign of illness
♦ Also heavy burdens in young horses cause massive pasture contamination
♦ Larvae are long-lived on pasture

Program on breeding farms
♦ Mechanical feces collection from pasture twice weekly
♦ Phenothiazine (1–2 g daily) in feed every second month or
♦ Periodic (variable but 6–8 weeks theoretical optimum, usually 6–8 treatments per year; down to 4 per year where ivermectin used) treatment of all horses with recommended anthelmintic (see treatment above)

♦ Mares 2 months before foaling, at foaling, then periodic
♦ Foals commence treatment at 10 weeks
♦ Periodic treatments at shorter intervals in spring and summer
♦ Introduced horses isolated, treated
♦ Periodic egg counts to check worm load; occasional check on resistance to benzimidazoles

LUNGWORM INFESTATION IN CATTLE (VERMINOUS PNEUMONIA, VERMINOUS BRONCHITIS) [VM8 p. 1246]

Etiology

Dictyocaulus viviparus.

Epidemiology

Occurrence
♦ Widespread, temperate, cold climates, especially UK, western Europe
♦ Mostly in calves about 6 months old at pasture contaminated by previous grazing by infected animals
♦ Seasonal in fall
♦ Likely to be enzootic on individual farms

Life cycle
♦ Mature worms in bronchi, eggs coughed up, swallowed, hatch, larvae passed in feces
♦ Moisture, warmth promote larval maturation to infective stage, minimum time 3–7 days, but may survive for 12 months
♦ Ingested infective larvae migrate through intestine wall, to mesenteric lymph node, then lymphatic vessels to veins, through heart to lungs
♦ 3–6 weeks after infection worms commence laying eggs into alveoli

Risk factors
♦ Larval survival on pasture reduced by dryness, heat, severe cold
♦ Hypobiosis in some animals with larvae persisting in latent form over winter, commencing egg-laying in spring
♦ Heavily contaminated pasture in spring may cause massive invasion, acute disease within 2 weeks
♦ Set stocking on same pasture permits recycling of infection with multiplication of worm burden, development of chronic disease in 2–4 months
♦ *Pilobolus* spp. fungus, a common inhabitant of dung pats spreads larvae by explosive opening of sporangium; increases infection rate of calves
♦ Immunity causes discharge of adult worms, but short-lived, reinfection common; repeated infection maintains immune status

Clinical findings

Acute disease
♦ Usually a high proportion of group affected at one time
♦ History of moving to new pasture 7–12 days previously
♦ Bout of diarrhea, usually unnoticed
♦ Sudden onset rapid, shallow, abdominal breathing
♦ Frequent cough
♦ Nasal discharge
♦ Fever
♦ Tachycardia
♦ Loud breath sounds, crackles over all parts of lungs
♦ Patient bright, active, attempts to eat
♦ By 24 hours severe, grunting dyspnea, mouth breathing, head extended
♦ Cyanosis
♦ Death in most (case fatality rate 75%) in 2–14 days

Subacute disease
♦ The commoner syndrome
♦ Frequent coughing paroxysms
♦ Moderate dyspnea
♦ Loud crackling breath sounds, especially dorsal
♦ Severe weight loss
♦ Course of 3–4 weeks
♦ Secondary bacterial pneumonia accompanied by fever, toxemia, anorexia
♦ Some deaths, many survive with respiratory insufficiency, poor growth
♦ Complication is sudden dyspnea, death during week 7–8 due to proliferative, probably allergic, pneumonia

Clinical pathology

♦ Larvae in feces the critical feature
♦ Appear 12 days after clinical signs commence; 24 days after infection
♦ Few at first, building to 500–1500/g by week 4
♦ Eosinophilia common from first day of illness, peaks at 3 weeks in chronic cases
♦ Complement-fixing antibodies detectable at day 35 after infection, peak at day 75
♦ ELISA positive after week 5
♦ Pasture clippings examined for larvae; counts of 3 larvae per 500 g indicate a

lethal level of infection; greater than 3/500 g indicate acute syndrome; count very variable with environmental conditions

Necropsy findings

Acute cases
- Enlarged lung, edema, emphysema, widespread dark pink collapsed areas
- Hemorrhagic bronchitis
- Fluid filled bronchi
- Regional lymph nodes enlarged

Subacute cases
- Total adult worm counts in bronchi exceed 3000; may be 200 000
- Gross interstitial emphysema
- Consolidated areas in all lobes, especially diaphragmatic
- Froth in bronchi
- Enlarged lymph nodes
- If self-cure has occurred, no adults, only larvae

Diagnosis

Resembles:
- Bacterial bronchopneumonia
- Interstitial pneumonia
- Acute pulmonary edema, emphysema
- *Heavy Ascaris suum infection*
- Viral pneumonia

Treatment

- Ivermectin 0.2 mg/kg I/M gives residual protection up to 28 days
- Benzimidazoles effective against all stages also
- Dramatic effect in early stages but no effect on lung damage; some deaths in severe case
- In acute cases treat with combination of anthelmintic, antihistamine, antibacterial

Control

- Reduce larval contamination of pasture; a few cause immunity
  - Separate grazing for young, adults
  - Avoid lush, swampy grazing for young
  - No comingling with deer
  - Control gastrointestinal parasites
  - Treat yearling cattle on turning out of barn
  - Turn barn manure several times before spreading on pasture
- Calves at pasture in enzootic area treated periodically or vaccinated
- **Periodic treatment** – ivermectin at 3, 8, 13

weeks after turning out; benzimidazoles every 3 weeks or in pulse-release bolus
- **Oral vaccination** with attenuated, e.g. irradiated, larvae, 2 doses in housed calves at 8 weeks, 12 weeks old, confined indoors for further 2 weeks; calves at pasture can be vaccinated at 3 weeks old
- Prevents clinical disease but calves can be carriers of infection
- Housing calves to protect against lungworm presents serious risk of enzootic calf pneumonia; best results from running at pasture

LUNGWORM INFESTATION IN
SHEEP AND GOATS [VM8 p. 1251]

Etiology

- *Dictyocaulus filaria*
- *Muellerius capillaris*
- *Protostrongylus rufescens*
- *Cystocaulus ocreatus, Neostrongylus linearis* doubtful pathogenicity

Epidemiology

Occurrence
- All countries
- All ages, 4–6 month lambs worst affected
- Moderate disease only in lambs, highly pathogenic in kids

Life cycle
- *D. filaria* direct, larvae long-lived, can overwinter
- Last year's lambs the main source of infection
- *M. capillaris* indirect. intermediate host snails, slugs
- *P. rufescens* indirect with land snail the intermediate host

Risk factors
- Warm, wet summers but acute cases due to massive infestations do not occur
- Immunity strong after exposure

Clinical findings

- Chronic cough, no dyspnea
- Weight loss
- Secondary bacterial bronchopneumonia, toxemia in some

Clinical pathology

First stage larvae in feces.

Necropsy findings

♦ D. filaria, P. rufescens adult worms in bronchi cause blockage, lung consolidation but lesions not extensive
♦ M. capillaris adults in sheep are in small fibrous, often calcified nodules under pleura; in goats lesions diffuse interstitial pneumonia
♦ Bronchiolar exudate, scattered patches of consolidation

Diagnosis

Resembles:
♦ Viral pneumonia
♦ Bacterial pneumonia
♦ Maedi-visna
♦ Jaagsiekte

Treatment

♦ Ivermectin 0.2 mg/kg
♦ Benzimidazoles effective also

Control

♦ Lungworms with direct life cycle susceptible to control program for D. viviparus
♦ Worms with indirect cycle can be limited in occurrence by avoidance of intermediate snail hosts

LUNG INFESTATION IN OTHER SPECIES

Lungworm infestation in pigs [VM8 p. 1252]

Etiology Metastrongylus apri, M. salmi, M. pudendodectus.
Epidemiology Commonest in 4–6 months pigs.
Life cycle Indirect, earthworm intermediate host.

Clinical findings:
♦ Bouts of harsh coughing
♦ Weight loss
Clinical pathology Larvae in feces.

Necropsy findings:
♦ Small areas of lung consolidation
♦ Bronchitis, emphysema, peribronchial lymphoid hyperplasia bronchiolar muscle hypertrophy
Diagnosis Resembles other causes of pneumonia.

Treatment Ivermectin and benzimidazole effective.
Control Avoidance of contact with earth worms.

Lungworm infestation of horses [VM8 p. 1252]

Etiology Dictyocaulus arnfieldi.

Epidemiology:
♦ Common in donkeys, rare in horses
♦ Clinical illness uncommon; rare cases in foals
♦ Direct lifecycle
Clinical findings Illness rare in field cases; experimental disease causes cough, hyperpnea, forced expiration for several months.
Clinical pathology Larvae in feces; not in horses because worms do not mature.
Necropsy findings Bronchi blocked with worms, mucus.
Diagnosis Resembles equine influenza.
Treatment Ivermectin 0.2 mg/kg; benzimidazoles also effective.
Control Program for control of D. viviparus would apply if control thought necessary.

ESOPHAGOSTOMIASIS (NODULE WORM DISEASE, PIMPLY GUT) [VM8 p. 1253]

Etiology

♦ Species-specific infections but some cross-infection
♦ Sheep and goats – Oesophagostomum columbianum, Oe. venulosum, Oe. asperum
♦ Cattle – Oe. radiatum, Oe. venulosum
♦ Pigs – Oe. dentatum, Oe. quadrispinulatum, Oe. brevicaudum

Epidemiology

Occurrence
♦ Commonest in subtropical, temperate climates with summer rainfall
♦ Chronic disease occurs in winter after infection the previous summer

Life cycle
♦ Direct, larvae susceptible to cold, dryness
♦ Infection by ingestion of larvae
♦ Invasion of small intestine wall, followed by re-emergence, invasion large intestine wall, C. columbianum commence egg-laying 6 weeks after infection
♦ Many larvae undergo hypobiotic stage

with longer prepatent period, nodule development
- Larvae leave nodule during periods of stress

Clinical findings

Sheep
- Persistent diarrhea, or intermittent semi-soft droppings, much mucus, occasionally blood
- Rapid weight loss
- Hollow back
- Stiff gait
- Tail elevated
- Intestinal nodules may be palpated rectally
- Rarely outbreaks of intussusception

Calves
- Anorexia, emaciation
- Diarrhea, dark, fetid, continuous
- Anemia in some

Pigs
- Rare primary cause of death in pigs
- Diarrhea
- Weight loss

Clinical pathology

Egg count may be low in early or in heavy, hypobiotic infections; heavy in active stages of disease; few in chronic stage.

Necropsy findings

- Acute cases – mild catarrhal enteritis, larvae in intestine scrapings
- Chronic cases – adult worms in thick mucus overlays catarrhal enteritis
- When nodules present are at all levels of intestine; up to 6 mm dia., contain yellow—green—brown, pasty or crumbly, partly calcified pus; local wall thickening, peritonitis
- 200 adult female worms regarded as heavy infestation

Diagnosis

In sheep resembles:
- Trichostrongylosis
- Malnutrition

In pigs resembles thin sow syndrome

Treatment

Sheep and cattle
- Ivermectin e.g. as pour-on at 0.5 mg/kg
- Benzimidazoles relatively inefficient against immature forms; can be used as controlled release capsules

Pigs
- Fenbendazole, flubendazole, pyrantel tartrate effective in feed or as single treatment

Control

Sheep
- Strategic dosing pastured sheep early spring, summer, late fall
- Removal to clean pasture after dosing
- Housed sheep single treatment each year 1–2 months before lambing

Pigs
- Housed pigs affected
- Treat all pigs before turning out to pasture in very cold climates
- In temperate climates pigs treated twice in fall
- Periparturient rise in infectivity at parturition means special care for piglets to be treated at 5–6 weeks, repeated 30 days later

STEPHANURIASIS (KIDNEY WORM DISEASE) [VM8 p. 1255]

Etiology

Stephanurus dentatus.

Epidemiology

Occurrence
- In mild climates permitting survival eggs, larvae
- Pigs only
- Low case fatality rate

Life cycle
- Direct by ingestion of feed contaminated by larvae, *or*
- Penetration of skin
- Larvae derived from eggs voided in urine
- Adult females lodged in cysts opening into renal pelvis
- Migration to kidney from intestine is via liver
- Egg-laying may commence 6 months, up to several years, after infection

♦ Migrating larvae may be misdirected, cause lesions in aberrant sites, eg. fetus

Clinical findings

♦ Poor growth, emaciation
♦ Ascites in some
♦ Stiffness, lameness hind limbs
♦ Paresis, paralysis in a few
♦ In early cases may be cutaneous, lymph node nodules

Clinical pathology

♦ Eggs in urine
♦ Eosinophilia, no anemia
♦ ELISA test available but necropsy diagnosis preferred

Necropsy findings

♦ Young pigs with heavy infestations may have no visible adult worms or lesions
♦ Fibrosis, perirenal abscesses
♦ Adult worms in perirenal tissue, renal pelvis
♦ Infarcts, scars in kidney
♦ White tracks, fibrosis, hemorrhage, abscess in liver parenchyma
♦ Worm larvae in nodules in many organs
♦ Peritoneal, pleural adhesions

Diagnosis

Poor condition syndrome resembles:
♦ Ascariasis
♦ Hyostrongylosis
♦ Necrotic enteritis
♦ Chronic swine dysentery

Posterior weakness syndrome resembles:
♦ Nutritional deficiency of vitamin A
♦ Osteodystrophia
♦ Brucellosis
♦ Spinal cord abscess
♦ Lumbar vertebral fracture

Treatment

♦ Ivermectin 0.3 mg/kg S/C
♦ Benzimidazoles effective against all stages

Control

♦ Repeated treatment with ivermectin at 4 month intervals can eradicate worm
♦ Randomly infected earthworms may perpetuate the infection
♦ Management programs devised when effective treatments unavailable also effective but costly in labor, capital investment

BUNOSTOMIASIS (HOOKWORM DISEASE) [VM8 p. 1257]

Etiology

Cattle
♦ *Bunostomum phlebotomum* the common one
♦ *Agriostomum vryburgi* in South America Asia

Sheep
♦ *Bunostomum trigonocephalum*
♦ *Gaigeria pachyscelis*
Pigs   An unimportant infection.

Epidemiology

Occurrence
♦ Serious disease only in tropics
♦ Only in cattle, sheep

Life cycle
♦ Direct, eggs in feces, larvae in 7 days
♦ Free-living larvae susceptible to desiccation
♦ Infective larvae enter host through intact skin; *B. phlebotomum* also via mouth to intestine
♦ To lungs via blood stream
♦ Up air passages to pharynx, swallowed, to intestine
♦ Prepatent period until egg-laying commences at 7–10 weeks

Risk factors
♦ Only young calves 4–12 months old
♦ Infestation greatest in winter months
♦ Percutaneous infection favored by wet conditions, e.g. housing without adequate bedding

Clinical findings

♦ Fidgeting, stamping, licking feet
♦ Mild abdominal pain
♦ Bouts of diarrhea
♦ Weight loss
♦ Mucosal pallor
♦ Submandibular, belly wall edema
♦ Staggery gait
♦ Recumbency
♦ Death after 2–3 day course
♦ Prolonged convalescence in survivors

Clinical pathology

♦ Heavy egg counts in feces; may not be evident in acute stages of heavy infestation
♦ Occult blood in feces
♦ Erythrocyte count, hemoglobin concentration, packed cell volume low

Necropsy findings

♦ Only small numbers of worms needed; 100 cause clinical illness, 500 often fatal; in first few feet of small intestine
♦ Intestinal contents blood stained

Diagnosis

Resembles:
♦ Haemonchosis
♦ Hepatic fascioliasis
♦ Eperythrozoonosis
♦ Nutritional deficiency of copper, cobalt
♦ Chronic molybdenosis

Treatment

♦ Ivermectin, benzimidazoles effective
♦ Convalescence shortened by dietary supplements iron, copper, cobalt, high quality protein

Control

♦ Avoid wet conditions
♦ Ample bedding, clean pens for housed animals
♦ Periodic treatment with active anthelmintics

TRICHOSTRONGYLIASIS,
OSTERTAGIASIS, COOPERIASIS,
NEMATODIRIASIS (SCOUR WORMS,
HAIR WORMS) [VM8 p. 1259]

Etiology

♦ The common infections and their anatomical preferences in the gut included in Table 26.1
♦ *Trichostrongylus axei* occurs in horse stomach

Epidemiology

Occurrence
♦ Worldwide; prevalence varies in different climates
♦ Sheep, goats, cattle, horses
♦ Infection morbidity very high; case fatality rate low, slow, few deaths each day over extended period

Life cycle
♦ Direct; eggs in feces, hatch on pasture in most; infective larvae ingested, populate abomasum and intestine
♦ Larvae migrate into intestine wall, re-emerge to commence egg-laying
♦ Larvae may be retained in wall in hypobiotic state for long periods
♦ Prepatent period 2–3 weeks, longer in *Nematodirus* spp.; much longer in hypobiotic larvae

Risk factors
♦ Most infections are of mixed species
♦ Particular species dominate in particular environments
♦ *Ostertagia* spp. dominant in winter rainfall areas, disease worst in winter
♦ *Haemonchus* spp. dominate in summer rainfall zone, disease worst in spring/summer
♦ Host specificity relative to cattle versus sheep
♦ Young animals most susceptible, lambs, yearling cattle
♦ Nutritionally stressed animals susceptible
♦ Wet weather favors prevalence
♦ Eggs, larvae resistant to cold but not to hot, dry conditions
♦ Larvae need wetness to migrate up grass, emerge from dung pat
♦ Infection leads to immunity; number of resident worms, number of eggs laid per worm, diminishes
♦ Immunity low compared to that of *Dictyocaulus viviparus*, overcome by nutritional stress
♦ Periparturient rise (increased egg production lambing to peak at 6–8 weeks)
♦ *Nematodirus* spp. infestation carried over winter in young lambs rather than on pasture
♦ Capacity for hypobiosis varies; pronounced in *Ostertagia* spp; negligible in *Trichostrongylus* spp.

Clinical findings

Lambs
♦ Insidious onset in lambs, yearlings
♦ Weight loss, growth retardation
♦ Anorexia
♦ Dark green, almost black, soft feces, foul breech,
♦ Few deaths each day

Calves
♦ Intake reduced but keep eating
♦ Weight loss

Table 26.1 Anatomical distribution of trichostrongylid worms in ruminants [VM8 p. 1259]

	Cattle		Sheep and goats	
Parasite	Abomasum	Small intestine	Abomasum	Small intestine
Trichostrongylus spp.				
T. axei	×		×	
T. colubriformis, T. longispicularis		×		×
T. falculatus, T. vitrinus, T. capricola, T. rugatus,				
T. probolurus				×
Ostertagia spp.				
O. ostertagi	×			
O. circumcincta			×	
O. trifurcata			×	
Cooperia spp.				
C. punctata, C. oncophora		×		×
C. pectinata		×		
C. curticei				×
Nematodirus spp.				
N. spathiger, N. battus, N. filicollis, N. abnormalis		×		×
N. helvetianus		×		

Trichostrongylus axei occurs in the stomach of horses.

● Soft feces, becoming thin, dark green to yellow,
● Dehydration
● Persistent diarrhea
● Treatment with anthelmintic often ineffective
● Long dry hair coat
● Tachycardia, mild fever
● Mucosa pale but no anemia
● Submandibular edema in some
● Emaciation, recumbency
● Occurs also in 2–3 year olds

Clinical pathology

● Fecal egg count best indicator of presence of disease but worm egg count not a good indicator of severity of the disease
● Larval culture of feces to identify worm species
● Plasma pepsinogen levels elevated

Necropsy findings

● Adult worms in abomasum, intestine (see Table 26.1)
● Surest diagnosis a total worm count at necropsy, including peptic digest of mucosa
● Counts >100 000 in heavy, counts >500 000 encountered
● Emaciation, dehydration, evidence of scouring
● Mucosa of abomasum, upper small intestine may be hyperemic, swollen with fibrinocatarrhal gastritis
● In chronic cases morocco leather appearance of mucosa due to hyperplastic gastritis

Diagnosis

Resembles:
● Secondary nutritional copper deficiency
● Coccidiosis
● Johne's disease
● Chronic fascioliasis

Treatment

● Ivermectin, moxidectin
● Benzimidazoles; multiple resistance to these drugs and levamisole in many areas, only ivermectin, moxidectin effective there
● Choice of drugs may depend on efficiency against lungworms, fluke and arthropods; cost, and availability as an injection are also major criteria
● Efficiency against hypobiotic larvae an essential criterion in choice of anthelmintic to use against *Ostertagia* spp. Fenbendazole, oxfendazole, albendazole, febantel, ivermectin, moxidectin effective
● Treated animals must be moved to clean paddock if value to be obtained from the medication

Control

● Overall plans not very much use because of variability in epidemiology in different areas
● Objectives are:
  • Cost-effectiveness
  • Avoidance of resistance to anthelmintic
  • Optimum growth, production rates
  • Reduction of pasture contamination
● Use locally recommended dosing strategy monitored by periodic:
  • Fecal egg counts
  • Total worm counts
  • Consultation of suitable computer simulation model
● Strategy should include:
  • Dosing of valuable animals whenever they are mustered for other reasons
  • Dosing during hot, dry periods damaging to larval survival to maximise larval kill
  • In-housed animals regular treatments after turning out to pasture
  • Counter periparturient rise by dosing ewes before and after lambing
  • Alternative grazing of paddocks with sheep, cattle if available
  • Move dosed animals to clean pasture or ensure use of drug effective against hypobiotic larvae

HEMONCHOSIS (BARBER'S POLE WORM) [VM8 p. 1265]

Etiology

● Cattle – *Haemonchus placei, H. contortus, Mecistocirrus digitatus*
● Sheep and goats – *Haemonchus contortus, H. placei, Mecistocirrus digitatus*
● Buffalo – *Mecistocirrus digitatus*

Epidemiology

Occurrence
● Worldwide
● Most severe disease in temperate, tropical climates with good summer rainfall
● Uncommon in semi-arid regions
● Can occur in humid summers in cold countries
● *H. contortus* the principal infection in sheep, *H. placei* in cattle; other infections

cause less severe disease, occur mostly when the two animal species comingle
- Outbreaks during massive infestations due to optimum climate and pasture conditions *or* in sheep with heavy worm burden stressed by feed shortage, possibly in winter
- Infections build up in spring, summer with most outbreaks in late summer and autumn

Life cycle
- Direct life cycle
- Infection by ingestion of infective larvae from pasture contaminated with eggs by donor
- Eggs hatch well, larvae migrate extensively in warm, moist conditions, warm nights
- Hypobiotic larvae may carry infection over winter

Risk factors
- Overcrowding
- Lush pasture
- Hot, humid climate
- Clinical disease precipitated by fall in nutrition
- Strong immunity develops causing self-cure by worm expulsion of *H. contortus* infections in sheep; partial, similar response in calves infected with *H. placei*

Importance
- Acute disease causes heavy death losses
- Subacute, chronic wasting disease cause poor production, growth

Clinical findings

- Lambs, young sheep
- Many found dead without prior signs
- Pale mucosae, conjunctivae
- Submandibular, belly wall edema
- Poor exercise tolerance
- Staggery gait
- Recumbency
- Hyperpnea
- Constipation
- Anorexia
- Death after course of few days
- Survivors, especially adults show:
  - Severe weight loss
  - Break in wool, fleece shed later
  - Lethargy
  - Long convalescence

Clinical pathology

- High fecal egg count (>5000 eggs/g in sheep, 500 eggs/g in cattle) but count may be low in fatal cases if all infecting worms are larvae

- Fecal larval culture to identify *Haemonchus* spp.
- Often part of mixed infections

Necropsy findings

- Severe anemia, pallor of tissues, thin blood
- Large numbers of worms in abomasum
- Abomasal wall hyperemic, with hemorrhages in mucosa
- Small ulcers at attachment points for worms

Diagnosis

Resembles other causes of sudden death:
- Anthrax
- Enterotoxemia

Other causes of anemia include:
- Coccidiosis
- Acute hepatic fascioliasis
- Eperythrozoonosis
- Snakebite

Treatment

- Ivermectin; in the case of resistance to it use moxidectin, nemadectin
- Benzimidazoles but resistance common
- For specific effect against *Haemonchus* spp. an organophosphate or fasciolicide, e.g. closantel, disophenol adequate

Control

- Based on strategic drenching to minimise pasture contamination
- Sheep – drench at end of winter; in mild climates repeat doses during spring, summer, intervals determined by degree of risk
- Mix treatments with ivermectin, closantel to avoid resistance
- Pre-lambing drench of ewes
- Drench lambs at 3 months, repeat at further 3 months
- Drenching at 2–4 week intervals in high risk seasons

PARASITIC GASTRITIS OF PIGS
[VM8 p. 1268]

Etiology

- *Hyostrongylus rubidus*
- *Ollulanus tricuspis*
- *Ascarops strongylina, A. dentata*
- *Physocephalus sexalatus*
- *Simondsia paradoxa*

Epidemiology

Occurrence

Infection common, clinical illness uncommon, reduced production rare.

Life cycle

♦ *H. rubidus*, direct life cycle
♦ *Ascarops, Physocephalus* spp. have indirect cycles with dung beetles intermediate hosts

Clinical findings

Young pigs

♦ Poor weight gain
♦ Diarrhea
♦ Anorexia
♦ Excessive water intake

Sows

♦ Emaciation
♦ Pallor
♦ Pica
♦ Poor reproductive efficiency
♦ Sporadic sudden deaths due to gastric ulcer hemorrhage or peritonitis from ulcer rupture
♦ *H. rubidus* may play a role in **thin sow syndrome**

Clinical pathology

Fecal egg counts >500 eggs/g positive but egg-laying very erratic.

Necropsy findings

♦ High total worm count, usually several thousand worms
♦ Gastric mucosal hyperemic, thickened, edematous, excessive gastric mucus, diphtheritic pseudomembranes, ulcers in some

Diagnosis

Poor weight gain syndrome resembles:
♦ Swine dysentery
♦ Necrotic enteritis caused by *Salmonella* spp.
♦ *Oesophagostomum dentatum*
♦ Malnutrition

Treatment

Ivermectin (0.3 mg/kg), levamisole, dichlorvos, benzimidazoles effective.

Control

♦ Pasture rotation
♦ House on concrete, frequent manure removal, avoid deep litter
♦ Treat sows just before farrowing, piglets at 8 weeks

HABRONEMIASIS (SUMMER SORES, SWAMP CANCER, BURSATTEE) [VM8 p. 1270]

Etiology

♦ *Habronema muscae, H. majus*
♦ *Draschia megastoma*

Epidemiology

♦ Widespread; important only in warm, wet climates
♦ Horses only, mostly in adults
♦ Lesions common; skin tumors a nuisance; stomach lesions cause sporadic deaths but illness uncommon

Life cycle

Indirect, flies are intermediate hosts:
• *Musca domestica* for *H. muscae, D. megastoma*
• *Stomoxys calcitrans* and others for *H. majus*
♦ Worm eggs passed in manure, infect maggots, horses eat dead flies or infected by larvae from fly proboscis to horse lip, wounds
♦ Larvae in wounds cause skin lesions
♦ Swallowed larvae cause gastritis, stomach tumor

Clinical findings

Gastric habronemiasis

♦ Variable appetite
♦ Poor coat
♦ Complications of:
• Acute gastric dilation due to pyloric obstruction
• Perforation to peritonitis, splenic abscess

Cutaneous habronemiasis

♦ On skin where lesions common, flies congregate, on:
• Face below eyes
• Abdomen midline
• Prepuce, penis
• Fetlock, coronet
• Withers
♦ Commence as papules, erodes, scab-covered center
♦ Rapid enlargement up to 30 cm dia.
♦ Center depressed, granulation tissue, edges raised, thickened

Conjunctival habronemiasis
* Granulation tissue lesions on third eyelid, eyelid
* Small, yellow, necrotic masses under conjunctiva, lacrimation, blepharospasm

Clinical pathology

* Skin biopsy contains larvae
* Larvae difficult to find in feces in cases with gastric lesions

Necropsy findings

* Granulomatous lesions containing small, yellow, caseous areas, larvae
* Rarely similar lesions in lung

Diagnosis

Gastric form resembles:
* Gasterophilosis
* Strongylosis

Cutaneous form resembles:
* Cutaneous pythiosis
* Sarcoid
* Infected skin wounds

Treatment

* Single treatment with ivermectin (0.2 mg/kg)
* Dienbendazole, fenbendazole also effective

Control

* Careful manure disposal
* Fly control
* Skin wound care

OXYURIASIS [VM8 p. 1272]

Etiology

Oxyuris equi.

Epidemiology

* In stabled horses
* Direct life cycle
* Inhabit cecum, colon; mature females migrate to anus, lay eggs on skin
* Eggs ingested by bites at irritation or contamination of feed
* Eggs resistant, airborne in dust

Clinical findings

Intense irritation perianal region causes annoyance, hair loss: rubbing, biting tail.

Clinical pathology

Eggs in scrapings made around anus.

Treatment

Ivermectin, benzimidazoles, piperazine effective.

STRONGYLOIDOSIS [VM8 p. 1272]

Etiology

* Sheep and cattle – *Strongyloides papillosus*
* Pigs – *S. ransomi*
* Horses – *S. westeri*

Epidemiology

* In most countries
* Cause minor problems
* May be parasitic or non-parasitic in a free-living life cycle
* Infection orally, by skin penetration, in milk
* Larvae reach lung via blood vessels, up trachea to pharynx, swallowed, mature in small intestine

Clinical findings

* Anorexia, depression
* Diarrhea
* Dermatitis of belly wall, lower limbs, including local swelling, bouts of frenzy in foals
* Mucosal pallor
* Lameness, susceptibility to footrot in sheep

Clinical pathology

Eggs in feces.

Necropsy findings

* Enteritis
* Pulmonary hemorrhage
* Larvae in damaged skin

Treatment

Ivermectin, benzimidazoles.

Control

Repeated treatment of dam, or continuous feeding.

RHABDITIS DERMATITIS
[VM8 p. 1272]

Etiology

Larvae of the nematode *Peloderma strongyloides*.

Epidemiology

♦ Principally disease of dogs; rare occurrences in cattle, horses
♦ A facultative parasite, usually free living; sporadic infections of animals
♦ Encouraged by bedding cattle on warm, wet bedding

Clinical findings

♦ Marked alopecia neck, flanks, belly
♦ **Severe cases** – skin patches swollen, raw, exude serum, severe irritation
♦ **Moderate cases** – skin thick, wrinkled, scurfy; pustules on belly wall, udder; contain thick yellow caseous material, larvae or mature worms

Clinical pathology

Parasites in skin scrapings, biopsy, bedding samples.

Treatment

Ivermectin or benzimidazole should cure.

Control

♦ Keeping cattle clean of manure in hair
♦ Frequent topping up or removal of bedding

TRICHURIASIS (WHIPWORM INFESTATION) [VM8 p. 1273]

Etiology

♦ Ruminants – *Trichuris ovis*, *T. discolor*, *T. globulosa*
♦ Pigs – *T. suis*.

Epidemiology

♦ Uncommon innocuous infection
♦ Life cycle direct
♦ Eggs can survive 6 months in piggery, 2 years on pasture
♦ Infection by ingestion
♦ Cases in pigs and lambs
♦ Can be heavy mortality in piglets

Clinical findings

♦ Anorexia, weight loss
♦ Diarrhea, some with excessive mucus, some blood

Clinical pathology

Easily identifiable eggs, occasionally worms, in feces.

Necropsy findings

♦ Worms in cecum
♦ Evidence of typhlitis

Treatment

Ivermectin, benzimidazoles.

CHABERTIASIS [VM8 p. 1273]

Etiology

Chabertia ovina.

Epidemiology

♦ Direct life cycle, infective larvae ingested, invades small intestine wall; histotrophic stage, then migrates to cecum, to colon
♦ Most cases in sheep, in colder areas, winter months

Clinical findings

♦ Soft feces, excess mucus, blood flecks
♦ Weight loss, some deaths

Clinical pathology

♦ Protein-losing enteropathy
♦ High fecal egg count; may be normal in early cases before egg-laying commences

Necropsy findings

♦ Colon wall thick, edematous, petechiation of wall
♦ Worms in first part of coiled colon
♦ Only 5–10 worms needed for infection to be pathogenic

Diagnosis

Resembles oesophagostomiasis.

Treatment

All broad spectrum anthelmintics effective.

NEUROFILARIASIS [VM8 p. 1274]

Etiology

Parelaphostrongylus tenuis.

Epidemiology

♦ Primarily a parasite of white-tailed deer
♦ Sheep and goats, in North America
♦ Eggs or larvae in deer feces, slugs, snails are
  intermediate hosts, eaten by sheep and
  goats migrates through nervous system

Clinical findings

♦ Lameness, incoordination
♦ Weakness, paralysis, recumbency
♦ Same disease in moose and deer called
  moose sickness with signs of:
  • Weakness, incoordination
  • Circling
  • Impaired vision
  • Abnormal head carriage
  • Aggressiveness
  • Paralysis

Necropsy findings

Worms in spinal cord and brain.

Diagnosis

Resembles:
• Cerebrospinal nematodiasis
• Micronema deletrix
• Other disruption of spinal cord

Treatment

Ivermectin at double dose ineffective.

Control

Avoid comingling with others.

CEREBROSPINAL NEMATODIASIS
(LUMBAR PARALYSIS, KUMRI)
[VM8 p. 1274]

Etiology

Setaria labiatopapillosa.

Epidemiology

♦ Microfilariae taken up from blood of
  patient
♦ Infective larvae develop in mosquitoes
  Aedes spp., *Armigeres* spp., *Anopheles* spp.
♦ Pass to atypical recipient by insect bite
♦ Congenital infection recorded
♦ Commonest in summer when vectors
  active

Clinical findings

♦ Paresis with stumbling gait, recumbency
  mostly in hind limbs
♦ Many die, some have permanent disability

Clinical pathology

Microfilariae in blood stream.

Necropsy findings

♦ Focal malacia, microcavitation
♦ Tracks of migrating larvae, larvae in
  section

Diagnosis

Resembles:
♦ Enzootic equine ataxia
♦ Paralytic rabies
♦ Spinal cord abscess
♦ Spinal cord trauma
♦ Spinal cord invasion by *Micronema dela-
  trix*, *Hypoderma* spp.

Treatment

None effective once lesions established.

Control

Periodic dosage with diethylcarbamazine.

MICRONEMA DELETRIX
GRANULOMATA [VM8 p. 1273]

Etiology

Free-living nematode *Micronema deletrix.*

Epidemiology

Sporadic cases in horses.

Clinical findings

→ Granuloma in nares, maxilla
→ May cause hard palate bulging displacing molars, prevents mastication
→ Lethargy, ataxia, recumbency death

Clinical pathology

Worms in biopsy of granuloma.

Necropsy findings

♦ Enormous numbers of worms in granuloma
♦ Microscopic granuloma in brain, kidney

Diagnosis

Resembles cerebrospinal nematodiasis.

THORN-HEADED WORM OF PIGS
[VM8 p. 1275]

Etiology

Macracanthorhyncus hirudinaceus.

Epidemiology

♦ Disease of pigs
♦ Indirect life cycle: inhabit pig small intestine, eggs passed in feces, larvae invade June bug larvae, eaten by pigs to set up new infection

Clinical findings

♦ Slow growth, weight loss
♦ Occasional fatal case caused by gut wall perforation

Clinical pathology

Eggs in feces.

Necropsy findings

♦ Worms in small intestine
♦ Nodules in small intestine wall at site of attachment

Treatment

Ivermectin effective.

Control

♦ Frequent manure disposal
♦ Prevention of contact with beetle larvae

THELAZIASIS (EYEWORM)
[VM8 p. 1276]

Etiology

Thelazia lacrymalis.

Epidemiology

♦ Worldwide distribution in all animal species
♦ Indirect life cycle; *Musca* spp. flies intermediate hosts
♦ Larvae deposited in conjunctival sac by fly while feeding
♦ Commonest in summer months

Clinical findings

♦ Excessive lacrimation
♦ Blepharospasm
♦ Corneal inflammation, ulcer
♦ Abscess in eyelid

Clinical pathology

Worms, eggs in lacrimal swab.

Diagnosis

Resembles:
♦ Infectious keratoconjunctivitis
♦ Foreign body in eye

Treatment

Levamisole orally or as 1% eye lotion.

Control

♦ Control face flies
♦ Treat clinical cases

ONCHOCERCIASIS (WORM NODULE DISEASE) [VM8 p. 1276]

Etiology

♦ Cattle – *Onchocerca gibsoni*, *O. gutterosa*, *O. linealis*, *O. ochengi*, *O. armillata* (also buffalo, goats)
♦ Horse – *O. cervicalis*, *O. reticulata*

Epidemiology

♦ Tropical, subtropical countries, and UK where vectors live
♦ Incidence increases with age

Life cycle

Microfilariae in blood stream ingested by midges, sandflies, blackflies (*Culicoides, Simulium* spp.) during feeding, undergo development in the intermediate host, deposited in skin of recipient while feeding
♦ Transported to preference site for females to mature, and fibrous tissue lesions include:
  • *O. armillata* – aortitis
  • *O. cervicalis* – ligamentum nuchae, eye, dermatitis
  • *O. gibsoni* – nodules in skin, subcutis, especially brisket
  • *O. gutterosa* – ligamentum nuchae
  • *O. lienalis* – gastrosplenic ligament
  • *O. ochengi* – dermatitis
  • *O. reticulata* – around flexor tendons
♦ Adult females lay microfilariae, remain in skin; some carried to eyes

Clinical findings

♦ Local nodules (*O. gibsoni*)
♦ Swelling around flexor tendons (*O. reticulata*) causing lameness
♦ Dermatitis with alopecia, scaling, pruritus on ventral abdomen, between fore limbs, inside thighs; also forehead, face, neck, thorax (*O. cervicalis*)
♦ Dermatitis of scrotum, udder (*O. ochengi*)

Clinical pathology

♦ Worm in fibrous tissue in biopsy specimen
♦ Microfilariae in blood; sample needs to be taken at optimum time

Necropsy findings

Worms in nodules, fibrous tissue at preference sites.

Diagnosis

Dermatitis lesions resemble:
♦ Demodectic mange
♦ Skin tuberculosis
♦ Ulcerative lymphangitis

Treatment

Ivermectin drug of choice in horses; local swelling, pruritus reaction at lesions 24 hours after treatment.

Control

♦ Insect control, housing at night.

ELAEOPHORIASIS (FILARIAL DERMATITIS) [VM8 p. 1277]

Etiology

♦ Sheep – *Elaeophora schneideri*
♦ Cattle – *E. poeli*
♦ Horses – *E. bohmi*

Epidemiology

♦ Patchy distribution Africa, Austria, Italy, USA
♦ *E. schneideri* primarily parasite of mule deer
♦ Clinical disease only in sheep
♦ Adults grazing at high altitudes in summer
♦ Transmission of microfilaria by *Tabanus, Hybomitra* spp. horse flies
♦ Morbidity about 1%

Clinical findings

♦ *Sheep* – severe dermatitis on poll, forehead, face, feet
♦ Small, intensely itchy areas of dermatitis quickly extended by rubbing, scratching to form bleeding, granulation tissue, small abscesses
♦ Local swelling lower limbs
♦ Recurrent quiescent periods with scab formation
♦ Long course 7 months up to 3 years
♦ Signs in elk include blindness, antler deformity, muzzle necrosis

Clinical pathology

Microfilariae in skin biopsy.

Necropsy findings

Worms free in blood; no lesions.

Diagnosis

Resembles:
♦ Photosensitization
♦ Ecthyma
♦ Mycotic dermatitis
♦ Strawberry foot rot

Treatment

♦ Parenteral bismuth, arsenic preparations used
♦ Ivermectin suggests itself

Control

Graze cattle instead of sheep in high-risk areas.

FILARIAL DERMATITIS
(CUTANEOUS PARAFILAROSIS)
[VM8 p. 1278]

Etiology

♦ Horses — *Parafilaria multipapillosa*
♦ Cattle – *P. bovicola*
♦ Pigs – *Suifilaria suis*

Epidemiology

♦ Tropical regions in most countries
♦ Filarid worms in nodules lay eggs, bearing microfilariae, on skin
♦ Transmitted by blood-sucking flies, house flies
♦ Occurs summer months

Clinical findings

♦ Nodules in skin ulcerate, bleed, heal spontaneously
♦ Cause inconvenience to harness

Clinical pathology

Eggs bearing microfilariae in bloody exudate.

Necropsy findings

Internal lesions in all tissues in some cases.

Diagnosis

Resembles onchocerciasis.

Treatment

Ivermectin 0.2 mg/kg I/M.

Control

♦ Treatment of clinical cases
♦ Fly control

MISCELLANEOUS FILARIAL
DERMATIDITES (CUTANEOUS
STEPHANOFILAROSIS)
[VM8 p. 1279]

Etiology

Stephanofilaria dedoesi, S. kaeli, S. assamensis, S. zaheeri, S. stilesia, S. okinawaensis.

Epidemiology

♦ In cattle, buffalo, goat
♦ Tropical, subtropical regions in most countries
♦ Transmission of microfilariae by biting insects, some by implantation in abrasions

Clinical findings

♦ Dermatitis in various anatomical locations, especially on the ventral abdomen, around dewclaws, base of the ears or horns, on the hump of humped cattle, around muzzle, on teats
♦ Raised, circumscribed, hairless, intensely pruritic lesions
♦ Thick scabs with bloodstained fluid in cracks
♦ Lesions coalesce to form lesions up to 25 cm diameter
♦ Healed lesions leave scars

Clinical pathology

Worms in cysts in skin scrapings.

Treatment

Ivermectin, levamisole effective.

Control

♦ Fly control
♦ Early treatment abrasions

27 DISEASES CAUSED BY ARTHROPOD PARASITES

GASTEROPHILUS SPP.
INFESTATION (BOTFLY)
[VM8 p. 1280]

Etiology

Larvae of the botflies *Gasterophilus nasalis, G. intestinalis, G. hemorrhoidalis, G. pecorum, G. inermis.*

Epidemiology

- Worldwide distribution in horses
- Flies active in summer months

Life cycle
- Hovering fly lays eggs in specific locations:
  - *G. intestinalis* on lower front limbs
  - *G. nasalis* on intermandibular space
  - Remainder on cheeks, lips
- Eggs hatch in 5–10 days
- Enter mouth by:
  - Biting or licking
  - Migration through cheeks
  - Migration in tissues around mouth
- Swallowed into stomach, locate in:
  - Cardiac region – *G. intestinalis*
  - Fundic region – *G. hemorrhoidalis, G. pecorum*
  - Pyloric region – *G. nasalis*
- Larvae pass out in feces 10–12 months later, in spring, early summer
- Pupate in ground, emerge as adult flies after 3–5 weeks

Clinical findings

- Slow weight gain, weight loss
- Poor coat
- Anorexia
- Occasional mild colic
- Shying, baulking, bad temper, disinclined to work when flies bother

Clinical pathology

- Eggs on hairs
- Larvae observed in feces after treatment

Necropsy findings

- Variable number of larvae in stomach
- Mucosal pitting at attachment site
- Gastric wall thickened
- Adhesive peritonitis, attachment to spleen, splenic abscessation rarely

Diagnosis

Easily coexist, confused with helminth infestations, especially *Strongylus* spp.

Treatment

- Ivermectin 0.2 mg/kg efficient
- Organophosphates, e.g. trichlorphon, usually administered with a benzimidazole to control helminths

Control

- Treat after fly activity ceased, 2 doses, one in winter, one in spring
- Watch for, treat, foals with painful mastication
- Fly control ineffectual

OESTRUS OVIS (NASAL BOTFLY)
[VM8 p. 1282]

Etiology

Oestrus ovis.

Epidemiology

Sheep, occasionally goats.

492

Life cycle

♦ Flies emerge late spring, mate, deposit larvae around nostrils
♦ Larvae migrate to dorsal turbinates, frontal sinuses
♦ After several months larvae migrate to nostrils, sneezed out
♦ Pupate in ground, adult flies may emerge in few weeks or after winter in cold climates

Importance

♦ Minimal effect on production
♦ Eye, upper respiratory tract infection common in humans in some countries

Clinical findings

♦ Sneezing
♦ Mucopurulent nasal discharge
♦ Stertorous, snoring respiration
♦ Fly worry causes stamping, head shaking, bunching with noses in each others fleeces; interferes with grazing

Treatment

Ivermectin, rafoxanide, closantel, nitroxynil effective.

Control

Treat twice – late summer and winter – to reduce future population.

HYPODERMA SPP. INFESTATION
(WARBLE FLY) [VM8 p. 1282]

Etiology

♦ Cattle – *Hypoderma bovis, H. lineatum*
♦ Sheep and goats – *H. aeratum, H. crossi, H. silenus*
♦ Horses – rarely infested by ruminant flies
♦ Deer – *H. diana*
♦ All species – *Dermatobia hominis*, a parasite of humans, rarely in all species

Epidemiology

♦ Common in northern hemisphere
♦ Young animals most susceptible
♦ Fly and grub seasons, critical to control program, vary between fly species, and with climate

Life cycle

♦ Adult flies active spring, summer
♦ Eggs laid on hairs on lower limbs, ventral abdomen (*H. lineatum*), or upper hind limb, rump (*H. bovis*)
♦ Hatching in few days, penetrate skin, migrate to esophagus (*H. lineatum*), epidural fat in spinal canal (*H. bovis*), local skin (*H. aeratum, H. crossi*)
♦ Further migration to subcutaneous tissue of back (*H. lineatum, H. bovis*)
♦ After several months emerge through breathing hole in skin, fall to ground, pupate
♦ Adult flies emerge in spring

Importance

♦ Severe damage to hides
♦ Fly worry an inconvenience

Clinical findings

Cattle

♦ Interference with grazing by fly worry
♦ Soft, fluctuating 3 cm dia. lumps on back
♦ Heavy infestations cause many painful lumps on back but attendant weight loss usually due to concurrent helminth infestation
♦ Sudden onset of paraplegia when larvae damage cord

Horses

♦ Rare infection
♦ Lumps on back interfere with riding
♦ Spinal cord injury by larvae causes sudden paraplegia

Clinical pathology

ELISA test for *H. bovis, H. lineatum* valuable in control program.

Necropsy findings

Early stage larvae in red, green discolored tissue; mature ones in cyst-like cavity with cloudy, yellow fluid.

Diagnosis

Resembles inherited subcutaneous cysts.

Treatment

♦ Ivermectin effective against all stages; larvicidal effect persists for 4 weeks
♦ Long-standing treatment has been with organophosphates but these have disadvantages of needing to be used at precisely

the correct stage, toxic effects are common
+ With any treatment timing in the life cycle is critical; treatment when grubs are in subcutaneous site, but not mature, is the objective; timing will vary with climate, species of fly

Control

+ Systemic treatment in fall and spring
+ Eradication has been achieved in some countries

SCREW-WORM INFESTATION
[VM8 p. 1284]

Etiology

Cochliomyia hominivorax, Chrysomyia bezziana.

Epidemiology

+ Major cause of livestock loss in tropical, subtropical regions in western hemisphere, Asia, Africa
+ Attacks all species, including humans
+ Lay eggs only in fresh wounds including surgical sites, excoriations, tick bite sites, perineum soiled by fetal fluids
+ Intact periorbital fossa, vulva in sheep attacked
+ Spread via fly migration, including on ships, in aircraft, long distances on strong wind
+ Dies out in winter, remigrates in warmer months

Life cycle

+ Eggs laid on wound edge
+ Larvae burrow into surrounding viable tissue
+ Mature in about a week, leave wound, fall to ground
+ Pupation length can be as short as 3 days, as long as 2 months
+ In best circumstances lifecycle complete in 3 weeks

Risk factors

+ Pupae susceptible to cold, heat, dryness
+ Attack favored by hot, humid weather

Clinical findings

+ Patient restless, wanders, seeks shade and foliage to brush against
+ Extensive wounds; patient 'eaten alive'

+ Profuse, brown exudate, objectionable odor
+ Many maggots

Clinical pathology

Larvae confirm diagnosis:
+ 1–2 cm long
+ Pink
+ Pointed front end, blunt posterior
+ 2 dark lines from posterior to mid point
+ Rows of fine, dark spines on anterior part of each segment

Necropsy findings

Extensive, raw, maggot-infested wounds

Diagnosis

Resembles:
+ Blow-fly infestation
+ *Callitroga macellaria* infestation; similar fly, attacks only advanced, necrotic lesions, dead cadavers

Treatment

+ Ivermectin (0.2 mg/kg S/C) kills all young larvae, some older ones; has residual effect for 16–20 days
+ Closantel 15 mg/kg effective, protects 8–15 days
+ Older methods included local application larvicide with antiseptic

Control

+ Objective to break life cycle by:
  • Avoiding surgery during danger season
  • Prompt protective action to wounds e.g. protective ivermectin injection, topical larvicide, antiseptic
  • Twice-weekly examination of all animals on farm
  • Arrange for parturition in non-danger period
+ Release of sterile male flies has eradicated disease
+ Screw-worm adult suppression system includes a synthetic bait plus an insecticide in a trap

CUTANEOUS MYIASIS (BLOWFLY STRIKE) [VM8 p. 1286]

Etiology

+ North America – *Phormia regina, P. terrae-novae*

- Britain – *Calliphora erythrocephala, C. vomitoria, P. terraenovae, Lucilia cuprina, L. sericata*
- New Zealand – *L. sericata, L. cuprina, C. stygia*
- Australia – *L. cuprina, L. sericata, C. stygia, C. novica, C. augur, C. hilli, C. albifrontalis, Chrysomyia rufifacies, C. varipes*

Epidemiology

Occurrence
- A problem in most countries where sheep kept
- Flock mortality rate up to 30% per annum

Life cycle
- Eggs, larvae deposited near source of smell, wound edge
- First larvae feed on exudate, later larvae burrow into, feed on skin
- Migrate laterally to set up new sites
- Larvae drop off to ground, pupate to adult fly in life cycle as short as 8 days
- Secondary flies attracted

Risk factors
Factors making sheep more susceptible, multiplying the number of flies in environment include:
- Primary fly species, e.g. *Lucilia cuprina* very effective initiators of strike
- Warm, moist weather
- Summer rainfall areas worst affected
- Odor created by:
  - Prolonged wetting of skin, wool, mycotic dermatitis, lumpy wool
  - Urine staining at perineum or prepuce
  - Perineum staining with fetal fluids
  - Feces accumulation in breech wool
  - A long tail encourages soiling
  - Foot rot
  - Wounds caused by head-butting, docking, castration
  - Sheep with fleece characteristics, e.g. Merinos with heavy skin wrinkles, conformation, conducive to easy wetting of wool, skin
- Availability of carcases for secondary flies to breed in

Importance
Death losses, loss of fleece, costs of treatment, control all high cost items.

Clinical findings

- Restless, will not feed, move about with head close to ground
- Bite, kick at struck area
- Continual tail wriggling
- Wool slightly lifted over area of strike
- Characteristic smell
- Wool moist, brown, other colors in very wet wools
- Skin inflamed, ulcerated, maggots burrowing into it
- Skin destruction more marked with secondary flies
- After several days fever, anorexia, tachycardia, hyperpnea, recumbency, some deaths
- Survivors may shed fleece, have a break in wool

Clinical pathology

Identification of species by inspection of larvae requires specialist knowledge

Treatment

- Powders or liquids containing organophosphates, e.g. diazinon, chlorfenvinphos have the advantage that the wool need not be clipped, a laborious task in difficult circumstances when done in the field with hand shears
- Insect growth regulators, e.g. cyromazine also extensively used but slow-acting

Control

Three objectives:
1. Reduce fly numbers:
   - Trapping
   - Early treatment clinical cases
   - Disposal of carcases, wool clippings, crutchings
2. Prophylactic application of larvicide before fly wave
   - When environmental conditions suitable, sheep susceptible, apply prophylactic treatment by application of:
     - Larvicide, e.g. organophosphate (diazinon, chlorfenvinphos), ivermectin
     - Oviposition suppressants, e.g. synthetic pyrethroids
     - Insect growth regulators, e.g. vetrazin, triflubenzuron
   - Application may be by:
     - Dipping, plunge or spray
     - Tip spray
     - Pour-on
     - Intraruminal slow release bolus
     - Crutching of wool over posterior aspect of thighs from above tail to hocks, application by jetting

3. Reducing sheep susceptibility:
   ♦ Mules operation – surgical extension of woolless area of perineum, modified by removing woolled skin from the sides of the tail, docking so as to leave enough tail to cover vulva tip
   ♦ Effecting same extension of woolless skin of crutch by selective breeding
   ♦ Reducing pizzle susceptibility by use of testosterone implants, pizzle-dropping, shearing around pizzle
   ♦ Selectively breed away from sheep with withers susceptible to fleece rot

KEDS   [VM8 p. 1291]

Etiology

Melophagus ovinus.

Epidemiology

♦ Worldwide in sheep and goats
♦ Heavy infestations in winter
♦ A problem in cool, wet areas

Life cycle

♦ Entire life spent on host
♦ Single larvae deposited, pupate in a few hours, adults emerge in 20–35 days; population increase is slow
♦ Spread is by direct contact between sheep
♦ Most keds in fleece removed by shearing

Importance

♦ Itching, scratching causes fleece damage
♦ Fouling by ked feces reduces fleece value
♦ Heavy infestations can cause blood loss anemia

Clinical findings

♦ Keds readily visible

Treatment and control

♦ Dipping with parasiticide with long residual time soon after shearing of all sheep on farm will eradicate insect
♦ Organophosphates, synthetic pyrethroids, ivermectins effective dips
♦ Power dusting with coumaphos, diazinon effective

LOUSE INFESTATIONS
[VM8 p. 1291]

Etiology

♦ Cattle – *Linognathus vituli, Solenoptes capillatus, Haematopinus eurysternus, H.* *quadripertusus, H. tuberculatus, Damalinia bovis*
♦ Sheep – *Linognathus ovillus, L. africanus, L. stenopsis, L. pedalis, Damalinia ovis*
♦ Goat – *Linognathus stenopsis, L. africanus, Damalinia caprae, D. limbata, D. crassipes*
♦ Pigs – *Haematopinus suis*
♦ Horses – *Haematopinus asini, Damalinia equi*

Epidemiology

♦ Worldwide distribution
♦ Young most susceptible
♦ Thin animals carry heaviest burdens
♦ Very low numbers in summer, peak in spring
♦ Shearing, loss of winter coat, removes bulk of infestation

Life cycle

♦ Direct, on host
♦ Egg, 3 nymph stages, mature lice completed in 2–4 weeks
♦ Transmission by direct contact
♦ Inert objects including pasture infective for a few hours
♦ Infestation between flocks by introduction infected sheep; over a year before most sheep in flock infected

Clinical findings

♦ Scratching, rubbing, restlessness,
♦ Pityriasis
♦ Coat rough, shaggy
♦ Hairballs causing indigestion in calves
♦ Dermatitis in pigs
♦ Deterioration in wool, mohair quality
♦ Foot lice cause nibbling, stamping of feet
♦ Weight loss, reduced milk production debated results of louse infestation, probably result of neglectful malnutrition

Clinical pathology

Search for lice best done on back, sides of neck, head, in mane, tail switch; after shearing on ventral neck; foot lice on haired lower limbs.

Diagnosis

Resembles:
♦ Itchmite
♦ Ked

Table 27.1 Single and multiple host ticks [VM8 p. 1294]

ONE-HOST TICKS
Boophilus spp.
Margaropus winthemia
Otobius megnini (adults are not parasitic)
Dermacentor albipictus

TWO-HOST TICKS
Rhipicephalus evertsi
R. bursa
Hyalomma spp. (most have two or three hosts)

THREE-HOST TICKS
Ixodes spp.
Rhipicephalus spp. (except *R. evertsi* and *R. bursa*)
Haemaphysalis spp.
Amblyomma spp.
Hyalomma spp. (most have two or three hosts)
Ornithodorus spp. – many hosts
Dermacentor spp.

Table 27.2 Ticks reported to cause paralysis [VM8 p. 1295]

Animal	Tick	Country
Sheep, calves, goats	*Dermacentor andersoni*	United States
	D. occidentalis	United States
Calves, lambs, foals, goats	*Ixodes holocyclus*	Australia
Sheep, goats, calves	*I. pilosus*	South Africa
Sheep, goats, calves, antelopes	*I. rubicundus*	South Africa
Lambs	*Rhipicephalus evertsi*	South Africa
Calves, sheep, goats	*Haemoaphysalis punctata*	South Africa, Europe, Japan
Sheep	*Ornithodorus laborensis*	Central Asia
Sheep	*Hyalomma aegyptium*	Yugoslavia
Sheep, goats	*Ixodes ricinus*	Crete, Israel
Cattle, sheep and goats	*Amblyomma cajannense*	Central and S. America
Cattle	*Rhipicephalus evertsi*	Africa

♦ Photosensitive dermatitis
♦ Scrapie

Treatment

♦ Ivermectin, moxidectin remove sucking lice, incomplete effect on biting lice
♦ Many topical preparations used in plunge dips, shower dips, jetting races; must be used in shorn sheep; careful jetting of long-woolled sheep reasonably effective; pour-ons, spot-ons used but expensive —
  • Arsenic, chlorinated hydrocarbons still used but increasingly banned because of residues
  • Organophosphates, carbamates widely used
  • Synthetic pyrethroids e.g. cypermethrim, alphamethrim, deltamethrim effective as pour-ons used immediately after shearing

Control

♦ Seasonal treatment of all sheep in fall
♦ Simultaneous spraying of housing
♦ Eradication achievable by single treatment if used correctly

TICK INFESTATION [VM8 p. 1293]

Etiology

Tick control depends on whether ticks are single or multiple host ticks; the common ticks of animals are listed in these categories in Table 27.1.

Epidemiology

♦ Worldwide distribution
♦ Commonest in tropics, semitropics in high rainfall zones

Life cycles
♦ Ticks may pass all their life on one host, or pass successive stages of life cycle on successive hosts
♦ Single host ticks are much easier to control
♦ Adult, engorged females drop to ground, lay eggs
♦ Larval ticks attach to passing host
♦ Successive nymphal stages may persist on original host or drop off and attach to further hosts

Clinical findings

Tick infestations can cause:
♦ Tick worry – interference with grazing, loss of condition, skin, hair coat problems
♦ Some are active blood suckers, cause anemia
♦ Tick paralysis (Table 27.2)
♦ Transmission of infectious diseases (Tables 27.3 and 27.4)

Treatment and control

Control measures include:
♦ Pasture-resting
♦ Breeding of tick resistant animals, e.g. Brahman cattle breeds
♦ Spraying or dipping with acaricide

Choice of acaricide
There are too many acaricides available, their advantages and disadvantages are too variable to make a recommendation suited to all circumstances.
♦ Characteristics of the most desirable acaricide —
  • Most effective, longest duration of effect
  • Least residue likely to be toxic to humans
  • Lowest probability of resistance developing in ticks
  • Lowest cost, especially when frequent treatments required
♦ The commonly used acaricides are listed in Table 27.5
♦ Some of the popular, current products are:
  • Amitraz, as a spray or dip, 0.025%
  • A synthetic pyrethroid e.g. flumethrin, cyhalothrin

  • Synthetic pyrethroids combined with organophosphate, e.g. cypermethrin plus chlorfenvinphos, deltamethrin plus ethion
  • Acaricides in feed or in impregnated ear-tags not effective
  • Ivermectin still under investigation
♦ **Control programs** should be based on principles:
  • Area eradication has been achieved but there have been many failures and reinfection common
  • Designed around the lifecycle of the target tick
  • Treatments early in tick season to prevent gross increase in numbers
  • Complete tick eradication disrupts immunity maintenance
  • Too many treatments encourages development of resistance

STABLE FLIES   [VM8 p. 1298]

Etiology

Stomoxys calcitrans, S. nigra.

Epidemiology

♦ In most countries
♦ Attacks cattle, horses, pigs
♦ Life cycle favored by:
  • Warm, moist conditions
  • Supply of urine-soaked straw, feces in which eggs laid

Clinical findings

♦ Bites are painful, cause insect harassment, interfere with grazing, cause weight loss
♦ Sores on lower fore limbs of cattle
♦ Possible allergic dermatitis in horses
♦ Mechanical transmission of anthrax, equine infectious anemia, bovine virus disease, surra, habronemiasis

Treatment and control

♦ Repellent spray ensures freedom for only a few hours
♦ Organophosphate, pyrethroid applied as spray, or pour-on can protect against infection for 4 days
♦ Similar spray on sun-warmed walls
♦ Weekly removals manure, bedding, compost piles, silage stacks where flies breed

HORSE FLIES, MARCH FLIES OR
BREEZE FLIES; DEER FLIES
[VM8 p. 1299]

Etiology

♦ Horse fly – *Tabanus* spp.
♦ Deer fly – *Chrysops, Haematopota, Pangonia* spp.

Epidemiology

♦ Widespread in most countries
♦ Affect horses, cattle
♦ Lifecycle – eggs laid on plants in or near water, larvae, pupae in water, mud

Clinical findings

♦ Worry may limit grazing, reduce productivity
♦ Mechanically transmit:
  • Equine infectious anemia
  • *Trypanosoma evansi, T. virax*
  • Bovine leukemia virus
  • Anthrax
  • Summer mastitis

Treatment and control

♦ Drain surface water or move patients away from water
♦ Repellent spray of o-diethyl toluamide reduces infestation for a few days
♦ Permethrin dust or solution on animals kills flies for 2 weeks

BUFFALO FLIES; HORN FLIES
[VM8 p. 1299]

Etiology

Haematobia irritans exigua, H. i. irritans, H. minuta.

Epidemiology

♦ In Australia, south-east Asia, continental USA, Hawaii, Africa
♦ Harass cattle, buffalo, horses, humans
♦ Brahman type cattle less affected
♦ Flies stay on host, leaving them only to lay eggs in fresh feces
♦ Eggs, larvae susceptible to dryness, cool temperatures
♦ Transmission of insect by movement of cattle, possibly strong wind

Clinical findings

♦ Flies congregate on withers, shoulders, flanks, around eyes
♦ Horses develop sores at these sites; may lead to cutaneous pythiosis, cutaneous habronemiasis, infection with *Onchocerca cervicalis*, transmit *Stephanofilaria* spp.

Treatment and control

♦ Ivermectin in anthelmintic dose controls horn flies in feces for 4 weeks but kills other arthropod enemies to the flies e.g. dung beetle
♦ Diflubenzuron or methoprene boluses have same effect for 20 weeks
♦ Back rubbers or ear tags impregnated with organophosphatic insecticides, dust bags containing them, can limit fly numbers but encourages development of resistance in flies

HORSE LOUSE FLIES [VM8 p. 1300]

Etiology

Hippobosca equina, H. maculata.

Epidemiology

♦ In horses in most countries with warm climate
♦ Fly lives on host, deposits puparia in dry humus

Clinical findings

♦ Flies congregate on perineum, between hind limbs
♦ Mechanical vectors for infectious disease

Treatment and control

No specific remedies; recommended procedures for *Haematobia* spp. should apply.

BITING MIDGES [VM8 p. 1300]

Etiology

Culicoides spp.

Epidemiology

♦ Worldwide distribution
♦ Prevalent in warm, moist weather
♦ Most active early morning, dusk

Table 27.3 Ticks reported to transmit protozoan diseases [VM8 p. 1296]

Disease	Protozoan	Vector ticks	Country
BABESIOSIS			
Cattle	Babesia bigemina	Boophilus annulatus	Africa
		B. microplus	
		B. (annulatus) calcaratus, B. decoloratus, Rhipicephalus appendiculatus, R. bursa, R. evertsi, Ixodes ricinus	
		Haemaphysalis punctata	Former USSR
	Babesia bovis	Ixodes persulcatus	Europe
		I. ricinus	Iran
		Boophilus annulatus	Australia
		B. microplus	Africa
	Babesia berbera	B. annulatus (calcaratus), Rhipicephalus bursa	
Sheep and goats	Babesia motasi	Dermacentor silvarum, Rhipicephalus bursa, Haemaphysalis punctata, Ixodes ricinus	Europe
	Babesia ovis	Rhipicephalus bursa	Former USSR
		Haemaphysalis bispinosa	India
	Babesia ovata	Haemaphysalis longicornis	Japan
Horses	Babesia caballi	Hyalomma dromedarii	Africa
		Dermacentor (reticulata), marginatus, D. pictus, D. silvarum, Hyalomma (excavatum) anatolicum, H. marginatum, H. volgense, Rhipicephalus bursa, R. sanguineus	Former USSR and the Balkans, S. America and Florida, United States
	Babesia equi	Hyalomma dromedarii, Rhipicephalus evertsi, R. sanguineus, Dermacentor marginatus, D. pictus, Hyalomma anatolicum, H. marginatum, H. uralense, Rhipicephalus bursa, R. sanguineus	Africa, the Balkans, S. America, Australia
Pigs	Babesia trautmanni	R. sanguineus (turanicus)	Former USSR

THEILERIOSIS

Cattle	*Theileria parva*	*Rhipicephalus appendiculatus*	Africa
	Theileria annulata	*Hyalomma anaticolicum*	Africa, Asia, former USSR, Europe, China, India
	Theileria sergenti	*Haemaphysalis sergenti*	Japan, Asia
	Theileria mutans	*Amblyoma variegatum*	Africa, Asia
		Haemaphysalis spp.	Europe, former USSR, North America, Australia
	Theileria buffeli	*Haemaphysalis* spp.	
Sheep	*Theileria ovis*	*Rhipicephalus bursa*	Africa, Asia
		Rhipicephalus evertsi	Europe
		Hyalomma spp.	
	Theileria hirci	*Rhipicephalus* spp.	Africa, Middle East
		Hyalomma anatolicum	Former USSR

Table 27.4 Diseases caused by bacteria, viruses and rickettsia and reported to be transmitted by ticks [VM8 p. 1297]

Disease	Causative agent	Vector ticks	Country
Tick pyemia (lambs)	Staphylococcus aureus	Ixodes ricinus	Great Britain
Tularemia (sheep)	F. tularense	Haemaphysalis leporispalustris, H. otophila, Dermacentor andersoni, D. variabilis, D. pictus, D. marginatus, Ixodes luguri	United States, Norway, Europe, former USSR
anaplasmosis Cattle	Anaplasma marginale	Boophilus annulatus, Argas persicus, Dermacentor albipictus, D. andersoni, D. occidentalis, D. variabilis, Ixodes scapularis, Rhipicephalus sanguineus Boophilus microplus B. decoloratus, Hyalomma excavatum, Rhipicephalus bursa, R. simus Haemaphysalis punctata, Ixodes ricinus Boophilus (annulatus) calcaratus	North America Australia and S. America Africa Europe Former USSR
Sheep and goats	Anaplasma ovis	Dermacentor silvarum, Rhipicephalus bursa, Ornithodorus laborensis	Former USSR
Brucellosis	Brucella abortus and Br. melitensis	Many ticks may be infected but infection of host appears to occur only if ticks or their feces are eaten	Former USSR
Heartwater	Cowdria ruminantium	Amblyomma spp.	Africa & Caribbean
African swine fever	Virus	Rhipicephalus appendiculatus (lab only) Ixodes ricinus	Africa England
Tick-borne fever	Rickettsia spp.	I. ricinus Rhipicephalus haemaphysaloides	Great Britain, Norway India
Caseous lymphadenitis of sheep	Corynebacterium pseudotuberculosis	Dermacentor albipictus	North America
Epizootic bovine abortion	Spirochete	Ornithodorus coriaceus	United States
Nairobi sheep disease	Virus	Rhipicephalus appendiculatus	Africa
Lyme disease	Borrelia burgdorferi	Ixodes dammini, I. pacificus, I. ricinus	United States, Europe, Australia

502

Table 27.5 Names of commonly used insecticides [VM8 p. 1298]

Generic names	Trade names
alphamethrin	Duracide
avermectin	Bastion, Avomec, Ivomec, Duotin
amitraz	Tactic, Triatox, Amidaz
bromophos ethyl	Nexagon, Nexajet
carbaryl	Sevin, Arylan, Seffein
carbophenothion	Trithion
chlorfenvinphos	Supona, Suprex
chlormethiuron	Dipofene 60
chlorpyrifos	Dursban, Dowco 109
closantel	Seponver
coumaphos	Asuntol, Baymix, Bayer 21/199, Muscatox, Resitox, Co-Ral, Melane
crotoxyphos	Ciodrin
crufomate	Ruelene, Montrel, Dowco 132
cyfluthrin	Bayofly
cyhalothrin	Grenade
cypermethrin	Ripcord, Barricade, Cypafly
cyromazine	Vetrazin
deltamethrin	Decis, Clout, Takfly, Butox
diazinon	Diazinon, Nucidol
dimethoate	Rogor, Roxion, Cygon, Fostion
dioxathion	Delnav, Navadel
ethion	Nialate
famphur	Warbex, Famophos
fenchlorphos	Ronnel, Nankor, Korlan, Ectoral
fenthion	Tiguvon, Baytex, Bayer S 1752
fenthion ethyl	Lucijet, S 1751
fenvalerate	Sumifly
flumethrin	Bayticol
methoxychlor	Marlate, Metachlor
moxidectin	Cydectin, Vetdectin
phosmet	Imidan, Phthalophos, Prolate
phoxim	Sebacil, Bay 9053, Sarnadip (S. Africa), Sarnacuran (S. America)
promacyl	Promacide
propetamphos	Safrotin, Ectomort
propoxur	Baygon, Aprocarb, Baygole
temophos	Lypor
tetrachlorvinphos	Stirophos, Gardona, Rabon
trichlorfon	Neguvon, Dylox, Dipterex, Chlorophos

♦ Can spread long distances on strong wind
♦ Horses, cattle, sheep

Clinical findings

♦ Restlessness, switching tail, stamping feet
♦ Transmit:
  • Bluetongue
  • African horse sickness
  • Bovine ephemeral fever
♦ Act as intermediate hosts for *Onchocerca* spp.
♦ Cause hypersensitivity of Queensland itch

Treatment and control

♦ Repellents e.g. dimethyl phthalate or *o*-diethyl tolumide effective for 1–2 days
♦ Fly screens ineffective
♦ Back-line pour-on of permethrin 3 times weekly reasonably effective

BLACK FLIES, BUFFALO GNATS, SANDFLIES [VM8 p. 1300]

Etiology

Cnephia pecuarum, Simulium arcticum, Austrosimulium pestilens, A. bancrofti.

Epidemiology

♦ In warm climates in North America, UK, Australia
♦ Prevalent with abundant fresh water, shade of trees, especially after flooding
♦ Cause problems when flies in enormous numbers, attack in swarms
♦ Attack all animal species

Clinical findings

♦ Actively restless, mill about, kick up dust, wallow in mud
♦ Young may be trampled to death
♦ Throat swelling may cause asphyxia
♦ Sudden deaths suspected caused by anaphylaxis
♦ Intermediate hosts for nematodes
♦ Transmit *Onchocerca* spp.

Treatment and control

♦ Difficult in the environments in which these insects thrive
♦ Widespread spraying with organochlorines is no longer an option
♦ Measures recommended for control of *Culicoides* spp. should apply

MOSQUITOES [VM8 p. 1301]

Etiology

Aedes, Anopheles, Culex, Mansonia, Psorophora spp.

Epidemiology

♦ Worldwide distribution
♦ Summer prevalence in wet environments providing breeding waters for larvae

Clinical findings

♦ Restlessness
♦ Milk yield, weight gain reduced
♦ Anemia in some
♦ Transmit the infectious causes of:
  • Equine encephalomyelitis
  • Japanese B encephalitis
  • Rift Valley fever
  • *Dermatobia hominis*
  • *Setaria digitata*

Treatment and control

♦ Mosquito screens
♦ Insect repellents e.g. dimethyl phthalate

♦ Insecticides especially synthetic pyrethroids e.g. permethrin provide protection for 3 days
♦ Large-scale insecticide spraying over water no longer an option

HOUSEFLIES [VM8 p. 1301]

Etiology

Musca domestica.

Epidemiology

♦ Universal occurrence
♦ Eggs laid in any decaying organic matter; fresh horse manure preferred
♦ Most prevalent in warm weather

Clinical findings

♦ Mechanical transmission of:
  • Ovine keratoconjunctivitis
  • Contagious bovine ophthalmia
  • Summer mastitis
  • Possibly anthrax, brucellosis, erysipelas
♦ Intermediate host for:
  • *Habronema muscae*
  • *Draschia megastoma*

Treatment and control

Remove or spray with insecticide, organic matter serving as breeding ground.

BUSH FLIES [VM8 p. 1301]

Etiology

Musca vestutissima.

Epidemiology

♦ Tropical Australia
♦ Prevalent in summer
♦ Congregates on wounds, any exposed mucosa, conjunctiva, so thick around eyes, lips

Clinical findings

♦ Intermediate host for:
  • *Habronema muscae*
  • *Draschia megastoma*
  • *Thelazia* spp.
♦ Mechanically transmits —
  • Ovine keratoconjunctivitis
  • Contagious bovine ophthalmia

Treatment and control

♦ Insect repellents e.g. dimethyl phthalate
♦ insecticides especially synthetic pyrethroids, e.g. permethrin provide protection for 3 days
♦ Large-scale insecticide spraying over water no longer an option

FACE FLY [VM8 p. 1302]

Etiology

Musca autumnalis.

Epidemiology

♦ Europe, Asia, North America
♦ Prevalent outdoors in summer

Clinical findings

♦ Congregate on face
♦ Feed on nasal exudate, ocular discharge, saliva
♦ Cause mild insect worry
♦ Transmit bovine infectious keratoconjunctivitis

Treatment and control

♦ Disposal or spraying with insecticide of manure, the fly's breeding ground
♦ Dust bags containing organophosphate insecticides placed to apply dust to heads
♦ Syrup baits containing organophosphates applied to forehead every 48 hours
♦ Diflubenzuron boluses fed to cattle achieve high kill of larvae in feces over period up to 20 weeks; problem is kill of beneficial insects in feces, e.g. dung beetle

HEAD FLY [VM8 p. 1302]

Etiology

Hydrotoea irritans

Epidemiology

♦ In UK, Europe
♦ Swarms around animals, humans in summer
♦ Breeds in litter, soil
♦ Only one life cycle per year

Clinical findings

♦ Restlessness, head shaking
♦ Lacerations to head caused by actions to ease fly worry
♦ May transmit summer mastitis

Treatment and control

♦ Ear tags impregnated with synthetic pyrethroids effective but predispose to resistance in flies
♦ Pour-ons recommended but need frequent application
♦ Dust bags containing organophosphate insecticides placed to apply dust to heads
♦ Syrup baits containing organophosphates applied to forehead every 48 hours
♦ Diflubenzuron boluses fed to cattle achieve high kill of larvae in feces over period up to 20 weeks; problem is kill of beneficial insects in feces, e.g. dung beetle

HARVEST MITE INFESTATION
(CHIGGER MITES) [VM8 p. 1302]

Etiology

Larvae of *Tyroglyphus* spp., *Pyemotes ventricosus*, *Trombicula sarcina*, *Neotrombicula autumnalis*, *Eutrombicula alfreddugesi*, *E. splendens*, *E. batatas*, *Leptotrombidium* spp., *Schoengastia* spp.

Epidemiology

♦ Natural hosts small rodents; nymphs, adults also parasitise arthropods in grain, hay
♦ Animals at pasture or fed new hay, grain infected

Clinical findings

Horses
♦ Lesions on lips, lower face
♦ On feet, lower limbs, especially flexures
♦ Lesions itchy, scaly, fragile scabs, hair loss
♦ Infested parts bitten, rubbed
♦ Stamping when stabled on infested bedding

Sheep
Leg skin erythematous, weeping.

Pigs (*Tyroglyphus* spp.)
♦ 3 cm dia. scabs over body
♦ Skin not damaged
♦ Lesions mildly itchy

♦ Commences 2 weeks after new feed begun, disappears spontaneously 3 weeks later

Clinical pathology

Mites in scrapings.

Diagnosis

Horses
Resembles:
♦ Lesions on white faced horse caused by photosensitization
♦ Lesions on limbs – chorioptic mange, greasy heel

Pigs
Resembles:
♦ Sarcoptic mange
♦ Swine pox

Treatment and control

♦ Disease self-limiting in a few days
♦ Any good insecticide wash, e.g. maldison
♦ Pasture spraying with chlorpyrifos

SHEEP ITCHMITE [VM8 p. 1303]

Etiology

Psorergates ovis.

Epidemiology

♦ Southern hemisphere countries, USA
♦ Life cycle entirely on sheep
♦ Spread by direct contact especially shorn sheep packed together in yards; from ewe to lamb during sucking
♦ Slow spread; several years after introduction before clinical cases in any number
♦ Clinical morbidity up to 15%
♦ Tolerance develops in individuals, signs disappear after several years, mites remain
♦ Merinos most susceptible
♦ In areas with cold, wet winters
♦ Skin irritation due to hypersensitivity

Clinical findings

♦ Rubbing, biting of sides, flanks, thighs
♦ Ragged, sometimes shed, fleece
♦ Wool in affected areas thready, tufted, contains dandruff scales

Clinical pathology

♦ Hyperkeratosis, epithelial desquamation
♦ Mites seen in skin scraping with hand lens
♦ Peak numbers in spring; lowest in summer
♦ Numbers decline after shearing

Diagnosis

Resembles:
♦ Lice infestation
♦ Scrapie

Treatment and control

♦ Two treatments, in summer, 1 month apart with ivermectin eradicates
♦ Phoxim, rotenone plus piperonyl butoxide reduce mite numbers

DEMODECTIC MANGE
(FOLLICULAR MANGE)
[VM8 p. 1304]

Etiology

Species-specific *Demodex bovis, D. ovis* etc., or *D. folliculorum* var. *bovis*, etc.

Epidemiology

♦ All species in most countries
♦ Most cases in thin, adult, dairy cattle in late winter, early spring; rare in sheep
♦ Life cycle on host; adults in hair follicles, sebaceous glands
♦ Spread by contact, probably while sucking; possibly spread by grooming in horses

Clinical findings

♦ Not readily visible clinically; often seen first when holes found in hides during curing
♦ No irritation
♦ Palpable, seen with difficulty, 3 mm dia. nodules or pustules in skin
♦ General skin thickening, hair loss in area in some
♦ Pustule contents white, cheesy, fluid in larger abscesses
♦ Cattle and goats – lesions on brisket, lower neck, shoulder, forearm, on back behind withers
♦ May be extensive in goats, combined with other skin disease
♦ Horses — on face, around eyes
♦ Pigs – on face, down neck to belly

Clinical pathology

Mites easy to find in pus from skin scrapings.

Diagnosis

In horses resembles:
♦ Non-specific staphylococcal dermatitis
♦ Deep ringworm

Treatment and control

♦ Ivermectin (3 mg/kg) cures cattle
♦ Acaricides generally moderately effective

SARCOPTIC MANGE (BARN ITCH)
[VM8 p. 1305]

Etiology

Sarcoptes scabiei var *bovis*, *S. scabiei* var *ovis*, etc. but host specificity not absolute, spread between species can occur.

Epidemiology

♦ Worldwide distribution
♦ All species, most serious in pigs, also in cattle, camels, rarely sheep
♦ In overcrowded, poorly fed animals
♦ Most active in winter
♦ Life cycle on the host; adults burrow in skin, hypersensitivity develops 8–10 weeks later
♦ No hypersensitivity in some pigs; become chronic carriers
♦ Spread by contact, grooming tools, bedding, rugs, sows to suckers
♦ Sows often clinically normal but large numbers of mites in ears
♦ Adults survive 3 weeks away from host
♦ Some effect on weight gain

Clinical findings

♦ Erythema, papules, intense pruritus
♦ Traumatic alopecia
♦ Thick, brown scabs over raw surface
♦ Skin thick, wrinkled
♦ Lesions over most of body in 3–6 weeks
♦ Lesions very extensive in neglected patients; become anorexic, emaciated, die
♦ Lesions located in —
  • Pig – trunk
  • Sheep and goat – face
  • Cattle – inside thighs, neck, brisket, root of tail
  • Horses and camels – head, neck

Clinical pathology

♦ Mites may be difficult to find in skin scrapings
♦ Best site is ear canal

Diagnosis

Resembles:
♦ Chorioptic mange
♦ Psoroptic mange
♦ Ringworm
♦ Chlorinated naphthalene poisoning
♦ Trombidiform mite infestation
♦ Photosensitization

Treatment and control

♦ Ivermectin a complete treatment; bad cases may require second treatment at 14 days
♦ Acaricide to buildings, clothing, equipment
♦ Acaricide spray with close attention to ears, under tail, between limbs
♦ All animals in group must be treated
♦ Sprays or pour-ons of organophosphates widely used

PSOROPTIC MANGE (SHEEPSCAB,
BODY MANGE, EAR MANGE)
[VM8 p. 1306]

Etiology

Body mites
♦ *Psoroptes ovis* on sheep, cattle horses (sheep scab)
♦ *P. natalensis* on cattle, water buffalo
♦ *P. equi* on horses, donkeys, mules

Ear mites
♦ *P. cuniculi*
♦ *P. cervinus*, ear and body mite of wildlife

Epidemiology

♦ Major disease in sheep and cattle but now eradicated from most progressive countries
♦ Life cycle on host; eggs laid at scab edge, cycle complete in 10–11 days
♦ Survive up to 3 weeks away from host
♦ Cool, moist climate encourages proliferation
♦ Fall–winter disease, especially in housed livestock
♦ Spread by contact; between farms by animal movement or infected fomites, e.g. wool

Clinical findings

Sheep
♦ Lesions anywhere, most obvious on sides
♦ Biting, scratching at part
♦ Small papules ooze serum, then yellow crusts
♦ Wool sheds, fibers bound together in scab
♦ Emaciation, weakness in severe cases
♦ Many mild, clinically inapparent cases in well-fed sheep
♦ Special search for lesions concentrates on ears, base of horns, infraorbital fossa, perineal, scrotal areas

Goats
♦ Varies from small dry scab on ear canal to widespread lesions, fatal outcome
♦ Ear site most common with thick scabs in meatus, spread to poll, pasterns
♦ Common in kids of infected does

Horses
♦ Thick crusts at mane, tail, udder, prepuce, axilla
♦ Itching, alopecia, skin thick

Cattle
♦ Lesions on withers, neck, root of tail
♦ Spread to whole body in bad cases
♦ Papules, scabs, spread, coalesce
♦ Alopecia, skin thick
♦ Intense itching

Ear mites
♦ Head-shaking
♦ Ear discharge
♦ Head-rubbing
♦ Touchiness around head

Clinical pathology

Mites easy to see in scrapings.

Diagnosis

General skin lesions resemble:
♦ Mycotic dermatitis
♦ Ked
♦ Lice
♦ Itchmite
♦ Harvest mite infestation
Ear mites need to be differentiated from *Raillietia* spp

Treatment and control

♦ A notifiable disease in most countries with treatments specified in legislation; quarantine, movement restriction compulsory dipping
♦ Thorough dipping, spraying in organophosphate or synthetic pyrethroid acaricide solution cures, provides continuing protection
♦ Ivermectin by injection effective, continuing protection, in cattle, not in sheep unless 2 treatments used
♦ In horses ears need to be cleaned of wax, topical application of suitable acaricide or
♦ Ivermectin systemically very effective

CHORIOPTIC MANGE (TAIL MANGE, LEG MANGE, SCROTAL MANGE) [VM8 p. 1308]

Etiology

♦ *Chorioptes bovis* the common infection on all species
♦ *C. texanus* in cattle, goats, Canadian reindeer

Epidemiology

♦ Mites most active in late winter
♦ Disappear in cattle at pasture
♦ Life cycle completed on host in 3 weeks
♦ Transmission by direct contact, grooming, possibly in bedding; lamb to ewe

Clinical findings

Cattle
♦ Small nodules, exude serum, scabs amongst hairs
♦ Skin thick, wrinkled
♦ Lesions on perineum, back of udder; cause no irritation but unsightly
♦ In bad cases down limbs, causing coronitis, onto rump, around muzzle intense irritation, fall in milk yield

Sheep
♦ Lesions on woolless parts, scrotum, lower hind limbs
♦ Severe scrotal lesion causes testicular degeneration

Horse
♦ Lesions in long hair on lower limbs
♦ Violent stamping hind feet, rubbing pas-

terns on wire, fence rails, especially at night or when resting
♦ Skin scabby, swollen, cracked, greasy

Clinical pathology

Mites in scrapings.

Diagnosis

♦ In horses resembles: greasy heel
♦ In cattle resembles: mucosal disease
♦ In sheep resembles:

- Strawberry footrot
- Ecthyma

Treatment and control

♦ Ivermectin effective in horses if accompanied by clipping of hair, topical acaricidal application, scab removal
♦ Effective topical insecticides include crotoxyphos, phoxim, flumethrin, fenvalerate, amitraz
♦ Recurrence common; 2 treatments at 10 day intervals recommended

28 METABOLIC DISEASES

PARTURIENT PARESIS (MILK FEVER) [VM8 p. 1314]

Etiology

Hypocalcemia.

Epidemiology

Occurrence
♦ Occurs universally
♦ Dairy cows, very rarely beef breeds, recorded in late pregnants fed very poor roughage diet
♦ Few cases hours before, during parturition; most in 48 hours afterwards; significant number up to 8 days after; rare cases up to 8 weeks after
♦ Many late cases are relapses
♦ Area morbidity 3.5–8%; in individual herds may reach 30% of susceptible cows; uncomplicated recovery after treatment in 75–85%

Risk factors
♦ High producing cows, including cows fed heavily before parturition to maximise production
♦ Any aged puerperal cow, mostly in 5–10 year group
♦ All breeds, Channel Island most susceptible
♦ High incidence in some families
♦ High recurrence rate in individual cow
♦ Complete udder emptying during first 48 hours after parturition
♦ Diets containing:
  • Excessive (>100 g daily) calcium
  • Excessive phosphorus (>80 g daily)
  • Excessive other cations, sodium, potassium,
  • High alkalinity
  • High crude protein
♦ Late cases, relapses increased by fatigue, excitement, estrus, low feed intake for 24–48 hours, bouts of diarrhea
♦ Subclinical hypocalcemia occurs in most puerperal dairy cows; risk factors listed above may exaggerate the hypocalcemia

♦ Bovine puerperal subclinical hypocalcemia may occur cyclically

Importance
Death losses, serious sequels which reduce productive life, cause serious losses in high-producing stud cattle.

Clinical findings

In absence of complication or concurrent disease immediate response to intravenous injection of calcium salt solution; complete recovery in 15–30 minutes depending on severity of disease.

Prodromal stage
♦ Anorexia, milk yield reduced
♦ Rumen stasis
♦ Scant feces
♦ Normal temperature, heart, respiratory rates

Excitement stage
♦ Restlessness
♦ Hypersensitivity
♦ Tremor, tetany
♦ Head shaking, tongue protrusion, teeth grinding in some
♦ Slight fever
♦ Stiff gait, falls easily

Sternal recumbency
♦ Depression, drowsy
♦ Sternal recumbency, unable to rise
♦ Limbs flexed normally
♦ Lateral neck kink, or head turned into flank
♦ Fear gesture when approached – head extended, mouth open, tongue protruded
♦ Hypothermia, skin cool
♦ Heart sound intensity decreased
♦ Heart rate elevated to 80/minute
♦ Pulse small amplitude
♦ Difficulty raising jugular vein
♦ Breathing normal, may be a little grunt or groan with each expiration

510

* Muzzle dry
* Eyes dry, staring
* Pupillary light reflex diminished to absent
* Pupil dilated
* Ruminal stasis, secondary bloat
* Constipation
* Anal relaxation, no anal reflex

Lateral recumbency
* Cow almost comatose
* Lateral recumbency, limbs stuck out but limbs flaccid, cow unable to sit up
* Hypothermia, heart inaudible, pulse impalpable, heart rate up to 120/minute
* Animal dies quietly after course of 12–24 hours

Complications
* **Hypomagnesemia** – tetany, hypersensitivity, restlessness persist after early episodes of:
  * Tremor, eyelid twitching, trismus, tetanic convulsions
  * Heart sounds loud, heart rate fast, dyspnea
  * Death during a convulsion
* **Dystokia** – in cows with milk fever at or before calving
  * Cervix incompletely dilated
  * Uterus atonic
  * Treatment with calcium relieves dystokia
* **Uterus prolapse**

Clinical pathology
* Total serum calcium levels below 8 mg/dl (2.0 mmol/l), usually below 5 mg/dl, sometimes below 2 mg/dl
* Total serum magnesium levels elevated to 4– 5 mg/dl (1,62–2.06 mmol/l)
* Serum inorganic phosphorus levels depressed to 1.5–3.0 mg/dl (0.48–0.97 mmol/l)
* Serum levels of creatine kinase elevated in some

Necropsy findings

No significant lesions unless concurrent disease, e.g. food aspiration into trachea, lungs.

Diagnosis

Needs to be differentiated from:
* Downer cow syndrome
* Non-parturient hypocalcemia
* Parturition syndrome
* Acetonemia
* Hypomagnesemic tetany
* Coliform mastitis

* Acute diffuse peritonitis
* Acute septic metritis
* Aspiration pneumonia
* Radial paralysis
  * Makes strong rising efforts
  * Stands when assisted
  * Unable to extend a fore limb
  * Limb takes no weight
* Gastrocnemius muscle rupture:
  * Makes strong efforts to rise
  * Unable to extend hock, limb
  * Stands when assisted
  * Hock close to ground
  * May be bilateral
* Maternal obstetric paralysis:
  * Makes strong rising effort
  * When lifted in sling cannot take much or any weight on limb
  * Least defect is weakness of limb, repeated kicking with limb, fetlock knuckling
  * Usually signs of difficult labor
* Sciatic nerve injury
  * Makes strong rising efforts
  * Stands when assisted
  * Unable to flex affected hind limb
  * Limb takes no weight
* Obturator nerve injury
  * Makes strong rising efforts
  * Stands when assisted
  * Involuntary hind limb abduction, goes down
  * Can remain standing if hocks tied together
* Coxofemoral joint dislocation
  * Strong rising effort
  * May sit like a dog
  * Affected limb not flexed
  * Extreme lateral mobility of limb
  * Limb abnormally placed laterally or posteriorly
  * Crepitus in hip joint
  * May be bilateral
  * May stand with assistance but limb not flexed nor extended, goes down easily
* Ischemic muscle necrosis (degenerative myopathy)
  * History of recumbency for more than 24 hours
  * Makes strong rising efforts
  * May stand when assisted in sling
  * Unable to flex affected hind limb
  * Limb takes no weight, fetlock knuckles
  * High creatine kinase, alanine, aspartase aminotransferase

Treatment

Basic
* Calcium borogluconate 25% solution:

- Small cow 350–500 ml
- Large cow 800–1000 ml
- Half dose intravenously, half subcutaneously
- Underdosing by farmer a common error

Response
▸ **Positive response** syndrome includes:
- Belching
- Muscle tremor, may shake body
- Muzzle sweating
- Heart rate slows, sounds louder, pulse amplitude increases
- Defecation of firm, mucus-covered turds
- Voluminous urination

▸ **Incomplete reaction**, i.e. improvement in pulse, heart beat, rumen movement, defecation, muzzle sweat but patient unable to rise due to:
- Prolonged recumbency before treatment
- Downer cow syndrome
- Hypophosphataemia
- Muscle, nerve, bone conditions listed above under diagnosis

▸ **Adverse reaction** indicating need to slow or stop injection, reconsider diagnosis:
- Serious heart rate increase
- Serious heart irregularity
- Sudden death

▸ Causes of adverse reaction include:
- Too rapid injection
- Overdosing, as in repeated subcutis injections by farmer before intravenous injection by veterinarian
- Presence of toxemia, e.g. coliform mastitis
- Cow excited, frightened, hyperthermic, e.g in early stages of milk fever

▸ **Relapse** due to:
- Extreme susceptibility of individual cow; usually a mature, high-producing Jersey with history of disease in previous lactations; often first attack will be before or at parturition
- Inadequate dose of calcium, failure to give some injection subcutaneously
- Complete milking out

Supplementary treatment
▸ To avoid adverse reactions, relapses, incomplete recoveries supplements to the basic treatment (above) include —
- Compound parenteral injections including glucose, magnesium, phosphorus; many variations available commercially; choice often based on satisfaction provided in a particular area
- Incomplete milking out for 48–72 hours

- Frequent turning from side to side, massage of upper limbs
- Early treatment
- Farmer education about the need to get early rising
- Slinging, by hips, mobile slings for use in pasture
- Pharmacological, electrical stimulants widely used

Control

▸ In low-incidence herds monitor cows closely at parturition time, treat cases early
▸ In high-incidence herds:
- Consider genetic selection
- Adjust feeding program
- Institute a prophylaxis procedure

Feeding management
▸ Because of practical difficulties in manipulating dietary concentration of calcium phosphorus content and ratio in diet use supplement of ammonium sulfate or ammonium chloride, each at 100 g/head/day significantly reduces milk fever incidence
▸ Reduced feed intake in dry period is also used, and will reduce milk fever incidence but creates risk of acetonemia, pregnancy toxemia
▸ Calcium intake should not be excessive (<100–125 g/head/day) in dry period

Calcium gel treatment
Before calving treat by stomach tube with **calcium gel** (containing 150 g calcium per dose for 3 doses, 24 hours before, 2 hours before, 12 hours after calving), plus dietary supplement to give calcium content of 1% of diet thereafter; if hypomagnesemia a possibility 60 g magnesium oxide in daily ration.

Vitamin D analogs
▸ Most commonly used is a single intramuscular injection of vitamin D_3 2–8 days before calving; results are variable but generally effective; alternative preparations used include
- 25-hydroxycholecalciferol
- 1,25-dihydroxyvitamin D_3
- 24-F-1,25-dihydroxyvitamin D_3
- 1-α hydroxyvitamin D_3

▸ Protocols for administration of these preparations are often complicated, principally by the need to predict date of calving; calving induction with corticosteroid plus the vitamin D analog is used but care needed to avoid other losses

BOVINE NON-PARTURIENT HYPOCALCEMIA [VM8 p. 1322]

Epidemiology

♦ Usually history of grazing green cereal crop
♦ Bout of diarrhea
♦ Rumen stasis due to high grain diet not severe enough to cause carbohydrate engorgement

Clinical findings

♦ Recumbency
♦ Recovers with standard calcium treatment for milk fever

Clinical pathology

Total serum calcium levels below 8 mg/dl (2.0 mmol/l).

OVINE HYPOCALCEMIC PARESIS [VM8 p. 1319]

Etiology

Depression of tissue fluid levels of ionized calcium occurs as a result of imbalance between calcium input, from diet plus resorption from bones, relative to calcium output in deposition in fetuses or secretion in colostrum or milk.

Epidemiology

♦ As outbreaks in pregnant (last 6 weeks) or lactating (first 10 weeks) ewes exposed to:
• Forced exercise
• Long-distance transport
• Sudden feed deprivation
• Grazing on oxalate-rich plants, green cereal crops, luxuriant, low-calcium-content pasture, after drought
♦ Outbreaks in dry sheep up to 1 year old on green oat grazing or short pasture
♦ Feedlot sheep on diets supplemented with magnesium as prophylaxis against hypomagnesemia

Clinical findings

♦ Early cases stilted, proppy gait
♦ Tremor of shoulder muscles
♦ Recumbency in some, not all
♦ Sternal recumbency, legs underneath or stretched out behind
♦ Head rested on ground
♦ Rumen flaccid

♦ Nostrils plugged with dried mucus
♦ Breathing fast
♦ Pulse impalpable
♦ Terminally flaccid paresis, somnolence
♦ Death in 6–12 hours without treatment
♦ Dramatic recovery with calcium treatment

Additional syndrome
Young sheep may also show poor growth, lameness, bone fragility (see calcium nutritional deficiency).

Clinical pathology

Total serum calcium level <4.6 mg/dl.

Necropsy findings

No lesions apart from those of concurrent, complicating disease.

Diagnosis

Can be confused with:
♦ Pregnancy toxemia
♦ Carbohydrate engorgement
♦ Soluble oxalate poisoning

Treatment

♦ 50–100 ml 25% calcium borogluconate I/V or S/C.

Control

♦ Avoid high calcium diets in late pregnancy
♦ Avoid alimentary tract stasis, feed deprivation, excitement, stress, exposure to inclement weather, transport, sudden changes of feed

CAPRINE PARTURIENT PARALYSIS [VM8 p. 1319]

Similar to bovine parturient paresis in all respects.

'DOWNER COW SYNDROME' [VM8 p. 1328]

Etiology

A complication of hypocalcemic parturient paresis encouraged in its development by:
♦ A dystokia
♦ Slippery footing
♦ Delay in treating patient with milk fever

- Excessive body weight of patient
- Concurrent hypophosphatemia
- Concurrent hypokalemia in **creeper** cows
- Inadequate dose of calcium in treatment of milk fever

Epidemiology

- Variable, low incidence
- Case fatality rate from death, euthanasia 60%
- Commonest in high producers, concurrent with milk fever
- Just before or in few days after calving most common

Clinical findings

- Prior history of milk fever in most
- Recumbency, unable to rise for 24 hours
- Bright, alert: appetite, water intake, urination, defecation normal
- Most patients make repeated attempts to rise
- Most can lift hindquarters a few centimeters only
- Progress forwards by crawling with fore limbs, hind limbs drag out behind in frog-like posture, the **creepers**
- Patient tends always to end up lying on affected limb: normal limb pushes rear end over when attempting to rise
- On good, rough footing, with cow lying on normal limb, energetic manual lift on tail head enables some cows to get to feet; inclined to go down again when weight put on affected limb
- Some patients assume lateral recumbency with opisthotonous but sit normally when raised to sternal recumbency but soon lapse back into lateral position
- Patients still recumbent at 7 days unlikely to rise but some can continue for weeks if light in weight, placid temperament, carefully nursed
- Euthanasia usually necessary in laterally recumbent cases

Complications
- Acute mastitis
- Decubitus ulcers at major limb joints
- Further injury to limbs

Clinical pathology

- No biochemical differences between milk fever cows that become downers and those that do not
- Serum levels of creatine kinase, serum glutamic oxaloacetic acid transaminase, alanine, aspartase aminotransferase elevated, reducing to normal by day 7
- Marked proteinuria (unexplained) in most

Necropsy findings

- Variable degrees of skeletal myopathy in upper hind limbs
- Variable damage to sciatic, peroneal nerves
- Unexplained acute, focal myocarditis

Diagnosis

Other causes of similar syndrome include:
- Radial paralysis
- Gastrocnemius muscle rupture
- Maternal obstetric paralysis
- Sciatic nerve injury
- Obturator nerve injury
- Coxofemoral joint dislocation
- Ischemic muscle necrosis (degenerative myopathy)

Treatment

Common, inconsistently successful, treatments include:
- Parenteral injections of solutions containing magnesium, phosphate, calcium
- Corticosteroids
- Vitamin E and selenium mixtures
- Slinging of cows which have some motor function remaining
- Repetitive electrical stimulation with cattle prod of upper thigh muscles in laterally recumbent patient

Control

- Early treatment of all recumbent cows; objective of getting them up by 24 hours
- Frequent turning to other side
- Provide rough, dry footing
- Plenty of bedding
- Early use of sling

TRANSIT RECUMBENCY OF RUMINANTS [VM8 p. 1332]

Etiology

Physical exhaustion with/without hypocalcemia.

Epidemiology

Occurrence

Widespread

Occurs after prolonged transport of any class or age of livestock but especially in:
- Late pregnant ewes and cows as replacement stock
- Lambs consigned to feedlots
- Cows and sheep to abattoirs
- Morbidity variable, case fatality high

Risk factors
- Severe physical stress
- Prolonged deficiency of feed and water
- Hot weather
- Overcrowding

Importance
Serious death losses.

Clinical findings

- Signs while still on train; may have to be manhandled off
- Restlessness
- Trismus, teeth grinding
- Complete anorexia
- Rumen stasis
- Staggering
- Hind limb paresis, paralysis
- Lateral recumbency in lambs
- Recumbency
- Coma, death after 3–4 day course

Clinical pathology

- Mild hypocalcemia, hypophosphatemia in cattle
- Hypocalcemia, hypomagnesemia, hypoglycemia in some sheep; many patients have no abnormality

Necropsy findings

- No significant lesion
- Ischemic myonecrosis in a few

Diagnosis

Can be confused with:
- Vitamin E and selenium nutritional deficiency
- Heat exhaustion
- Exertional myopathy

Treatment

- Some cases respond to intravenous fluids containing calcium, magnesium salts, phosphates, glucose
- Large volumes isotonic fluids intravenously recommended but impractical in the usual circumstance of a group problem; rehydration by oral fluid alimentation effective
- Corticosteroids as support therapy

Control

- Provide feed and water before and during transport
- Tranquilizer before travel in nervous animals
- Minimum feed and water for first 24 hours after episode
- Minimum exercise for 3 days

LACTATION TETANY OF MARES
(ECLAMPSIA, TRANSIT TETANY)
[VM8 p. 1332]

Etiology

Hypocalcemia.

Epidemiology

- In lactating mares at about:
  - 10 days after foaling
  - 2 days after weaning
- Stallions, geldings, dry mares subjected to feed deprivation, physical stress
- Can be outbreaks with high morbidity, many recover spontaneously but case fatality rate may be 60% especially lactating mares at foal heat or weaning

Risk factors
- Mares with heavy milk flow
- Mares on lush green pasture
- Session of hard physical work
- Trapping, confinement of wild ponies
- Prolonged transport

Clinical findings

- Profuse sweating
- Limb tetany causes unwillingness to move, stiff gait, elevated tail
- Dyspnea
- Wide nostril dilation
- Diaphragm spasm causes thumping hiccough in some

- Masseter muscle fibrillation, trismus, no third eyelid prolapse
- Patient anxious, hypersensitive to movement, touch
- Transient temperature elevation
- Heart rate fast, irregular
- Unable to prehend or chew but tries persistently
- Gut sounds reduced
- No urination, defecation
- At 24 hours recumbency, tetanic convulsions
- Death after course of 48 hours
- Prompt, complete recovery after intravenous calcium therapy

Clinical pathology

- Hypocalcemia (4–6 mg/dl, 1.0–1.5 mmol/l)
- Serum magnesium levels variably increased, decreased

Necropsy findings

No specific lesions.

Diagnosis

Resembles:
- Tetanus
- Colic
- Laminitis

Treatment

Slow intravenous calcium borogluconate solution to effect.

Control

Avoid transport, physical stress in lactating mares.

HYPOMAGNESEMIC TETANY
(LACTATION TETANY, GRASS
TETANY, GRASS STAGGERS,
WHEAT PASTURE POISONING)
[VM8 p. 1333]

Etiology

Hypomagnesemia caused by a combination of nutritional deficiency and metabolic factors which reduce magnesium's availability or increase its loss by the body.

Epidemiology

Occurrence

- Important disease in UK, northern Europe, North America, Australia, New Zealand
- Commonest in 4–7 year old cows in early lactation
- Occurs principally in well-defined management circumstances:
  - Lactating cows turned out from barn onto lush grass-dominant pasture in spring – **classical lactation or grass tetany**
  - Any type of cattle grazing young green cereal crops – **wheat pasture poisoning**
  - Beef or dry dairy cattle running at pasture in winter with inadequate nutrition and changeable, inclement weather
  - Housed cattle on poor feed
- Morbidity variable, up to 12%; case fatality rate high, 30–100%

Risk factors

- Grass-dominant pastures – low magnesium content
- Cool-season grasses most hazardous
- Grasses with high potassium content relative to calcium, magnesium, e.g. *Dactylis glomerata, Phalaris arundinacea*
- Pasture top-dressed with nitrogen dangerous, more so if potash added
- Early growing season, especially during rapid growth after cold wet weather
- Cereal crop grazing has high potassium, low magnesium content
- Local soil types influence electrolyte content of pasture
- Bouts of diarrhea, as on lush pasture, reduce sojourn in colon, reduces magnesium absorption
- Preserved feed made from low magnesium content pasture fed to housed, lactating animals
- Partial starvation reduces magnesium intake
- Cold, wet, windy weather without shelter

Clinical findings

Acute

- Sudden onset of anxiety, extreme alertness
- Muscle tremor, ear twitch
- Extreme hypersensitivity; slight disturbances precipitate bouts of bellowing, frenzied galloping
- Staggering gait, easy falling
- Tetanic-clonic convulsions with opisthotonus, nystagmus, jaw champing, frothy salivation, ear pricking, eyelid retraction,
- Quiet periods between convulsions

◆ Hyperthermia
◆ Heart, respiratory rates high
◆ Heart sounds very loud
◆ Response to treatment with magnesium solutions intravenously very good but untreated cases die after a course of 30–60 minutes

Subacute

◆ 3–4 day onset
◆ Slight inappetence, milk yield reduced
◆ Wild expression
◆ Exaggerated movements
◆ Throws head about
◆ Frequent urination, defecation
◆ Ruminal movement decreased
◆ Tremor
◆ Mild tetany of hind limbs and tail
◆ Unsteady, straddling gait
◆ Trismus, opisthotonus
◆ Convulsion easily stimulated
◆ Spontaneous recovery in few days, *or*
◆ Good response to treatment with magnesium solution intravenously; tendency to relapse, *or*
◆ Continuous convulsions, death

Hypomagnesemic milk fever syndrome

◆ Paresis–recumbency–circulatory collapse syndrome but hyperesthesia, tetany instead of somnolence, flaccidity
◆ Poor response to treatment with calcium alone, good with combined calcium and magnesium solutions

Chronic

◆ Many subclinical cases in herd
◆ Some sudden deaths
◆ Dullness, indifferent appetite
◆ Depressed milk yield of herd as a whole
◆ Occasional cases of acute, subacute hypomagnesemia or the hypomagnesemic parturient paresis syndrome

Clinical pathology

◆ Serum magnesium levels below 1.2 mg/dl (0.4 mmol/l)
◆ Lower levels of serum magnesium encountered in clinically normal animals in high-risk herds
◆ Serum calcium levels often reduced to 5–8 mg/dl
◆ Hyperkalemia common in acute disease and in wheat pasture poisoning
◆ Ventricular cerebrospinal fluid magnesium levels reduced, normals are same as in serum; levels unchanged at death until 12 hours later
◆ Urinary magnesium levels reduced; can be used as herd guide; creatinine-corrected urinary magnesium concentration a more sensitive indicator of herd magnesium status than serum levels

Necropsy findings

◆ Blood extravasations in subcutis, under pericardium, endocardium, pleura, peritoneum, intestinal mucosa in some cases
◆ Magnesium content vitreous humor up to 48 hours after death is accurate indicator of patient's premortal magnesium status, provided external temperature dies not exceed 23°C (73°F)

Diagnosis

Similar diseases:
◆ Lead poisoning
◆ Bovine spongiform encephalopathy
◆ Rabies
◆ Nervous acetonemia
◆ *Claviceps paspali* poisoning

Treatment

◆ 500 ml intravenous injection solution containing:
  • Calcium borogluconate 25%
  • Magnesium hypophosphite 5%
◆ Followed by a subcutaneous injection of 200 ml of 50% magnesium sulfate
◆ Magnesium sulfate (200–300 ml of 20% solution) alternatively to the combined solution recommended in some areas but is likely to be cardiotoxic
◆ All animals in the group to receive dietary magnesium supplement (see below)

Control

◆ Dietary supplementation of magnesium as oxide, carbonate, sulfate, phosphate at daily rate of at least 60 g magnesium/day by:
  • Foliar dusting in intensive grazing systems
  • Mixing with molasses into hay
  • Drenching
  • Magnesium-rich pellets
  • Heavy, reticulum retention bullets
  • Pasture top-dressing with magnesium-rich fertilizers
  • Supplement in drinking water
◆ Managing pastures by:

- High-risk pastures to be grazed by low-risk animals
- Feeding high-risk animals on rough pasture plus magnesium-treated hay
- Including legumes in seeding mixture
- Avoiding use of potash fertilizers or using only in fall
- Use of magnesium-rich fertilizers
♦ Providing shelter sheds or trees
♦ Postpone calving season

HYPOMAGNESEMIC TETANY OF
SHEEP [VM8 p. 1336]

♦ Recorded in any class of sheep, including wethers grazing young green cereal crops
♦ Also in ewes with heavy milk yield, raising fat lambs
♦ Clinical syndrome similar to ovine hypocalcemic paresis
♦ Serum magnesium levels 0.5 mg/dl
♦ Resembles acute *Phalaris aquatica* poisoning
♦ Treatment is 50 ml intravenous injection solution containing calcium borogluconate 25%, magnesium hypophosphite 5%
♦ Prophylaxis is target of 7 g magnesium intake/day by methods described under cattle disease

HYPOMAGNESEMIC TETANY OF
CALVES [VM8 p. 1341]

Etiology

Dietary deficit of magnesium causes hypomagnesemia.

Epidemiology

Occurrence
♦ Recorded only in calves; produced experimentally in foals
♦ Poor calf rearing practices in winter housing; usually milk-only diets for calves older than 2 months
♦ Sporadic cases, occasional outbreaks

Risk factors
♦ A milk diet for calves heavier than 50 kg
♦ Roughage low in magnesium
♦ Chronic diarrhea, reducing magnesium absorption

Importance
♦ Uncommon disease
♦ Serious death losses on affected farms

Clinical findings

♦ Constant ear-flicking first sign
♦ Hyperesthesia to touch
♦ Apprehensive when approached, retraction eyelids
♦ Exaggerated tendon reflexes
♦ Head-shaking, droopy ears
♦ Opisthotonus
♦ Ataxia
♦ Difficulty getting to bucket interferes with drinking
♦ Tremor
♦ Kicking at belly
♦ Frothing at mouth
♦ Limb tetany
♦ Convulsions with trismus, apnea, clonic–tonic limb movements, defecation, urination, alternating retraction, protrusion of eyeballs, extreme tachycardia
♦ Cyanosis, death after course of 20–30 minutes, *or*
♦ Recovery to normal with subsequent recurrences

Clinical pathology

♦ Serum magnesium levels below 0.8 mg/dl (0.33 mmol/liter)
♦ Depressed serum calcium levels
♦ Bone calcium:magnesium ratio greater than 90:1 indicates severe magnesium depletion; normal is 55:1
♦ Urine magnesium levels depressed

Necropsy findings

♦ Calcification spleen, diaphragm, calcified plaques in aorta, endocardium in some cases
♦ extensive congestion in all organs, hemorrhages in gall bladder, under endocardium, in pericardial fat, aorta, mesentery, intestinal wall, all associated with terminal venous necrosis, in some cases

Diagnosis

Similar diseases are:
♦ Acute lead poisoning
♦ Tetanus
♦ Strychnine poisoning
♦ Polioencephalomalacia
♦ Enterotoxemia due to *Clostridium perfringens* type D
♦ Hypovitaminosis A
♦ Encephalitis
♦ Meningitis

Treatment

ntravenous magnesium sulfate solution 100 ml of 10%) corrects deficit for 24 hours; upplement with dietary magnesium.

Control

* Dietary supplementation beginning at 7 days old; after that skeletal attrition will have occurred; continued to 10 weeks old
* Magnesium 1 g/day to 5 weeks, 2 g/day to 10 weeks, 3 g/day after 10 weeks
* 2 sheep magnesium-rich bullets effective
* Indoor calves on milk diet need calcium, magnesium, vitamin D supplement

ACETONEMIA OF CATTLE
[VM8 p. 1343]

Etiology

Negative nutritional balance caused by inadequate nutrition.

Epidemiology

Occurrence
* Disease of dairy cattle
* Occurs all countries, especially in intensive dairy industries
* Commonest in housed cows in winter
* 90% of cases in first 60 days, most in first 30 days, of lactation
* Cows of any age, rare at first lactation, peak at fourth
* Morbidity low, usually about 5%; case fatality nil

Risk factors
* Low energy intake
* High protein intake
* Excessively fat cows
* Intercurrent disease limiting feed intake, e.g. milk fever, foot rot,

Importance
Production loss during illness; poor return to full lactation in untreated cases.

Clinical findings

Wasting syndrome
* Gradual, moderate decreased milk yield, appetite during 2–4 days
* Grain not eaten, hay is
* Pica in some
* Weight loss
* Cutaneous elasticity lost
* Feces firm, dry
* Moderate depression, disinclined to move
* Temperature, pulse, respiratory rates normal
* Ruminal movements decreased in amplitude, number
* Ketone odor on breath, in milk
* May be transient bouts staggering, blindness
* Spontaneous recovery but milk yield not regained

Nervous syndrome
* Sudden onset 1–2 hour episodes of bizarre syndrome
* Circling
* Straddling or legs-crossed posture
* Head-pressing, leaning into stanchion
* Blindness
* Aimless wandering
* Vigorous licking of self or fixed objects
* Depraved appetite
* Chewing movements with excessive salivation
* Hyperesthesia; bellows on stroking, pinching
* Moderate tremor, tetany in some
* Gait incoordinated
* Self injury in some
* Bouts recur at 8–12 hour intervals

Subclinical disease
* Ketonuria
* Milk yield depressed
* Reduced fertility, ovarian dysfunction, endometritis

Clinical pathology

* Hypoglycemia – 20–40 mg/dl; severity of clinical signs closely related to severity of hypoglycemia
* Ketonuria – 80–1300 mg/dl; basis for field-test using tablets, paper strips; positive test purple color in 30 seconds; primary ketosis cases give deep purple, secondary cases give mauve color
* Ketonemia 10–100 mg/dl
* Milk ketone levels increased – up to 40 mg/dl
* Liver glycogen levels low, glucose tolerance curve normal
* Blood volatile fatty acid levels very high
* Ruminal butyric acid elevated relative to acetic, propionic acids
* Mild hypocalcemia – 9 mg/dl

Necropsy findings

♦ Not a fatal disease
♦ Fatty degeneration of liver

Diagnosis

Wasting syndrome may be confused with:
♦ Traumatic reticuloperitonitis
♦ Bovine pyelonephritis
♦ Indigestion
♦ Left abomasal displacement

Nervous syndrome may be confused with:
♦ Listeriosis
♦ Rabies
♦ Sporadic bovine encephalopathy
♦ Hepatic encephalopathy
♦ Polioencephalomalacia

Treatment

♦ **Replacement therapy** – I/V injection 500 ml 50% glucose solution; rapid improvement, relapse common
♦ Subcutaneous injection concentrated glucose solutions **not** recommended
♦ Plus oral propylene glycol or glycerin (225 g twice daily for 2 days, then 110 g daily for 2 days) by drench or in feed but some cows refuse to eat it
♦ Alternatives to propylene glycol, sodium propionate, lactates, also effective but response slow
♦ **Hormonal therapy** — glucocorticoids, e.g. dexamethazone, produce hyperglycaemic effect within 24 hours, lasting 4–6 days
♦ Insulin used in cases unresponsive to corticosteroid, glucose therapy

Control

Procedures vary in their applicability to particular situations in which the disease occurs.
♦ Cows should be in moderate condition at calving (<10% with body condition score 4)
♦ Best preventive feed in late pregnant cows is ground maize
♦ Housed cows should get some exercise every day; herd turned out at first opportunity in spring
♦ Adequate cobalt, copper, phosphorus, iodine in ration
♦ Prophylactic feeding sodium propionate (110 g/day), propylene glycol (150 ml/day), glycerin, from calving for 6–8 weeks
♦ Monensin has prophylactic effects but needs care to avoid side effects
♦ Monitoring of blood glucose or betahyd-

roxybutyrate, or urine ketones and improvement in herd diet, or individual cow treatments instituted when indicated may be profitable in problem herds

EWE PREGNANCY TOXEMIA
[VM8 p. 1348]

Etiology

Negative nutritional balance due to inadequate nutrition in late pregnancy in twin or large single pregnant ewes.

Epidemiology

Occurrence
♦ Widespread in all sheep industries, especially in intensive systems
♦ Morbidity very variable; outbreaks due usually to management error, e.g penning ewes without feed for a day, change to different kind of feed
♦ Case fatality rate with or without treatment close to 100%

Risk factors
♦ Late pregnant ewes, last month
♦ Adult ewes carrying multiple lambs or large singles
♦ Decline in plane of nutrition during last 2 months of pregnancy in previously well-fed ewes; sudden further deprivation during management procedures, e.g. crutching, transport, often precipitates severe outbreak 48 hours later
♦ Overfat ewes
♦ Intercurrent disease, e.g. foot rot, reducing feed intake

Importance
Severe death losses, usually in studs or intensively managed farms.

Clinical findings

Early stages
♦ Separation from flock, alert bearing, disinclination to move (all indicating blindness)
♦ Walks into objects, head-presses
♦ May lap water continuously
♦ Constipation
♦ Teeth-grinding
♦ Brief convulsive episodes, often missed
  • Lip-twitching
  • Jaw-champing with salivation
  • Cog-wheel dorsiflexion, or lateral deviation of head

- Circling in either direction
- Recumbency, tonic–clonic convulsion

Later stages
- Somnolence
- More visible convulsive episodes
- Star-gazing posture
- Incoordination, easy falling
- Ketone smell on breath
- Recumbency
- Fetal death common; followed by toxemia in ewe
- Death in coma after course of 6–8 days

Clinical pathology

- Hypoglycemia early; terminally blood glucose levels normal to high
- Ketonemia, ketonuria
- Severe metabolic acidosis
- Terminal uremia
- Dehydration
- Elevated plasma cortisol levels (>10ng/ml terminally

Necropsy findings

- Severe fatty degeneration of liver
- Twin lambs or large single; usually dead
- Poorly defined renal lesion

Diagnosis

Needs to be differentiated from:
- Hypocalcemic paresis
- Listeriosis
- Rabies
- Brain abscess
- Coenurosis
- Otitis media
- Louping-ill

Treatment

- Response to treatments recommended for bovine acetonemia unsatisfactory
- In ewes still able to stand 25 mg dexamethazone effective; may be due to birth induction resulting
- Good results recorded with anabolic steroids, e.g. 30 mg trenbolone acetate
- Other expensive, complicated treatments reported
- Removal of fetus by hormonal induction, caesarean but only in early stages before condition irreversible

Control

- Avoid management errors; especially ensure nutrition plane rising, no forced inanition; ensure weight gain of 10% in ewes carrying single lambs, 18% for those with twins, during last 2 months of pregnancy
- Examine flock daily, treat suspects with propylene glycol orally; start supplementary feeding

GOAT DOE PREGNANCY
TOXEMIA [VM8 p. 1346]

- Both acetonemia type (as in cows) and pregnancy toxemia type (as in ewes) syndromes occur
- Exaggerated dominance/submissive attitudes in goats may lead to inadequate feed intake by some does where herd fed heavily on grain in self-feeders

FATTY INFILTRATION OF THE
LIVER IN CATTLE (FAT COW
SYNDROME, PREGNANCY
TOXEMIA OF CATTLE)
[VM8 p. 1354]

Etiology

Mobilization of excessive quantities of fat from body depots and their deposition in the liver because of:
- Deprivation of feed in fat, heavily pregnant beef cows, *or*
- Sudden demand for energy in early lactating dairy cows

Epidemiology

- Dairy and beef herds
- Increased occurrence in farms with erratic or high risk management
- Morbidity about 1%; case fatality rate about 100%

Risk factors
- A disease caused in dairy cows by the management practices aimed at maximizing milk yield per cow, e.g. **challenge feeding** in which feed intake is maximized during late pregnancy and increments of feed are added to the diet as milk yield increases; some very fat cows result
- Young cattle most affected
- Cows carrying twins
- Abnormally long dry periods
- Feeding in groups

♦ Sudden reduction of feed in last 6 weeks of pregnancy to reduce dystokia rate, especially in cows with twins

Clinical findings

Puerperal dairy cows
♦ Usually a history of intercurrent disease, e.g. retained placenta, left abomasal displacement
♦ Incomplete recovery from primary disease
♦ Complete anorexia
♦ Recumbency
♦ Staring gaze, opisthotonus, tremor in some
♦ Severe ketosis
♦ Terminal tachycardia, coma
♦ Death in 7–10 days

Late pregnant beef cows
♦ Aggression
♦ Restlessness, excitement
♦ Stumbling gait, fall easily
♦ Terminally recumbency
♦ Scant, firm feces; yellow diarrhea terminally
♦ Tachycardia
♦ Anorexia
♦ Depression
♦ Respiration rapid, expiratory grunt
♦ Clear, profuse nasal discharge
♦ Flaking muzzle skin
♦ Cows die quietly after 10–14 days

Clinical pathology

♦ Hypoglycemia, ketonemia, ketonuria
♦ Serum non-esterified fatty acids increased
♦ Increased blood levels β-hydroxybutyrate
♦ Elevated serum bilirubin, liver enzyme levels
♦ Liver fat levels in biopsy specimens assessed by estimates of triglyceride content

Necropsy findings

♦ Liver grossly enlarged, pale yellow, friable, greasy
♦ May be intercurrent disease, usual cause of death in fatal cases

Diagnosis

Lactating dairy cows differentiate from:
♦ Left abomasal displacement
♦ Downer cow
♦ Acetonemia, wasting syndrome
♦ Parturition syndrome

Late pregnant beef cows, disease resembles:
♦ Abomasal impaction
♦ Vagus indigestion
♦ Chronic peritonitis

Treatment

♦ Prognosis guarded, especially for anorexic cows
♦ Intensive intravenous fluid, electrolyte therapy, or water plus balanced electrolytes intraruminally
♦ Intraruminal infusion of 5–10 liters rumen juice from normal cow
♦ Corticosteroids, e.g. dexamethazone 20 mg, every second day, or anabolic steroids

Control

♦ Avoid overfatness during dry period or third trimester of pregnancy, by sorting cows into groups on basis of body score, feeding appropriately
♦ Treat puerperal diseases early

EQUINE HYPERLIPEMIA
[VM8 p. 1358]

Etiology

Deficient metabolizable energy in pony mares during late pregnancy, early lactation.

Epidemiology

♦ Widespread occurrence
♦ Pony mares, mostly obese Shetlands; rarely in geldings, stallions secondary to other disease
♦ All ages
♦ Sporadic cases, some outbreaks
♦ Most cases occur 4–8 weeks after foaling
♦ Case fatality rate 65%

Risk factors
♦ Recent transport
♦ Concurrent sand colic, parasitism
♦ Falling nutritional plane during late pregnancy, early lactation

Clinical findings

♦ Depression, anorexia, weight loss
♦ Muscle fasciculation limbs, trunk, neck
♦ Ventral edema in some
♦ Compulsive walking, mania in some
♦ Continuous lapping or attempts to drink but unable to swallow
♦ Heart and respiratory rates increased

♦ Persistent diarrhea terminally
♦ Thick, porridgy, fetid feces
♦ Somnolence, coma
♦ Abortion, may precede recovery
♦ Death after course of 6–8 days

Clinical pathology

♦ Milk-like opalescence of serum, plasma
♦ Total lipids greatly increased up to 4–8 g/dl of serum
♦ Blood glucose normal
♦ Leukocytosis, neutrophilia
♦ Renal, hepatic function tests abnormal
♦ Irreversible metabolic acidosis in late stages

Necropsy findings

♦ Fatty change in most internal organs
♦ Enlarged, yellow–orange liver
♦ Widespread vascular thrombosis, generalized skeletal muscle degeneration

Diagnosis

May be confused with:
♦ Mare hypocalcemia
♦ Congestive heart failure
♦ Hepatitis

Treatment

♦ Identification, treatment of primary disease
♦ Parenteral administration of glucose valuable in very early stages
♦ Insulin 30 iu parenterally with 100 g glucose orally, then 15 iu insulin plus 100 g galactose orally on alternate days
♦ Correction of acidosis

Control

♦ Control program for nutrition, parasite control near parturition for pony mare bands
♦ Periodic blood sample examination for hyperlipemia

STEATITIS [VM8 p. 1360]

♦ Uncommon foal disease, rare in adults
♦ Firm, soft, 2–4 cm dia. plaque-like swellings in adipose tissues
♦ Recognizable most easily in subcutis of belly wall, back, upper neck
♦ Biopsy shows fat necrosis with mineralization

NEONATAL HYPOGLYCEMIA
(BABY PIG DISEASE) [VM8 p. 1360]

Etiology

Inadequate milk intake due to:
♦ Sow's milk supply failure
♦ Piglet nursing failure
♦ Malabsorption due to enteropathy

Epidemiology

Occurrence
♦ Mostly UK, USA
♦ Piglets less than 4 days old
♦ Twin and triplet lambs
♦ Morbidity 30–70%; case fatality rate 100%, many weak piglets overlaid

Risk factors
♦ Immature or undersized neonates
♦ Exposure to cold
♦ Piglets with diseases causing anorexia and malabsorption, e.g. coliform septicemia, transmissible gastroenteritis, streptococcal infection, myoclonia congenita, neonatal hemolytic disease
♦ Diarrheic disease in calves which receive insufficient milk, milk replacer in convalescence
♦ Mismothering by ewes

Clinical findings

♦ Piglets younger than 1 week
♦ Stumbling gait, easy falling
♦ Shivering, dullness, anorexia
♦ Weak squeal
♦ Hypothermia, cold skin
♦ Ruffled hair
♦ Heart rate slow, cardiac impulse weak
♦ Marked pallor
♦ Recumbency
♦ Convulsions in some:
  • Aimless head, fore limb movements
  • Galloping movements all limbs, opisthotonus, jaw champing
  • Tortuous movements, head, neck rigidity
♦ Coma, death after 24–36 hour course
♦ Rapid response to treatment

Clinical pathology

♦ Blood glucose levels fall to below 50 mg/dl, often to 7 mg/dl in piglets, below 40 mg/dl in calves
♦ Elevated blood urea nitrogen levels

Necropsy findings

♦ No visible lesions
♦ Little or no milk curd in stomach
♦ Liver glycogen levels low

Diagnosis

Resembles:
♦ Viral encephalomyelitis
♦ Pseudorabies
♦ Streptococcal meningoencephalitis
♦ Listeriosis

Treatment

♦ Piglets – 15 ml 20% glucose solution I/P every 4–6 hours till sucking returns
♦ Lambs – 10 mg/kg body weight glucose as 20% solution I/P
♦ Protection from cold (environment temperature should be 27–32°C (80–90°F)

Control

♦ Close surveillance of piglets during first week
♦ Maintain environmental temperature
♦ Ensure adequate colostrum (200 ml/kg in first 18 hours) to lambs

POSTPARTURIENT
HEMOGLOBINURIA [VM8 p. 1362]

Etiology

Hemolytic anemia caused by agents in feed of cattle made susceptible by low phosphorus, copper or selenium intake.

Epidemiology

Occurrence
♦ Widespread
♦ Adult cows calved 2–4 weeks previously
♦ High producing cows in lactations 3–6
♦ Morbidity low, usually sporadic cases; may be outbreak; case fatality 50%

Risk factors
♦ Diets deficient in phosphorus or copper, or possibly selenium
♦ Rape, other cruciferous plants in diet
♦ Lush spring pasture
♦ Very cold drinking water

Importance
Uncommon disease, with severe losses in some herds; easily prevented.

Clinical findings

♦ Anorexia, mild cases may continue to eat
♦ Weakness, stumbling gait, unwilling to move
♦ Serious drop in milk yield
♦ Red-black, slightly turbid urine
♦ Mucosal pallor; possibly jaundice in late stages
♦ Tachycardia, loud heart sounds
♦ Exaggerated cardiac impulse, jugular pulse
♦ Deep respiration, dyspnea in some
♦ Recumbency, death after 3–5 day course

Sequel
♦ 3 week convalescence
♦ Pica
♦ Gangrene in digits, ear tips in some
♦ Acetonemia

Clinical pathology

♦ Erythrocyte counts and hemoglobin levels greatly reduced
♦ Heinz bodies in erythrocytes reported in copper deficiency induced disease
♦ Hemoglobinuria
♦ Serum inorganic phosphorus levels often normal; may be as low as 0.4–1.5 mg/dl
♦ Blood, liver copper levels may be subnormal

Necropsy findings

♦ Blood thin
♦ Carcase jaundiced
♦ Hemoglobinuria

Diagnosis

Similar to other causes of hemoglobinuria:
♦ Bacillary hemoglobinuria
♦ Babesiosis
♦ Leptospirosis
♦ Rape, kale poisoning

Treatment

♦ Avoid excessive restraint, harassment
♦ Blood transfusion with minimum of 5 liters
♦ Sodium acid phosphate solution (60 g in 300 ml water) I/V, same dose subcutaneously; subcutaneous dose repeated 12 hourly for 3 occasions
♦ Sodium acid phosphate or bone meal subsequently as permanent addition to ration or in lick or salt block

Control

◊ Adequate phosphorus supplementation in diet
◊ Copper supplementation in copper deficient areas

PARALYTIC MYOGLOBINURIA (AZOTURIA) [VM8 p. 1364]

Etiology

Skeletal muscle necrosis caused by lactic acid resulting from anaerobic metabolism of muscle glycogen.

Epidemiology

◊ Sporadic cases in performance horses
◊ Horses maintained on full grain rations during period (2–14 days) of sudden cessation of exercise; due usually to minor injuries, riding pleasure horses only at weekends
◊ After general anesthesia
◊ Occasional outbreaks in horses at pasture
◊ Sporadic cases in cattle after release from housing in spring (see nutritional deficiency of selenium and vitamin E)

Clinical findings

◊ Signs commence 15 minutes to 1 hour after exercise, which need be mild only
◊ Profuse sweating
◊ Stiff gait
◊ Reluctant to move
◊ Mild cases, without hemoglobinuria, if rested completely at this stage, may recover
◊ Lateral recumbency
◊ Struggling, attempts to rise
◊ Dyspnea
◊ Temperature elevated
◊ Usually both hind limbs involved; may be only one
◊ Rump, thigh muscles hard, soreness over the area
◊ Urination suspended
◊ Urine brown-red
◊ Death after course of 24–48 hours

Clinical pathology

◊ Myoglobinuria
◊ Casts, protein in urine
◊ Serum creatine kinase markedly elevated for several days

Necropsy findings

◊ Myonecrosis in gluteal, quadriceps, iliopsoas, vastus muscles causing pale discoloration, with a waxy, cooked appearance
◊ Dark brown urine in bladder

Diagnosis

Similar to:
◊ Laminitis
◊ Nutritional deficiency of selenium
◊ Generalized or local myositis
◊ Exertional rhabdomyolysis
◊ Iliac thrombosis
◊ Tying-up

Treatment

◊ Immediate cessation of all exercise; horse moved by motor transport
◊ Avoid recumbency; sling if necessary
◊ Analgesic if pain severe
◊ Corticosteroids I/V
◊ Thiamin hydrochloride (0.5 g I/M daily), selenium and vitamin E preparations, widely used
◊ Intensive intravenous fluid–electrolyte therapy to prevent renal tubular blockage with myoglobin; alkalinization of urine preferred

Control

◊ Reduce grain ration when horses skip training
◊ In high-risk situations commence exercise with gentle walking, increased gradually

HYPERKALEMIC PERIODIC PARALYSIS [VM8 p. 1366]

Etiology

◊ A probable inherited metabolic defect; autosomal dominance of the defect proposed
◊ Resembles hyperkalemic periodic paralysis in humans

Epidemiology

◊ in Quarter Horses
◊ 1–5 years old

Clinical findings

◊ May be history of bouts of muscle fasciculation or involuntary recumbency
◊ Intervals between bouts months or years
◊ bouts of:

- Muscle twitching in neck, trunk, spreading to other areas
- Muscle weakness, swaying, staggery gait
- Dog-sitting posture
- Recumbency in some
♦ Generalized sweating in some
♦ Some patients apprehensive
♦ Temperature normal, heart and respiratory rates may be elevated
♦ Inspiratory stridor in some
♦ Third eyelid prolapse common
♦ During attack percussion of muscle with plexor causes sustained muscular contraction
♦ Spontaneous recovery after course of 30–60 minutes, rarely some hours

Clinical pathology

♦ Serum potassium levels elevated to 5.0–11.7 mEq/liter
♦ Packed cell volume, total plasma protein concentration increased
♦ Electromyographic abnormalities in clinically normal patients is sensitive test for the disease
♦ Disease reproduced in sensitive horses by nasal tube administration of KCl (88–140 mg/kg body weight in 6 liters warm water) 1–2 hours later

Diagnosis

Similar to:
♦ Exertional rhabdomyolysis

♦ Abdominal colic
♦ Esophageal obstruction
♦ Upper respiratory tract obstruction

Treatment

♦ Recovery spontaneous
♦ Recommended treatments during attack include:
  - Sodium bicarbonate 2% solution I/V at 1 mEq/kg *or*
  - Dextrose solution 5% (4.4–6.6 ml/kg) *or*
  - Calcium borogluconate solution (23% at 0.2–0.4 ml/kg) diluted in 1–2 liters of 5% dextrose

Control

♦ Acetazolamide (2.2 mg/kg) orally every 8–12 hours controls subsequent episodes
♦ Feed oaten instead of alfalfa hay, grain 2–3 times daily, free access to salt
♦ Cull affected animals identified by electromyography

LOW MILK FAT SYNDROME
[VM8 p. 1367]

♦ Milk fat reduced, often to less than 50% normal, in normal milk yield
♦ Caused by low fiber diets, lush pasture, finely ground grain, as meal or pelleted

29 DISEASES CAUSED BY NUTRITIONAL DEFICIENCIES

DISEASES CAUSED BY NUTRITIONAL DEFICIENCIES OF MINERAL NUTRIENTS

DEFICIENCIES OF ENERGY AND PROTEIN

(See Starvation and Inanition)

COBALT DEFICIENCY
[VM8 p. 1374]

Etiology

A deficiency of cobalt in the diet causes a deficiency of vitamin B_{12} (cyanocobalamin).

Epidemiology

Occurrence
♦ Many parts of the world; major problem in North America, UK, Australia, New Zealand
♦ Mostly in pastured animals
♦ Sheep more susceptible than cattle
♦ Horses and pigs unaffected

Soil and feed content
♦ Occurs only on soils deficient in cobalt; good relationship between soil and plant contents but not always consistent
♦ Critical soil level <0.25 mg/kg cobalt
♦ Critical feed content/kg dry matter in clinical disease cases:
  • Sheep <0.07 mg/kg
  • Cattle <0.04 mg/kg
♦ Recommended daily intake —
  • Sheep 0.08 mg/kg
  • Growing lambs 0.10 mg/kg
  • Growing cattle >0.04 mg/kg

Risk factors
♦ Young animals
♦ Seasonal variation in pasture content, lowest in spring

♦ Lower content in grasses than legumes
♦ Factors reducing soil content of cobalt:
  • Heavy annual rainfall
  • Heavy liming
  • High soil content of manganese

Importance
♦ Poor ruminant productivity limits use of large areas of land for animal agriculture
♦ Contributes to white liver disease

Clinical findings

♦ Signs commence 6 months after access
♦ Gradual onset of inappetence
♦ Poor growth, milk, wool yield, weight loss
♦ Mucosal pallor
♦ Profuse lacrimation, wool matted on face
♦ Break in wool
♦ Pica
♦ Exercise intolerance
♦ Parturition exacerbates syndrome
♦ Terminal emaciation, weakness, recumbency in presence ample green feed
♦ Abortion
♦ Death after course of 3–12 months

Clinical pathology

♦ All tests difficult to interpret, some chance of error; most reliable test is liver cobalt, vitamin B_{12} content at necropsy
♦ Serum vitamin B_{12} indicative of cobalt deficiency in animals – <0.20–0.25 μg/liter
♦ Plasma cobalt levels of 0.03–0.41 μmol/L
♦ Elevated plasma levels, or simple presence in urine, of methyl-malonic acid (MMA) indicate state of cobalt deficiency
♦ Forminimoglutamic acid in urine indicates cobalt deficiency but occurs only in late stages

◆ Affected animals anemic but hemoglobin, erythrocyte levels normal because of hemoconcentration
◆ Hypoglycemia, low serum alkaline phosphatase
◆ **Dose response trial** and construction of **dose response curve** are critical to diagnosis of cobalt deficiency and monitoring of response in area diagnosis

Necropsy findings

◆ Extreme emaciation
◆ Heavy hemosiderin deposits in spleen, liver
◆ Liver cobalt levels <0.05 mg/kg dry matter
◆ Liver vitamin B_{12} <0.1 mg/kg dry matter

Diagnosis

Resembles other causes of weight loss.

Treatment

◆ Oral dosing sheep with cobalt (1 mg/day) as cobalt sulfate; may be accumulated, administered at 1 week intervals; cattle 10 mg/day
◆ Vitamin B_{12} by injection to sheep 100–300 μg at weekly intervals effective but expensive; effect lasts longer at preferred regimen of 1 mg injection to lambs lasts 14 weeks; lasts 40 weeks in weaners
◆ Overdosing (45 mg/50 kg body weight daily) calves with cobalt causes:
  • Listlessness, anorexia, weight loss
  • Incoordination

Control

◆ Safe minimal cobalt content in feed 0.11 mg/kg dry matter
◆ On deficient pasture all ages, including calves before weaning, require supplement
◆ Pasture top-dressing 400–600 g/ha cobalt sulfate annually *or* 1.2–1.5 kg/ha every 3–4 years; treat animals to cover for period before pasture content elevated
◆ In salt mixture, lick or drinking water; objective is providing 0.1 mg cobalt/day for sheep, 0.3–1.0 mg/day for cattle
◆ Heavy pellets containing 90% cobalt oxide, 5 g pellet for sheep, 20 g pellet for cattle, by mouth to lodge in reticulum; ineffective in preruminant lambs; some failures, require repeat dosing, area problem of mineral coating of pellets countered by supplying abrasive metal pellet
◆ Supply of cobalt, and selenium, in anthel-mintic drench a suitable vehicle if repeated drenching used in worm control

OVINE WHITE LIVER DISEASE
[VM8 p. 1375]

Etiology

Probably a toxic hepatopathy, adequate cobalt intake protective.

Epidemiology

◆ New Zealand, Australia, UK, Norway
◆ Sheep only, usually lambs
◆ Deficient cobalt in pasture

Clinical findings

Acute – photosensitization
Chronic – anemia, emaciation

Clinical pathology

◆ Hepatic function tests depressed
◆ High serum copper

Necropsy findings

Liver gray in color.

Treatment

Vitamin B_{12} curative.

COPPER DEFICIENCY [VM8 p. 1379]

Etiology

◆ Primary – diet contains inadequate copper because:
  • Soil content deficient
  • Soil content adequate but copper unavailable to plants
◆ Secondary – diet contains adequate copper which is unavailable due to:
  • High molybdenum content of diet
  • Dietary inorganic sulfate in combination with molybdenum; heavy superphosphate applications can add sulfate to soil
  • Dietary zinc, iron, lead, calcium carbonate possibly conditioning agent
◆ Supplementary selenium may enhance copper absorption

Epidemiology

Occurrence
◆ Primarily young ruminants
◆ Minor occurrences in horses and pigs

In many large areas in many countries nutritional deficiency of copper causes defined locally as:

♦ **Primary deficiencies:**
  • Lamb **enzootic ataxia** – Australia, New Zealand, USA
  • Cattle **licking sickness** (liksucht) – Netherlands
  • Cattle **falling disease** – Australia
  • Piglet anemia
  • Foal abnormal joints, limbs
♦ **Secondary deficiencies**
  • Sheep **swayback** – UK, USA
  • Sheep *renguerra* – Peru
  • Sheep, cattle **peat scours, teart** – UK, New Zealand, Netherlands, Canada
  • Cattle **salt sick** – USA
  • Cattle **pine** – Scotland
  • Cattle **yellow calf disease** – Hawaii
♦ **Combined copper, cobalt deficiencies**
  • Cattle, sheep **coast disease** – Australia
  • Cattle, sheep **salt sickness** – USA

Soil and feed content
♦ Critical level copper in pasture – <3 mg/kg dry matter
♦ Soil content copper in primary deficiency – <2 mg/kg
♦ Soil content copper in secondary deficiency may be normal (18–22 mg/kg)
♦ Critical molybdenum content in feed <3 mg/kg dry matter safe; disease may occur at 3 mg/kg if copper level also low
♦ Dangerous soil levels of molybdenum include 10 mg/kg and up; naturally occurring or overdosing to promote legume growth

Risk factors – soil
♦ Sandy, organic matter poor soils; heavily weathered coastal sands, low in copper
♦ Marine, river silts, marine black shales, with high molybdenum content
♦ Peat or muck soils reclaimed from swamps; limit copper availability by unknown mechanism

Risk factors – feed
♦ Copper content of pasture lowest in spring and summer
♦ Low blood copper levels in cattle coincide with high rainfall
♦ Availability of copper low in fresh forage, increased in stored hay, silage, high in low fibre cereals, brassicas
♦ Pasture molybdenum content highest in periods of maximum legume growth
♦ Molybdenum effect reduced in hay compared with fresh grass

♦ Housed animals tend to receive imported grain, supplementary feeds containing copper; can be at risk if local stored feed has low copper, high molybdenum

Risk factors – host
♦ Young more susceptible (except falling disease)
♦ Placental transfer of copper less efficient in lambs than calves; more likely to have low liver copper levels at birth
♦ Milk a poor source of copper; weaning lambs enhances copper status
♦ Some sheep breeds genetically influenced to absorb copper more efficiently, e.g. Welsh Mountain superior to Scottish Blackface, and have less susceptibility to copper deficiency

Importance
♦ Some mortalities in falling disease, enzootic ataxia
♦ Massive wastage due to production limitation over large areas

Clinical findings

Bovine subclinical copper deficiency
♦ Blood copper levels <57 mg/dl
♦ Production suboptimal
♦ Increased occurrence no-visible estrus in dairy cows
♦ Improved growth rate, productivity generally after dietary supplementation with copper; wide, unexplained variability in response

Bovine primary copper deficiency
♦ Weight loss
♦ Poor milk production
♦ Anemia in adult cows
♦ Increased occurrence postparturient hemoglobinuria (New Zealand)
♦ Red, black coat color bleached to rust-red, gray
♦ Coat rough, dry
♦ Poor growth in calves
♦ Chronic diarrhea in some but not persistent as in secondary copper deficiency
♦ Bones tend to fracture, including limbs
♦ Ataxia, collapsing after exercise; normal after rest
♦ Itching, hair-licking in some outbreaks
♦ Stiffness, joint enlargement, standing on toes due to flexor tendon contraction; present at birth or develop after weaning

Bovine secondary copper deficiency

♦ As for primary disease except anemia rare
♦ Chronic diarrhea

Bovine falling disease

♦ Normal cows suddenly throw up heads, bellow, fall dead
♦ Some may struggle feebly on sides, bellow intermittently
♦ Rarely survive 24 hours
♦ Sudden death during episode of pivoting on front limbs

Bovine and ovine peat scours

♦ Signs develop within several weeks of going onto pasture
♦ Persistent diarrhea
♦ Watery, yellow–green to black feces, inoffensive odor
♦ Defecation precipitate without lifting tail
♦ Appetite good but emaciation
♦ Hair rough, depigmented, rusty black or gray flecking, especially around eyes
♦ Rapid recovery after oral copper treatment

Bovine pine

♦ Stiff gait
♦ Weight loss
♦ Enlargement of fetlocks, painful on palpation in some
♦ Pasterns upright
♦ Severe lameness in some
♦ Graying of hair
♦ Diarrhea in a few patients
♦ Death after course of 4–5 months

Ovine primary copper deficiency

♦ Syndrome associated with marginal deficiency
♦ More frequent in Merinos
♦ Fine wool is limp, glossy (steely), straight without crimp,
♦ Wool depigmentation, often in bands to match copper-deficient episodes; may be break in wool
♦ Extreme cases have anemia, diarrhea, weight loss, infertility
♦ Easy bone fracture, enzootic ataxia in lambs

Ovine swayback

♦ Primary copper deficiency in breeds genetically susceptible to copper deficiency
♦ Lambs, kids
♦ Some at birth; most at 3–6 weeks old
♦ Born dead, or weak, unable to stand, suck
♦ Spastic incoordination

♦ Blindness in some
♦ Paralysis

Ovine enzootic ataxia

♦ Only unweaned lambs, kids
♦ Some cases at birth
♦ Most at 1–2 months
♦ Hind limb incoordination when driven
♦ Respiratory, heart rates greatly increased with exercise
♦ Progressive excessive joint flexion, fetlock knuckling
♦ Hindquarter wobbling, falling
♦ Lamb may drag itself in sitting posture
♦ Fore limbs affected in some
♦ Recumbency, death due to starvation
♦ Strong limb movement persists until end
♦ Course varies; the lambs affected later live longer, may survive with nervous deficit
♦ Neonatal cases die after course of 3–4 days

Cervine enzootic ataxia

♦ In young, mature adults
♦ Ataxia, hindquarter swaying
♦ Dog-sitting posture, hind limb paralysis

Porcine enzootic ataxia

♦ Rare
♦ Pigs 1–2 months old
♦ Ataxia
♦ Nystagmus
♦ Posterior paresis, recumbency, paddling movements
♦ Death in 3–5 days
♦ Pigs 4–6 months old; posterior paresis to paralysis in 1–3 weeks

Equine limb deformity

♦ Foals at birth or develop up to weaning
♦ Findings lack laboratory confirmation
♦ Slow growth, poor body weight
♦ Limbs stiff, joint enlargement
♦ Stands on toes, flexor tendons contracted
♦ No ataxia, nervous deficit
♦ Slow recovery after weaning; convalescence up to 2 years

Clinical pathology

♦ Measuring blood copper levels of individual animals can be misleading because animals which do not respond subsequently to a diet supplement test may be:
   • Clinically normal animals with marginal levels
   • Thin animals with subnormal levels

A definitive diagnosis requires:

- Estimates of blood copper levels on a sample of the group; size of sample determined statistically
- Determination of copper content of feed, soil, water supply
- Treatment response trial with variables of calf growth rate, calf mortality, reproductive efficiency
♦ Interpretation of plasma, liver copper levels needs to take into account whether patient is in the depletion, marginally deficient, functionally deficient or disease stage of the deficiency
♦ Plasma copper levels indicating:
  - Marginal deficiency: 19–57 μg/dl
  - Hypocuprosis: <19 μg/dl
♦ Normal liver copper levels are:
  - >200 mg/kg dry matter in adult sheep
  - >100 mg/kg dry matter in adult cattle
♦ Low liver copper levels are:
  - <80 mg/kg dry matter in adult sheep
  - <30 mg/kg dry matter in adult cattle
♦ Liver copper levels in neonates and fetuses much higher than in adults
♦ Liver biopsy is a satisfactory source of material for estimation of copper status
♦ Copper content of hair an acceptable measure
♦ Estimation of plasma caeruloplasmin (copper/protein complex) simpler than for blood copper; the estimation is a reliable guide to blood copper levels
♦ Needles, containers used for collection of samples for copper estimation need to be free of copper contamination
♦ Low blood hemoglobin concentrations, erythrocyte counts in advanced cases

Necropsy findings

♦ Emaciation, anemia
♦ Extensive hemosiderin deposits in liver, spleen, kidney
♦ Osteoporosis in lambs, normal appearance in cattle
♦ Epiphyseal plate widening in secondary deficiency
♦ Degeneration elastic fibers in arterial, aortic walls in copper deficient pigs
♦ Low liver copper levels (see above)
♦ In secondary deficiency may be high copper levels in kidney, high molybdenum in liver, kidney, spleen

Swayback

♦ Softening, cavitation cerebral white matter in most cases
♦ Spinal cord demyelination

Enzootic ataxia

♦ Spinal cord demyelination
♦ Softening, cavitation cerebral white matter in a few extreme cases

Falling disease

♦ Flabby, pale myocardium
♦ Muscle fiber atrophy, fibrous tissue replacement

Diagnosis

General copper deficiency syndrome resembles:

♦ Helmintic disease
♦ Inanition, malnutrition

Enzootic ataxia resembles:

♦ Cerebellar agenesis
♦ Enzootic muscular dystrophy
♦ Spinal cord abscess

Peat scours resembles:

♦ Johne's disease
♦ Winter dysentery
♦ Salmonellosis
♦ Mucosal disease
♦ Ostertagiasis, trichostrongylosis

Falling disease resembles:

♦ Enzootic muscular dystrophy
♦ Plant cardiac glycosides
♦ Inherited cardiomyopathy

Treatment

♦ Response to treatment with copper salts dramatic except in advanced cases with irreversible lesions, e.g. nervous tissue demyelination, myocardial fibrosis
♦ Copper sulfate orally; calves to 6 months old 4 g; adults 8–10 g, weekly for 3–5 weeks for primary, secondary deficiency
♦ Other preparations, dose rates in control (below)
♦ Supplementation of diet by addition 3–5% copper sulfate to mineral mixture

Control

♦ Diets protective against primary copper deficiency contain copper at greater than the following levels:
  - Cattle 10 mg/kg dry matter
  - Sheep 5 mg/kg dry matter
  - Mature ponies 3.5 mg/kg dry matter
♦ Diets with copper:molybdenum less than 5:1 conducive to secondary hypocuprosis

Supplementation methods include the following; dose rates are for primary deficiency,

may need to be higher with secondary deficiency, requiring a dose response test:
- **oral dosing** with copper sulfate, by drench:
  - Cattle: 5 g weekly
  - Sheep: 1 g weekly
  - Lambs: 35 mg every 2 weeks
- **Mineral mixture** incorporated into ration to make at least 10 ppm in total ration
- **Salt lick, mineral mixture** free access, containing copper sulfate:
  - Sheep: 0.25–0.5%
  - Cattle: 2%
- **Pasture top-dressing** 10 kg/ha copper sulfate annually; amount needed very variable depending on soil type and rainfall
- Poisoning likely unless rain washes forage clean
- **Drinking water** supplementation has too many difficulties relating to pipes and troughs to be practicable
- **Injectable, slow-release copper preparations** can be used regularly or at potential danger times:
  - Copper calcium ethylenediamine tetraacetate
  - Copper methionate
  - Copper heptonate
  - Copper glycinate
  - Copper oxyquinoline sulfonate
- Some risk of precipitating blackleg in cattle; severe local reaction needs to be hidden in purebred animals by using I/M injection; for meat animals S/C injection gives removable blemish
- Severe overdosing causes heavy mortality; some unexplained deaths; some preparations less hazardous (methionate) than others (calcium edetate, oxyquinoline sulfonate)
- Neonates have copper stores sufficient for about 6 weeks; milk is not a good source, so they need the supplement at about 6 weeks old
- Most injections maintain good blood copper status for 3 months
- **Controlled release glass boluses** administered orally have more prolonged delivery time, up to 1 year
- **Copper oxide needles**, fragments of oxidized copper wire orally, for deposition in forestomachs, provide good blood copper levels for 5 months

IODINE DEFICIENCY [VM8 p. 1395]

Etiology

- Primary – deficient intake in water supply and feed

- Secondary due to:
  - High calcium diet
  - Goitrogenic plant glucosinolates, some of which impede iodine uptake; commonest source *Brassica* spp., meals made from seeds of these plants

Epidemiology

- Primary goiter occurs on all large continental land masses where soil continually leached by heavy rainfall, iodine not replaced by usual onshore wind causing deposition of oceanic iodine
- Florid disease uncommon now because of ease of recognition, prevention
- Major concern is subclinical disease in marginally deficient areas

Risk factors

- Young dams more likely to bear goitrous offspring
- Some breeds more susceptible, e.g. Dorset Horn
- Limestone, low-humus soils easily leached of iodine
- High dietary intake of calcium, heavy liming of pasture
- High mineral content water
- Marked variation between plants in tendency to accumulate iodine; *Holcus lanatus* (Yorkshire fog grass) always has very low content

Clinical findings

General syndrome – Adults

- Loss of bull libido
- Anestrus
- High incidence of aborted, stillborn young in cattle
- Prolonged gestation in mares, ewes, sows

General syndrome – neonates

- High incidence stillbirths, weak neonates
- Partial or complete thinning, loss of hair
- Goiter, palpable, visible in some
- Too weak to stand, suck
- High mortality
- Survivors normal except thyroid enlargement persists
- Thyroid thrill palpable over gland

Cattle – adults

Little thyroid enlargement.

Calves

- Thyroid enlargement, may obstruct respiration
- Weakness in neonates
- High mortality at range; recovery if nursed
- Rarely partial alopecia

Sheep and goats – adults

- Thyroid enlargement
- Otherwise clinically normal

Lambs and kids

- Weak at birth
- General alopecia
- Thyroid gland enlargement

Piglets

- Hairless, especially limbs, stillborn or weak
- Neck myxoedema
- Non-visible thyroid enlargement
- Most die within few hours of birth
- Survivors lethargic, waddling gait, poor growth
- Weak ligaments, joints cause leg weakness

Horses – adults

Thyroid gland enlargement.

Foals

- Weak at birth; do not suck
- Normal hair coat
- Little thyroid enlargement
- Flexion lower fore limbs, extension lower hinds
- Lameness, hock deformity; collapse of central, third tarsal bones

Clinical pathology

- Blood and milk iodine levels good indicators of thyroxine status
- Normal range is 2.4–14 μg protein-bound iodine/100 ml plasma
- In ewe milk iodine concentration <8 μg/liter indicates iodine deficiency

Necropsy findings

- Thyroid enlargement, alopecia, myxedema
- Thyroid weight increased
- Thyroid iodine content low
- Thyroid hyperplasia
- Hypoplastic hair follicles
- Delayed osseous maturation

Diagnosis

Resembles:
- Inherited goiter
- Continuous, low-level cyanogenetic glucoside poisoning
- Unidentified goitrogens suspected in *Glycine max* (soybean meal), *Arachis hypogaea* (ground or peanuts)
- Goiter due to gross bacterial pollution of feedstuffs, e.g. by sewage, feeding sewage sludge

Treatment and control

- Recommended daily intake:
  - Lactating, pregnant females: 0.8–1.0 mg/kg dry matter in feed
  - Other cattle 0.1–0.3 mg/kg dry matter in feed
- Supply by salt lick or fertilizer; salt mixture needs protection against leaching by rain
- Individual oral dosing of ewes at 4 and 5 months pregnant 280 mg potassium iodide (or 370 mg potassium iodate) prevents goiter in lambs
- Weekly anointing inside thigh with iodine tincture (4 ml cattle, 2 ml sheep and pigs)
- Injection of 40% iodine in poppy seed oil; 1 ml S/C 8 weeks before lambing protects lamb

IRON DEFICIENCY [VM8 p. 1398]

Etiology

Primary nutritional deficiency of iron.

Epidemiology

- Neonates of any species reared on milk diet with no contact with earth
- Mostly in sucking piglets; very low iron stores at birth; rarely lambs, kids
- Maintained indoors, no contact with earth, disease appears in 2–3 week old piglets
- Incidence up to 90%
- Signs may be present at birth, usually at 3–6 weeks
- May occur in calves on ration containing iron <19 mg/kg dry matter, but not normally in veal calves reared indoors in crates
- Dietary iron requirement of fast growing lambs is 40–70 mg/kg; growth suboptimal on rations containing iron at <25 mg/kg
- Piglets have lower liver iron at birth than other species
- Piglets increase body weight very quickly;

daily iron requirement 15 mg/day; milk supplies only 1 mg/day
♦ Birth levels of hemoglobin in piglets decline physiologically to day 8–10, commence to rise if there is access to iron; without it severe anemia develops

Risk factors
♦ Black pigs more susceptible than white ones
♦ Addition of calcium carbonate and manganese to ration causes conditioned iron deficiency in young pigs but not adults

Importance
Failure to thrive, some deaths; important cause of loss in enclosed rearing units designed to control earth-borne parasitic diseases.

Clinical findings

♦ High incidence of anemia at 3 weeks, some cases up to 10 weeks
♦ Growth rate slower than normal
♦ Diarrhea
♦ Severe dyspnea
♦ Lethargy
♦ Skin, mucosae very pale; skin in white pigs often yellow
♦ Lean, white, hairy appearance
♦ Fat, puffy appearance due to edema in head, forequarters in some
♦ Marked increase in apex beat after exercise
♦ High mortality rate without treatment; often sudden death
♦ Survivors thin, unthrifty

Complications
♦ Enteric colibacillosis
♦ Streptococcal pericarditis

Clinical pathology

♦ Microcytic, hypochromic anemia
♦ Hemoglobin levels fall to 2–4 g/dl in week 3
♦ Serum iron <67 yg/dl at day 50
♦ Clinical signs at 4 g/dl
♦ Erythrocyte counts depressed to 3–4 × $10^6/\mu l$

Necropsy findings

♦ A thin, pale carcase with watery blood, anasarca
♦ Dilated, hypertrophic, heart
♦ Mottled, enlarged liver

Diagnosis

Resembles:
♦ Eperythrozoonosis
♦ Isoimmunization hemolytic anemia
♦ Navel bleeding

Treatment and control

Overdosing with iron; at level higher than body can bind it, susceptibility to infectious diseases, diarrhea increases.

Diet supplement
♦ Feeding sows 2 g iron/kg feed prevents anemia in piglets because they eat sow feces
♦ Iron concentration of sow's milk cannot be increased by feeding iron; injection in sow elevate milk iron level but not enough to prevent anemia in her piglets
♦ Milk replacers for calves should contain 100 mg iron /kg of dry matter
♦ Veal calf diets should contain 15–30 mg soluble iron /kg dry matter
♦ Iron-deficient anemic adult horses and cattle require 3–4 g ferrous sulfate daily in feed for 2 weeks

Oral dosing
♦ Single oral treatment with iron-dextran or iron-galactan **provided** administered to piglet before 12 hours after birth when passage possible through immature intestinal mucosa **and** high quality creep feed available
♦ Reduced iron 0.5–1.0 g once weekly
♦ Painting sow's udder daily with syrup containing ferrous and copper sulfates
♦ Overdosing causes diarrhea
♦ Diarrhea reduces absorption of orally administered iron

Intramuscular iron injections
♦ One injection between day 3 and 7
♦ 200 mg of rapidly absorbed, readily utilizable form of iron (commonly the dextran, fumarate or glutamate, or Heptomer); preparations containing 200 mg in 1 ml preferred
♦ Creep feed should also contain 240 mg iron /kg
♦ Acute poisoning, sudden death after iron-dextran administration if dam deficient in vitamin E and selenium during gestation
♦ Combined iron, selenium preparations available
♦ Iron-dextran preparations usually too expensive for adults of other species
♦ Iron-dextran solutions by intramuscular

injection to horses can cause death within a few minutes

SODIUM CHLORIDE (SALT) DEFICIENCY [VM8 p. 1401]

Etiology

Requires a combination of:
- High demand during rapid growth
- When intake poor on deficient diet
- Heavy loss in milk
- Excessive loss in sweat in high environmental temperature

Epidemiology

Rare disease; occurs only in special combination of circumstances.

Risk factors
♦ Young, rapidly growing, lactating cattle
♦ Horses unaffected
♦ Alpine pastures
♦ Heavily fertilized leys with low dry matter (<0.1 g/100 g dry matter)
♦ Heavy milkers

Clinical findings

♦ Haggard appearance
♦ Lusterless eyes
♦ Rough coat
♦ Anorexia
♦ Rapid weight loss, milk yield drops
♦ Polyuria, polydipsia
♦ Pica, especially salt hunger, licking dirt, each other
♦ Drinking urine
♦ Severe cases collapse, die
♦ Rapid response to sodium chloride treatment

Clinical pathology

♦ Low specific gravity urine
♦ Urine concentration sodium, chloride decreased, potassium increased
♦ Salivary sodium content decreased (to 70–100 mmol/liter), potassium increased; saliva the best indicator
♦ Serum sodium (to 137 mmol/liter), chloride concentration decreased
♦ Low sodium, chloride content, feed, water

Diagnosis

Resembles:
♦ Acetonemia

♦ Fatty liver syndrome
♦ Left abomasal displacement
♦ Toxic nephrosis

Treatment and control

♦ 0.5% salt in diet adequate in most circumstances
♦ 0.7% may be necessary for lactating gilts

MAGNESIUM DEFICIENCY [VM8 p. 1402]

Occurs in:
♦ Ruminant hypomagnesemia, milk tetany of calves
♦ Experimentally-induced deficiency in young growing pigs causes limb deformity, arched back, tremor, hyperirritability, recumbency, tetany, death
♦ Osteoporotic disease, cattle on high grain, low roughage diets, Japan; characterized by high serum calcium, alkaline phosphatase levels, low serum magnesium levels

ZINC DEFICIENCY [VM8 p. 1403]

Etiology

Secondary deficiency due to:
♦ High phytic acid content of diet; zinc bound to phytic acid unavailable to monogastric animals
♦ High calcium content in pig diet (0.5–1.5%); disease prevented by zinc supplementation

Epidemiology

♦ Principally a disease of pigs; also calves, goats, sheep
♦ Morbidity 20–80%

Risk factors

Pigs
♦ Fast-growing pigs; especially those fed growth promotants
♦ Most common in 7–10 week pigs, fast growth phase after weaning
♦ Pigs on dry feed; pasture preventive, curative
♦ Excess sulfur in diet

Ruminants:
♦ Soil pH >6.5
♦ Heavy dressings of nitrogen, phosphorus fertilizers
♦ Heavy legume content in pasture

- Plant ageing, e.g. late cut hay
- Pasture containing <10 mg/kg zinc causes disease in sheep; diet requirement for spermatogenesis 32 mg/kg
- Inherited susceptibility assumed; common in some cattle breeds, families; see adema disease

Clinical findings

Pigs
- Reduced weight gain
- Areas of erythema on belly wall, inside thighs
- Symmetrically distributed lesions 3–5 mm dia. papules, to covering of scales, thick scab
- Crumbly, non-greasy scab thickens (5–7 mm), easily detached
- Little scratching, rubbing
- Lesions most plentiful around joints, ears, tail
- Parakeratosis lesions vanished by 10–45 days if ration corrected
- Moderate diarrhea
- Complication – secondary skin abscesses

Cattle
- Severe cases show alopecia, parakeratosis over 40% skin area
- Lesions on muzzle, vulva, anus, tail head, ears, backs of hind limbs, knee folds, flanks, neck
- Subnormal weight
- Small stature
- After treatment recovery complete in 3 weeks
- Pregnant cows may have difficult parturition

Sheep
Mild cases – inappetence, slight weight loss

Severe cases:
- Wool shed
- Wool-eating
- Reduced growth rate
- Salivation
- Swollen hocks
- Thick, wrinkled skin
- Parakeratotic skin lesions around eyes, hooves; hooves may be shed
- Impaired testicle growth, cessation of spermatogenesis
- Zinc-associated infertility in ewes

Goats
- Zinc-responsive alopecia, hyperkeratosis
- Pruritus, hyperemia,
- Reproductive inefficiency

Clinical pathology
- Serum zinc levels low (<39 μg/dl indicates deficiency; may be as low as 18 μg/dl sheep, cattle)
- Serum levels labile, e.g. precipitate fall in serum zinc levels just before parturition in cows, not in sheep
- Parakeratosis in biopsy

Diagnosis

Resembles:
- Sarcoptic mange
- Exudative epidermitis
- Mycotic dermatitis

Treatment

Pigs
- Diet supplemented with 50 mg/kg (200 mg zinc sulfate/kg)
- Calcium content of diet to be 0.65–0.75%
- Injection 2–4 mg/kg zinc daily for 10 days
- Zinc oxide in olive oil as intramuscular injection (200 mg for adult sheep, 50 mg for lambs) for long-term treatment
- Oral dosing 250 mg zinc sulfate daily for 4 weeks

Control

- Pig rations for growing pigs to contain:
  - <0.5 % calcium
  - Zinc sulfate up to 50 mg/kg; compound has low toxicity
- Cattle rations supplemented with zinc sulfate 2–4 g daily
- Pasture top-dressed with zinc fertilizer
- Subcutis zinc depots of zinc metal dust show promise

MANGANESE DEFICIENCY
[VM8 p. 1406]

Etiology

- Primary deficiency in plants due to deficiency in local soil and rock formations
- Excess dietary calcium, phosphorus reduces availability of manganese

Epidemiology

Risk factors
- Pasture on soils with levels <3 mg/kg manganese create bovine infertility problems
- Secondary hypomanganesemia when soil

highly alkaline; the critical pH varies with soil type: may be as low as 5.5, as high as 7
♦ Herbage containing <20 mg/kg manganese causes cow infertility
♦ Herbage containing >200 mg/kg manganese prevents congenital deformities
♦ Important variations between grains in manganese content; maize, barley low, wheat, oats high, bran very high
♦ Cow's milk very low

Clinical findings

Cattle
♦ Cow infertility (delayed estrus, poor conception rate, subnormal ovary size, weak estrus)
♦ Congenital limb deformity, fetlock knuckling, joint pain, hopping gait, reluctant to move
♦ Calves with poor growth, dry coat, loss of coat color

Clinical pathology

♦ Low levels of manganese in blood, liver, hair but lack reliability for accurate diagnosis
♦ Hair levels <8 mg/kg hair associated with infertility
♦ No laboratory test available on which to base diagnosis
♦ Dose response trial needed to confirm diagnosis

Necropsy findings

Congenital enlarged joints, twisted limbs, short bones.

Diagnosis

Resembles:
♦ Other causes of infertility including phosphorus deficiency, energy deficiency
♦ Other causes of congenital limb deformity:
  • Akabane virus disease
  • Inherited defects

Treatment and Control

♦ Diet supplementation of 2–4 g manganese sulfate daily
♦ Excessive feeding causes secondary deficiency of cobalt, zinc in ruminants

POTASSIUM DEFICIENCY
[VM8 p. 1408]

♦ Naturally occurring deficiency rare
♦ Calves fed roughage grown on deficient soils develop syndrome of poor growth, anemia, diarrhea; diet supplement of potassium salts cures
♦ Experimental deficiency in pigs causes syndrome of poor appetite, emaciation, rough coat, incoordination, marked cardiac impairment and significant electrocardiographic changes
♦ Optimum dietary levels are:
  • Ruminants 0.5%
  • Growing pigs 0.26%

SELENIUM AND/OR VITAMIN E
DEFICIENCIES [VM8 p. 1408]

Etiology

♦ Selenium deficiency dealt with here to include:
  • Well-defined diseases caused by known deficiencies of selenium and/or vitamin E in the diet, and
  • Less well-defined syndromes which respond to selenium administration but which are not necessarily caused by selenium deficiency
♦ Selenium deficiency occurs in animals fed plant material grown on soils poor in the element
♦ Vitamin E deficiency may be caused by a primary deficiency of the vitamin in the feed, or by the presence in the diet of polyunsaturated fatty acids which destroy the vitamin

NUTRITIONAL MUSCULAR
DYSTROPHY [VM8 p. 1414]

Epidemiology

Occurrence
♦ All farm animal species, including foals
♦ Morbidity 15%, case fatality rate 100%

Risk factors
♦ Mostly in young (2–4 months) of deficient dams
♦ Also in grain-fed yearling beef cattle, heifers at parturition
♦ Occurs in 7 month foals, rare cases in adult horses but no evidence vitamin E or selenium involved in paralytic myoglobinuria or tying-up
♦ Dams fed for long periods on diets deficient in selenium, and/or vitamin E
♦ Precipitating factors may convert an asymptomatic deficiency state to one of clinical disease of skeletal muscle:
  • Myopathic agents in feed

- Sudden, unaccustomed exercise a common precipitant but disease can occur without it
- Prolonged transport, driving
- Increased activity at weaning
- Climatic stress
- Intercurrent disease
- The myopathic agents are not identified but could include:
  - Unidentified substances in fish and vegetable oils
  - Possibly cyanogenetic glucosides

Selenium deficiency
- Most countries have areas of selenium-deficient soils, those derived from igneous rocks and pumice, and areas of selenium-rich, usually sedimentary, rocks
- Forage, grain of crops grown on soil derived from selenium-deficient rocks are deficient in selenium (<0.1 mg/kg)
- Soils containing <0.5 mg/kg selenium classified as deficient
- Alkalinity of soils enhance selenium uptake by plants
- High sulfur content of soil, as after heavy applications of superphosphate, inhibits selenium uptake by plants
- Legumes take up much less selenium than grasses
- Specific **converter** or **selector** plants take up more selenium than do other plants (see selenium poisoning)
- Heavy rainfall reduces selenium uptake

Vitamin E deficiency
- Occurs on diets of:
  - Inferior hay, straw
  - Root crops
- Factors decreasing vitamin E content of feeds:
  - Maturation of plant; decreases by up to 90%
  - Further fall after harvesting and storage; may fall to zero; falls greater in hay than silage
  - Propionic acid-treated grain
  - High-moisture grain
  - Rations rich in unsaturated fatty acids, e.g. cod liver, other fish oils, fishmeal, lard, linseed, corn, soybean oils; milk replacers containing these substances,
  - Fresh spring grass containing a sufficient concentration of linolenic acid

Clinical findings – cattle and sheep

Acute enzootic muscular dystrophy

- Sudden death, without prior illness, often after exercise, excitement *or*
- Sudden onset of dullness
- Dyspnea, frothy, sometimes blood-stained nasal discharge in some
- Many cases laterally recumbent
- Heart rate 150–200 /minute, often grossly irregular
- Death, in spite of treatment, after 6–12 hour course

Subacute enzootic muscular dystrophy (white muscle or stiff lamb disease)
- Sternal recumbency
- Patient anxious to stand but most unable to do so
- Standing patients have rigidity, tremor, stumbling gait, easy falling
- Calf gait has hock rotation
- Lamb gait stiff, goose-stepping
- Large, upper limb muscle masses symmetrically swollen, firm
- Dyspnea in many
- Transient fever in some
- Heart rate moderately elevated, no irregularity
- Rapid response to treatment, may be walking in 3–5 days

Sequels
- Scapula protruding above vertebral column, shoulders widely separated from chest, toes spread, fetlock knuckling, standing on tip-toe, carpal and metacarpal joint sagging
- Difficulty swallowing, inability to use tongue, choking when drinking

Bovine paralytic myoglobinuria
- Acute or subacute enzootic muscular dystrophy in yearling cattle recently (within 1 week) turned out to pasture after winter housing, plus
- Myoglobinuria in older animals

Clinical findings – horses

Foals
- First week of life to first few months
- Fail to suck
- Difficulty rising, unsteady, tremor
- Recumbency
- Polypnea, tachycardia

Adults
- Depression
- Stiff gait
- Head hung low

♦ Head, neck edema
♦ Unable to eat
♦ Myoglobinuria

Clinical findings – pigs

♦ Occurs rarely as a specific syndrome in pigs
♦ After farrowing in gilts:
  • Stumbling gait
  • Tremor
  • Recumbency
  • Dyspnea, cyanosis
♦ Some cases of mulberry heart disease complex show staggery gait, incoordination suggesting muscular dystrophy

Subclinical findings – all species

♦ Usually when clinical cases occurring in group
♦ Many are cases in a preclinical stage
♦ Serum creatine kinase levels elevated
♦ Electrocardiographic changes
♦ Good treatment response

Clinical pathology

♦ Creatine kinase levels elevated, good guide to muscle damage for 3 days; levels usually 1000 iu/l, often 5000–10 000
♦ SGOT levels elevated for 1–10 days, not as specific
♦ Selenium estimations expensive; not usually performed unless problem widespread
♦ Glutathione peroxidase (GSH-Px) activity in blood directly related to selenium content of tissues; delay of 4–6 weeks to equilibrate in blood after treatment, plasma responds more quickly; commercial spot test using blood samples places patients in deficient, marginal or adequate groups
♦ Blood tocopherol levels difficult to estimate, result interpretation also difficult so not usually used as clinical pathology tests
♦ Anemia due to selenium deficiency due probably to increased susceptibility to hemolysis

Necropsy findings

♦ Bilateral lesions of skeletal, diaphragm muscles
♦ Local areas white, grey discoloration, fish flesh appearance
♦ Lesions are streaks through a muscle mass or peripheral to a core of normal muscle

♦ Affected muscle friable, edematous, may be calcified
♦ Secondary pneumonia associated with throat, chest muscle lesions
♦ Myocardial involvement indicated by white, degenerative areas under left ventricular endocardium in calves, both ventricles in lambs; also interventricular septum, papillary muscles
♦ Cardiac hypertrophy, pulmonary congestion, calcified lesions in some

Diagnosis

Acute muscular dystrophy resembles:
♦ Pneumonia
♦ Septicemia
♦ Toxemia

Subacute muscular dystrophy resembles other causes of paresis, paralysis, especially:
♦ Spinal cord compression
♦ Polyarthritis
♦ Poisoning by organophosphates
♦ Tetanus
♦ *Hemophilus* spp. meningoencephalitis
♦ Those characterized by myositis, myopathy

PORCINE MULBERRY HEART
DISEASE AND HEPATOSIS
DIETETICA [VM8 p. 1418]

Epidemiology

♦ Rapidly growing pigs during postweaning period; 1–4 months old
♦ Uncommon occurrences in gilts, sows
♦ On high energy diets containing soybeans, high moisture corn, cull peas, cereal grains grown on soils deficient in selenium
♦ Mulberry heart disease can occur in presence of adequate vitamin E and selenium intakes
♦ Common component of diet is coconut meal, fish liver oils, fish scraps, flaxseed
♦ Morbidity up to 25%, case fatality 90%

Clinical findings

Mulberry heart disease
♦ Usually a number found dead
♦ Severe dyspnea, cyanosis
♦ Recumbency
♦ Heart rate fast, irregular

Hepatosis dietetica
♦ Most found dead
♦ Severe depression

- Dyspnea
- Vomiting
- Staggering
- Diarrhea
- Jaundice in some
- Recumbency
- Sudden death on exercise

Clinical pathology

- Elevated blood levels of muscle enzymes, especially creatine kinase, are diagnostic but not commonly used because of the acuteness of the disease and the early availability of necropsy material
- Blood levels of selenium, vitamin E can be used with similar reservations

Necropsy findings

Mulberry heart disease
- Excess fluid, fibrin shreds or as lacy net in all body cavities
- Liver enlarged, mottled, nutmeg appearance
- Lungs edematous, distended interlobular septa, ventral parts collapsed
- Multiple subepicardial, subepicardial hemorrhages
- Marked myocardial hemorrhage, parenchymatous degeneration
- Cerebral white matter lysis in some cases
- Nutritional muscular dystrophy lesions common

Hepatosis dietetica
- Swollen, mottled liver
- Hemorrhage, degeneration, necrosis in liver
- Nutritional muscular dystrophy lesions common

MISCELLANEOUS SELENIUM-RESPONSIVE DISEASES
[VM8 p. 1419]

Selenium-responsive unthriftiness in sheep and cattle

Epidemiology
- In New Zealand, Australia, USA
- Sheep and cattle
- Occurs in selenium-deficient areas
- All ages, mostly lambs and calves
- Mostly in fall and winter

Clinical findings
- Low growth rate
- Poor wool yield
- Chronic diarrhea, calves
- Responds to selenium supplementation

Clinical pathology
- Diagnosis based on laboratory estimations of selenium content of soil, pasture plants, animal tissues
- Glutathione peroxidase activity in blood a good medium for monitoring selenium status of patient or test animal

Selenium-responsive reproductive inefficiency

Reported as a field observation in sheep and cattle but experimental evidence inconclusive.

Selenium-responsive retained placenta

Extensively reported as a field observation in cows but not confirmed experimentally.

Selenium-enhanced resistance to infectious disease

- Laboratory studies suggest the involvement of selenium in immunological functions
- Preliminary observations suggest that higher blood selenium levels in neonates are associated with greater resistance to infections
- Selenium supplementation is known to enhance resistance to experimental parainfluenza virus infection in sheep and infectious bovine rhinotracheitis virus infection in cattle
- There is no evidence that naturally occurring selenium and vitamin E deficiency is associated with increased incidence or severity of infectious diseases
- There may be a relationship between blood levels of selenium in cattle and the prevalence of mastitis and mammary gland health

Equine degenerative myeloencephalopathy

Suspicions that this disease might be vitamin E deficiency-induced seem not to have been substantiated.

Generalized steatitis

Steatitis, including fat necrosis, yellow fat disease and polymyositis often ascribed to vitamin E/selenium deficiency but there is no obvious relationship

Treatment

- Single I/M treatment of combined alpha-tocopherol-selenium preparations recommended (2 ml/45 kg body weight of solution containing 3 mg selenium as sodium or potassium selenite plus 150 iu/ml of DL-alpha-tocopherol acetate/ml)
- Patients with myocardial involvement unlikely to respond
- In-contact animals treated similarly as prophylaxis

Control

- Both selenium and vitamin E should be provided; vitamin E is less stable, more expensive
- Selenium can be provided to young directly or via the dam during pregnancy
- Administration of selenium and vitamin E before expected occurrence of disease is effective strategy
- Selenium a potent toxin; control program needs careful surveillance
- Care needed to avoid any chance of poisoning humans with residues in animal products
- Proper supplementation of livestock in an area dependant on assay of selenium content of locally produced feeds; requirement of selenium is 0.1 mg/kg of feed
- High sulfate diets increase the requirement of selenium
- The most reliable index of selenium status in ruminants is whole blood level of glutathione peroxidase

Techniques for supplying selenium and vitamin E

- **Pasture top dressing**, where this permitted by law, can be effective for 12 months, have low toxicity risks at 10 g/ha selenium, as selenate, dose rate annually, used on very deficient pumice soils
- **Diet supplements** the exact amounts of supplement depending on the degree of deficiency determined locally, the concentration of polyunsaturated fatty acids, sulfur-containing amino acids; care needed because of the risk of toxicity with long-term provision of selenium; general recommendation for all species is daily intake of 0.1–0.3 mg/kg body weight selenium, daily intake of alpha-tocopherol 1 g daily for cows, 150 mg for yearlings, 75 mg for ewes
- **Salt mixtures**, the amount of selenium depending on the degree of deficiency and the average intake of salt; local legislation may also control the amount of selenium that can be fed
- **Slow-release subcutaneous injection** barium selenate 1.0 mg/kg body weight maintains adequate glutathione peroxidase levels for 5 months, piglets of treated sows for 3 months
- **Slow-release rumen pellets** of elemental selenium plus finely divided metallic iron persist for up to 4 years but absorption rate varies widely; combination pellets containing selenium, cobalt, potassium, zinc, manganese, sulphate, vitamins A, D, E also available; an osmotic pump-type slow release bolus provides adequate selenium for 3 months
- **Oral dosing** with selenium combined with anthelmintics or vaccines are useful when regular drenching is practised at appropriate time intervals and at strategic times
- **Individual prophylactic injections of vitamin E and selenium** injected recommended doses of sodium selenite (0.1 mg/kg body weight) maintains elevated levels for 23 days in calves, 14 days in lambs and piglets; commercial preparations often contain insufficient vitamin E; sodium selenate injections (0.1–0.15 mg/kg body weight) to adults maintains adequate blood levels for 5–6 months

CALCIUM DEFICIENCY
[VM8 p. 1426]

Etiology

- Rarely primary
- Uncommon secondary deficiency due to marginal calcium intake plus high phosphorus in diet

Epidemiology

Occurrence

- Horses in top racing training fed high-grain, grain byproduct diets plus cereal, grass hay
- Pigs fed high grain diets without calcium supplement in grain-producing areas; causes:
- Osteodystrophia fibrosa
- Possibly slipped femoral head of sows
- May contribute to development of atrophic rhinitis

- Cattle in feedlots on high-grain diets
- Sheep on long-term feed deprivation due to poor pasture growth
- In sheep on cereal crop grazing; calcium intake may be 3–5 g/week; requirement is 3–5 g/day
- Greater risk in late pregnant, early lactating mares when calcium balance likely to be negative

Importance
Wastage due to disabling bone, joint lesions.

Clinical findings

Specific syndromes
- Rickets
- Osteomalacia
- Osteodystrophia fibrosa
- Bovine degenerative arthropathy
- Ovine hypocalcemic paresis

General syndrome
- More marked in young sheep
- Growth retardation, unresponsive to anthelmintic treatment
- Poor incisor development, gum deformity
- Eruption of permanent teeth delayed to as long as 27 months
- Permanent teeth excessive wear due to defective enamel, dentine
- Inappetence
- Stiff gait
- Lameness
- Bones soft, ribs bendable, cranial bones depressed by pressure, easy fracture
- Reduced fertility
- Difficult parturition
- Tetany in pigs, young cattle, responsive to calcium borogluconate parenteral treatment

Clinical pathology

- Serum calcium levels usually normal; may be low (3.5 mg/dl) in long-standing cases in sheep
- Radiographic detection of osteoporosis variable
- Diagnostic response to diet supplementation with calcium

Necropsy findings

- Osteoporosis
- Parathyroid hyperplasia
- Low ash content of bone

Diagnosis

Resembles:
- Phosphorus deficiency
- Vitamin D deficiency
- Copper deficiency
- Fluorosis
- Chronic lead poisoning

Treatment and control

- Calcium borogluconate solution injection (as in milk fever) for tetany
- Supplement diet with calcium:
  - Ground limestone, animal feed quality
  - Bone meal more expensive; additional phosphorus may be undesirable
  - Alfalfa, clover, molasses good sources
- Reduce excessive phosphorus intake
- Aim at calcium:phosphorus ratio of 2:1 (optimum) up to 1:1; if urolithiasis a problem ratio should be 2.5:1
- Ensure adequate vitamin D intake

PHOSPHORUS DEFICIENCY
[VM8 p. 1428]

Etiology
- Usually primary due to diet low in phosphorus
- May be partly secondary due to:
  - Deficiency of vitamin D
  - Excess calcium in diet
  - High intake vitamin A

Epidemiology

Occurrence
- Widespread
- Geographical distribution related to deficiency in local soil, rocks
- Primary deficiency only in cattle
- At pasture lactating cows worst affected
- Amongst housed cattle dry and young stock likely to be neglected, receive no supplement
- Lactating sows most susceptible amongst pigs
- Sheep, horses much less susceptible than cattle; disease rarely occurs in them

Risk factors
- Critical soil level <0.002% citrate–soluble phosphorus
- Critical pasture level <0.1% below which rickets and osteomalacia occur
- Recommended daily intake: dairy cattle 25 g, beef cattle 12 g

♦ Suboptimal levels of vitamin D increase requirement
♦ Local soil factors reducing availability of phosphorus to plants:
  • High phosphate retention soils
  • High calcium
  • High magnesium intake, e.g. grass tetany prophylaxis
  • Aluminium pollution
  • High iron in rock salt
  • Excessive leaching by heavy rainfall
♦ Plant phosphorus content low in bad droughts
♦ Phosphorus deficient farms where regular superphosphate dressing suspended, usually as an economy
♦ Poor quality superphosphate
♦ High diet content of phytic acid reduces phosphorus availability in feed to pigs, not to herbivores

Importance
♦ Wastage due to slow maturation of animals
♦ Reduced productivity meat, wool, milk
♦ Bone injuries
♦ Reproductive inefficiency
♦ Botulism
♦ Contributes to development of postparturient hemoglobinuria

Clinical findings

Cattle – specific syndromes
♦ Rickets in calves, yearlings
♦ Osteomalacia in adults

Cattle – general syndrome
♦ Inappetence
♦ Retarded growth
♦ Low milk yield
♦ Associated non-specific reduction in fertility, e.g. calving percentage reduced to 20%
♦ Possibly dental malocclusion but no excess wear
♦ Characteristic conformation associated with phosphorus deficiency:
  • Long legs, small trunk, abdomen
  • Narrow chest, small girth
  • Small pelvis
  • Slab-sided
♦ Fine bones
♦ Hair coat, rough, diluted pigmentation
♦ Osteophagia, botulism common
♦ Late-pregnant cows recumbent, continue to eat

Pigs
Posterior paralysis in sows.

Sheep and horses
♦ No osteodystrophy
♦ Poor stature
♦ Unthrifty
♦ Pica

Clinical pathology

♦ Serum phosphorus levels normal unless deprivation has been serious, prolonged
♦ Serum inorganic phosphorus levels of 1.5–3.5 mg/dl usually associated with clinical signs

Necropsy findings

Findings listed under rickets, osteomalacia, osteodystrophia.

Diagnosis

General syndrome resembles:
♦ Malnutrition
♦ Helmintic infestation
♦ Chronic toxemia due to infection
♦ Cobalt deficiency
See also rickets, osteomalacia, osteodystrophia

Treatment and Control

♦ Urgent treatment is 30 g sodium dihydrogen phosphate in 300 ml water I/V for cattle
♦ Daily supplementation for cattle of 15 g phosphorus minimal, 40–50 g optimal; as bone meal, rock phosphate, soft (colloidal clay) phosphate in form of:
  • Free-access lick, block
  • Mineral mix fed in concentrate or hay
  • Pasture topdressing
  • In drinking water by automatic dispenser, e.g. monosodium dihydrogen phosphate 10–20 g/liter
  • Superphosphate supernatant – **superjuice** sprinkled on feed

VITAMIN D DEFICIENCY
[VM8 p. 1433]

Etiology

♦ Lack of ultraviolet irradiation of skin
♦ Lack of preformed vitamin in diet

Epidemiology

♦ Widespread recognition of need to provide supplementary vitamin D has reduced incidence of deficiency to very low level

- Sun-dried mature grass pasture has high vitamin D precursor; modern harvesting of immature green chop, or rapid, mechanical drying reduce vitamin content
- Grazing on lush, green pasture, especially in winter, leads to high incidence of musculoskeletal disease

Risk factors
- Areas distant from equator
- Persistently cloudy, overcast sky
- Winter months
- Animals with dark skin, long fleece
- Animals kept indoors without diet supplement
- High carotene intake has antivitamin D potency
- When calcium:phosphorus ratio is wider than the optimum (1:1 to 2:1) the requirement for vitamin D to enhance bone mineralisation increases

Clinical findings

- Reduced productivity, poor weight gains
- Inappetence, inefficient feed utilisation
- Infertility

Late stages
- Rickets in young
- Osteomalacia in adults

Clinical pathology

- Pronounced hypophosphatemia early
- Hypocalcemia later
- Elevated plasma alkaline phosphatase
- Vitamin D levels in body tissues low

Necropsy findings

Necropsy findings of rickets, osteomalacia.

Diagnosis

General syndrome resembles:
- Malnutrition
- Helmintic infestation
- Chronic toxemia due to infection
- Cobalt deficiency

See also rickets, osteomalacia, osteodystrophia.

Treatment and control

- Arrange exposure to solar irradiation
- Include sun-dried hay in diet

- Total daily intake of vitamin D 7–12 iu/kg body weight by diet supplementation as:
  - Irradiated yeast
  - Stable, water soluble vitamin D
- Massive oral doses also used, e.g. 2 million iu to 2 month old lambs
- Depot I/M injections 11 000 iu/kg body weight calciferol in oil lasts 3–6 months; administered just before risk period, e.g. during late pregnancy to protect lamb

VITAMIN D TOXICITY

- Poisoning occurs after oral, parenteral dosing of excessive amounts of vitamin D_3
- 15 million iu to cattle parenterally, similar oral doses to lambs, cause signs in 3 weeks of:
  - Anorexia
  - Weight loss
  - Dyspnea
  - Tachycardia, loud heart sounds
  - Torticollis
  - Weakness, recumbency
  - Fever
  - High case fatality rate
- Horses poisoned by 12 000 iu/kg body weight in feed (1 million iu/kg feed):
  - Anorexia
  - Stiffness
  - Weight loss
  - Polyuria, polydipsia
  - Soft tissue calcification including endocardium, large blood vessels
- Pigs poisoned by 50 000 iu/kg body weight:
  - Anorexia, vomiting, diarrhea
  - Dyspnea
  - Aphonia
  - Emaciation, death
  - Gastritis, interstitial pneumonia at necropsy

RICKETS [VM8 p. 1436]

Etiology

- Deficiency of calcium, phosphorus or vitamin D, or a combination, exacerbated by nutritional needs of bone growth
- Inherited susceptibility in pigs

Epidemiology

Occurrence
- No longer a common disease
- Occurs mostly in management systems which do not provide replacement supplements, e.g.

- Exploitative range grazing
- Intensive fattening units
- Heavy dependence on lush grazing in winter months
- Morbidity up to 50%; case fatality rate nil but some euthanasias necessary

Risk factors
- Only in young, growing animals
- Fast growers worst affected

Calves
- Phosphorus deficient range-type grazing
- Grazing in winter at latitudes where solar irradiation deficient, e.g. southern New Zealand
- Long-term indoor raising on pasture hay, roots deficient in calcium, phosphorus, vitamin D

Lambs
- Green cereal or lush grass grazing in winter, eliciting carotene antivitamin D effect
- Grazing where solar irradiation inadequate

Pigs
High cereal diets containing excess phosphate, deficient calcium, vitamin D.

Clinical findings

Subclinical signs of the nutritional deficiency plus:
- Stiff gait, lameness
- Increased tendency to fracture
- Limb joint, costochondral junctions enlargement
- Curved limb bones, forward, outward at carpus
- Back arched
- Pelvis contracture, collapse
- Teeth eruption delayed, irregular
- Teeth irregularly calcified, pitted, grooved, pigmented
- Teeth malaligned, wear quickly
- Jawbones thick, soft
- Inability to close mouth
- Tongue protrudes
- Saliva drools
- Eating difficult
- Chest deformity causes dyspnea, ruminal tympany in some
- Terminal recumbency
- Hypersensitivity, tetany in some
- Death due to inanition

Clinical pathology

- Serum calcium and phosphorus variable
- Serum alkaline phosphatase elevated
- Serum levels of 25-hydroxyvitamin D_3, 25-hydroxyvitamin D_2 decreased in vitamin D-deficient rickets
- Bone radiological density lacking, bone ends woolly in appearance, flat or concave
- Biopsy of costochondral junction shows diagnostic lesion

Necropsy findings

- Bone shafts soft, large diameter
- Joints enlarged, soft to cut, thick epiphyseal cartilage
- Typical rickets histology of distal metacarpal, metatarsal cartilages
- Normal bone ash:organic matter ratio of 3:2 is 1:2, even 1:3; reduction below 45:55 suggests osteodystrophy

Diagnosis

Resembles:
- Copper deficiency
- Epiphysitis
- *Mycoplasma* spp. arthritis/synovitis
- *Erysipelas* spp. arthritis
- *Chlamydia* spp. arthritis
- Arthritis
- Inherited rickets in pigs

Treatment

Recovery usual with treatment as listed under vitamin D deficiency etc., but gross deformity persists.

Control

Repair of nutritional deficiency (see above).

OSTEOMALACIA [VM8 p. 1438]

Etiology

Nutritional deficiency of calcium, phosphorus or vitamin D, exacerbated by strains of pregnancy, lactation, in mature animals.

Epidemiology

- Area occurrence due to local nutritional deficiency, especially of phosphorus, less commonly vitamin D
- More common in cattle than in sheep at pasture

- In feedlots most common cause is high phosphorus intake without complementary calcium and vitamin D increases
- Sows on calcium deficient diets after long lactation

Clinical findings

Cattle – early stages
- Reduced productivity, weight loss
- Reproductive inefficiency
- Licking, chewing inanimate objects, **osteophagia** leads to:
  - Oral, pharyngeal, esophageal obstruction
  - Traumatic reticuloperitonitis
  - Lead poisoning
  - Botulism

Cattle – later stages
- Stiff gait
- Shifting lameness, especially hind limbs
- Crackling sounds while walking
- Arched back
- Disinclined to move
- Recumbent for long periods
- Colloquial, descriptive names include **creeps, stiffs, cripples, pegleg, bog-lame; milk-leg, milk-lame** in heavily milking cows
- Pathological fractures, tendon separations during exercise, transportation
- Dystokia when pelvis deformed
- Bone deformity only in extreme cases, e.g. facial bones in pigs
- Terminal recumbency, death due to starvation

Sows
- Dog-sitting posture or lateral recumbency, unable to rise
- Femoral shaft or neck fracture common
- Often after moving to new pen, fighting amongst sows

Clinical pathology

- Serum calcium and phosphorus variable
- Serum alkaline phosphatase elevated
- Serum levels of 25-hydroxyvitamin D_3, 25-hydroxyvitamin D_2 decreased in vitamin D-deficient osteomalacia
- Bone radiological density lacking

Necropsy findings

- Bone shafts soft, large-diameter osteoid deposits

- Some joint cartilage erosions in cattle with phosphorus deficiency
- Normal bone ash:organic matter ratio of $3:2$ is $1:2$, even $1:3$; reduction below $45:55$ suggests osteodystrophy

Diagnosis

Resembles:
- Chronic fluorosis
- Magnesium deficiency
- Spinal cord compression, especially in sows

Treatment and control

See under calcium, phosphorus, vitamin D deficiency.

OSTEODYSTROPHIA FIBROSA
[VM8 p. 1439]

Etiology

Secondary calcium deficiency due to excess dietary phosphorus.

Epidemiology

- Horses, pigs commonly; reported in goats
- Affected horses are those on unbalanced heavy grain/light roughage diets in transport and racing

Risk factors
- Horse diets with calcium:phosphorus ratios $1:2.9$ or greater, irrespective of total calcium intake
  - Ratio $1:13$ cause disease in 5 months
  - Diets with $1:5$ ratio and normal calcium intake cause disease in 1 year, shifting lameness in 3 months
- Pig diets similar; optimum ratio $1.2:1$; optimum calcium intake 0.6–1.2% of ration
- Diets heavy in grain, low in roughage
- Cereal roughage instead of legume hay
- Army horses in foreign terrain fed imported feed at most risk
- Long-term ingestion oxalate-rich plants, especially palatable grasses causing oxalate-induced equine secondary hyperparathyroidism

Clinical findings

Horses – early stages
- Shifting lameness
- Reduced racing performance

- Arched back
- No physical lesion at lameness site
- Creaking in joints at walk in many

Horses – late stages
- Severe lameness
- Tendon sprains, small bone fractures, including vertebrae
- Swelling of lower edge, alveolar margins of mandible
- Soft, symmetrical swelling facial bones; may interfere with respiration
- Ribs flattened, fractured during work
- Long bone curvatures
- Joint swellings
- Emaciation
- Anemia

Pigs
- Similar lesions to horses
- Often unable to walk, or may balance on nose as well as four limbs
- Mandible distortion, long bone curvatures, joint swellings often gross

Clinical pathology

- Blood changes in calcium, phosphorus, alkaline phosphatase inconclusive
- Radiographically distinguishable bone translucence

Necropsy findings

- Whole skeleton osteoporosis
- Large deposits of fibrous osteoid
- Articular erosions
- Displacement of bone marrow by osteoid

Diagnosis

In horses resembles:
- Traumatic limb injury
- Parathyroid adenoma
- Inherited multiple exostosis

In sows resembles:
- Hypovitaminosis A
- Manganese deficiency
- Polyarthritis

Treatment and control

- In horses to treat and prevent, adjust calcium:phosphorus ratio to 1:1 to 1:1.4
- Calcium supplementation with finely ground limestone, legume hay

'BOWIE' OR 'BENTLEG'
[VM8 p. 1440]

Etiology

- Specific cause uncertain, probably phosphorus deficiency
- Similar clinical syndrome occurs naturally caused by ingestion *Trachymene glaucifolia* (wild parsnip)
- Produced experimentally by diet low in calcium and phosphorus

Epidemiology

- Occurs only in sucking lambs on unimproved pasture in New Zealand, in 3–12 month ram lambs in South Africa
- Morbidity up to 40%
- Spontaneously recovering similar disease in Saanen goat bucks

Clinical findings

- Hoof tenderness early
- Lateral fore limb curvature at knees, rarely medial curvature
- Lateral aspects of hooves badly worn
- Lameness
- Do not feed properly

Clinical pathology

- Low blood phosphorus levels
- Plasma calcium:phosphorus ratio lower than normal

Necropsy findings

- Limb curvature; no osteoporosis, nor osteoid
- Epiphyseal cartilages thick
- Articular erosions

Diagnosis

Resembles rickets.

Treatment and Control

- Diet supplement of phosphorus, or pasture improvement generally reduces incidence
- Vitamin D, trace elements ineffective

DEGENERATIVE JOINT DISEASE
[VM8 p. 1441]

Etiology

Inherited susceptibility, because of shallow acetabular cup, exacerbated by rapid weight gain, high phosphorus diet.

Epidemiology

♦ Sporadic disease of young bulls
♦ All breeds, especially beef cattle

Risk factors
♦ Most serious in calves making rapid weight gains
♦ Long-term housing, little exercise
♦ High grain (i.e. high phosphorus, high phosphorus:calcium ratio) diet
♦ Supplementing dam's milk by use of foster (nurse) cows
♦ Inherited shallow acetabulum, possibly straight hind limb; animals with inherited defect run at pasture develop joint disease much later if at all
♦ Early use in mating, fighting, violent exercise may initiate clinical signs

Clinical findings

♦ Lameness in one or both hindlimbs
♦ Usually gradual onset over 6 months; may be acute after sudden movement
♦ Eventually very severe, hopping lameness
♦ Crepitus over affected hip joint, detected by palpation, auscultation while walking or rocking animal from side to side, passive movement
♦ Moderate lesions other joints, especially stifles, rarely front fetlocks
♦ Reluctant to walk, recumbency
♦ Local muscle atrophy accentuates joint enlargement

Necropsy findings

♦ Extensive erosion hip joint cartilages with penetration to cancellous bone
♦ Deformity femoral head, femoro-tibial epiphyses
♦ Increased, brownish, turbid joint fluid
♦ Thick, calcified joint capsule
♦ Multiple periarticular exostoses
♦ Stifle joint cartilages small or absent

Diagnosis

Resembles:
♦ Inherited osteoarthritis
♦ Milk-leg (osteomalacia) in adult cows
♦ Copper deficiency

Treatment and Control

♦ Ensure adequate calcium and vitamin D intake
♦ Reduce feeding intensity in young cattle

DISEASES CAUSED BY DEFICIENCIES OF FAT-SOLUBLE VITAMINS

VITAMIN A DEFICIENCY
(HYPOVITAMINOSIS-A)
[VM8 p. 1442]

Etiology

♦ Primary disease as absolute deficiency of carotene in diet
♦ Secondary to:
  • Poisoning with highly chlorinated naphthalenes
  • Long-term ingestion of mineral oil and other indigestible oils

Epidemiology

♦ Universal occurrence in specific circumstances
♦ All animal species
♦ Occurs in nomadic animal-based cultures, winter housed beef cattle
♦ Long-keep beef feedlots feeding poor quality, long storage, late cut, rain-leached hay, straw instead of hay

Risk factors
♦ Lack of carotene in diet due to:
  • Confined housing with feed limited to poor quality hay, beet pulp, grains, especially if preceding summer feed drought-stricken
  • Prolonged drought with no green feed available to pastured animals
♦ Neonates born with no stored vitamin A; depend on colostrum content; deprivation leads to hypovitaminosis-A
♦ Long-term deprivation depletes liver storage; cattle off green pasture protected 6–18 months; pigs safe for 6 months, horses for 3 years
♦ Commercial mixed feeds may lose carotene of original feed during processing, storage:
  • Oxidation losses of vitamin A in oil-containing feeds rich in unsaturated fatty acids
  • Pelleting of feed
  • Exposure to heat, humidity, light
  • Contact with mineral mixture

♦ Prevention of carotene to vitamin A conversion, e.g. by chlorinated naphthalene poisoning
♦ Failure to absorb carotene because solution in indigestible oil, e.g. mineral oil used in bloat control

Importance
♦ Rare in developed countries now
♦ Some losses in pastoral beef systems, especially in winter-housing period
♦ Serious losses in nomadic animal-based cultures; also vitamin A deficiency in dependent human community

Clinical findings

♦ Night blindness
♦ Corneal changes including:
  • Thin, seromucoid ocular discharge, clouding, ulceration in some
  • Xerophthalmia in calves
♦ Rough, dry, coat, pityriasis
♦ Seborrheic dermatitis in some pigs
♦ Dry, scaly, cracked hooves
♦ Sperm numbers reduced
♦ Abortion, stillbirths, weak young
♦ Placental retention
♦ Staggery, incoordinated gait beginning in hind limbs in young, especially pigs followed by:
  • Fetlock knuckling
  • Sagging hindquarters
  • Recumbency
♦ Convulsions, especially beef calves of 6–8 months, sometimes congenital, plus:
  • Increased cerebrospinal fluid pressure
  • Response to vitamin A therapy in early cases
♦ Blindness in both eyes 1–2 year old cattle, sometimes congenital, plus:
  • Dilated pupils
  • Menace reflex absent
  • Papilledema, peripapillary retinal detachment, hemorrhage
♦ Congenital defects, only in piglets, attributed to vitamin A deficiency include:
  • Cleft palate, harelip
  • Cardiac defects
  • Abnormally located kidneys
  • Cardiac defects
  • Diaphragmatic hernia
  • Genital hypoplasia
  • Internal hydrocephalus
  • Spinal cord herniations
  • Anasarca

Clinical pathology

♦ Minimally adequate plasma vitamin A level 20 μg/dl

♦ Clinical signs appear at plasma vitamin A levels below 5 μg/dl
♦ Clinical signs appear in cattle at plasma carotene levels of 9 μg/dl
♦ Plasma carotene levels very low in normal sheep
♦ Liver carotene, vitamin A measurable on biopsy specimen; levels at which clinical signs occur include:
  • 2 μg/g vitamin A
  • 0.5 μg/g carotene
♦ Cerebrospinal fluid pressures above 200 mm water in calves, pigs, above 150 mm in sheep

Necropsy findings

♦ No gross changes
♦ Transient squamous metaplasia of interlobular ducts of parotid salivary gland is diagnostic

Diagnosis

Convulsive disease in calves resembles:
♦ Hypomagnesemic tetany
♦ Polioencephalomalacia
♦ enterotoxemia due to Clostridium perfringens type D
♦ Acute lead poisoning
♦ Rabies
♦ Sporadic bovine encephalomyelitis

Paraplegic convulsive disease in pigs resembles:
♦ Pseudorabies
♦ Viral encephalomyelitis
♦ Salt poisoning
♦ Organic arsenical poisoning
♦ Organic mercurial poisoning

Treatment

♦ Immediate parenteral treatment with water-soluble preparation at a dose of 440 iu/kg body weight
♦ Overdosing toxicity unlikely; sudden death recorded in pigs, bone, cartilage lesions in calves

Control

♦ Supply minimal daily vitamin A requirement 40 iu/kg body weight; commonly supplied level 60–80 iu; 50% added during pregnancy, lactation
♦ Supplementation may be by:
  • Daily or weekly in grain or concentrate feed

- Intramuscular injection at 60 day intervals at rate of 3000–6000 iu/kg body weight; in late pregnancy to protect calves

VITAMIN K DEFICIENCY [VM8 p. 1448]

Epidemiology

◆ Sporadic cases due to faulty absorption in cases of impaired fat digestion–absorption caused by reduced bile flow
◆ Outbreaks of hemorrhagic disease due to:

- Mouldy *Melilotus alba* (sweet clover) poisoning
- Poisoning by warfarin or its analogues
- Suspected use of antibacterial drugs in pig feed

Treatment

◆ Minimum daily requirement 5 μg/kg body weight
◆ Treatment dose vitamin K_1 20 μg/kg body weight

DISEASES CAUSED BY DEFICIENCIES OF WATER–SOLUBLE VITAMINS

VITAMIN C DEFICIENCY [VM8 p. 1449]

◆ Synthesized by all species; not a dietary essential in domestic animals
◆ Possible occurrence of deficiency-induced dermatosis in calves characterised by:
- Low plasma ascorbic acid levels
- Pityriasis, waxy crusts, alopecia, dermatitis on ears, cheeks, neck, shoulders
- Spontaneous recovery or response to ascorbic acid injection

THIAMIN DEFICIENCY (HYPOTHIAMINOSIS) [VM8 p. 1449]

Epidemiology

◆ Naturally occurring primary deficiency rare; reported in sheep transported long distances by sea and subjected to special feeding regimes before and during transport
◆ Secondary deficiency due to thiaminases occurs in —
- Amprolium poisoning
- Plant poisoning due to *Pteridium aquilinum* (bracken), *Equisetum arvense* (horsetails), *Marsilea drummondii*, *Cheilanthes* spp., *Dryopteris* spp., *Malva parviflora*
◆ Polioencephalomalacia

Clinical findings, clinical pathology, necropsy findings
(see Thiaminase poisoning)

Treatment

Injection 5 mg/kg body weight every few hours to effect, usually 2–4 days, followed by oral supplement for 10 days; dietary error corrected.

PANTOTHENIC ACID DEFICIENCY (HYPOPANTOTHENOSIS) [VM8 p. 1451]

Epidemiology

Seen in pigs on corn-based rations.

Clinical findings

◆ Anorexia, weight loss
◆ Periocular dermatitis, patchy alopecia
◆ Diarrhea
◆ Goose-stepping gait

Necropsy findings

◆ Severe colitis, sometimes ulcerative
◆ Myelin degeneration

Treatment

Calcium pantothenate 500 μg/kg body weight, daily.

BIOTIN DEFICIENCY (HYPOBIOTINOSIS) [VM8 p. 1452]

Epidemiology

◆ Cereal-based diets will be marginal or deficient
◆ Continuous feeding of sulfonamides, antibiotics may induce deficiency

Clinical findings

♦ Lameness in pigs due to deep cracks, fissures in hooves at the heel–sole junction, and the sidewalls and white line, and in foot-pad
♦ Hunched-up appearance with hind legs under (kangaroo-sitting appearance)
♦ Alopecia over back, tail base, hindquarters
♦ Serum biotin levels below 400 ng/ml
♦ Long convalescence, heavy culling

Treatment

♦ Pigs: 350–400 μg/kg feed recommended (4–5 mg/sow/day)
♦ Horses: 10–30 mg/horse/day for 6–9 months recommended for weak hoof horn

FOLIC ACID DEFICIENCY
(HYPOFOLICOSIS) [VM8 p. 1453]

♦ Equine nutritionists have a particular interest relative to improving racing performance

♦ Racing horses, especially stabled ones may need oral supplement

VITAMIN B$_{12}$ DEFICIENCY
(HYPOCYANOCOBALAMINOSIS)
[VM8 p. 1453]

♦ Probably an essential dietary ingredient in pigs and young calves on diets which do not contain animal protein
♦ Sows on deficient diets may show reproductive inefficiency
♦ Used empirically in horses to alleviate parasitic, dietary anemia (2 μg/kg body weight)
♦ Cyanocobalamin zinc tannate provides effective tissue levels for 2–4 weeks

RIBOFLAVIN, NICOTINIC ACID,
PYRIDOXINE, AND CHOLINE
DEFICIENCIES [VM8 p. 1451, 1453]

♦ Not known to occur naturally
♦ Syndromes produced by experimental deprivation

30 DISEASES CAUSED BY PHYSICAL AGENTS

ENVIRONMENTAL POLLUTANTS AND NOISE [VM8 p. 1454]

Chemical pollutants

♦ Major pollutants are cadmium, lead, mercury, arsenic, fluorine
♦ Less common agents with high hazard potential are silver, gold, chromium, copper, tin, thallium, antimony, zinc
♦ Organic compounds including polybrominated, polychlorinated biphenyls, chlorinated hydrocarbons generally

Physical agents

♦ Smoke, as in bushfire injury
♦ Dust, as in volcanic eruption
♦ Animal manure disposal is now an environmental issue; errors in handling can cause manure gas poisoning, copper poisoning, botulism, wide dissemination of feces-borne infectious disease

Noise

♦ An important legal issue; specific effects appear minimal
♦ Most impact is initial fear reaction causing losses by suffocation, cannibalism of young, trampling during flight

RADIATION INJURY [VM8 p. 1455]

Etiology

♦ Damage caused by exposure to radioactive material
♦ Animals may act as reservoirs, conduits for transmission of radioactivity to humans

Epidemiology

♦ Source may be atomic bomb injury, leakage from atomic energy plants, research laboratories, X-ray machines
♦ Major effect is spread of radioactive material from the blast, carriage of the material long distances by wind as **fall-out**

Clinical findings

Acute, after high somatic dose
♦ Intense, refractory diarrhea
♦ Dehydration, electrolyte depletion
♦ Focal depilation, skin necrosis
♦ Death in a few days

Subacute, median somatic dose
♦ Initial **radiation sickness** stage:
  • Anorexia, profound lethargy
  • Vomiting
  • Lasts few hours to few days
♦ Normal phase for 1–4 weeks
♦ Terminal phase of:
  • Fever
  • Diarrhea, melena, dysentery, with tenesmus in some
  • Limb swelling, fetlock knuckling
  • Anorexia, intense thirst
  • Weakness, recumbency
  • Easily excited
  • Profuse nasal discharge, blood-stained in some
  • Dyspnea
  • Severe anemia
  • Terminal septicemia in some
  • Death after course of 1 week
♦ Long convalescence in survivors includes:
  • Poor weight gains
  • Alopecia
  • Lens opacity blindness
  • Temporary or permanent infertility
  • Mutant offspring in some
  • Hemopoietic, cutaneous tumors

Chronic exposure over several years
Lens opacity.

Clinical pathology

Cattle – median somatic dose

- Precipitate leukopenia after irradiation, peak at day 15 – 25; most effect on neutrophils and platelets
- Erythrocyte count, hematocrit decreased, prothrombin times prolonged
- Return to normal leukon takes over 1 year in survivors

Necropsy findings

- Hemorrhagic, necrotic gastroenteritis
- Pharynx ulceration
- Pulmonary edema
- Extensive petechiase gross hemorrhages
- Assay of radioactive material in tissues
- Degenerative lesions in all organs

Diagnosis

Resembles other causes of hemorrhagic disease.

BRISKET DISEASE (ALTITUDE, MOUNTAIN SICKNESS) [VM8 p. 1457]

Etiology

- Alveolar hypoxia of high altitude, exacerbated by:
  - Myocardial dystrophy
  - Anemia
  - Pulmonary disease
  - Hypoproteinemia

Epidemiology

- Disease of cattle, all ages; rarely in other ruminants
- Morbidity high; case fatality close to 100%
- Indigenous cattle <1% morbidity
- Horses, mules lose weight, fatigue easily at high altitude but no congestive heart failure

Risk factors

- Commonest in young, and recently introduced cattle
- Permanent pasturing at >1800 m for months; serious disease at >2200 m
- Spontaneous recovery in early cases moved to low altitude
- Cattle ingesting *Oxytropis sericea* (locoweed)

Clinical findings

- Depression, rapid weight loss
- Rough, lusterless coat
- Hyperpnea, dyspnea, poor exercise tolerance
- Elbows abducted
- Jugular vein engorgement, edema of brisket, neck, submandibular space, ventral thorax, abdomen
- Ascites, abdominal distension
- Mucosa cyanotic
- Loud, crackling breath sounds or absent sounds
- Heart sounds loud, rapid early, muffled as hydropericardium develops; hemic murmur, cardiac impulse enlarged

Clinical pathology

- Central pulmonary artery pressure elevated
- Erythrocyte counts, hemoglobin concentration increased early; subsequent depression

Necropsy findings

- Cardiac enlargement; gross dilation, hypertrophy right ventricle
- Anasarca, edema of all cavities
- Pulmonary emphysema
- Congestive changes in liver, especially enlargement

Diagnosis

Resembles other causes of right congestive heart failure.

Treatment

- Move affected cattle to lower altitude
- Avoid exercise
- Digoxin as a temporary measure
- Diuretics to aid removal excess fluid

Control

- Keep only cattle which adapt to alpine pasture conditions
- Prompt treatment early cases
- Select for resistance to disease

LIGHTNING STROKE, ELECTROCUTION [VM8 p. 1459]

Etiology

- Linear lightning during thunderstorms; large number close together can be killed instantly

- Fallen overhead electrical transmission wires carrying high voltages
- Faulty electrical installations in animal housing, milking sheds
- Wire fences, pools of water, metal structures in sheds, trees may become electrified

Epidemiology

- All species, especially cattle and horses
- Lightning stroke commonest summer
- Case fatality rate approximates 100%

Risk factors

- Animals sheltering under trees and other hazardous locations
- Trees with spreading growth pattern, surface roots, e.g. oak
- Wire rails, stanchions, metal feed, water troughs likely to become electrified
- Faulty installation of electrical equipment close to animals, e.g heat lamps over piglets, milking machines, water pumps
- Electrical transmission wires able to contact shed guttering

Clinical findings

- Some fall dead without a struggle; most bellow once or twice
- Hair singed, skin burned at point of contact, e.g. feet, muzzle
- Some fall unconscious with a struggle
- Spontaneous recovery in few minutes to several hours
- Survivors may be blind, have local paralyses, e.g. monoplegia, facial paralysis
- In pigs continued recumbency and lameness due to bone fracture, e.g. vertebra

Minor shocks

- Restless, kicking intermittently as contact made with electrified point
- Farmer protected by rubber boots

Necropsy findings

- Ensure carcase no longer electrified
- Rarely singe marks on skin
- Rapid onset and disappearance of rigor mortis, rapid decomposition
- Blood from orifices
- Pupils dilated, anus relaxed
- All viscera congested
- Generalized petechiation
- Fractures commonly in pigs

Diagnosis

Resembles other causes of sudden death.

Treatment

- No treatment applicable in most cases
- Artificial respiration in those observed to collapse

Control

- All electrical equipment and constructions properly earthed
- Minimum amperage safety fuses to protect against short-circuits

STRAY VOLTAGE [VM8 p. 1460]

Etiology

Electrical voltage between two points that can result in a current flow through an animal when it contacts them; voltage low, not usually sensed by humans; called also tingle or transient voltage, free electricity.

Epidemiology

- All electrified housing and feeding systems potentially hazardous
- Common in new buildings where system not properly connected to earth
- Great variation between cows in sensitivity to stray voltage
- Many farms affected where insufficient cows disturbed to arouse suspicion

Clinical findings

Cattle

- Reluctance to enter milking parlour
- Reluctance to cross metal grid
- Restless in parlour, anxious to leave, may stampede
- Cow experiencing current flow:
  - Anxious, trembling
  - Back arched, head elevated, ears laid back
  - Frequent urination, defecation
  - Lapping water; crowd at waterer
- Stray voltage at milking causes:
  - Incomplete, slow letdown
  - Increased milking time
  - Elevated somatic cell count, mastitis incidence

Pigs
♦ Aggressiveness
♦ Disturbed drinking pattern
♦ Reduced productivity

Clinical pathology

Measurement of stray voltage with sensitive voltmeter; interpretation of results requires engineering skills

Diagnosis

Resembles herd restlessness in:
♦ Water deprivation
♦ Subacute hypomagnesemic tetany

Treatment and control

♦ Correct the installation error
♦ Fit a tingle voltage filter

VOLCANIC ERUPTIONS [VM8 p. 1461]

Etiology

Damage to land, plants by:
♦ Lateral blast
♦ Rock fragment, lava, mud flows
♦ Ash and rock fallout at a distance

Epidemiology

♦ Pasture feed may be hidden under dust; food deprivation leads to starvation, acetonemia, pregnancy toxemia, hypocalcemia
♦ Fluorine poisoning at some volcanoes
♦ Selenium, magnesium deficiency common sequels

Clinical findings, clinical pathology, and necropsy findings

Syndromes and lesions caused by the sequels listed above.

BUSHFIRE INJURY [VM8 p. 1463]

Etiology

♦ Softwood forest fires create intense heat, smoke; few animals survive the asphyxiation
♦ Hardwood forest fires move very quickly, leaving tree trunks little harmed, capable of immediate regeneration; suffocation prob-

lem not as bad, many animals may survive but badly burned
♦ Grass, prairie fires; many animals survive but burned ventrally

Epidemiology

Importance is the need to decide whether to:
♦ Destroy burned animals for humane reasons
♦ Salvage burned animals via abattoirs
♦ Treat or allow to recover spontaneously

Clinical findings

Burn damage to eyelids, conjunctiva, lips, udder, teats, perineum, coronets, penis with urethral obstruction.

Treatment

Astringent lotions, protective, healing ointments, fly prophylaxis.

WETNESS [VM8 p. 1464]

Constant wetting by heavy rainfall causes:
♦ Dorsal dermatosis (**scald**) in horses
♦ Fleece rot in sheep
♦ Standing in water or urine leads to:
  • mycotic dermatitis behind the pastern
  • Greasy heel in horses
  • Sporadic lymphangitis in horses

FLEECE ROT OF SHEEP [VM8 p. 1464]

Etiology

Continuous wetting of skin; does not dry out because of insulation by wool, causes dermatitis, plus infection by *Pseudomonas aeruginosa*.

Epidemiology

♦ Sheep only
♦ Australia and UK
♦ Wet seasons
♦ Susceptible sheep

Risk factors
♦ Young sheep
♦ Inherited susceptibility:
  • Long wool
  • Dense fleece resists wetting, but if it wets takes a long time to dry
  • High, irregular fiber diameter

- Low wax content of wool
- Wool with high suint (water soluble fraction of wool yolk) content
- When rainfall sufficient to keep skin wet for at least one week

Clinical findings

- Lesions over withers and along back
- Wool wet, top of tip open
- Wool leached, dingy, plucks easily
- Matted layer of wool on purple skin; matted lump or distant wool may be brightly discolored green, brown, orange, pink, blue
- Provides starting point for mycotic dermatitis
- Attractive to blow fly strike
- Self-limiting when wool dries

Clinical pathology

Culture for *Pseudomonas* spp.

Diagnosis

Resembles mycotic dermatitis.

Treatment

Limit loss by shearing sheep as soon as matted wool lifts

Control

- Select sheep for resistance to wetting
- Shear just before wet season
- Drying living fleece by spraying with mixture of zinc, aluminium oxides, with sterols, fatty acids dries fleece for up to 3 months
- Vaccine containing *Pseudomonas aeruginosa* reduces severity

NEAR DROWNING [VM8 p. 1465]

Etiology

Near-drowning, survival following asphyxia and aspiration of fluid, while submerged, can be a veterinary medical problem.

Epidemiology

- Sporadic cases only
- Overenthusiastic plunge dipping
- Drenching through wrongly placed nasal tube

- Recumbent animals with heads in water
- Horses swum too long during exercise

Clinical findings

- Hyperpnea, dyspnea,
- Tachycardia
- Loud breath sounds
- Crackles in some areas of lung
- Mucosae congested, cyanotic or muddy

Clinical pathology

- Hypoxia
- Metabolic acidosis

Necropsy findings

Aspiration pneumonia.

Diagnosis

Resembles pneumonia.

Treatment and control

Near-drowning requires aggressive treatment:
- Forced standing
- Nasal insufflation humidified oxygen
- Correction of acidosis
- Bronchodilators
- Non-steroidal anti-inflammatories
- Pulmonary infusion with a surfactant transplant
- Broad-spectrum antibacterial

COLD INJURY (FROSTBITE)
[VM8 p. 1465]

Etiology

Exposure to below freezing temperatures.

Epidemiology

Mostly neonates up to several weeks old.

Risk factors
- Absence of shelter
- Weak animals with impaired circulation

due to dehydration, toxemia; most cases associated with concurrent disease
◆ Prolonged sternal recumbency

Clinical findings

◆ Ear tips, distal limbs especially hinds, tail affected
◆ Not readily visible
◆ Calf recumbent, dehydrated, diarrheic, extremities cold, clammy
◆ Lesion swollen, edematous, well demarcated upper limit
◆ Gangrenous sloughing of skin and hooves several days later

◆ Ears stiff, skin separates, curls at edges, sloughs eventually
◆ Teats of milking cows swollen, cold, skin blisters, peels; teat may be permanently damaged; mastitis, thelitis sequels
◆ Scrotum freezing occurs in young bulls

Diagnosis

Resembles gangrene of extremities caused by ergot alkaloid poisoning.

Treatment

Symptomatic treatment.

31 DISEASES CAUSED BY INORGANIC AND FARM CHEMICALS

Indicators for a **presumptive diagnosis** of poisoning:
♦ Illness in previously healthy animals in circumstances not suggestive of infectious or nutritional deficiency disease
♦ Concurrent occurrence of clinically and pathologically similar cases
♦ A suspected poison is locally accessible

A **definitive diagnosis** requires laboratory analysis of biopsy or postmortem tissues. Supportive evidence includes the toxin in gut contents and feed materials. Inhalation or cutaneous absorption are rare portals of entry. Specimens submitted should include:

♦ Liver, kidney, gut wall, gut contents
♦ Blood and urine
♦ Bone and teeth from suspect lead, fluorine cases
♦ Ingesta in a filled, airtight container for HCN and NO_2 suspects
♦ Complete clinical, epidemiological, clinical pathology, necropsy reports, with nomination of suspected poison, based on local experience
♦ In cases where litigation or compensation claim likely, specimens to be collected, packaged, sealed before witnesses, with duplicates

DISEASES CAUSED BY INORGANIC POISONS

LEAD POISONING (PLUMBISM)
[VM8 p. 1469]

Etiology

♦ Accidental ingestion of lead compounds on farm
♦ Environmental pollution over wide area

Epidemiology

Occurrence
♦ One of the commonest poisonings in farm animals
♦ Commonly cattle, uncommonly horses, sheep; pigs very tolerant
♦ Morbidity 10–30%; case fatality rate about 100%, reducible by vigorous treatment
♦ Ingestion common source; inhalation in environmental pollution

Toxic doses – acute single, lethal dose
♦ Calves 400–600 mg/kg body weight
♦ Adult cattle 600–800 mg/kg body weight

♦ Goats 400 mg/kg
♦ Horse >1000 mg/kg
♦ Much variability between physical or chemical composition of substance, e.g lead sheeting less toxic than lead paint

Chronic poisoning – daily dose for extended period
♦ Cattle 6–7 mg/kg body weight (100–200 mg/kg in feed)
♦ Sheep 4–5 mg/kg body weight
♦ Horses 15–30 mg/kg body weight (100–300 mg/kg in feed)
♦ Pigs 33–66 mg/kg body weight

Common sources
♦ Farm rubbish dumps provide most cases
♦ Car batteries
♦ Sump, crankcase oil
♦ Lubrication grease
♦ Television screens
♦ Linoleum
♦ Roofing felt
♦ Putty
♦ Lead in paint from rusted pots, licked,

chewed from boards, farm gates, burlap, canvas, silo interiors
- Boiled linseed oil used as laxative
- Solder, lead shot, leadlight windows, soft water stagnant in lead pipes
- Animals grazing fields, eating hay or silage made from herbage polluted by lead smelters, car exhausts, lead arsenate insecticide, defoliant spray

Risk factors
- Spring in northern hemisphere, when housed cattle let out to pasture
- Summer in southern hemisphere, when feed in pasture short, cattle fossick
- Sweet taste of lead acetate, lack of oral discrimination, chewing reflex, osteophagia, pica, dietary curiosity encourage ingestion lead compounds
- Milk diet

Importance
- Heavy death losses on individual farms
- Very small risk of possible entry to human food chain

Clinical findings

Cattle – acute
- Common in calves, rare in adults
- Many found dead
- Sudden onset
- Tremor head, neck
- Staggery gait
- Jaw champing, saliva frothing
- Eyelid snapping, eye rolling
- Pupil dilation, palpebral eye reflex absent
- Ear flicking, facial and neck twitching
- Bellowing
- Recumbency in **calves** plus
  - Bouts of paddling convulsions until death
  - Between bouts opisthotonus, hyperesthesia
- Most **adults** remain standing, show
  - Blindness, mania; blind charging, climbing walls, strong head pressing
  - Aggression in some
  - Gait stiff, jerky
- Death after 12–24 hour course

Cattle – subacute
- Common syndrome in adults
- Extreme depression, immobility
- Complete anorexia
- Blindness
- Palpebral eye reflex absent
- Staggery gait
- Intermittent circling in either direction
- Tremor, hyperesthesia in some
- Salivation
- Teeth grinding
- Kicking at belly in some
- Complete ruminal atony
- Initial constipation followed by fetid, black diarrhea
- Death often by misadventure, e.g. walking into waterhole, *or*
- Recumbency, quiet death after 3 – 4 day course

Sheep
- Subacute syndrome as in cattle, *or*
- Two chronic syndromes in 3–12 week old lambs on old lead mine sites:
Syndrome 1
  - Always fatal
  - Stiff gait
  - Lame
  - Paralysis, recumbency
  - Lambs unthrifty
  - Osteoporosis leading to spinal cord compression
  - High blood lead levels
Syndrome 2
  - Most recover, some die of intercurrent disease
  - Incomplete limb joint flexion
  - Feet drag
  - Recumbency
  - No osteoporosis
  - High blood lead levels
- Abortion, temporary infertility with chronic ingestion

Goats
- Anorexia
- Fetid diarrhea
- Tenesmus, bloating in some

Horses
Acute   As for subacute in cattle.
Chronic   Caused by pasture pollution
- Inspiratory dyspnea
- Pharyngeal paralysis, choking during eating, regurgitation through nostrils in some cases
- Aspiration pneumonia
- Lip paralysis in a few
- General muscle weakness, joint stiffness in most cases
- Hair coat dry, rough

Pigs
- Depression, anorexia, weight loss
- Tremor, incoordination
- Blindness

- Teeth grinding, squealing as though in pain, salivation, mild diarrhea
- Carpal joints enlarged; disinclined to stand on fore feet
- Recumbency, convulsions terminally
- Death after long course

Subclinical lead poisoning
Cattle subjected to chronic ingestion due to pasture pollution show decreased growth rate.

Clinical pathology

- Blood lead levels elevated but significance difficult to interpret
- Elevated fecal levels indicate lead ingested in preceding 2–3 weeks; availability, toxicity indicated by accompanying high blood levels
- Urine lead levels too erratic to be valuable diagnostically
- Blood levels of δ-aminolaevulinic acid dehydratase (ALA-D) decrease sharply, quickly after lead intake
- Urine levels of ALA (aminolaevulinic acid) increase concurrently
- Blood ALA-D decrease, urine ALA increase detectable well before clinical signs
- Problem with ALA-D estimations is values rise in normal calves up to 6 months
- Recommended procedure is assessment of blood ALA-D *and* blood lead, *plus* erythrocyte protoporphyrin content in cases of long-term exposure
- Hair lead content also a good indicator of chronic poisoning

Necropsy findings

- No gross lesions in acute cases
- Particular lead-bearing material, e.g. paint flakes in reticulum, rumen
- Chronic cases in cattle may show cerebro-cortical softening, cavitation, yellow discoloration, especially in occipital lobes
- Diagnostic tissue lead levels:
  - Cattle 25 mg/kg in wet kidney cortex; liver 10–20 mg/kg
  - Pigs 40 mg/kg liver
  - Horse 4 – 7 mg/kg; up to 250 mg/kg
- Clinically normal animals resident in polluted areas have much higher tissue levels than animals in clean areas

Diagnosis

Acute, subacute disease in cattle resembles:
- Hypomagnesemic tetany

- Nervous acetonemia
- Tetanus
- Arsenic poisoning
- Mercury poisoning
- *Claviceps paspali* poisoning
- Brain abscess
- Cerebral edema-hemorrhage
- Encephalitis
- Encephalomalacia
- Hypovitaminosis A

Chronic form in sheep resembles:
- Polyarthritis
- Enzootic ataxia
- Enzootic muscular dystrophy

Treatment

Results of treatment poor because of difficulty of elimination of poison, combined with the usual very large dose taken.
   The following treatments are used singly or in combination
- Immediate relief of acute nervous signs in calves by intravenous pentobarbital sodium
- Emptying of rumen/reticulum of particulate material via a rumenotomy; emptying of contents must be complete, supplemented by wash-out, careful dredging of reticular mucosal cells, subsequent frequent treatment with magnesium or sodium sulfate to precipitate residual lead
- Removal of lead from deposit site in bone then indirectly from parenchymatous sites by parenteral calcium versenate recommended; hospitalization required for a 5 day course of prolonged, intermittent intravenous infusions
- Parenteral thiamin hydrochloride (2 mg/kg body weight daily) may reduce deposition of lead in tissues and may be a valuable adjunct to calcium versenate therapy

Control

- Adequate nutrition to prevent scavenging, pica
- Proper disposal of garbage
- Only lead-free paints used

ARSENIC POISONING [VM8 p. 1480]

Etiology

- Inorganic arsenicals as
  - Arsenites in herbicides, ectoparasite dips, oral LD50 10–25 mg/kg

♦ Arsenates in herbicides, pasture insecticides, oral LD50 30–100 mg/kg
♦ **Aliphatic organic arsenicals** as herbicides (methanearsonates), and pharmaceuticals (cacodylic, phenarsonic acids) oral LD50 25 mg/kg for 1 week
♦ **Aromatic organic arsenicals** as pharmaceuticals (thiacetarsamide, arsphenamine, arsanilic acid, roxarsone, nitarsone) LD50 2–4 × therapeutic dose.

Epidemiology

Occurrence
♦ Rare poisoning because of declining use as agricultural chemical and more care with industrial effluents
♦ Case fatality rate with alimentary tract syndrome 100%, negligible in nervous syndrome

Source
♦ Herbicide-treated plants
♦ Topical insecticides on animals or pasture or as baits
♦ Effluents from industrial plants treating iron, copper and gold ores
♦ Wood preservatives, including ash from burnt timber
♦ Pharmaceuticals injected, orally, in feed as additive, as growth promotant, antibacterial, antiprotozoal

Route of intake
♦ Usually oral
♦ Skin rarely due to overdosing or treatment when skin hot, in dips, sprays, jets

Agent risk factors
♦ Arsenic persists in environment indefinitely
♦ Not unpalatable, no immediate effect so intake unlimited
♦ Water-soluble compounds most toxic

Environment risk factor
Common problem is pasture contamination by smoke drift from factory, spray drift from neighboring farm.

Importance
♦ Occasional farm or area animal wastage due to deaths or unthriftiness
♦ Can be sentinel for human poisoning via drinking water

Clinical findings

Acute alimentary syndrome
♦ Delay of 24–50 hours after ingestion before illness
♦ Severe diarrhea
♦ Severe dehydration
♦ Abdominal pain, grinding teeth
♦ Rarely vomiting
♦ Ruminal stasis
♦ Tachycardia
♦ Recumbency
♦ Death after 3–4 hour course

Subacute alimentary syndrome
♦ Similar signs to acute disease plus:
♦ Anorexia, thirst
♦ Dehydration, weight loss
♦ Reluctance to move
♦ Tremor
♦ Incoordination
♦ Convulsions, terminal coma
♦ Death after 2–7 day course

Chronic
♦ Unthrifty low body weight, poor milk yield
♦ Dry, thin hair coat
♦ Loss of vigour
♦ Capricious appetite
♦ Muzzle, buccal mucosal reddening, ulceration
♦ Eyelid edema

Skin application
Slow-healing ulceration.

Nervous syndrome
♦ Arsanilic acid
  • Incoordination, blindness in lambs, pigs
  • Recovery if feeding stopped
♦ **Roxarsone and nitarsone**
  • Restless when disturbed
  • Frequent urination, defecation
  • Incoordination, frequent falling
  • Shrill 'screaming'
  • Tremor, convulsions

Clinical pathology

Urine
♦ Level may be as high as 16 mg/kg
♦ Normal levels 10 (inorganic compounds), 5 (organic) days after intake ceases

Hair
- Good source, arsenic level remains till hair shed
- Normal animals may have high levels

Blood
Arsanilic acid causes elevated levels of urea nitrogen, alkaline phosphatase, gamma-glutamyl transpeptidase.

Necropsy findings

- Arsenic levels >10 mg/kg wet weight in kidney or liver diagnostic
- Assay stomach and intestinal wall recommended
- Patient may die before maximum tissue levels achieved; ingesta levels will be high, average 36 mg/kg

Alimentary form
- Pronounced hyperemia, patchy hemorrhage stomach (or abomasum), duodenum and cecum
- Gut contents fluid, contain mucosal shreds, mucous
- Severe degeneration parenchymatous organs

Nervous form
- No gross lesions
- Axonal degeneration peripheral nerves, optic nerves

Diagnosis

Resembles:
- Lead poisoning
- Bovine malignant catarrh
- Bovine virus diarrhea
- Salmonellosis
- Many poisonous plants causing diarrhea

Treatment

- Dimercaptopropanol (BAL), dimercaptosuccinate, sodium thiosulfate, ferric hydrate all rational, specific treatments, but tissue destruction too advanced for significant effect
- Supportive treatment of dehydration plus charcoal orally 1–5 g/kg

Control

- Careful disposal all arsenic residues
- Consult geological data on ore bodies to identify local hazards
- Use alternative insecticides, herbicides

SELENIUM POISONING   [VM8 p. 1484]

Etiology

Acute Poisoning by overdosing (oral or parenteral injection) with selenium compounds.
Chronic Poisoning by ingestion selenocompounds in selenium-containing plants.

Toxic dose rates
Acute Single oral dose:
- Sheep 2.2 mg/kg body weight
- Cattle 9 mg/kg
- Horses 2.2 mg/kg
- Pigs 15 mg/kg

Chronic Daily in diet:
- Ruminants 0.25 mg/kg body weight
- Pigs 11 mg/kg of feed
- Horse 44 mg/kg of feed
- Sheep 2 mg/kg of feed marginally toxic

Epidemiology

Occurrence
- Increasing incidence because of popularity as a ration supplement or 'shotgun' remedy
- Widespread natural occurrence where soil selenium content high
- Morbidity and case fatality rates very high

Source
- Ingestion in plants containing excess absorbed selenium from high-content soil
- Plants dusted or sprayed with selenium
- Oral dosing or injection pharmaceutical selenium-containing compounds used in therapy, prevention of myopathy or growth stimulant
- Aerial pollution from coal treatment works

Environment risk factors
- High rock content in enzootic areas
- Selenium content in overlying soil may contain 1 200 mg/kg
- Poisoning occurs on soils containing 0.01 mg/kg
- Selenium content in 'indicator' (converter plants), listed in selenocompounds, reach 10 000 mg/kg; non-indicator plants <100 mg/kg
- Concurrent selenium and monensin administration
- Selenium in anthelmintic mixtures settles out
- Diets deficient in cobalt or protein
- Low rainfall

Agent risk factors
- Selenite more toxic than selenate, more toxic than selenium dioxide
- Inorganic preparations less toxic than organic, in other than ruminants

Host risk factor
Cattle more tolerant than sheep.

Importance
Large areas of otherwise fertile land not available for farming.

Clinical findings

Acute
- Dyspnea
- Restlessness
- Anorexia
- Salivation
- Diarrhea
- Tachycardia
- Incoordination
- Recumbency, death after short course
- In pigs, additional signs of walking on tiptoe, tremor, vomiting

Chronic (blind staggers)
- Blindness
- Stumbling gait
- Aimless wandering
- Circling
- Head-pressing
- Pica
- Abdominal pain in some
- Recumbency, death

Chronic (alkali disease)
- Dullness
- Emaciation
- Stiff gait, lameness,
- Rough coat, hair loss at tail head and switch, general alopecia in pigs, horses
- Hoof abnormalities (may be congenital) – coronary band swelling, deformity, separation, sloughing of hooves

Miscellaneous pig syndromes
- Paralysis due to poliomyelomalacia
- Low conception rate plus neonatal mortality

Clinical pathology

Critical levels diagnostic of chronic selenosis:
- 3 mg/kg in blood
- Urine levels >4 mg/kg
- Hair 5–10 mg/kg borderline, >10 mg/kg positive

Necropsy findings

Acute poisoning
- Hepatic, renal medullary congestion
- Epicardial petechiation, hyperemia and necrosis
- Some ulceration, abomasum, small intestine

Chronic poisoning
- Skeletal, cardiac myopathy
- Symmetrical myelomalacia
- Pulmonary edema
- Hepatic fibrosis, atrophy
- Glomerulonephritis
- Articular erosion
- Hoof deformity

Selenium levels in tissues
- 20–30 mg/kg in kidney, liver in chronic cases
- Wool 1–2 mg/kg, horse hair >5 mg/kg

Diagnosis

Resembles:
- Subacute lead poisoning
- Hepatic encephalopathy
- Hypovitaminosis A

Treatment and control

- No effective treatment available
- Arsanilic acid in diet (0.01–0.02 %) gives some protection
- Other protection possibly provided by linseed oil, high protein diet or pretreatment with copper compound

PHOSPHORUS POISONING [VM8 p. 1486]

- Elemental phosphorus used (very rarely) as rodenticide
- Causes severe gastroenteritis, with abdominal pain, diarrhea, salivation and vomiting, immediately
- Survivors for 4–10 days develop hepatic necrosis and nephrosis, with jaundice, anorexia, recumbency, oliguria

MERCURY POISONING [VM8 p. 1487]

Etiology and epidemiology

- Mercury compounds used as antifungal agents in stored grain
- Rubefacient topical applications
- All uses of mercury have declined so mercury poisoning rare
- Currently popular phenylmercury fungicides excreted rapidly causing less toxicity and less residue
- Ethyl and methyl compounds retained in tissues, cause nephrosis if fed to pigs at heavy doses for long periods with treated grain more than 10% of diet; can poison humans eating contaminated meat

Clinical findings

Acute inorganic mercury
- Diarrhea
- Vomiting
- Dehydration
- Death in few hours
- Survivors for several days are anorectic, depressed, recumbent, die of uremia due to nephrosis

Chronic inorganic mercury
- Depression
- Anorexia, emaciation
- Alopecia, scabby dermatitis, pruritus
- Mucosae petechiated and tender, teeth shed
- Chronic diarrhea
- Stiff gait
- Incoordination, recumbency
- Convulsions

Chronic organic mercury
After 10 days on feed:

Pigs:
- Blind
- Staggering gait
- Willing but unable to eat

Cattle:
- Tiptoe stance
- Paretic, staggering gait
- Recumbency
- Eat well

Clinical pathology and necropsy findings

- High levels of mercury in feed, urin blood, feces
- High serum alkaline phosphatase, gamm glutamyl transpeptidase
- Necropsy lesions include gastroenteriti nephrosis in inorganic poisoning
- In organic mercury poisoning also neu onal necrosis vacuolation and gliosis brain and spinal cord
- Toxic mercury concentration in kidne 100 mg/kg in organic poisoning, 2000 m; kg in organic mercury poisoning.

Diagnosis

- Acute poisoning resembles arsenic poisor ing
- Chronic poisoning resembles lead poisor ing

Treatment and control

- Dimercaptopropanol (BAL), dimercapto succinate probably rational, specific trea ments, but tissue destruction too advance for significant effect
- Supportive treatment of dehydration plu charcoal orally 1–5 g/kg
- Avoid feeding mercury-treated grain

FLUORINE POISONING [VM8 p. 1489]

Etiology

- Sodium fluoride most toxic, 50 ppm in dr ration causes teeth pitting, 100 ppm sever bone lesions
- Cryolite or rock phosphate less toxic, 10(ppm in dry feed causes only minor teet lesions. Calcium fluoride, sodium fluorosi licate least toxic
- Standard recommendation for dairy cow: is <40 ppm in feed to avoid fall in milk production; lifetime threshold should b lower still

Epidemiology

Occurrence
- Widespread but sporadic, related tc specific local hazards
- Mostly an insidious chronic disease likely to irreversibly affect large numbers of grazing ruminants before detection

Source

♦ Pasture contaminated by superphosphate factory fumes
♦ Volcano ash
♦ Water leached through high fluorine soil into deep wells or artesian bores
♦ High content fluorine rock salt used as feed supplement or pasture top-dressing

Importance

♦ Deaths rare except in acute poisoning
♦ Wastage due to failure to gain weight on apparently good pasture

Clinical findings

Most records refer to disease in cattle; similar clinical signs occur in all other species.

Acute poisoning

♦ Anorexia
♦ Diarrhea, vomiting, ruminal stasis
♦ Tremor
♦ Easily startled, constant chewing, tetany, convulsions
♦ Pupil dilation
♦ Death after few hours

Chronic poisoning ('Fluorosis')
Includes **dental fluorosis** and **osteofluorosis**

Dental fluorosis:
♦ Temporary teeth affected in utero and permanent teeth while still growing
♦ Develop horizontal bands of mottling, then pitting, across all teeth, unless period of exposure is very short
♦ Teeth painful, wear rapidly, easily fractured, mastication difficult, animals lose weight

Osteofluorosis:
♦ Stiff gait
♦ Lameness mostly hind, upper limbs, hip lameness, *or*
♦ Herd-scale sudden onset lameness due to fore limb third phalanx fracture
♦ Bones (mandible, sternum, lower limbs) thickened

Clinical pathology

♦ In diseased cattle blood fluorine levels elevated to 0.6 mg/kg
♦ Urine fluorine levels elevated
♦ Serum alkaline phosphatase levels elevated to 3–7 times normal

♦ Radiological examination of affected bones shows porosity, thickening, frequent fractures

Necropsy findings

Acute poisoning
Gastroenteritis.

Fluorosis

♦ Bones brittle, old fractures, exostoses, some bridging and spurring of joints
♦ Defective, irregular calcification, active periosteal bone formation
♦ Tooth enamel and dentine hypoplasia
♦ Fluorine concentration in bone or teeth elevated from high normal of 1200 to over 4000 mg/kg
♦ Mandibles and ends of the long bones have highest concentrations
♦ Bone ash a good indicator:
  • Normal bone contains up to 0.15% fluorine
  • 1.5% indicates high intake, usually no lesions present
  • Clinical signs associated with 2% fluorine

Diagnosis

Resembles:
♦ Nutritional deficiency of phosphorus
♦ Nutritional deficiency of vitamin D

Treatment

♦ No practical effective treatments available
♦ In acute cases injections of calcium salts and oral administration of aluminium salts to neutralise the fluorine intake.

Control

♦ Feed supplement content of fluorine not to exceed:
  • Milking cows 0.2%
  • Fattening cattle 0.3%
♦ Toxic rock phosphate to be defluorinated
♦ Adequate calcium and phosphorus intakes necessary
♦ Aluminium salts fed as 'alleviators' but unpalatable
♦ Precipitation of fluorine in drinking water possible in large storage tanks

ALUMINIUM POISONING [VM8 p. 1493]

Source

♦ A pasture contaminant from 'acid rain'
♦ Dust in factory effluent
♦ May suppress absorption of phosphorus, cause secondary phosphorus deficiency

MOLYBDENUM POISONING [VM8 p. 1493]

Etiology

♦ Daily intake 120–250 mg molybdenum toxic for cattle
♦ High sulfate, low copper intakes enhance toxicity

Epidemiology

Occurrence
♦ On diets of pasture or hay grown on molybdenum-rich soil
♦ An area problem in most countries

Source
♦ Soils containing 10–100 mg molybdenum/kg potentially dangerous
♦ Forage containing 3–10 mg/kg dangerous
♦ Signs may appear at 1 mg/kg of forage if sulfate content high and copper low
♦ Industrial fumes; aluminium, steel alloy, oil refineries
♦ Overuse of molybdenum fertilizers to promote nitrogen-fixing bacteria

Risk factors
♦ Mostly ruminants, especially cattle
♦ Young animals
♦ Spring
♦ Legumes, especially *Trifolium hybridum* (alsike clover)

Clinical findings

♦ Persistent diarrhea within 10 days of access to pasture
♦ Appetite good
♦ Emaciation, milk production drops
♦ Dry, staring coat
♦ Black hair turns gray, noticeably around eyes
♦ Stiff gait, reluctant to move

Clinical pathology

♦ Blood copper decreases from 15 μmol/l to 2.5 μmol/l
♦ Blood molybdenum rises, 0.05 mg/kg to 0.10 mg/kg; up to 1.4 mg/kg on industrial contaminated pasture
♦ High molybdenum levels in feed, feces, urine, blood, milk.

Necropsy findings

♦ No lesions; no enteritis
♦ Tissue copper levels reduced

Diagnosis

Resembles:
♦ Johne's disease
♦ Intestinal parasitism
♦ Intestinal parasitism and molybdenum poisoning often occur together

Treatment and control

♦ Oral dosing with copper sulfate:
  • Cattle 5 g/week
  • Sheep 1.5 g/week
♦ Long-term prevention is to increase copper content in diet by 5 mg/kg

COPPER POISONING [VM8 p. 1495]

Etiology

The toxicity of copper salts variable depending on other dietary risk factors; causes several forms of poisoning:
♦ **Primary** – excess copper intake
♦ **Secondary** – normal copper intakes but high retention:
  • **Phytogenous** – due to plant intake without liver damage
  • **Hepatogenous** – due to plant-induced liver damage

PRIMARY COPPER POISONING
[VM8 p. 1495]

Epidemiology

Occurrence
♦ Sporadic outbreaks due to accidental ingestion toxic amounts
♦ Rarely enzootic due to copper rich soils
♦ Case fatality rate approximates 100% in acute or chronic forms

Source

- Plants on soil naturally rich in copper
- Plant contamination by:
  - Fungicidal spray
  - Molluscicide
  - Fertilizer
  - Industrial fall-out
  - Drippings from overhead copper cables
  - Manure from pigs fed copper-supplemented ration used as fertilizer
- Grain dusted with copper antifungal agent used as feed
- Overdose parasiticide drench
- Overdose of oral or injectable therapeutic copper agent
- Copper-supplemented pig ration fed to cattle
- Chicken litter from birds fed high copper diet
- Pigs fed diet containing excess or improperly mixed copper
- Pelleted rations containing 8 – 11 mg/kg can be toxic if molybdenum content low

Agent risk factors

Variation in toxicity of injectable preparations – paste preparations and copper methionate non-toxic; soluble compounds, e.g. copper edetate and copper diethylamine oxyquinoline sulfonate toxic.

Host risk factor

- Only ruminants susceptible to low level intakes
- Sheep have varied susceptibility; Texel, Finnish Landrace resistant, Ronaldsay, Orkney very susceptible
- Pigs and horses resistant

Clinical findings

Acute copper poisoning, ingested dose

- Abdominal pain
- Severe diarrhea
- Vomiting
- Green feces, vomitus
- Severe shock, dehydration, death in 24 hours
- Survivors show dysentery, jaundice

Acute poisoning, injected copper salts

- Anorexia, depression, dehydration
- After day 3 massive ascites, hydrothorax, hydropericardium
- Hemoglobinuria
- Extensive hemorrhages
- Dyspnea

- Head-pressing, aimless wandering, circling, ataxia

Chronic copper poisoning

- Intake of copper over long period but disease acute in onset
- Anorexia, thirst
- Hemoglobinuria, pallor, jaundice
- Death in 24–48 hours

Clinical pathology

Acute poisoning

- High copper levels in feces
- Blood and liver levels not elevated for several days

Chronic poisoning

- Blood copper levels 78–114 μmol/l (normal 15 μmol/l)
- Liver biopsy about 16 mmol/kg (normal 5.5 mmol/kg) in sheep, higher in calves and pigs
- Kidney levels rise before liver
- Low blood PCV (40% decreases to 10%)
- Large rise in serum enzymes before hemolytic crisis; SGOT, aspartate aminotransferase, sorbitol dehydrogenase, diethyl succinate carboxylesterase all elevated

Necropsy findings

Acute poisoning, oral intake

Severe gastroenteritis.

Poisoned by injection

- Massive hepatic necrosis
- Fluid accumulations in body cavities.

Chronic poisoning

- Swollen yellow liver, enlarged soft spleen, gunmetal colored kidneys
- Hemoglobinuria, jaundice, pallor
- High liver copper levels (as above).

Diagnosis

Resembles other acute hemolytic diseases:
- Poisoning by plants containing S-methyl-L-cysteine-sulfoxide
- Bovine bacillary hemoglobinuria
- Postparturient hemoglobinuria
- Acute leptospirosis in calves
- Other causes of hepatogenous jaundice

Treatment and control

♦ Poor prognosis in sheep with acute or chronic poisoning
♦ Can be treated symptomatically for gastroenteritis, and hemolytic anemia respectively
♦ Normal lambs with high copper loads prevented from crisis with daily 100 mg ammonium molybdate plus 1 g anhydrous sodium sulfate, or repeated intravenous injections of ammonium tetrathiomolybdate
♦ To prevent uptake of copper additional molybdenum provided in diet (7 mg/kg/day) in superphosphate dressing to pasture, in lick or mineral mixture, or spray on pasture

SECONDARY COPPER POISONING
('TOXEMIC JAUNDICE' COMPLEX)
[VM8 p. 1499]

The following three diseases can occur singly and in any of a series of combinations in parts of Australia; known collectively as **toxemic jaundice.**

Phytogenous copper poisoning
[VM8 p. 1499]

♦ Occurs in sheep grazing pasture with low copper content
♦ Liver copper accumulates, hemolytic crisis occurs as in chronic copper poisoning
♦ Related to pasture domination by *Trifolium subterraneum* (subterranean clover)
♦ British breeds and crosses with merinos most susceptible
♦ Control by daily molybdenum administration

Hepatogenous copper poisoning [VM8 p. 1499]

♦ Hepatic cells damaged by toxins of *Heliotropum europaeum*, *Senecio* spp., *Echium plantagineum*
♦ No occurrence of clinical hepatic insufficiency
♦ Accumulate copper to point of hemolytic crisis

Heliotropum europaeum poisoning [VM8 p. 1499]

♦ Cumulative effects of hepatoxin from plant cause hepatic insufficiency
♦ No copper accumulates

♦ Hepatic jaundice instead of hemolytic jaundice

SODIUM CHLORIDE POISONING
[VM8 p. 1499]

Etiology

♦ Cattle drinking water containing 1.25% salt show decreased milk yield
♦ At 1.5% gain weight suboptimally
♦ At 1.75% show clinical illness
♦ Toxic single dose of salt is 2.2 g/kg body weight

Epidemiology

Occurrence
♦ A minor disease except where bore (artesian and subartesian) waters used for drinking water for livestock
♦ Sporadic deaths only

Source
♦ Thirsty cattle get access to saline bore water
♦ Animals on low salt diet allowed access to *ad lib* salt
♦ Animals on normal salt intake (2% of ration) temporarily deprived of water
♦ Prepared feeds to housed cattle contain excess salt
♦ Swill to pigs contains brine, salted whey
♦ Oil field residues

Host risk factor
Lactating females most susceptible.

Clinical findings

Acute poisoning – cattle and sheep
♦ Rare syndrome – single massive dose can cause vomiting, diarrhea, mucus in feces abdominal pain, anorexia
♦ Uusual syndrome:
  • Opisthotonus
  • Nystagmus
  • Tremor
  • Blindness
  • Paresis, fetlock knuckling, recumbency
  • Convulsions
  • Death after course of 24 hours

Acute poisoning – pigs
♦ Muscle tremor
♦ Weakness, prostration
♦ Convulsions
♦ Death after course of 48 hours

Chronic poisoning – pigs
- Constipation
- Thirst
- Pruritus for 2–4 days then
- Blindness
- Deafness
- Aimless wandering, head-pressing, circling, pivoting intermittent epileptiform convulsions at regular intervals
- Death after course of 2–4 days

Chronic poisoning – cattle and sheep
- Anorexia
- Thirst
- Bawling
- Weight loss
- Hypothermia, dehydration
- Incoordination, convulsions

Topical salt poisoning in pigs
Severe eosinophilic dermatitis when salt rubbed into skin.

Clinical pathology

In pigs serum sodium levels in chronic poisoning elevated from normal (135–145 mmol/l) to 170–210 mmol/l.

Necropsy findings

Acute, single-dose poisoning Gastritis, abomasitis.

Chronic poisoning:
- No gross lesions
- Acute cerebral edema in all species
- **Pigs** – eosinophilic meningoencephalitis
- Sodium levels >150 mg/dl in brain or liver, plus
- Chlorides >180 mg/dl in brain, 70 mg/dl in muscle, 250 mg/dl in liver diagnostic for salt poisoning

Diagnosis

Resembles:
- Encephalomyelitis
- Polioencephalomalacia
- Gut edema, mulberry heart disease

Treatment

- Immediate change of feed and water supply
- Restrict access to unsalted water
- Cerebral decompression by diuretic

Control

- Salt and water available at all times
- Not more than 1% salt in pig diets
- Ensure adequate water available when using feeds, e.g whey with high salt content, or highly salted grain rations to reduce occurrence of urolithiasis
- Drinking water for all livestock to contain not more than 0.5% sodium chloride, or total salts; animals can survive on much higher salinities

ZINC POISONING [VM8 p. 1502]

Etiology

Large intakes necessary, e.g. 6–8 mg/kg in drinking water, 1.5–1.7 g/kg in feed.

Epidemiology

Rare poison in farm animals.

Sources
- Galvanized pipes, tanks or drinking utensils eroded by lactic acid in fermenting milk, pig swill
- Fumes from galvanizing plant
- Common industrial pollutant
- Zinc-based paint
- Excessive supplement to rations for prevention swine parakeratosis, ovine facial eczema, lupinosis
- Thirsty sheep drinking footrot footbath solution

Clinical findings

Pigs
- Anorexia, lethargy, unthriftiness, rough coat
- Subcutaneous hematomas
- Stiffness, lameness
- Joint enlargement, arthritis, especially distal end of tibia
- Recumbency

Cattle
- Chronic constipation, diarrhea
- Somnolence, paresis
- Fall in milk yield

Clinical pathology

Zinc levels in feces and serum elevated.

Necropsy findings

♦ Degenerative lesions in liver and pancreas (obligatory sample for zinc poisoning)
♦ Arthritis, osteoporosis in pigs
♦ Zinc content of liver, bones, kidney and spleen in chronic poisoning 3–4 times normal

Diagnosis

In pig resembles:
♦ Erysipelas
♦ Rickets
    In cattle resembles chronic constipation (not a critical sign in any other disease).

Treatment

Calcium supplementation in diet, short of causing parakeratosis.

SULFUR POISONING [VM8 p. 1504]

Etiology

Very large amounts of flowers of sulfur (horse 0.2–0.4 kg single dose to a horse, 100–400 g to cattle, 45 g to ewes) fed as treatment or prophylaxis, e.g. ovine enterotoxemia.

Clinical findings

♦ Dullness
♦ Abdominal pain
♦ Black diarrhea
♦ Hydrogen sulfide smell on breath
♦ Dyspnea
♦ Tremor, recumbency, convulsions, coma, death

Necropsy findings

Severe gastroenteritis.

SULFUR DIOXIDE POISONING
[VM8 p. 1504]

Exposure to atmosphere containing SO_2 causes salivation, conjunctivitis, coughing due to tracheitis in pigs.

POISONING BY ORGANIC IRON
COMPOUNDS [VM8 p. 1504]

Horses
♦ Fatal, acute hepatitis injected with organic iron prophylactics against juvenile anemia

♦ Newborn **foals** die after oral dosing with iron fumarate causing acute hepatitis; two days after dosing depression, ataxia, recumbency, jaundice, nystagmus
♦ Some sudden deaths minutes after intramuscular iron compound

Piglets
♦ 1–2 hours after injection sudden death or death after vomiting and diarrhea; skeletal but not cardiac, muscle necrosis; 2-day old pigs more susceptible than 8-day olds
♦ Iron injections possible cause of **asymmetric hindquarters**

Cattle
Fatal, acute hepatitis after organic iron prophylactic injection against juvenile anemia; yearling bulls have died 24 hours after iron injection.

IODINE POISONING [VM8 p. 1505]

♦ Rare poison
♦ Occurs only with overdose as medication for goitre, long-term in feed for footrot prophylaxis; 10 mg/kg body weight daily needed to kill calves

Cattle, sheep, and horses
♦ Anorexia
♦ Heavy, large-scaled dandruff, hair loss, dry coat
♦ Lacrymation, nasal discharge, hypersalivation
♦ Hyperthermia
♦ Coughing due to bronchopneumonia
♦ Serum iodine levels elevated, vitamin A levels reduced
♦ Heavy dosing mares and foals may cause goiter in foals

CADMIUM POISONING [VM8 p. 1505]

Etiology

Rare poisoning in farm animals. Caused by:
♦ Improper use as anthelmintic
♦ Environmental pollutant, e.g. sewage sludge or sewage, cadmium paint

Clinical findings

Cattle – chronic poisoning

♦ Anorexia
♦ Weakness
♦ Dry, brittle horns, hair matting
♦ Skin hyperkeratosis
♦ Forestomach wall hyperkeratosis
♦ Congenital defects, abortion in pregnant cows

Pigs
♦ Reduced growth rate
♦ Anemia

Horse
♦ Colic
♦ Ataxia

CHROMIUM POISONING [VM8 p. 1506]

♦ In protein supplement of tannery waste fed to pigs
♦ Tremor, diarrhea, dyspnea

BROMIDE POISONING [VM8 p. 1506]

♦ Accidental access by goats
♦ Somnolence, recumbency, dribbling urine

COBALT POISONING [VM8 p. 1506]

♦ Accidental overdosing to calves
♦ Weight loss, rough coat, listlessness, anorexia, incoordination
♦ Sheep and pigs resistant

BORON POISONING [VM8 p. 1506]

♦ Solubilized boron preparations used as additives to fertilizers
♦ **Cattle** – depression, weakness, tremor, ataxia, spastic gait, seizures, opisthotonus, tremor of periorbicular muscles, backwards stumbling, recumbency, death
♦ **Goats** – similar plus head-shaking, oral champing, phantom-dodging, restlessness, frequent urination, sham eating and drinking

DISEASES CAUSED BY FARM CHEMICALS

Many farm chemicals have potential as poisons but are safe if used in accordance with manufacturer's instructions. Most of the following poisonings occur as a result of ignorance of the poisonous nature of the chemical or its improper use. Subjects dealt with are the clinical illnesses that occur. More important are the pollutions of the human food chain that can occur.

POISONING BY ANTHELMINTICS
[VM8 p. 1507]

See Table 31.1.

INSECTICIDES [VM8 p. 1511]

See Table 31.2.

HERBICIDES AND DEFOLIANTS
[VM8 p. 1517]

See Table 31.3.

FUNGICIDES [VM8 p. 1519]

Used on plants and as seed dressings:
♦ Hexachlorobenzene (HCB), organic mercury compounds, popular seed fungistats
♦ **Zineb,** used on growing plants; can cause thyroid hyperplasia, hypofunction, cardiac and skeletal muscle degeneration, testicular weight reduction, decreased germ cell volume
♦ **Thiram,** general agricultural fungistat; causes conjunctivitis, rhinitis, bronchitis on local contact; suspected teratogen and abortifacient.

RODENTICIDES [VM8 p. 1519]

See Table 31.4.

MOLLUSCICIDES [VM8 p. 1520]

See Table 31.5.

WOOD PRESERVATIVES [VM8 p. 1521]

See Table 31.6.

SEED DRESSINGS [VM8 p. 1521]

Used as baits for insects and birds, bird repellents, grain fumigants against weevils, fungistats in grain, see Table 31.7.

ADDITIVES IN FEED [VM8 p. 1522]

Used mostly as growth promotants and feed substitutes; see Table 31.8.

MISCELLANEOUS FARM
CHEMICALS [VM8 p. 1527]
See Table 31.9

Table 31.1 Poisonous anthelmintics

Substance	Use	Species	Clinical signs, clinical pathology	Necropsy lesions	Treatment
Carbon Tetrachloride or Tetrachloroethylene [VM8 p. 1507]	Fasciolicide	All	**Acute** Immediate narcosis, collapse, convulsions **Subacute** Day 3–4 Anorexia, depression, jaundice, photosensitisation, liver enzymes in serum elevated	Pulmonary, hepatic, renal damage, abomasitis	Artificial respiration
Phenothiazine [VM8 p. 1508]	Anthelmintic	Cattle, sheep, pig, goat	Photosensitive conjunctivitis, keratitis, dermatitis	Cutaneous lesions	Protect from sunlight
Hexachloroethane [VM8 p. 1509]	Fasciolicide	Cattle, sheep	Narcosis, tremor, falling, recumbency especially emaciated animals. Some show abdominal pain, dyspnea, bleat, diarrhea	Nil	Treat as for milk fever. Calcium solutions
Hexachlorophane (=Hexachlorophene) [VM8 p. 1509]	Fasciolicide, detergent	All	Nystagmus, tremor, opisthotonus, anorexia, diarrhea, recumbency. Seminiferous tubule atrophy	Repeated dosing – periportal hepatic fatty degeneration	Nil
Rafoxanide, Closantel [VM8 p. 1509]	Anthelmintic	All	Overdose – temporary or permanent blindness	Degeneration optic nerves and cerebral optic paths	Nil
Nicotine [VM8 p. 1509]	Anthelmintic	All	Rarely used. Immediate dyspnea, tremor, recumbency, convulsions: abdominal pain, salivation, diarrhea	Abomasitis	Respiratory stimulants, artificial respiration, oral tannic acid preparations
Toluene [VM8 p. 1509]	Anthelmintic	All	Vomiting, purgation, incoordination, tremor	Bone marrow depression	Nil

Continued

573

Table 31.1 Continued

Substance	Use	Species	Clinical signs, clinical pathology	Necropsy lesions	Treatment
Piperazine [VM8 p. 1509]	Anthelmintic	Horse	Incoordination, pupil dilation, tremor, hyperaesthesia, somnolence, recumbency	Nil	Spontaneous recovery
Cadmium salts [VM8 p. 1509]	Ascaricide	Pig	Rarely used. Vomiting, uremia	Tissue accumulation, gastroenteritis, nephrosis	Nil
Thiabendazole [VM8 p. 1509]	Anthelmintic	Cattle, sheep	Rare occurrence – **Acute** Aggression, incoordination collapse **Delayed** Uremia	Nephrosis	Nil
Levamisole [VM8 p. 1510]	Anthelmintic	Cattle, sheep, goat and pig	Liplicking, salivation, headshake, tremor, excitable, compulsive running, cough. Higher dose – diarrhea, continuous skin twitch, teeth grind, ptosis, frequent micturition, straining. High mortality after injection	Nil	Nil
Parbendazole, Cambendazole (Albendazole?) [VM8 p. 1510]	Anthelmintic	Cattle, sheep	Teratogens at high dose rates in early pregnancy. Abnormal gait and posture, limb deformity, cranial asymmetry (Albendazole possibly similar at very high doses)	Vertebral fusion. Cerebral hypoplasia, hydrocephalus	Contra-indicated use in pregnant females
Fenbendazole plus bromsalans [VM8 p. 1510]	Simultaneous or close use anthelmintic and fasciolicide	Cattle, sheep	Found dead	Nil	Nil

574

Substance	Use	Species	Clinical signs	Post-mortem	Notes
Ivermectin [VM8 p. 1510]	Anthelmintic	Horse	I/V cattle preparation (forbidden) collapse, coma, nystagmus. I/M injection: edema ventral midline, limbs, eyelids, dyspnea, disorientation, colic, sudden death	Nil	Nil
Ivermectin [VM8 p. 1510]	Anthelmintic	Cattle, Murray-Grey only	Sporadic outbreaks of incoordination, knuckling, swaying gait, tremor, ear droop, blind, salivation, within 24 hours. All die	Very high concentration Ivermectin in brain. No lesions	Suspected genetic susceptibility
Hygromycin B [VM8 p. 1510]	Ascaricide	Pigs	Prolonged dosings causes cataracts in sows	Nil	Nil
Organophosphorus compounds [VM8 p. 1510]			(See under Insecticides – Table 31.2)		
Tetrachlorodifluoroethane (FREON-112) [VM8 p. 1511]	Fasciolicide Some samples toxic	Sheep, cattle	Marked prolongation clotting time	Kidney, liver, myocardium damage. Extensive haemorrhages, anasarca	Nil
Sumicidin (Fenvalerate) [VM8 p. 1511]	Anthelmintic (synthetic pyrethroid) Single oral dose	All	Non-fatal, restless, yawn, froth at mouth, dyspnea, ear and tail erection. Pupil dilation, regurgitation, incoordination, tremor, convulsions, recumbency. Repeated doses fatal	Nil	Nil

Table 31.2 Poisonous insecticides

Substance	Use	Species	Clinical signs, clinical pathology	Necropsy findings	Treatment
Chlorinated Hydrocarbons (DDT, benzene hexachloride, lindane, aldrin, dieldrin, chlordane, toxaphene, methoxychlor, DDD, isodrin, endrin, heptachlor [VM8 p. 1511]	General insecticide	All	Formidable threats as pollutants to meat industry. Use forbidden on animals in most countries. Can be ingested after agricultural use. Minutes or hours after administration: anorexia, excitability, hyperaesthesia, tremor, recumbency, salivation, vomiting. Teeth grinding, salivation, vomiting. Most severe cases show frenzy, frequent urination. Toxin estimation done on tail/head fat pad	Liver damage in some. Nephrosis in some	Sedation. 3–6 months to clear toxin from body fat
Organophosphorus compounds and carbamates. Many commercially available products. [VM8 p. 1514]	Spray, pour-on, oral insecticides. Big risk is kerosene-based formulations for buildings applied to animals	All	*Cholinesterase inactivation syndrome* **Cattle** Salivation, lacrymation, restless, cough, dyspnea, stagger, frequent urination, stiff gait, pupil constriction. Signs at 30 mins, peak at 90 mins, death at 24–28 hours. **Horse** Plus colic, diarrhea	Nil	Atropine, double doses repeated as needed. Oximes useful if used early. Atropine and oximes recommended
		All	**Delayed neurotoxicity** 3 weeks after dosing. Knuckling of hind fetlocks, completely flaccid paralysis. Bright and alert	Distinctive degenerative lesions in spinal cord and peripheral nerves	Nil
		Pigs	**Teratogenicity** Ataxia, tremor, in piglets. **Clinical pathology** Blood cholinesterase levels reduced for long periods. Estimation of DETP in urine useful guide	Nil	Nil
Rotenone [VM8 p. 1517]	Insecticide	Pigs	Very high accidental doses. Salivation, tremor, vomiting, ascending paralysis, incoordination, quadriplegia, coma, death	Nil	Nil
Amitraz [VM8 p. 1517]	Anti-tick spray prohibited for use in horses	Horse (accidental use)	Somnolence, incoordination, reduced gut sounds, large bowel impaction colic	Nil	Hose to remove Amitraz spray. Anti-impaction treatment with oral oil and fluids oral and I/V. Some

576

Table 31.3 Poisonous herbicides, defoliants

Substance	Use	Species	Clinical signs, clinical pathology	Necropsy findings	Treatment
Arsenical herbicides [VM8 p. 1517]	Herbicide	All	See Arsenic poisoning (p. 560)		
Sodium Chlorate [VM8 p. 1518]	Herbicide	All	Accidental heavy doses. Diarrhea, haemoglobinuria, anaemia, methemoglobinemia. Somnolence, dyspnea	Abomasal, duodenal ulcers. Blood, muscles, viscera very dark	Copious blood transfusions
Dinitrophenols (Dinitrophenol DNP; dinitro-orthocresol DNOC, dinoseb) [VM8 p. 1517]	Herbicide dinitrophenols	All	Inhalation, ingestion or percutaneous absorption. Restless, sweating, dyspnea, fever, collapse. In ruminants also intravascular hemolysis, methemoglobinemia, hypoproteinemia. Death in 24–48 hours	Nil	Nil
2, 4-D, Silvex, MCPA, 2, 4, 5-T piclorum, clopyralid, barban [VM8 p. 1518]	Herbicides, hormonal substances	Cattle, sheep, pig	Only with large doses. **Cattle** Salivation, tachycardia, anorexia, dysphagia, tympanites, recumbency. **Pigs** Vomiting, incoordination, diarrhea	Long term administration to pigs – degenerative lesions liver and kidneys	Nil
Carbamate, triazine, propionanilide, diallylacetamide [VM8 p. 1518]	Herbicides	Sheep	Initial stomatitis, colic, vomiting Acute, large doses – death. Repeat small doses – alopecia	Nil	Nil
Paraquat [VM8 p. 1518]	Dipyridillium herbicide	Sheep, cattle, pig	At 7 days, dyspnea, diarrhea, death in pigs	**Pigs** – pulmonary edema, fibrosing pneumonitis. **Ruminants** – abomasitis, enteritis	Nil

Continued

577

Table 31.3 Continued

Substance	Use	Species	Clinical signs, clinical pathology	Necropsy findings	Treatment
Diquat [VM8 p. 1578]	Dipyridil herbicide	Cattle, sheep	Diarrhea, high mortality	Abomasitis, enteritis, pulmonary emphysema, enteritis, hepatitis, myocardial degeneration	Nil
Triallate	Herbicide	Sheep, pigs	Salivation, vomiting, bradycardia, dyspnea, tremor, convulsions, recumbency, death on day 3	Nil	Nil
Triazine (simazine, atrazine, prometone)	Triazine herbicides	Sheep, cattle	**Acute** Dyspnea, diarrhea, teeth grinding, exophthalmos, salivation, stiff gait, tenesmus, recumbency fatal. **Chronic** Tremor, tetany paraplegia	Nil	Activated charcoal
Simazine and aminonitrazole (Hormone weed killer)	Herbicide mixture	Sheep, horses	**Sheep** Incoordination, recumbency. **Horse** Colic	Nil	Nil
Trichlopyr	Post-emergence herbicide	Horses	Large doses only – colic, diarrhea, dyspnea, ataxia, tremor	Nil	Nil
Monochloracetate (SMCA)	Defoliant	Sheep, cattle	Diarrhea, colic, tremor, stiff gait, dyspnea, excitable, aggression, convulsions. Death in few hours	Nil	Nil
Tributyl phosphororithioite	Organophosphatic defoliant	Sheep, cattle	Dyspnea, diarrhea, bloat, tremor, pupil constriction	Nil	Atropine plus oximes
Thidiazuron	Defoliant for cotton plants	Sheep, cattle	Not toxic but serious potential human food chain pollutant	Nil	Nil

Table 31.4 Poisonous rodenticides

Substance	Use	Species	Clinical signs, clinical pathology	Necropsy findings	Treatment
Sodium Fluoroacetate (1080) [VM8 p. 1519]	Rodenticide bait, combined with cereal	All	**Herbivores** Sudden death without struggle or dyspnea; convulsions, cardiac arrhythmia, weak pulse. ECG abnormality. May appear only during activity. **Pigs** Hyperexcitability, tetanic convulsions	Multifocal myocardial injury	Nil
Alphanaphthylthiourea ANTU [VM8 p. 1519]	Rodenticide bait	All	Death within 24–48 hours	Pleural effusion, pulmonary edema, pericardial effusion	Nil
VALOR [VM8 p. 1519]	Rodenticide bait. No longer available	All	Too risky to be generally available. **Horse** Dehydration, abdominal pain, hind limb paresis, inappetent, fishy smell of urine	Nil	Empty stomach. Nicotinamide effective antidote if given early, within 1 hour
Warfarin [Including brodifacoum, pindone, diphacinone, coumatetralyl] [VM8 p. 1520]	Rodenticide bait	All	Mostly **pigs** Repeated doses cause sudden massive haemorrhage and death or subcutaneous haemorrhages with lameness over period of days. Prolonged prothrombin time	Massive haemorrhages	Blood transfusions. Vitamin K is complete antidote
Red Squills [VM8 p. 1520]	Rodenticide	All	Convulsions, gastritis, bradycardia	Gastritis	Nil
Zinc phosphide [VM8 p. 1520]	Rodenticide	Pig, horse	Anorexia, dullness	Haemorrhages, enteritis, liver damage	Nil

Table 31.5 Poisonous molluscicides

Substance	Use	Species	Clinical signs, clinical pathology	Necropsy findings	Treatment
Metaldehyde [VM8 p. 1520]	Snail bait in a bran base	All	Incoordination, hyperaesthesia, tremor, salivation, dyspnea, diarrhea, part blindness, cyanosis, coma, death in a few hours. Hyperthermia in some	Nil	Rumenotomy, tranquillizer, sedative. Mineral oil orally
Methiocarb [VM8 p. 1520]	Carbonate molluscicide	All	Depression, hypersalivation, diarrhea, dyspnea, ataxia, aimless wandering, tremor, sweating	Pulmonary edema	Atropine large dose, repeated as needed

Table 31.6 Poisonous wood preservatives

Substance	Use	Species	Clinical signs, clinical pathology	Necropsy findings	Treatment
Phenolic compounds, pentachlorophenol dinitrophenol, etc. [VM8 p. 1521]	Wood preservative used on accommodation. Dioxins may be contaminants	Pig, cattle	Depression, dermatitis, death; stillbirths, anorexia, weight loss, ventral edema, limb edema, anaemia, alopecia	Hepatic necrosis	Nil
Copper – chrome – arsenate [VM8 p. 1521]	Treated lumber used in yards/barns	All	Animals need to have chewing habit. Copper, arsenic poisoning	Nil	Nil

Table 31.7 Poisonous seed dressings

Substance	Use	Species	Clinical signs, clinical pathology	Necropsy findings	Treatment
Arsenic [VM8 p. 1521]	Bird bait	All	See text (p. 560)	Nil	Nil
Organophosphorus compounds [VM8 p. 1521]	Insect baits	All	See Table 31.2	Nil	Nil
Metaldehyde [VM8 p. 1521]	Snail baits	All	See Table 31.5	Nil	Nil
Methyl bromide [VM8 p. 1521]	Insect fumigant		See Table 31.9	Nil	Nil
Dibromoethane [VM8 p. 1521]	Insect fumigant	Sheep	Dyspnea. Death in 2–5 days	Pulmonary edema, epithelialization, fibrosis	Nil
Organic mercurials [VM8 p. 1522]	Seed fungistat	All	See text (p. 564)	Nil	Nil
Hexachlorobenzene [VM8 p. 1522]	Seed fungistat	All	Potent persistent human food chain pollutant	High doses cause hepatitis	Nil
4-amino-pyridine [VM8 p. 1521]	Bird repellent	Horse, cattle	Fright, sweating, convulsions, death in 2 hrs. Tremor, ataxia, erratic behaviour, walking backwards, anorexia, diarrhea, tenesmus	Nil	Nil
Sodium fluorosilicate [VM8 p. 1529]	Insect baits	Sheep, horses	Drowsy, anorexia, constipation, ruminal stasis, abdominal pain, diarrhea, teeth grinding, bradycardia	Nil	Nil

581

Table 31.8 Poisonous feed additives

Substance	Use	Species	Clinical signs, clinical pathology	Necropsy findings	Treatment
Copper salts [VM8 p. 1522]	Growth promotant pigs and poultry	All	Copper poisoning (p. 566)	Copper poisoning	Nil
Amprolium [VM8 p. 1522]	Antithiamine coccidiostat	Ruminants	Polioencephalomalacia (p. 668)	Polioencephalomalacia	Nil
Arsenilic acid [VM8 p. 1522]	Swine dysentery prophylaxis	Pigs	Arsenic poisoning (p. 560)	Arsenic poisoning	Nil
Iodinated casein [VM8 p. 1522]	Increase milk yield	Cattle	Cardiac irregularity, dyspnea, restlessness, diarrhea in hot weather	Nil	Nil
Estrogenic substances [VM8 p. 1522]	Growth stimulant. Also as implants contaminating animal residues used as feed additives	Cattel, sheep, goats, pigs	**Cattle** Steers mounting steers, head butting injuries, hole digging; prepuce prolapse, rectum and vagina prolapse, tail head elevation, pelvic fractures, hip dislocation. Retardation testicle and epididymis development. Pregnants – abortion, vulvar swelling; endometritis, irregular estrus. **Lambs** Prolapse rectum, vagina, obstructive urolithiasis. **Pigs** Tenesmus, rectum prolapse, anuria, uremia	Enlargement uterus. Male supernumerary teat length increased. **Pigs** Rectal wall necrosis, kidney enlargement, bladder distension, ureters thickened, prostate enlarged	Nil
Urea (and other industrial byproducts, e.g. diureido isobutane) [VM8 p. 1522]	Accidental feeding excess amounts used as protein supplement. Causes NH$_3$ poisoning	Ruminants, horse experimentally	**Acute** 10–30 minutes after feeding. Severe abdominal pain, frothing at nose and mouth, hyperexcitability, aggression, tremor, incoordination, dyspnea, bloat, recumbency, convulsions, bellowing. Death in a few minutes up to 4 hours. High case fatality rate	High rumen ammonia levels. Pulmonary edema	Oral weak acid, e.g. vinegar (4L/cow). Must be administered very early. Rumen lavage or rumenotomy

Substance	Source / Use	Species	Clinical signs	Lesions	Treatment
Propylene glycol [VM8 p. 1523]	Acetonemia preventive for cows fatal if accidentally fed to horses, or by tube	Horse	Short course; colic, sweating, salivation, staggery gait, depression, fetid faeces	Gastroenteritis, brain edema	Nil
Dried poultry wastes [VM8 p. 1523]	Manure feathers, spilt feeds, carcases as protein supplement	Ruminants	See Copper poisoning, Monensin poisoning (below), estrogen poisoning (p. 582). Also botulism (p. 285). Also syndrome in lambs of ascites, hypoalbuminemia, hepatic necrosis	Nil	Nil
Newsprint [VM8 p. 1524]	Roughage supplement	Ruminants	Lead residues in tissues without clinical signs	Lead residues	Nil
Sewage sludge [VM8 p. 1524]	Top dressing or feed supplement	Ruminants	Lead poisoning (p. 558), cadmium poisoning (p. 570)	Nil	Nil
Ionophores (e.g. monensin, lasolocid, maduromicin, marasin, salinomycin) [VM8 p. 1524]	Growth promotants. Contaminant in poultry wastes used as feed additive	All species. Especially horses	**Cattle** Feed refusal, diarrhea, tremor, tachycardia, ruminal atony (acute heart failure). Survivors show congestive heart failure. Deaths months later also at exertion, calving. **Sheep** Same plus hindquarters skeletal muscle atrophy, stiff gait. **Pigs** Same plus myoglobinuria, cyanosis, pruritus. **Horses** Very susceptible. Found dead or restless, dyspnea, diarrhea, mucosal congestion, profuse sweating, cardiac irregularity, tachycardia, red urine, difficulty rising, stiff gait, fetlock knuckling, recumbency. High serum CPK, LDA, AAT. Myoglobinuria	Cardiomyopathy, pulmonary edema, hepatic enlargement, skeletal muscle necrosis, myoglobinuric nephrosis. Cardiac and skeletal muscle fibrosis	Activated charcoal of limited value

Continued

Table 31.8 Continued

Substance	Use	Species	Clinical signs, clinical pathology	Necropsy findings	Treatment
Monensin and tiamulin, or Salinomycin and tiamulin [VM8 p. 1526]	Simultaneous administration of coccidiostats or growth promotants	Pigs	Anorexia, weight loss. Toxaemia only if manufacturer's recommendations about dose rates are exceeded	Myonecrosis of tongue, diaphragm, limbs	Avoided by using correct dose rates and lapse of 72 hours between the two substances
Pluronics [VM8 p. 1526]	Bloat preventive	Accidental feeding to calves	Dyspnea, ruminal tympany, bellow, tongue protrusion, nystagmus, recumbency, opisthotonus, convulsions. Death after 24 hours	Nil	Nil
Carbadox (mecadox, fortigro) or olaquindox [VM8 p. 1526]	Growth promotant, control of swine dysentery. Recommended dose exceeded	Pigs	Gaunt, emaciated, hard faecal pellets, long rough coat, pale skin, tachycardia, swaying walk, fetlock knuckling, recumbency. Death in 8–9 days. Pigs screech frequently. Sows agalactic, stillborn or weak piglets. Low serum Na, high serum K. High BUN	Adrenal zona glomerulosa necrosis. Renal tubular necrosis	Irreversible. May survive but grave disability
Bronopol [VM8 p. 1526]	Laboratory preservative for milk fed to calves or pigs	Calves, pigs	Salivation, depression, collapse, death by 24 hours	Necrotizing abomasitis and local peritonitis	Nil
Furazolidone [VM8 p. 1670]	Calf scour Prophylaxis in milk replacer	Calves	Septicemia in neonates. Mucosal petechial and granulocytosis	General petechiation	Blood transfusion. Intensive antibiotic program

Table 31.9 Poisonous miscellaneous farm chemicals

Substance	Use	Species	Clinical signs, clinical pathology	Necropsy findings	Treatment
Polybrominated Biphenyls [VM8 p. 1527]	Flame retardants, feed pollutants	All	Experimental with very heavy doses only. Anorexia, diarrhea, lacrimation, salivation, emaciation, dehydration, depression, abortion, contamination of meat, milk, etc. causes their condemnation for human use	Mucoid enteritis, degenerative lesions in kidney, cutaneous hyperkeratinization	Nil
Polychlorinated Biphenyls [VM8 p. 1528]	Industrial use chemicals, common environment and feed pollutants	All	Reduced reproduction efficiency, feed conversion rate. Experimentally diarrhea, anal and nasal erythema, abdomen distension, growth retardation, coma, death	Possibly hepatic hypertrophy, gastric erosion	Nil
Methylbromide [VM8 p. 1528]	Soil fumigant	Cattle, goat, horse	Ataxia, somnolence, drunken behaviour	Nil	Nil
Formalin [VM8 p. 1528]	In preserved colostrum, treated grain	Cattle	Severe diarrhea, salivation, abdominal pain, recumbency	Rumenitis, enteritis	Alimentary protectives
Sodium hydroxide [VM8 p. 1524]	Caustic treated grain	Cattle	No apparent illness	Focal interstitial nephritis, rumenitis, abomasal ulceration	Nil
Ammonia [VM8 p. 1524]	Ammoniated forage contains substituted imidazole	Cattle, sheep	'Bovine Bonkers' Hyperexcitability, restless, blinking, pupil dilation, earflicking, frequent urination and defecation, dyspnea, frothing at mouth, bellowing, charging, circling convulsions, tremor, opisthotonos	Nil	Sedation. Poor response

Continued

585

Table 31.9 Continued

Substance	Use	Species	Clinical signs, clinical pathology	Necropsy findings	Treatment
Oil, petroleum, kerosene, diesoline [VM8 p. 1528]	Accidental ingestion of oil products on farm	Cattle, sheep, goat	Incoordination, anorexia, regurgitation, short course, death. Pupil dilation, smell of oil, oil in feces, constipation to diarrhea. Poor condition for 6 months	Oil in gut contents for long periods. Aspiration, pneumonia	Nil
Dibutyl tin laureate [VM8 p. 1529]	Coccidiostat	Cattle	Short course, tremor, convulsions, recumbent, diarrhea for calves. Adults – chronic, diarrhea, weight loss, anorexia, polyuria	Nil	Nil
Highly chlorinated naphthalenes [VM8 p. 1529]	Lubricants, insulants, wood preservatives	Cattle	Antivitamin A. Cutaneous hyperkeratosis, emaciation, hairloss, conjunctivitis, cough, infertility, abortion	Nil	Nil
Coal tar pitch (toxic cresols) [VM8 p. 1530]	Tarred walls and floors of pens, clay pigeons	Pigs	**Acute** Anorexia, rough coat, weakness, depression. **Chronic** Plus anaemia, jaundice or just growth rate reduction. Low levels haemoglobin, RBC count	Jaundice, ascites, anaemia. Liver damage	Nil
Methyl alcohol [VM8 p. 1530]	Antifreeze or oilfield pumps	Cattle	Vomiting, recumbency, death	Nil	Nil
Ethylene glycol [VM8 p. 1530]	Automobile antifreeze	Cattle, goat, pig	Oxalate nephrosis. **Pig** Depression, recumbency. **Cattle** Dyspnea, incoordination, paresis, recumbency, death, uremia, hypocalcaemia	Edema in body cavities, nephrosis. Toxin in tissues	4-methyl pyrazole, or ethanol

Substance	Source/Use	Species	Signs	Lesions	Control
Industrial organophosphorus compounds [VM8 p. 1530]	Hydraulic fluids, lubricants, coolants	All	Several weeks after ingestion. Knuckling, leg weakness, posterior paralysis	Degenerative lesions in peripheral nerves, spinal cord (as for insecticide organophosphates)	Nil
Superphosphate [VM8 p. 1530]	Fertilizer, used as phosphate dietary supplement	Sheep, cattle	Anorexia, polydipsia, diarrhea, ataxia, recumbency. Uremia, death in 48 hours	Nephrosis	Nil
Manure gas (1) H_2S [VM8 p. 1531]	From holding pits under barn floors	Cattle, pig	Sudden death when pit agitated before emptying	Pulmonary edema, extensive haemorrhages muscles, viscera. Cerebral necrosis and edema	Oxidizing agent in holding pit
(2) NH_3 [VM8 p. 1531]		Pigs	Conjunctivitis, sneezing, coughing, reduced weight gain, increased incidence pneumonia	Pneumonia	Ventilation

32 DISEASES CAUSED BY TOXINS IN PLANTS, FUNGI, CYANOBACTERIA, CLAVIBACTERIA, INSECTS AND ANIMALS

DISEASES CAUSED BY MAJOR PHYTOTOXINS

Minor phytotoxins are listed in Table 32.1 (p. 602)

Establishing a diagnosis of plant poisoning requires as many of the following criteria as possible to be satisfied:
♦ Epidemiology, clinical signs, clinical pathology, necropsy lesions of the case match those of the suspected poison
♦ Patient had access to, preferably known to have eaten, suspect plant
♦ Suspect plant identified precisely
♦ Suspect plant in rumen
♦ Toxin of plant in gut or tissues
♦ Feeding trial to establish plant has observed effect

CYANOGENETIC GLYCOSIDE
POISONING (CYANIDE,
HYDROCYANIC ACID)
[VM8 p. 1533]

Etiology

Important plants containing cyanogenetic glycosides and liberate cyanide ions in rumen: *Acacia* spp. (wattle), *Amelanchier alnifolia* (Saskatoon serviceberry), *Brachyachne convergens*, *Chaenomeles* spp. (flowering quince), *Cynodon* spp. (couch grasses), *Eucalyptus* spp. (gum trees), *Glyceria maxima* (tall manna grass), *Linum usitatissimum* (linseed), *Lotus* spp. (birdsfoot trefoils), *Malus sylvestris* (common crabapple), *Nandina domestica* (nandina), *Photinia* spp. (Christmas berry), *Prunus* spp. (chokecherry, etc.), *Sorghastrum nutans* (Indian grass), *Sorghum* spp. (sorghums), *Suckleya suckleyana*, *Triglochin* spp. (arrowgrass), and many others.

Epidemiology

♦ Cyanide content greatest in plants growing rapidly after retardation period
♦ Greatest danger when animals hungry, eat quickly; signs may appear within 15 minutes of access

Clinical findings

Acute
Common syndrome:
♦ Dyspnea
♦ Pupil dilation, nystagmus
♦ Weak, irregular pulse
♦ Salivation
♦ Mucosal cyanosis
♦ Tremor, restless, moaning
♦ Stumble, recumbent
♦ Convulsions
♦ Terminal vomiting, aspiration into lungs
♦ Death after a course of a few minutes usually 2–3 hours

Chronic
♦ Ataxia–cystitis in horses, possibly cattle, sheep, grazing *Sorghum* spp.
  • Frequent urination, scalding perineum
  • Incoordination, worst when backing
♦ Arthrogryposis of foals and calves; dam grazing *Sorghum* spp. – dystokia

Clinical pathology

Field (Henrici) test for HCN in plants and rumen contents.

Necropsy findings

Acute
♦ No diagnostic lesions
♦ Critical test is high HCN content in rumen, liver (up to 4 hours after death) or muscle (up to 20 hours)

Chronic
♦ Degenerative lesions in spinal cord white matter, cystitis
♦ Arthrogryposis

Diagnosis

Resembles:
♦ Nitrite poisoning
♦ Cyanobacterial toxins
♦ Lightning stroke
♦ Vitamin E and selenium deficiency
♦ Inherited cardiomyopathy

Treatment

♦ Early treatment very effective
♦ Sodium nitrite–sodium thiosulfate mixture I/V, *or*
♦ Heavy doses thiosulfate alone, *or*
♦ With cobaltous chloride, *or*
♦ With *p*-aminopropriophenone, *or*
♦ *p*-aminopropriophenone alone

Control

♦ Avoid cyanogenetic glycoside-containing plants, especially fast-growing crops after retardation
♦ Care with hungry sheep and cattle
♦ Hay made from danger plants equally dangerous
♦ If in doubt, test plants with Henrici test, graze with pilot group

NITRATE POISONING
[VM8 p. 1536]

Etiology

Nitrate in:
♦ Salt curing mixtures from meat plants
♦ Effluent from rubber processors
♦ Residues of blasting powders in dams
♦ Water from deep surface wells

Clinical findings

♦ Salivation
♦ Abdominal pain, vomiting, diarrhea
♦ Dehydration, death
♦ Nitrite poisoning

NITRITE POISONING [VM8 p. 1536]

Etiology

♦ Preformed nitrite in feed due to conversion of nitrate, present as contaminant or due to high soil content, by bacterial action or heating
♦ Conversion of nitrate as feed component by rumen bacteria
♦ Safe content in pasture is 2% of dry matter as nitrate

Epidemiology

♦ Commonest in cattle because ready conversion nitrate
♦ Sheep readily convert nitrite to ammonia
♦ Pigs very susceptible but poisoned only when nitrite preformed in feed
♦ High nitrate in soil/plant when:
  • Heavy application of nitrate fertilizer
  • After drought allows accumulation of nitrate
  • Plant growth retarded because of disease, herbicide application, cold spell
♦ Monensin promotes nitrate-nitrite conversion
♦ Access to specific plants, e.g. *Amaranthus* spp. (redroot), *Arctotheca calendula* (capeweed), *Atriplex muellerius* (annual saltbush), *Avena sativa* (oats), *Beta vulgaris* (beets), *Brassica* spp. (rape, turnip, etc.), *Carduus* spp. (winged thistle), *Chenopodium* spp. (goosefoot), *Lolium* spp. (ryegrasses), *Pennisetum* spp. (kikuyu, Napier grasses), *Salvia reflexa* (mintweed), *Silybum marianum* (variegated thistle), *Sorghum* spp., *Urochloa panicoides* (liverseed grass) and many others

Clinical findings

Acute
♦ Dyspnea, gasping respiration
♦ Tremor, stumbling gait
♦ Mucosal cyanosis, then blanching
♦ Fast, weak pulse
♦ Severe cases:

- Mucosa brown due to high blood content of methemoglobin
- Recumbency
- Terminal convulsions
- Death after course of minutes to an hour

Subacute
Abortion reputed to occur.

Clinical pathology

- Diphenylamine test to estimate blood nitrite content
- Blood methemoglobin level unreliable indicator unless analysis shortly after collection
- Diphenylamine test useful also to estimate plant nitrite content

Necropsy findings

- Hemorrhages, congestion most tissues
- Blood brown color
- Methemoglobin level in blood elevated
- Estimate metHb in cerebrospinal fluid and aqueous humor, failing other fluids available

Diagnosis

Resembles:
- Cyanogenetic glycoside poisoning
- Acute anaphylaxis
- Acute bovine pulmonary edema and emphysema

Treatment and control

- Methylene blue I/V, 1–2 mg/kg as 1% solution
- Feeding chlortetracycline or sodium tungstate reduces nitrate to nitrite conversion
- Feed should not contain >1% nitrate.

OXALATE (SOLUBLE FORMS)
POISONING [VM8 p. 1539]

Etiology

- Pasture containing 2% soluble oxalate toxic for sheep
- High concentrations potassium oxalate in: *Amaranthus* spp. (red amaranth), *Atriplex* spp. (saltbush), *Bassia hyssopifolia* (red burr), *Chenopodium album* (fat hen), *Cenchrus ciliaris* (buffel grass), *Halogeton glomeratus* (halogeton), *Mesembryanthemum nosiflorum* (slender iceflower), *Oxa-*

lis spp. (soursob), *Portulacca oleracea* (pigweed), *Rumex* spp. (dock, sorrel), *Salsola kali* (tumbleweed), *Sarcobatus vermiculatus* (greasewood), *Setaria* spp., *Nechessia* (= *Threlkeldia*) *proceriflora* (soda bush), *Trianthema portulacastrum* (giant pigweed), leaves of rhubarb, mangels, sugar beet

Epidemiology

- Mostly sheep
- Cattle metabolize very large amounts

Risk factors
- Hungry animals
- Lush growth oxalate-rich plants

Clinical findings

Acute hypocalcemia sheep
- Anorexia, hyposensitivity
- Tremor, paresis
- Ruminal atony
- Dyspnea
- Stumbling, recumbency, head in flank
- Pupil dilation
- Coma, death

Acute nephrosis – cattle and pigs
- Hypocalcemia, recumbency
- Proteinuria, high BUN
- Coma, death

Chronic nephrosis – sheep
- Anorexia, poor body weight
- Ascites

Clinical pathology

- Hypocalcemia in acute cases
- Albuminuria, sometimes hematuria
- High BUN, serum potassium in nephrotic syndrome

Necropsy findings

- Acute – no lesions
- Chronic – nephrosis, perirenal edema, tubal crystalluria

Diagnosis

Resembles:
- Milk fever
- Lactation tetany
- Transport tetany

Treatment

♦ Parenteral injection calcium salts, as for milk fever
♦ Fluids I/V to prevent renal tubular blockage by oxalate crystals

Control

♦ Avoid grazing dangerous plants
♦ Prophylactic feeding dicalcium phosphate

OXALATE-INDUCED EQUINE
NUTRITIONAL SECONDARY
HYPERPARATHYROIDISM
[VM8 p. 1541]

Etiology

Pasture grasses containing prismatic or druse crystals of calcium oxalate are *Setaria sphacelata* (setaria), *Cenchrus ciliaris* (buffel grass), *Panicum maximum* (guinea grass), *Pennisetum* spp. (kikuyu, Napier grasses), *Brachiaria* spp., *Digitaria* spp.

Epidemiology

Horses and donkeys grazing pure stands of potent grasses affected after 2–8 months, mostly mares and foals.

Clinical findings

♦ Weight loss
♦ Bilateral, firm swellings of maxilla and mandibles
♦ Stiff gait at fast pace
♦ Then reluctant to move
♦ Finally recumbent
♦ Spontaneous recovery when taken off grass

Clinical pathology

♦ High blood parathormone levels
♦ Blood calcium and phosphorus normal
♦ Blood alkaline phosphatase may be elevated
♦ Jaw bone biopsy diagnostic lesion

Necropsy findings

♦ Jaw swelling
♦ Articular cartilages eroded, pitted
♦ Bone fractures common
♦ *Osteodystrophia fibrosa* in bone sections
♦ Parathyroid hyperplasia

Diagnosis

Identical to osteodystrophia caused by excessive phosphorus intake.

Treatment and control

♦ Remove horses to other pasture
♦ Allow grazing of toxic pasture for one month only
♦ Mineral supplement calcium and phosphorus (weekly 2 kg of 1 part calcium carbonate mixed with 2 parts dicalcium phosphate) for 6 months
♦ Add legume to pasture

OXALATE (INSOLUBLE FORMS –
CALCIUM) POISONING
[VM8 p. 1542]

♦ Rare poisoning in farm animals
♦ Toxic plants are horticultural specimens: *Arum italicum* (arum lily), *Dieffenbachia* spp. (dumbcane), *Monstera deliciosa* (monstera), *Philodendron* spp. (philodendron), *Zantedeschia* spp. (calla lily)
♦ Needle-shaped, raphide crystals of insoluble calcium oxalate cause oral mucosal erosions, salivation, tongue swelling, protrusion.

CALCINOGENIC GLYCOSIDE
POISONING (ENZOOTIC
CALCINOSIS) [VM8 p. 1543]

Etiology

Vitamin D analogues in: *Solanum malacoxylon, Nierembergia veitchii, Cestrum diurnum* (wild jessamine). Suspect plants include *Solanum linnaeanum, S. sodomeum, S. torvum, Trisetum flavescens* (yellow oat grass).

Epidemiology

♦ Affects all animal species after 3 years old
♦ *Solanum* spp. mostly in tropics
♦ *Trisetum* in Europe
♦ Hay, silage still potent

Clinical findings

♦ Chronic disease of several years duration
♦ Wasting
♦ Lame, reluctant to walk, stiff gait, restless feet
♦ Disinclined to rise or lie down
♦ Back arched, limbs stiff

- Cardiac murmurs
- Aortic calcification palpable per rectum
- Terminally recumbent
- Death unless removed from pasture, then spontaneous recovery

Clinical pathology

- High blood levels of calcium and phosphorus
- Tissue calcification visible radiologically
- Anemia common

Necropsy findings

- Emaciation, anasarca, ascites
- Blood vessels calcified
- All viscera, pleura, ligaments calcified
- Degenerative arthritis in limb joints

Diagnosis

Resembles repeated overdosing with vitamin D.

Treatment and control

No practicable measures.

CARDIAC GLYCOSIDE POISONING
[VM8 p. 1544]

Etiology

Two groups – **cardenolides** and **bufadienolides** – with identical actions in plants: *Acokanthera, Adonis, Apocynum, Asclepias, Bryophyllum, Carissa, Cerbera, Convallaria, Corchorus, Cotyledon, Cryptostegia, Digitalis, Diplarrena, Euonymus, Gomphocarpus, Homeria, Kalanchoe, Melianthus, Moraea, Nerium, Ornithoglossum, Scilla, Thesium, Thevetia, Tylecodon, Urginea* spp.

Epidemiology

- Mostly in ruminants, some horses
- Plants unpalatable, may not be eaten except in hay bales, or seeds in grain crop
- Horticultural specimens, e.g. oleander prunings cause sporadic deaths
- Mortality rate high

Clinical findings

Acute
- Apathy, head bowed
- Abdomen tucked up
- Salivation, teeth-grinding, groaning
- Tachycardia, arrhythmia
- Dyspnea
- Ruminal atony, bloat
- Diarrhea, tenesmus, dysentery in some
- Dribbling urine
- Pupil dilation
- Tremor, convulsions
- Posterior paresis

Chronic (cotyledonosis, krimpsiekte)
- Seen only in small ruminants in Africa
- Lag behind
- Head hangs loose, stand with feet under body, torticollis common
- Mandible droops, saliva drools, tongue protrudes, dysphagia, feed accumulates in mouth
- Horses may have colic
- Lie down a lot
- Tremor, tetanic spasms after exertion

Clinical pathology

- ECG's indicate ventricular fibrillation, ectopic foci in myocardium
- Parts of plants identifiable in rumen

Necropsy findings

Acute
- Multifocal myocardial degeneration, necrosis
- Lesions may not be visible if patient dies within 12 hours
- Pulmonary atelectasis, edema

Chronic
- Dehydration, emaciation
- Hemorrhages in myocardium

Diagnosis

Resembles other plant poisonings:
- Fluoroacetate poisoning
- *Albizia tanganyicensis, A. versicolor*
- *Fadogia homblei, F. monticola*
- *Galena africana*
- *Gossypium* spp.
- *Pavetta* spp.
- *Pseudogaltonia (Lidneria) clavata*
- *Urechites lutea*

Treatment and control

- Activated charcoal effective
- Arrhythmia combated with atropine or propanolol
- Early treatment essential

DICOUMAROL POISONING
[VM8 p. 1546]

Etiology

♦ Fungal activity in cut plants containing coumarin, 4-oxycoumarin, melilotin, converts them to dicoumarol, a potent anticoagulant
♦ Plants containing the precursors: *Anthoxanthum odoratum* (sweet vernal grass), *Ferula communis*, *Lespedeza stipulacea* (lespedeza), *Melilotus alba* (sweet or Bokhara clover), *M. altissima* (tall melilot), *M. indica* (King Island melilot, Hexham scent), *M. officinalis* (yellow sweet clover, ribbed melilot)
♦ Infecting fungi include *Aspergillus* spp., other unspecified fungi

Clinical findings

♦ Lameness, leg swelling
♦ Painless subcutaneous hematomas
♦ Pallor
♦ Persistent hemorrhage after injury, surgery, recent parturition, especially in the neonate
♦ Short course, high case fatality rate usual

SWEET CLOVER POISONING
[VM8 p. 1546]

Etiology

Ingestion of moldy sweet clover (*Melilotus alba*) hay containing usually >20 mg/kg dicoumarol highly toxic samples contain 60–70 mg/kg; toxicity varies with variety and coumarin content, degree of fungal contamination no indication.

Clinical findings

♦ Hemorrhagic syndrome, especially in neonates
♦ Cases continue for 6 days after feeding stopped

Clinical pathology

♦ Severe anemia
♦ Prolonged clotting and prothrombin times
♦ High blood and tissue levels dicoumarol

Necropsy findings

♦ Extensive hemorrhages at sites subject to mild contusion
♦ Pale tissues

Diagnosis

Resembles:
♦ Hemophilia
♦ Purpura hemorrhagica in horses

Treatment and control

♦ Blood transfusion
♦ Vitamin K
♦ Menadione sodium bisulfite (synthetic vitamin K) ineffective
♦ Intermittent feeding moldy hay mixed 1 part in 3 with good hay usually safe

DITERPENOID ALKALOID POISONING [VM8 p. 1548]

Etiology, Epidemiology

♦ Large number of alkaloids, including aconitine, methyllycaconitine, delphinine, elatine occurring in over 100 plant species, especially *Delphinium* spp. (rangeland larkspurs), *Aconitum* spp. (monkshood), *Erythrophloeum* spp. (ironwood)
♦ Heavy losses can occur in cattle and sheep but *Delphinium* spp. lose palatability with increasing toxicity

Clinical findings

♦ Salivation, ruminal atony, vomiting, constipation common
♦ Diarrhea common with *Aconitum* spp.
♦ Episodic weakness, tremor, staggery gait
♦ Then paralysis, recumbency
♦ Death due to respiratory paralysis or aspiration pneumonia

Clinical pathology and necropsy findings

No significant findings.

Treatment

Physostigmine an effective antidote against *Delphinium* spp. poisoning but has practical limitations.

GLUCOSINOLATE POISONING
[VM8 p. 1549]

Etiology

♦ Two groups in plants
  • **Goitrogens** (thiones and thiocyanates)
  • **Mustard oil glucosinolates,** alimentary tract irritants occur with enzyme (myrosinase) that hydrolyzes the glucosinolate to the toxic radicle
♦ Plants containing **goitrogens**: *Brassica napus* (rape, canola), *Brassica oleracea* (culinary brassicas, cabbage, cauliflower, etc.), *Brassica chinensis* (chinese cabbage), *B. campestris* (turnip rape), *B. napobrassica* (swede), *B. rapa* (turnip), *Raphanus sativa* (radish), *Rapistrum rugosum* (turnip weed), rapeseed oil cake
♦ Plants containing **mustard oil glucosinolates,** mostly isothiocyanates: *Armoracia rusticana* (horse radish), *Lepidium, Nasturtium, Tropaeolum* spp. (cress, mustard greens), *Raphanus raphanistrum* (wild radish), *Sinapis alba* (white mustard), *Sinapis nigra* (black mustard), *Brassica juncea* (oriental mustard), *Thlaspi arvense* (fanweed), *Sinapis arvensis* (charlock), *Erysimum cheiranthoides*

Epidemiology

♦ Outbreaks where animals have accidental access to plants
♦ Commonest is feed residues, e.g. seeds, residual cakes after oil extraction, fed to livestock in feedlots

Clinical findings

Goiter At any age including newborn.

Enteritis
♦ Abdominal pain
♦ Salivation, vomiting
♦ Diarrhea, dysentery
♦ Death

Rape blindness
♦ Blindness
♦ Head-pressing, mania in some (probably mild polioencephalomalacia)
♦ Spontaneous recovery

Acute pulmonary emphysema, interstitial pneumonia
♦ Dyspnea
♦ Subcutaneous emphysema
♦ Survivors persistently dyspneic

Digestive disturbances
♦ In steers on rape
♦ Anorexia
♦ Small, pasty, black stools
♦ Ruminal atony, rumen pack doughy

Clinical pathology

Blood glucosinolate levels high.

Necropsy findings

♦ Goiter, *or*
♦ Enteritis, *or*
♦ Pulmonary emphysema, interstitial pneumonia

Diagnosis

Goiter also caused by:
♦ Iodine deficiency
♦ Chronic cyanogenetic glucoside poisoning
Enteritis, polioencephalomalacia have many other, commoner causes.

Treatment and control

♦ Supportive treatments only
♦ Plant biproducts can be detoxified by alkali solutions

INDOLE ALKALOID POISONING
[VM8 p. 1552]

Includes groups of alkaloids in plants.

1. Beta-carboline indoleamine alkaloid poisoning
[VM8 p. 1552]

Etiology
In *Pegamum harmala* (African rue), *P. Mexicana* (Mexican rue), *Tribulus terrestris* (caltrops), *T. micrococcus* (yellow vine), *Kallstroemia hirsutissima* (hairy caltrop).

Clinical findings
♦ Hyper- or hypomotility
♦ Tremor, limb paresis, limb crossing, head swaying
♦ Walking backwards
♦ Sham eating
♦ Terminal convulsions
♦ Spontaneous recovery

Necropsy findings
No lesions.

2. Dimethyltryptamine poisoning [VM8 p. 1552]

Etiology

In *Phalaris aquatica* (Toowoomba canary grass), *P. angusta*, *P. arundinacea*, *P. caroliniana*, *P. brachystachys*, *P. minor* (canary grass) and rhompa grass.

Clinical findings

♦ **Sudden death** in sheep just put onto pasture, *or*
♦ **Incoordination** syndrome in sheep on pasture for 2–3 weeks
♦ Cases continue for long periods after removal from pasture
♦ Tremor, hyperexcitability
♦ Stiff gait, falling
♦ Tetanic convulsions, nystagmus
♦ Recumbency, death
♦ **Cattle** less severely affected
♦ Incoordination of tongue, lips, prehension difficult

Necropsy findings

♦ Greenish discoloration renal medulla, brain stem midbrain
♦ Degenerative lesions in spinal cord, cerebellum in some

Control

Affected pasture may be grazed if sheep dosed weekly, orally with cobalt.

3. Alstonines

Etiology

In *Urginea constricta* (bitter bark tree), *Gelsemium sempervirens* (yellow jessamine), *Urtica* spp. (stinging nettle).

Clinical findings

♦ Stagger syndrome
♦ Nettles also cause convulsions and death in some

INDOLIZIDINE ALKALOID POISONING [VM8 p. 1554]

Swainsonine and **castanospermine** the important members.

1. Swainsonine [VM8 p. 1554]

Etiology

In *Astragalus lentiginosus*, *A. emoryanus*, probably many others in the genus, *Oxytropis sericea*, *O. ochrocephala* plus others, in North America as 'loco', *Swainsona* spp., e.g. *S. galegifolia* (Darling pea).

Clinical findings

♦ Lose weight after several weeks on plant
♦ Incoordination, tremor
♦ Difficulty rising, eating, drinking
♦ Opisthotonus
♦ Spontaneous recovery if moved early
♦ Advanced cases recumbent, die
♦ Pregnant ewes poisoned by *Astragalus* spp. abort or have deformed, arthrogrypotic fetuses

Necropsy findings

♦ In *Swainsona* spp. poisoning vacuolation in circulating lymphocytes, high mannose-containing oligosaccharide content of urine
♦ Cytoplasmic vacuolation of cells, especially neurons and kidney cells

Diagnosis

Identical lesions to those of inherited mannosidosis.

2. Castanospermine [VM8 p. 1555]

In ripe fruits of *Castanospermum australe* (Moreton Bay fig). Affected cattle indistinguishable from heterozygotes for generalized glycogenosis type II (Pompe's disease).

NITROCOMPOUND POISONING (NITROTOXINS) [VM8 p. 1555]

Etiology

♦ **Miserotoxin** in *Astragalus* spp., e.g. *A. canadensis*, and probably *Oxytropis* spp.,
♦ **Corynocarpin** in *Corynocarpus* spp., e.g. *C. laevigatus*
♦ **Indospicine** in *Indigofera linnaei*
♦ Many plants in these genera, e.g. *Astragalus* spp., not poisonous, excellent feed

Clinical findings

Acute
See nitrite poisoning.

Chronic
♦ Lose weight, poor coat
♦ Low exercise tolerance

♦ Dyspnea
♦ Ataxia, paraplegia
♦ Temporary blindness, salivation in some
♦ Usually fatal after course of several months

Birdsville horse disease due to *Indigophera linnaei* – the above chronic syndrome after initial acute attack of incoordination, dyspnea

Treatment and control

Feed arginine-rich diet, e.g. peanut meal, gelatin, prevents *I. linnaei* poisoning.

PHYTOESTROGEN [VM8 p. 1557]

1. Phytoestrogens in pasture plants [VM8 p. 1557]

Etiology
Coumestans, isoflavones and isoflavan occur in *Medicago sativa* (alfalfa, lucerne), *Trifolium alexandrinum*, *T. alpestre*, *T. pratense* (red clover), *T. repens* (white clover), *T. subterraneum* (subterranean clover), *Glycine max* (soybean)

Clinical findings
♦ 'Clover disease' seen rarely now. Includes dystokia, uterus, vagina prolapse, severe infertility in ewes, teat elongation, mammary and bulbourethral gland enlargement in wethers
♦ Common syndrome in sheep is temporary infertility, recovering spontaneously
♦ Long-term intake, over 2 years, irreversible defeminisation
♦ Rams unaffected
♦ Cows – temporary infertility

Clinical pathology and necropsy findings
♦ Blood, fodder phytoestrogen levels elevated
♦ Severe, irreversible cases – cystic endometrial degeneration, cervicitis, tail head elevation, clitoridal hyperplasia, vulvar labial fusion

2. Unidentified phytoestrogen in *Pinus* spp. tree foliage [VM8 p. 1557]

♦ Ingestion of foliage of *Pinus ponderosa* (yellow pine), *P. cubensis, P. radiata* reduces serum progesterone levels, causes placental lesions, abortion in cows, not sheep
♦ *Cupressus macrocarpa* foliage also causes abortion in cows

PTAQUILOSIDE POISONING
[VM8 p. 1559]

Etiology

A norsesquiterpene glycoside in *Pteridium aquilinum* (bracken), *Cheilanthes* spp. (rockferns), e.g. *C. sieberi* causes the following four syndromes.

1. Bracken fern and rock fern poisoning [VM8 p. 1559]

Clinical findings
♦ Mostly cattle, rarely sheep
♦ Weight loss
♦ Dry, slack skin
♦ High fever
♦ Severe diarrhea, dysentery or melena in most
♦ Bleeding from orifices
♦ Salivation
♦ Nasolabial ulcers, petechiae in mucosae and skin
♦ Death after 1–3 days in most

Clinical pathology
♦ Platelet, leukocyte (especially polymorphs) counts greatly reduced
♦ Bone marrow biopsy conclusive indicator of platelet, leukocyte series

Necropsy findings
Multiple hemorrhages with associated ulcers.

Treatment
Broad-spectrum antibiotic cover used but limited value.

2. Enzootic hematuria [VM8 p. 1561]

Etiology and epidemiology
♦ In adult cattle due to long-term (years) access to *Pteridium aquilinum* or *Cheilanthes sieberi*
♦ High incidence of bladder carcinomas in isolated outbreaks in sheep grazing bracken

Clinical findings
- Intermittent high-volume hematuria
- Hemorrhagic anemia
- Discrete, firm lesions palpable rectally in bladder wall
- Entire wall thickened in advanced cases
- Cystitis a common complication

Clinical pathology
- Hematuria may be microscopic only
- Analysis of bracken for ptaquiloside requires rhizomes and croziers

Necropsy findings
- Emaciation
- Pale tissues
- Haemangioma-type lesions in bladder wall

Diagnosis
Resembles:
- Cystitis
- Other bladder neoplasm

Treatment and control

- Bladder lesions irreversible
- Blood transfusion may delay the inevitable death

3. 'Bright blindness' of sheep
[VM8 p. 1562]

- In sheep on bracken for years
- Blind but bright, alert
- Pupils dilated
- Poor light, menace reflexes
- Retinal degeneration
- Leucopenia

4. Alimentary tract neoplasia
[VM8 p. 1562]

- Carcinomas in sheep on long-term grazing bracken pasture
- Lesions in small intestine, liver, mandible, pharynx, esophagus of cattle

PYRROLIZIDINE ALKALOID (PA)
POISONING [VM8 p. 1563]

Etiology

- Very many PAs, up to 10 in the one plant
- Found in *Amsinckia intermedia* (tarweed), *Arnebia hispidissima*, *Crotalaria* spp., e.g. *C. anagyroides*, *Cynoglossum officinale* (hounds tongue), *Echium* spp., e.g. *E. plan-**tagineum* (Paterson curse), *Heliotropum* spp., e.g. *H. europaeum* (heliotrope), *Senecio* spp., e.g. *S. jacobea* (ragwort), *Symphytum officinale*, *Trichodesma* spp., e.g. *T. incanum*

Epidemiology

- Horses and cattle most susceptible
- Plants unpalatable, eaten when other feed short
- Pasture plants commonest source
- Hay, bedding, seeds in grain also toxic

Clinical findings

Common syndrome
- Sudden onset of hyposensitivity, anorexia, fall in milk yield
- Jaundice
- Photosensitization in some
- Uremia, dyspnea in some outbreaks
- Death the usual outcome

Cattle
Additional signs include:
- Outbursts of frenzy, aggression
- Diarrhea with tenesmus, rectal prolapse, abdominal pain
- Staggery gait, circling, blindness
- Death after course of 3 days to 3 weeks

Horses
Additional signs include:
- Profound somnolence, yawning
- Tremor
- Dysphagia, nasal regurgitation, aspiration pneumonia
- Severe inspiratory dyspnea due to laryngeal paralysis
- Blind, blunder into inaccessible places, headpressing
- Some have outbursts of frenzy

Pigs
- Uremia
- Interstitial pneumonia

Clinical pathology

- Blood pyrrolizidine levels high
- Serum levels of liver enzymes high; precede changes visible in biopsy specimens

Necropsy findings

- Hepatic megalocytosis
- Venoocclusive fibrosis
- Biliary hyperplasia the diagnostic lesions

♦ Spongy necrosis in brain
♦ Nephrosis, interstitial pneumonia in some

Diagnosis

Cattle and sheep
Resembles:
♦ Other hepatitis
♦ Primary photosensitization

Horses
Resembles:
♦ Viral encephalomyelitides
♦ Nigropallidal encephalomalacia
♦ Leukoencephalomalacia caused by *Fusarium moniliforme*

Treatment and control

♦ No practicable treatment
♦ Control may be possible by insects that parasitize only plants containing PAs

S-METHYL-L-CYSTEINE-SULFOXIDE
(SMCO) [VM8 p. 1566]

Etiology

♦ SMCO a hemolytic agent found in many members of *Brassica* spp., some of which also contain glucosinolates. SMCO occurs in *Brassica campestris* (turnip rape), *B. napobrassica* (swede), *B. oleracea* (vegetables such as cauliflower, calabrese), *Raphanus raphanistrum* (wild radish)
♦ Members of the Liliaceae family, e.g. *Allium canadense, A. cepa, A. validum*, the onions, also cause hemolytic anemia because they contain an agent, *n*-propyldisulfide, similar to the one in *Brassica* spp.

Epidemiology

♦ All parts of the plants are toxic, flowers, seeds more so than foliage
♦ Most poisonous in wet years
♦ Only ruminants affected
♦ Poisoning only after 3 weeks grazing

Clinical findings

♦ Sudden onset
♦ Hemoglobinuria
♦ Mucosal pallor
♦ Tremor
♦ Tachycardia
♦ Dyspnea
♦ Jaundice, diarrhea in some

Clinical pathology

♦ Erythrocyte count, hemoglobin concentration, PCV all decreased
♦ Heinz–Ehrlich bodies in all erythrocytes
♦ Hemoglobinuria
♦ High blood levels dimethyl disulfide

Necropsy findings

♦ Pallor
♦ Jaundice
♦ Hemoglobinuria
♦ Swollen spleen
♦ Hepatic necrosis

Diagnosis

Resembles:
♦ Postparturient hemoglobinuria
♦ Bacillary hemoglobinuria
♦ Chronic copper poisoning
♦ Babesiosis

Treatment and control

♦ Blood transfusion
♦ Dilute fodder crop with hay
♦ Feeding onions to livestock has similar hazards to *Brassica* spp. but risk avoided by mixing with other feeds in ratio of 1 to 3

THIAMINASE POISONING
[VM8 p. 1567]

Etiology

♦ Enzymes which catalyze destruction of thiamin present in *Pteridium aquilinum* (bracken), *Equisetum* spp., e.g. *E. arvense* (horsetails), *Marsilea drummondii* (nardoo), *Cheilanthes* spp., e.g. *C. sieberi* (rock fern), *Dryopteris* spp., e.g. *D. borreri* (male fern), *Malva parviflora* (marshmallow)
♦ The thiaminases in plants are methyl transferases
♦ Plants containing thiaminases usually thiamin deficient

Clinical findings

Horses
♦ Hyposensitive,
♦ Sway at rest and while walking
♦ Wide stance, back arched, head close to ground
♦ Tremor
♦ Cardiac irregularity, bradycardia

♦ Falls easily, recumbent
♦ Blind
♦ Whinnying, frequent pawing
♦ Dyspnea

Pigs
♦ Anorexia
♦ Dyspnea
♦ Convulsions
♦ Death after six hour course

Sheep
♦ Dyspnea
♦ Depression
♦ Recumbency, death, *or*
♦ Polioencephalomalacia, including blindness, incoordination

Cattle
♦ Hyposensitive
♦ Blind, recover but blindness persists

Clinical pathology

♦ Low blood levels of thiamin
♦ Transketolase, blood pyruvate levels elevated

Necropsy findings

♦ Congestive heart failure in horses
♦ Polioencephalomalacia in sheep and pigs

Diagnosis

Resembles:
♦ Hepatic encephalopathy
♦ Toxic encephalopathy
♦ Viral encephalomyelitides
♦ Staggers syndromes

Treatment

Thiamin (100 mg/kg parenterally, twice on day 1, single daily dose thereafter) plus removal source of thiaminase.

PLANT MATERIALS CAUSING
PHYSICAL DAMAGE [VM8 p. 1584]

Gut impaction or obstruction by phytobezoar
[VM8 p. 1584]

♦ **Horse**: *Senecio jacobea* (ragwort), *Sorghum* spp.
♦ **Cattle**: *Fraxinus excelsior* (ash tree), *Chrysocomia excelsior* (bitter weed), *Prosopis juliflora* (mesquite), *Eremocarpus setigerus* (turkey mullein), *Romulea rosea* (onion weed), cocoon silk of *Gonometa* spp. (Molopo moth)
♦ **Pig**: *Nicotiana* spp. stalks (tobacco)

Corneal ulcer [VM8 p. 1584]

Arctica lappa (burdock) bristles.

Mouth ulcers [VM8 p. 1584]

Setaria lutescens (yellow bristle grass) bristles, triticale seed awns.

Grass seed abscesses
[VM8 p. 1584]

Stipa, *Stipagrostis* spp. (spear grasses), *Tagetes* spp., *Aristida arenaria* (silver grass, kerosene grass), *Opuntia* spp. (prickly pear), *Hordeum jubatum* (barley grass).

Enteritis

Dittrichia graveolens (stinkwort) possibly.

PLANT POISONING DUE TO UNIDENTIFIED TOXINS
[VM8 p. 1584]

Plant poisonings in which the toxin has not been identified are listed below according to the syndrome they produce. Other plants in the main section of the chapter also cause similar syndromes.

Abortion
Cupressus macrocarpa (monterey cypress), *Iva angustifolia* (narrow-leafed sumpweed).

Cystitis
Didymotheca cupressiformis (double-seeded emu bush).

Dermatitis
Heracleum mantegazzianum (cow parsnip). *Vicia villosa* (hairy vetch), *V. dasycarpa* (woolly pod vetch), *V. villosa* × *V. dasycarpa* hybrid.

Diarrhoea without gastroenteritis as a lesion

Anredera cordifolia (lambs tail), *Bulbine bulbosa* (native leek), *Chaerophyllum sylvestre*, *Datisca glomerata*, (Durango root), *Juncus inflexus* (blue rush), *Ligustrum vulgare* (privet hedge), *Linum catharticum* (purging flax), *Mentha australis* (native mint), *Salvia coccinea* (red salvia).

Diarrhea with gastroenteritis, abdominal pain, incoordination, sometimes with dysentery, vomiting

Azadirachta indica, *Brunsfelsia bonodora* (yesterday, today and tomorrow), *Buxus sempervirens* (common box bush), *Centaurium beyrichii* (rock centaury), *Cissus quadrangularis*, *Dichrocephalia chrysanthemifolia*, *Dipcadi glaucum*, (poison onion), *Diplocyclos palmatus*, *Diplolophium africanum*, *Fagus sylvaticus* (European beech tree), *Gymnocladus dioica* (Kentucky coffee tree), *Iris* spp., e.g. *I. foetidissima* (stinking iris), *Ligustrum vulgare* (privet hedge), *Ludwigia peploides* (water primrose), *Ornithogalum longibracteatum* (chinkerinchee), *Sapium sebiferum* (Chinese tallow wood), *Scrophularia aquatica* (water betony), *Sisyrinchium* spp. (scour weed), *Siam angustifolium*, *Tulipa* spp. (tulips), *Turraea robusta*.

Dysphagia

Buxus sempervirens (box tree), *Descurainia pinnata* (tansy mustard).

Gestation prolonged

Salsola tuberculatiformis (cauliflower saltwort), *Lysichiton americanus* (skunk cabbage).

Heart failure with sudden death or congestive failure and cardiomyopathy

Fadogia homblei, *Galenia africana*, *Ixiolaena brevicompta* (button weed), *Pachystigma latifolium*, *P. pygmaeum*, *P. thamnus*, *Pavetta harborii*, *P. schumanniana*, *Urechites lutea*, *Persea americana* (avocado tree leaves, only the Guatemalan and hybrid varieties; Mexican strains not toxic.)

Hemolytic disease

Acacia nilotica subsp. *kraussiana* (scented thorn). *Acer rubrum* (red maple, wilted leaves only, to horses), *Secale cereale* (cereal rye), *Mercurialis* spp. (mercury).

Hemorrhagic disease

Dendrochium toxicum.

Hepatic injury plus dummy syndrome

Helichrysum argyrosphaerum, *H. blandowskianum* (woolly daisy), *Trema tomentosa (syn. T. aspera)*, *Matricaria nigellifolia*.

Hepatic injury with jaundice and/or photosensitization

Acanthospermum hispidum (star burr), *Capparis tomentosa*, *Chlorozoa plicata* (terba), *Ficus tsiela* (fig tree), *Kochia scoparia* (Monterey cypress), *Nolina texana* (sacahuiste), *Persicaria lapathifolia (syn. Polygonum lapathifolium)* (pale willow weed), *Pteronia pallens* (Scholtz bush), *Sartwellia flaveriae* (sartwell), *Sessea braziliensis*, *Stryphnodendron coriaceum*, *Tetradymia canescens* (spineless horsebrush), *Trifolium hybridum* (alsike clover), *Polygonum sagittatum*, *P. orientale*, (smartweeds), and *P. convolvulus*.

Incoordination of gait

Araujia hortorum (cruel vine), *Brachychiton populneus* (kurrajong tree), *Combretum platypetalum*, *Echinopogon* spp. (roughbearded grass), *Euphorbia mauritanica*, *Gomphrena celosioides* (soft khaki weed), *Idiospermum australiense*, *Pennisetum clandestinum* (kikuyu grass), *Romulea* spp. (onion weed), *Solidago chinensis*, *Stachys arvensis* (stagger weed), *Trachyandra laxa* and *T. divaricata*, *Romulea bulbocodium*, *Gomphrena celosioides*, *Echinopogon mauritanica*, *E. ovatus*, *Xanthorrhoea* spp. (grasstrees).

Mania with wild running, hyperexcitability, incoordination, circling, aimless wandering, blindness

Burrtia prunoides.

Mastitis with edema, reddening and clots in the milk but no infection and no cellular reaction in goats and mares

Persea americana (avocado leaves).

Myopathy with gait incoordination, recumbency, elevated serum creatine kinase

Karwinskia humboldtiana (coyotillo), *Cassia* spp., e.g. *C. occidentalis*.

Photosensitization primary; without hepatic lesion

Echinochloa utilis (Japanese millet), *Erodium cicutarium* (storksbill), *Holocalyx glaziovii*, *Mentha saturoides*, *Sphenosciadium capitellatum*, *Medicago denticulata* (burr trefoil).

Pulmonary edema with dyspnea, etc.
Eupatorium adenophorum (crofton weed), *E. riparium* (mist flower), *Glechoma hederacea* (ground ivy), *Gyrostemon* spp. (camel poison), *Lactuca serriola* (prickly lettuce).

Red urine due to a pigmented substance from the plant
Haloragis odontocarpa (raspwort), *Swartzia madagascariensis*, *Xanthorrhoea minor*.

Stomatitis
Puccinia graminis.

Sudden death without cardiomyopathy
Eupatorium wrightii, *Lamium amplexicaule* (dead nettle), *Viguiera annua* (annual goldeneye).

Uremia, nephrosis with high blood urea nitrogen
Dimorphandra gardneriana, *Psilostrophe* spp. (paperflowers), *Sapium sebiferum* (Chinese tallow tree), *Sarcolobus globosus*.

POISONING BY MYCOTOXINS

Identification of mycotoxins by sophisticated laboratory techniques is entering a phase where the investigation of a possible myco-intoxication can proceed in that way, rather than depending on visual evidence of a fungal infection in plant material, and the identifying it by botanical means. This section on poisonings by fungi is now arranged on that basis in Table 32.2. Sections dealing with fungal infections of tissues commence on p. 446.

MISCELLANEOUS FUNGI LACKING
IDENTIFIED MYCOTOXINS
[VM8 p. 1605]

Liver damage
Drechslera campanulata, *Helminthosporium* spp., e.g. *H. ravenelli*.

Incoordination, convulsions
Trichothecium roseum, *Penicillium cyclopium*, *Diplodia maydis*, unidentified fungi on standing crops of *Pisum sativum* (peas).

Reproductive dysfunction
Penicillium roqueforti, unidentified fungi on *Trifolium repens* (white clover), *Ustilago hordei* (barley smut fungus), *Helminthosporium biseptatum* on *Romulea rosea* (onion weed).

Uremia
Tilletia tritici (wheat smut fungus).

POISONING BY CYANOBACTERIAL TOXINS

CYANOBACTERIA IN
WATER BLOOMS
[VM8 p. 1606]

Etiology

Toxins found in cyanobacteria associated with blue–green algae on stagnant water containing high concentrations nitrogen, phosphorus. *Microcystis* spp. (= *Anacystis cyanea*), *Anabaena circinalis*, *A. spiroides*, *Aphanizomenon*, *Gloeotrichia*, *Gomphosphaeria*, *Coelosphaerium*, *Oscillatoria* spp., *Nodularia spumigena*.

1. Anatoxins (neurotoxic fast death factor) [VM8 p. 1606]

Clinical findings
♦ Within 15 minutes of exposure
♦ Tremor
♦ Depression, hypersensitivity
♦ Salivation
♦ Staggering gait
♦ Recumbent, convulsions
♦ Abdominal pain, diarrhea
♦ Dyspnea
♦ Death within a few minutes

Necropsy findings
♦ Massive hepatic necrosis
♦ General petechiation

Table 32.1 Minor phytotoxins

Toxin	Clinical	Necropsy	Plants
Aesculin [VM8 p. 1569]	**Ruminants** – stiff gait, recumbency, convulsions. **Monogastrics** – vomiting	Nil	Aesculus spp. e.g., Aesculus pavia (horse chestnuts, buckeyes)
Alcohols, complex, plant			
i). Cicutoxin [VM8 p. 1569]	Restless, stumbling, violent convulsions, bloat, dyspnea, teeth grinding, salivation, frequent urination and defecation, pupil dilation, die in minutes to several hours	Nil	Cicuta spp. (water hemlock)
ii). Oenanthotoxin [VM8 p. 1569]	As for cicutoxin	Nil	Oenanthe spp. (hemlock water dropwort)
iii). Tremetol [VM8 p. 1569]	**Ruminants** – stiff gait, tremor, salivation, recumbency, coma, death. **Horses** – sweating, regurgitation, congestive heart failure, ECG abnormality	Liver damage, nephrosis	Eupatorium glandulosum (snakeroot), Haplopappus heterophyllus (goldenrod).
Albizia pyridoxine analogue [VM8 p. 1569]	**Cattle** — hypersensitivity, hyperthermia, dyspnea, ataxia, convulsions	Cardiomyopathy, petechiation, pulmonary edema. Treat with pyridoxine	Albizia versicolor, A. tanganyicensis
Amines, Toxic [VM8 p. 1569]			
i). Cyclopamine [VM8 p. 1570]	**Ruminants** – cyclopian head deformities, prolonged gestation, gigantism, many other skeletal defects, when dams fed plant in early pregnancy	Skeletal defects, pituitary absent	Veratrum californicum (skunk cabbage)
ii). Tyramine [VM8 p. 1569]	Ataxia, recumbency, spontaneous recovery	Nil	Acacia berlandieri (guajillo), possibly Phoradendron villosum (a mistletoe)

Toxin	Clinical signs	Lesions	Plants
Amino acids, toxic [VM8 p. 1570]			
i). Canavanine [VM8 p. 1570]	Weight loss, anorexia, stiff gait, stumbling, recumbency, diarrhea	Gastroenteritis, nephritis, pulmonary emphysema	*Indigophera linnaei* (Birdsville indigo), *Canavalia* spp.
ii). Mimosine [VM8 p. 1570]	Both plants – alopecia. *Leucaena* spp.— ataxia, excitability, sometimes infertility, stillbirths, goiter, cataract	Alopecia, goiter, oral and esophageal ulcers, spontaneous recovery	*Leucaena leucocephala, Mimosa pudica* (sensitive plant)
Aminoproprionitrile [VM8 p. 1571]	**Cattle** — lameness, pain in feet, recumbency, convulsions	Nil	*Lathyrus* spp. (wild peas), e.g. *L. hirsutus*
Andromedotoxin (acetylandromedol, grayanotoxin) [VM8 p. 1571]	Dullness, salivation, vomiting, bloat, tenesmus, abdominal pain, ataxia, recumbency,	Aspiration pneumonia	*Agauria salifolia, Andromeda, Kalmia* (laurels), *Ledum* spp. (western Labrador tea), *Leucothoe davisiae* (sierra laurel), *Lyonia ligustrina, Menziesia ferruginea* (mock azalea), *Pieris japonica* (Japanese pieris), *Rhododendron* spp.
Anthraquinone [VM8 p. 1571]	Diarrhea, abdominal pain	Gastroenteritis, liver damage	*Cassia occidentalis* (coffee senna), *C. obtusifolia* (sicklepod), *C. roemeriana, C. italica, Frangula alnus* (alder buckthorn), *Rhamnus* spp. (buckthorn)
Apocynin [VM8 p. 1571]	Abdominal pain, diarrhea, vomiting	Gastroenteritis	*Apocynum* spp. (dogbanes)
Aristolochine [VM8 p. 1571]	**Goat** — alopecia, dyspnea, diarrhea, hind limb weakness. **Horse** — polyuria, straining to urinate, tachycardia	Nil	*Aristolochia clematitis* (birthwort), *A. bractea, A. densivenia*
Cannabinoids [VM8 p. 1572]	**Horse** — restless, hypersensitivity, tremor, sweating, salivation, Dyspnea, ataxia, death or spontaneous recovery	Nil	*Cannabis sativa* (marihuana)

Continued

603

Table 32.1 *Continued*

Toxin	Clinical	Necropsy	Plants
Carboxyatractyloside [VM8 p. 1572]	Hyperexcitability, restless herd, depression, stiff limbs, ears, aggression, stumble, recumbency, convulsions, opisthotonus, death usual in up to 48 hrs	Hepatic necrosis, nephrosis, fluid in body cavities	Sprouted seeds of *Xanthium strumarium* (cockleburr, Noogoora burr), other *Xanthium* spp., *Cestrum* spp., except for *C. diurnum*, *Atractylis gummifera*. *Wedelia asperrima* contains wedeloside a very similar toxin, causes same syndrome.
Colchicine [VM8 p. 1572]	Salivation, vomiting, tenesmus, diarrhea, abdominal pain,	Gastroenteritis, subserosal hemorrhages	*Colchicum autumnale* (autumn crocus) *Gloriosa superba* (flame or glory lily)
Crepenynic acid [VM8 p. 1572]	Staggery gait, recumbency	Myopathy	*Ixioloena brevicompta* (button weed)
Cycad glycosides [VM8 p. 1572] i). MAM (methylazoxymethanol) glycosides [VM8 p.1572]	Anorexia, weight loss, jaundice, photosensitisation, diarrhea	Liver damage, gastroenteritis	*Bovenia*, *Cycas*, *Encephalartos*, *Macrozamia*, *Zamia* spp.
ii). Unidentified cycad toxin [VM8 p. 1573]	Cattle — posterior ataxia, stiff goose-stepping gait	Muscle atrophy, degenerative lesions spinal cord	*Bovenia*, *Cycas*, *Macrozamia*, *Zamia* spp.
Cyclopamine [VM8 p. 1570]	Cyclopean deformity, prolonged gestation	Congenital cyclopean deformity, pituitary gland absent	*Veratrum californicum* (skunk cabbage, Western hellebore)
Cynanchoside [VM8 p. 1573]	Hypersensitivity, restless, tremor, stumbling, recumbency, convulsions, opisthotonus, vomiting, salivation, teeth grinding, dyspnea	Nil	*Cynanchum* spp. (monkey rope). Very similar toxin in *Sarcostemma australe* (caustic vine) *S. viminale* (caustic bush)
Dianthrone, e.g. Hypericin [VM8 p. 1573]	Photosensitive dermatitis, spontaneous recovery	Nil	*Hypericum perforatum* (Klamath weed, St Johns Wort), *H. triquetrifolium*

Toxin	Clinical signs	Plants
Dihydroxycoumarin glycoside [VM8 p. 1573]		
i). Alimentary tract syndrome [VM8 p. 1573]	Abdominal pain, diarrhea, dysentery, stomatitis, salivation, vomiting, some convulsions	Stomatitis, gastroenteritis	*Daphne* spp. some of the *Pimelea* spp. *Gnidia* spp.
ii). Hemorrhagic syndrome [VM8 p.1573]	Mucosal pallor, bounding pulse, nasal bleeding, dysentery, low blood erythrocyte count, hemoglobin content	Widespread hemorrhages, tissue pallor, gastroenteritis	*Wikstroemia* spp. (tiebush)
Diterpene [VM8 p. 1573]		
i). Simplexin [VM8 p. 1573]	**Cattle, ingestion** — congestive heart failure, diarrhea. **Inhalation** — congestive heart failure only	Congestive heart failure	*Pimelea simplex, P. trichostachya*, etc. (desert rice flower, flaxweed, wild flax, mustard seed, broom bush)
ii). 12-deoxyphorbol [VM8 p. 1573]	Stomatitis, diarrhea	Gastroenteritis	*Euphorbia* spp. (spurges)
Fluoroacetate [VM8 p. 1574]	Within few minutes to 12 hours sudden death or frenzy, dyspnea, cyanosis, heart rate up to 300/min, cardiac irregularity, ataxia, recumbency, convulsions.	Cardiomyopathy, pulmonary edema	*Acacia georginae* (Georgina gidgee), *Dichapetalum, Gastrolobium, Oxylobium* spp, *Palicourea macgravii*, possibly *Mascagnia rigida*
Furanocoumarins (Furocoumarin) [VM8 p. 1574]	Photosensitive dermatitis. Vesicles on swine snouts resemble foot and mouth disease, etc.	Dermatitis lesions	*Ammi majus, A. visnaga, Cymopteres longipes, C. watsoni* (wild parsley), *Thamnosma texana* (dutchman's breeches). *Pastinaca sativa* (parsnip root) infested with *Ceratocystis fimbriata* (rot fungus), *Apium graveolens* (celery) infested with *Sclerotinia* spp. (pink rot fungus). Related compounds in *Heracleum mantegazzianum* (giant hogweed), *Cooperia pedunculata*

Continued

Table 32.1 Continued

Toxin	Clinical	Necropsy	Plants
Galegin [VM8 p. 1575]	Dyspnea, nasal froth, convulsions, sudden death	Pulmonary edema, hydrothorax	*Galega officinalis* (French honeysuckle), *Schoenus asperocarpus* (poison sedge), *Verbesina encelioides* (crown beard)
Iforrestine [VM8 p. 1575]	Uremia, anorexia, depression, diarrhea, oliguria, recumbency, death. Proteinuria, glycosuria	Renal tubular necrosis	*Isotropis forrestii*, *I. cuneifolia*
Isoquinoline alkaloid [VM8 p. 1575]			
i). Berberine [VM8 p. 1575]	Weight loss, dyspnea, subcutaneous edema, diarrhea, abdominal pain, recumbency	Cardiomyopathy, congestive heart failure, some with gastroenteritis	*Argemone mexicana* (Mexican poppy), *A. ochraleuca*, *A. subfusiformis*, *Berberis* spp., *Mahonia* spp.
ii). Bulbocapnine [VM8 p. 1575]	Tremor, convulsions, frenzy, biting at objects, salivation, vomiting. Transient episodes. May die during an episode.	Nil	*Corydalis flavula* (fitweed, fumatory), *Dicentra spectabilis* (bleeding heart)
iii). Chelidonine [VM8 p. 1575]	Ataxia, dribbling urine, salivation, convulsions	Nil	*Chelidonium majus* (greater celandine, celandine poppy)
iv). Corydaline [VM8 p. 1575]	Diarrhea, frenzy, excitement, convulsions, increased by harassment, death, short course	Gastroenteritis in some	*Corydalis caseana* (fitweed), *Dicentra cucullaria*
Juglone [VM8 p. 1575]	**Horse** — lameness, edema lower limbs	Lower limb edema	*Juglans nigra* (black walnut) shavings as bedding
Juniperine [VM8 p. 1575]	Abdominal pain, diarrhea, proteinuria, abortion, high blood levels BUN	Nephrosis, cystitis, rumenitis	*Juniperus* spp. (juniper tree)
Lectin [VM8 p. 1575]	Anorexia, vomiting, diarrhea, sometimes dysentery, dyspnea, dehydration, rapid weight loss, recumbency, death. Elevated BUN, serum liver enzymes	Abomasal, intestinal erosions, hepatocyte and renal tubular injury, pulmonary hemorrhage, edema and emphysema	*Ricinus communis* (castor oil plant) contains ricin, *Abrus precatorius* (jequirity bean) contains abrin, *Phaseolus vulgaris* (kidney bean) contains phaseolus hemolytic agent, *Adenia digitata*

606

Lycorine [VM8 p. 1576]	Salivation, vomiting, diarrhea	Nil	*Amaryllis, Clivia, Lycoris, Narcissus, Nerine* spp.
Lysergic acid [VM8 p. 1576]	Exercise-induced ataxia	Nil	*Ipomoea muelleri* (convolvulus, glory vine)
Oil, irritant [VM8 p. 1576] i). Bryonin [VM8 p. 1576]	Depression, dyspnea, diarrhea, polyuria, stumbling, tremor, recumbency, convulsions. Also sweating, agalactia, sudden death	Nil	*Bryonia dioica* (white bryony, British mandrake)
ii). Unspecified irritant oil [VM8 p. 1576]	Salivation, oral mucosal lesions, abdominal pain, diarrhea, sometimes dysentery,	Nil	*Actaea spicata* (baneberry), *Artemisia filifolia, Barbarea vulgaris, Croton* spp. (croton), *Inula conyza* (ploughman's spikenard), *Dittrichia graveolens* (stinkwort), *Sambucus* spp. (elders, elderberry).
Phenol, plant [VM8 p. 1576] i). Gossypol [VM8 p. 1576]	After 1–3 months anorexia, dyspnea, cough, brisket edema, jugular vein distension, weak, poor exercise tolerance, hematuria in some. Death after few days. Low intakes may reduce fertility, stunt growth in males, stillbirths, premature deaths in sows. Serum sorbitol dehydrogenase elevated. ECG abnormalities	Anasarca, fluid in body cavities, congestive heart failure, degeneration skeletal and cardiac muscles. Liver centrilobular necrosis	*Gossypium* spp. (commercial cotton)
ii). Tannin, of oak trees [VM8 p. 1577]	Polyuria, ventral edema, abdominal pain, constipation, BUN elevated, proteinuria, low urine S.G.	Nephrosis, hepatic injury, intestinal wall and mesentery edema	Leaves and windfall acorns of *Quercus robur* (European oak), *Q. havardi* (sand shin oak), *Q. marilandica* (blackjack oak), *Q. garryanna*

Continued

607

Table 32.1 Continued

Toxin	Clinical	Necropsy	Plants
iii). Tannin of yellow-wood tree [VM8 p. 1577]	Cattle, acute – jaundice, photosensitisation, abdominal pain, dehydration, polyuria, urine low S.G. Chronic – polyuria, emaciation. Sheep – convulsive seizures when handled; spontaneous recovery	Cattle, acute – hepatic necrosis, nephrosis, abomasal hemorrhagic erosions. Cattle, chronic – nephrosis, renal cortical fibrosis	Terminalia oblongata (yellow-wood)
Piperidine alkaloids [VM8 p. 1577]			
i). Conium piperidine alkaloids [VM8 p. 1577]	Skeletal muscle paralysis – tremor, ataxia, fetlock knuckling, frequent belching, some vomit, frequent urination, defecation, salivation, pupil dilation, nictitating membrane prolapse, mousy odor milk and urine. Course few hours, recumbency, death usual, except sheep recover spontaneously. Congenital deformities in some	Congenital malformations – carpal flexure, limb and vertebral malalignments, permanent in calves, piglets, transitory in lambs. Also cleft palate, hare lip in calves and piglets	Conium maculatum (poison hemlock), possibly Trachymene spp. (parsnip, wild parsnip)
ii). Cynapine [VM8 p. 1578]	Dyspnea, ataxia	Nil	Aethusa cynapium (fools parsley, lesser hemlock)
iii). Nicotiana spp. piperidine alkaloids, nicotine, anabasine, anagyrine [VM8 p. 1578]	Acute due to nicotine sulfate – dyspnea, tremor, recumbency, convulsions, death. Survivors have abdominal pain, salivation, diarrhea. Long-term plant ingestion by pregnant females – neonates have arthrogryposis limb and vertebral joints, cleft palate	Acute – abomasitis, duodenitis. Long-term – congenital defects	Nicotiana spp. (commercial, wild tobacco)
iv). Lobeline [VM8 p. 1578]	Mouth erosions, salivation, diarrhea	Enteritis	Lobelia berlandieri
Podophyllin [VM8 p. 1579]	Salivation, severe diarrhea	Enteritis	Podophyllum peltatus
Protoanemonin [VM8 p. 1579]	Salivation, stomatitis, abdominal pain, diarrhea, dysentery, hematuria, blind, ataxia, convulsions	Enteritis	Anemone spp., Caltha palustris, Ceratocephalus testiculatus (bur buttercup), Clematis spp., Ficaria verna Pulsatilla spp., R. auricalus, Thalictrum

Quinolizidine alkaloid [VM8 p. 1579]

i). Alkaloids causing nervous disease, e.g. sparteine, lupinine, spathulatine. [VM8 p. 1579]	**Acute** – dyspnea, depression, coma, death, some with episodes of staggery gait, mouth frothing, convulsions. **Subacute** – anorexia, depression, eyelid edema, tremor, stiff gait, arched back, tucked-up abdomen, rough hair coat, recumbency. High blood levels SGOT, CPK, LDH.	Myopathy suggested but unconfirmed	*Lupinus angustifolius, L. cosentinii,* many others in which presence of these toxins assumed. Toxins concentrated in seeds. Other plant species in which toxins assumed to occur – *Cytisus* (syn. *Laburnum* spp.) (laburnum, broom), *Baptisia, Sophora, Thermopsis, Sarothamnus* spp.
ii). Anagyrine [VM8 p. 1579]	Congenital deformity of arthrogryposis, including limb and vertebral column deformity, cleft palate in some; dystokia. Mostly calves "crooked calf disease". Rarely lambs	Congenital arthrogrypotic deformities	*Lupinus sericeus, L. caudatus,* many others
Rhoeadine [VM8 p. 1580]	Restless, hypersensitive, ataxia, ruminal stasis, dyspnea, convulsions	Nil	*Papaver rhoeas* (field poppy), possibly *P. nudicaule, P. somniferum*
Saponins [VM8 p. 1580]			
i). Triterpene saponins [VM8 p. 1580]	Diarrhea, dysentery, abdominal pain; severe cases show vomiting, salivation	Enteritis, gastroenteritis	*Aleurites fordii* (tung oil tree), *Dialopsis africana, Gutierrezia microcephala* (perennial broomweed), *Hedera helix* (ivy), *Jatropha curcas* (purging nut), *Phytolacca* spp., *Saponaria officinalis* (soapwort), *Sesbania* spp. (rattlepods), *Bulnesia sarmientii* (palo santo tree).
ii). Steroidal saponins [VM8 p. 1580]	Jaundice, photosensitisation, hepatic insufficiency	Birefringent crystals accumulated in bile ducts, damage surrounding hepatocytes.	*Panicum* spp. grasses. Suspected plants – *Tribulus terrestris* (caltrops), *Narthecium ossifragum* (bog asphodel), *Avena sativa* (oats), *Kochia scoparia* (summer cypress), *Agrostemma githago* (cockles), *Brachiaria decumbens* (signal grass)

Continued

Table 32.1 *Continued*

Toxin	Clinical	Necropsy	Plants
Selenocompounds [VM8 p. 1580]	**Subacute** – aimless wandering, circling, blind, headpressing, dyspnea, lame, recumbent, teeth grinding, salivation. **Chronic** – alopecia, weight loss, coronitis, hoof deformity and shedding. High levels selenium in plants, tissues.	Non-specific hepatic, myocardial, renal injury	*Acacia cana, Aster* spp. (woody aster), *Astragalus bisulcatus, A. pattersonii, A. praelongus, A. pectinatus, A. racemosus* (poison vetches), *Atriplex canescens* (saltbush), *Castilleja* spp, *Comandra pallida* (bastard toadflax), *Grayia* spp., *Grindelia squarrosa* (gumweeds), *Machaeranthera ramosa, Morinda reticulata, Neptunia amplexicaulis, Oonopsis condensata* (goldenweed), *Penstemon* spp., *Sideranthus* spp. (ironweed), *Stanleya pinnata* (princes plume), *Xylorrhiza* spp. (woody aster)
Sesquiterpenes [VM8 p. 1581]			
i). Furanoid sesquiterpenes (furanosesquiterpenoids), e.g. ngaione, myodesmone [VM8 p. 1581]	Jaundice, photosensitisation	Liver damage	*Lasiospermum bipinnatum* (ganskweed), *Myoporum* spp. (boobialla, ellangowan poison bush)
ii). Ipomeanols [VM8 p. 1581]	Dyspnea, abdominal, grunting respiration, mouth breathing, nasal discharge, fever, death in most at 24 – 48 hours, up to 21 days	Pulmonary emphysema, edema, interstitial pneumonia	*Ipomoea carnea, Perilla frutescens* (purple mintweed), *Zieria arborescens* (stinkwood). Fungi including *Fusarium solani, F. javanicum, Ceratostomella fimbriata* infesting sweet potato tubers
iii). Sesquiterpene lactones [VM8 p. 1581]	**Cattle** – (not *Centaurea* spp.) spewing sickness of regurgitation, salivation, cough, dysphagia. **Horse** – (*Centaurea* spp.) depression, chewing, salivation, tongue flicking, dysphagia, intestinal	**Cattle** – nil. **Horses** – nigropallidal encephalomalacia, fluid in body cavities	*Centaurea picris, C. repens* (Russian knapweed), *C. solstitialis* (yellow star thistle), *Geigeria* spp. (vermeerbos), *Helenium* spp. (sneezeweeds),

Steroidal solanum alkaloids, e.g. solanidine, tomatodine [VM8 p. 1582]	**Acute** – very large doses; diarrhea. **Subacute** – exercise-induced incoordination, falling, nystagmus, convulsions, cardiac irregularity, diarrhea. Special entity is "crazy cow disease" (*S. dimidiatum*)	**Acute** – mucosal necrosis stomach, intestines **Subacute** – possibly encephalomalacia, cerebellar agangliosidosis. Teratogens in some plants but no lesions reported	*Solanum bonariensis, S. dimidiatum, S. dulcamara, S. eleagnifolium, S. esuriale, S. fastigiatum, S. kwebense, S. pseudocapsicum* (nightshades), sprouted *S. tuberosum* (potato), *Brunsfelsia pauciflora, Lycium halimifolium, Lycopersicon esculentum* (tomato)
Strychnine [VM8 p. 1582]	Increased reflex excitability, stiff limbs, tetanic convulsions, periods of relaxation. Death due to respiratory failure. Treat with tannic acid absorbents, sedative, and time for the alkaloids to be metabolized	Nil	*Strychnos* spp. Poisoning due usually to medicinal application
Stypandrol [VM8 p. 1583]	Blind, ataxia, flaccid paralysis, recumbency, pupil dilation, retinal hemorrhage, papilledema,	Generalised neuronal vacuolation, axonal degeneration optic nerve fibres, some cases a diffuse status spongiosis in brain	*Stypandra* spp. (blind grass, nodding blue lily), green shoots only, *Hemerocallis* spp. (day lily).
Triterpenes [VM8 p. 1583] i). Cucurbitacins [VM8 p. 1583]	Ripe fruits cause lethargy, dehydration, abdominal pain, diarrhea, dyspnea, death, course of a few hours	Ruminal epithelium necrosis, intestinal mucosal congestion, pulmonary edema, liver damage in some	*Cucumis africanus, C. myriocarpus* (prickly paddymelon), probably *Ecballium elaterium* (squirting cucumber), *Citrullus colocynthis*
ii). Lantadenes, icterogenins [VM8 p. 1583]	Ruminal stasis, jaundice, photosensitisation	Bile canaliculi damage, gall bladder paralysis, intrahepatic cholestasis	**Lantadenes** – *Lantana* spp. **Icterogenins** – *Lippia* spp.

Continued

Table 32.1 Continued

Toxin	Clinical	Necropsy	Plants
iii). Meliatoxins [VM8 p. 1583]	Diarrhea, melena, vomiting, dyspnea	Gastroenteritis, pulmonary edema	*Melia azederach* var. *australasica* (white cedar)
Taxine [VM8 p. 1583]	Dyspnea, tremor, bradycardia, hypothermia, recumbency, death. May be sudden death	Nil	*Taxus baccata* (yew tree), *T. cuspitata* (Japanese yew tree)
Tropane alkaloids (atropine, hyoscine, hyoscyamine, scopolamine) [VM8 p. 1583]	Restless, tremor, pupil dilation, blind, frenzy, convulsions, recumbency	Nil	*Atropa belladonna* (deadly nightshade), *Datura* spp. (thornapple, Jimson weed), *Duboisia* spp. (corkwood, pitury), *Hyoscyamus niger* (henbane)
Tutu [VM8 p. 1584]	Hypersensitive, restless, convulsions, short course, death	Nil	*Coriaria* spp. (tutu tree)
Vellein [VM8 p. 1584]	Hyposensitive, dyspnea, tachycardia, recumbency, death	Nil	*Velleia discophora*
Veratrine [VM8 p. 1584]	Dyspnea, salivation, vomiting, diarrhea, frequent urination, cardiac irregularity, convulsions	Nil	*Veratrum californicum* (skunk cabbage, Western hellebore)
Zigadine (zigadenine) [VM8 p. 1584]	Salivation, vomiting tremor, ataxia, dyspnea	Nil	*Zigadenus* spp. (death camas)

Toxin	Clinical	Necropsy	Fungi
Aflatoxins (Aflatoxicosis) [VM8 p. 1590]	Hepatic encephalopathy, photosensitive dermatitis and conjunctivitis, diarrhea, tenesmus, anal prolapse, abortion, terminally recumbency, convulsions, death at 48 hours. Serum levels liver enzymes high. Aflatoxin content of tissues elevated.	Hepatic necrosis, jaundice, swollen liver, fluid in body cavities, degenerative lesions in brain and spinal cord in some. Enterocolitis in some pigs	Aspergillus clavatus, A. flavus, A. parasiticus, Penicillium puberulum
Citrinin [VM8 p. 1591]	'Pyrexia-pruritus-hemorrhagic syndrome' of cows. Itching, alopecia, dermatitis, fever, petechiation on exposed mucosa, conjunctiva. A few die	Petechiae in all tissues	Penicillium citrinum, P. palitans, P. viridicatum, Aspergillus ochraceus, A. terreus
Cyclopiazonic acid [VM8 p. 1592]	Anorexia, weakness, food refusal, infertility in sows	Gastric ulceration, alimentary tract hemorrhages	Aspergillus flavus, Penicillium spp.
Ergot alkaloids (ergotoxins) [VM8 p. 1592]			
i). Fescue summer toxicosis [VM8 p. 1592]	Severe drop milk production or body weight increase, hyperthermia, dyspnea, salivation, anorexia, rough coat, low blood levels prolactin. Dosing thiabendazole, spraying pasture with fungistat, ammoniating hay prevents signs	Nil	Acremonium coenophialum on Festuca arundinacea (tall fescue grass), Claviceps purpurea
ii). Fescue foot [VM8 p. 1593]	2 weeks on pasture, severe lameness, 2 weeks later gangrene, sloughing digits, tail tip, new cases for 1 week after moving cattle	Gangrene of extremities	Acremonium coenophialum or Claviceps purpurea on Festuca arundinacea
iii). Mare dystokia [VM8 p. 1593]	Dystokia, prolonged gestation, low foal survival, small udder development, low milk yield	Nil	Acremonium coenophialum on Festuca arundinacea, Claviceps purpurea on Lolium multiflorum.
iv). Fat necrosis [VM8 p. 1593]	Fat necrosis masses palpable rectally in cattle	Fat necrosis in mesentery	Acremonium coenophialum on Festuca arundinacea

Continued

Table 32.2 Continued

Toxin	Clinical	Necropsy	Fungi
v). Ergotism [VM8 p. 1595]	**Chronic** – lame, recumbent, gangrene of digits, ear tips, tail tip in cattle, not sheep, pigs. Sows – agalactia, small piglets, small litters, heavy piglet mortality. **Acute** – episodic convulsions in cattle	Gangrene of extremities	*Claviceps purpurea* on *Secale cereale* (cereal rye), other cereals, grasses. Most cases in animals fed ergot infested grain
vi). Ryegrass staggers [VM8 p. 1593]	'Ryegrass staggers', all species gross incoordination on larrassment, fall, convulsions. spontaneous recovery. Rare deaths due to misadventure. Lolitrem content estimated by ELISA. Hyphae visible in plant histologically	Focal necrosis skeletal muscle, degenerative lesions in Purkinje cell neurone in chronic cases	*Acremonium lolii* (toxins are lolitrems) on *Lolium perenne* (perennial rye grass)
vii). Paspalum staggers [VM8 p. 1596]	Hypersensitivity to sound, movement; tremor, head shake, gross ataxia, falling, paddling convulsions. Spontaneous recovery	Nil	*Claviceps paspali* on *Paspalum dilatatum* (paspalum, Dallas grass), *P. distichum* (water couch), *P. notatum* (Argentine bahia grass), *P. commersonii*, *P. scrobiculatum*, *Claviceps cineraria* on *Hilaria mutica* (tobosa grass), *H. jamesii* (galeta grass), *Balansia epichloe* on *Cynodon* spp. and other grasses
Fumonisins [VM8 p. 1597]			
i). Equine leukoencephalomalacia [VM8 p. 1597]	Tremor, staggering, circling, dysphagia, depression; jaundice in some. Death in 48–72 hrs	Hemorrhagic softening of cerebral white matter	*Fusarium moniliforme* on moldy corn, often standing crop, *Diplodia maydis* also on corn
ii). Ovine, porcine pulmonary edema [VM8 p. 1597]	Dyspnea, cough, death	Pulmonary edema	*Fusarium moniliforme*
Fusaric acid [VM8 p. 1597]	Mostly pigs; depression, vomiting	Nil	*Fusarium moniliforme*
Ipomeanols [VM8 p. 1597]	Dyspnea, cough, death in 48–72 hrs	Pulmonary edema, emphysema, interstitial pneumonia	*Fusarium solani* (= *F. javanicum*), *F. semitectum*, *Oxysporum* spp. on

Ochratoxin [VM8 p. 1598]	Mostly pigs; diarrhea, polyuria, polydipsia, high BUN, proteinuria	Generalised edema, renal enlargement, fibrosis, renal tubular epithelial necrosis	Aspergillus spp., e.g. A. ochraceus, Penicillium spp., e.g. P. viridicatum
Patulin [VM8 p. 1598]	Mostly pigs; vomiting, salivation, anorexia, polypnea, weight loss, leucocytosis, erythropenia,	Hemorrhagic enteritis	Penicillium urticae, P. patulum, P. claviforme usually on fruit products
Phomopsin [VM8 p. 1598] i). Hepatic injury [VM8 p. 1599]	**Acute** – anorexia, constipation, hepatic encephalopathy syndrome, stumbling, recumbency, jaundice, photosensitisation in some. Serum enzymes elevated. **Chronic** – ill-thrift, subject to stress, bouts of photosensitisation	**Acute** – swollen liver, jaundice. **Chronic** – shrunken liver, fibrosed	Phomopsis leptostromiformis, P. rossiana on Lupinus spp. (lupins) stubble, or lupin seed.
ii). Equine skeletal myopathy [VM8 p. 1599]	Stiff gait, reluctant to walk, lame, humped back, difficult rising.	Skeletal muscle myopathy	Phomopsis leptostromiformis on lupin stubble
Peptide [VM8 p. 1599] i). Gastroenteritis [VM8 p. 1601]	Salivation, oral mucosal erosions, vesicular, necrotic lesions, matting of hair at anus, tenesmus at defecation, pain on abdominal palpation, vomiting	Gastroenteritis	Amanita verna, Scleroderma citrinum, Ramaria, Clavaria spp. macrofungi, mushrooms, toadstools
ii). Nephrosis [VM8 p. 1601]	Anorexia, polyuria, polydipsia, anorexia, depression, BUN elevated	Nephrosis	Cortinaria speciocissimus
Rubratoxin [VM8 p. 1601]	Anorexia, depression, vomiting, diarrhea, dysentery, recumbency, convulsions, jaundice in some, death on day 4 – 5	Liver damage, hemorrhagic enteritis	Penicillium rubrum, P. purpurogenum
Slaframine [VM8 p. 1601]	Lacrimation, polyuria, bloat, anorexia, diarrhea, spontaneous recovery	Nil	Rhizoctonia leguminicola on standing legumes
Sporidesmin [VM8 p. 1601]	'Facial eczema', acute dullness, anorexia, jaundice, photosensitisation. Many die. Survivors ill-thrifty, bouts of photosensitisation, susceptible to stress. Few develop hepatic encephalopathy. Serum liver enzymes high. Zinc in drinking water, drenched, or by spraying on pasture prevents disease	Liver damage, enlargement, thickening bile ducts. Spongy vacuolation in brain tissue. Long-standing cases have hepatic fibrosis, shrinking in liver size. Perilobular fibrosis obliterating bile ducts	Pithomyces chartarum on dead leaf litter, underneath pasture plants, especially Lolium perenne (perennial rye grass)

Continued

615

Table 32.2 Continued

Toxin	Clinical	Necropsy	Fungi
Sterigmatocystin [VM8 p. 1602]	A carcinogen. Not recorded in agricultural animals	Hepatic carcinoma	Bipolaris spp., Aspergillus nidulans, A. versicolor on groundnuts
Tremorgens (penitrems, verruculogen, roquefortine, fumitremorgens, flavus tremorgens) [VM8 p. 1602]	"Staggers syndrome". Tremor, ataxia, stiff posture, falls easily, recumbent, convulsions. Nystagmus, salivation in some	Neuronal degeneration in midbrain, medulla, spinal cord in some	Penicillium spp., e.g. P. cyclopium, P. crustosum, P. puberulum, P. simplicissimum, Aspergillus fumigatus, A. flavus, A. clavatus and others
Macrocyclic Trichothecenes [VM8 p. 1603]			
i). Stachybotrytoxicosis (satratoxins, roridin, verrucarin) [VM8 p. 1603]	Fever, ruminal atony, diarrhea, dysentery, hemorrhages and ulcers nasal and oral mucosae, dry, cracked skin around eyes, on face. Leucopenia. Immunosuppression.	Generalised hemorrhages, enteritis. Myositis (horses)	Stachybotrys atra (= S. alternans)
ii). Myrotheciotoxicosis (roridin) [VM8 p. 1603]	Sudden death	Abomasitis, liver damage, pulmonary edema	Myrothecium roridum, M. verrucaria.
Non-macrocyclic Trichothecenes (T2 toxin, deoxynivalenol, diacetoxyscirpenol etc.) [VM8 p. 1603]	Vomiting, feed refusal, anorexia, diarrhea, ataxia, mucosal hemorrhages, ulcerative stomatitis	Generalised hemorrhages, enteritis	Fusarium tricinctum, F. sporotrichoides, F. poae, F. roseum, F. culmorum, F. nivale, F. moniliforme, F. semitectum, F. sporotrichiella, Trichothecium spp., Trichoderma spp., Cephalosporium spp.
Zearalenone [VM8 p. 1604]	Mostly **pigs**; vulvovaginitis, mammary gland swelling, vagina, rectum prolapse, low serum progesterone levels, infertility due to low litter size, neonatal mortality, congenital defects. **Cattle**, sheep – irregular estrus, vaginitis	Enlarged ovaries, uterus hypertrophy	Fusarium roseum (= F. graminearum), F. culmorum on stored grain, standing herbage

2. Microcystin (hepatoxic slow death factor) [VM8 p. 1606]

Clinical findings
* Anorexia, ruminal atony
* Depression, hypersensitivity initially in some
* Jaundice, photosensitization
* Diarrhea, dysentery, dehydration in some
* Recumbency
* Serum levels of liver enzymes elevated

Necropsy findings
* Severe liver damage
* Gastroenteritis in some

Treatment
* Activated charcoal
* Contaminated water isolated, straw or hay immersed in it

CYANOBACTERIA ASSOCIATED WITH NEMATODE GALLS ON GRASSES (TUNICAMYCIN) [VM8 p. 1606]

Etiology

Plant nematode (*Anguina funesta*), accompanied by *Corynebacterium rathyi* (= *Clavibacter* spp.) on seed heads of *Lolium rigidum* (Wimmera or annual ryegrass) *L. temulentum* (darnel), *Festuca rubra commutata* (Chewings fescue), *Polypogon monspieliensis* (annual beard grass), *Agrostis avenacea* (blowaway grass). Tunicomycin in water damaged grain kills pigs [VM8 p. 1607]

Clinical findings

(Annual ryegrass toxicity – ARGT, flood-plain staggers)
* Mostly cattle affected, rarely sheep
* Sudden falling
* Convulsions, death when harassed, driven
* Death usual within 24 hours
* Recovered animals ataxic, fall, have convulsive episodes

Necropsy findings

* Perivascular edema in brain and meninges
* Liver damage
* General hemorrhages

Treatment and control

No practicable treatment or control program.

DISEASES CAUSED BY ZOOTOXINS (ANIMAL BITES AND STINGS)

SNAKEBITE [VM8 p. 1608]

Etiology

* Snake venoms contain varying proportions of a number pf toxins including:
  * Necrotizing
  * Anticoagulant
  * Coagulant
  * Neurotoxic
  * Cardiotoxic
  * Myolytic
  * Hemolytic
* Effects vary depending on concentration of each toxin; see Table 32.3 for world summary

Epidemiology

* Most cases in horses
* In summer
* Most bites about the head
* Deaths rare because of animal size

Clinical findings

* Rarely local, rapidly developing swelling at bite causing excitement, anxiety; sloughs later
* Pupil dilation, pupillary light reflex negative, menace reflex present
* Salivation
* May be local paralysis tongue, lips, eyelids, pharynx causing dysphagia in foals
* Tremor, hyperaesthesia, restless, lies down frequently
* Terminal paralysis, recumbency
* Convulsions with asphyxial death

Clinical pathology

Accurate ELISA for detection specific venoms in blood.

Necropsy findings

Serous, blood-stained fluid, fang marks, bacterial cellulitis, at bite site in a few.

Table 32.3 Important venomous snakes of the world. Adapted from Dorland's Illustrated Medical Dictionary. W. B. Saunders, 1988.

Family and type of fangs	Common names	Type of venom	Distribution	Remarks
Colubridae: rear, immovable, grooved	Colubrids	Mostly mild	Warm parts of both hemispheres	Over 1000 species, the few poisonous ones not dangerous
Example:	Boomslang	Hemorrhagin	South Africa	Arboreal, timid
Elapidae: front, immovable, grooved	Elapids	Predominantly neurotoxin	Mostly in Old World	Over 150 species, very poisonous
Examples	Cobras	Mostly neurotoxin	Africa, India, Asia, Philippines, Celebes	Spitting cobra in Africa aims at eyes
	Kraits	Strong neurotoxin	India, S.E. Asia, Indonesia	Sluggish, often buried in dust
	Mambas	Neurotoxin	Tropical W. Africa	Arboreal
	Blacksnake	Neurotoxin	Australia	Large snake, wet terrain
	Copperhead	Neurotoxin	Australia, Tasmania, Solomons	Damp environment
	Brown snake	Neurotoxin	Australia, New Guinea	Slender
	Tiger snake	Strong neurotoxin	Australia	Dry environment; aggressive; very dangerous
	Death adder	Neurotoxin	Australia, New Guinea	Sandy terrain
	Coral snakes	Neurotoxin	United States, tropical America	About 26 species, 2 in southern U.S.A.
Hydrophidae: front, immovable, hollow	Sea snakes	Some mild; others very toxic	Tropical, Indian and Pacific Oceans	Gentle, rudder-like tail. Over 50 species
Viperidea: front, movable, hollow	True vipers; viperines; viperids	Predominantly hematoxin	Entirely in Old World	About 50 species
Examples:	European viper	Hematoxin	Europe (rare), N. Africa, Near East	Dry rocky country
	Russell's viper	Hematoxin	S.E. Asia, Java, Sumatra	Mostly open terrain; deadly
	Sand vipers	Hematoxin	N. Sahara	Buried in sand
	Puff adder	Hematoxin	Arabia, Africa	Open terrain; sluggish
	Gaboon viper	Neurotoxin and hematoxin	Tropical W. Africa	Forests; deadly
	Rhinoceros viper	Hematoxin	Tropical Africa	Wet forests

Crotalidae: front, movable, hollow	Pit vipers; crotalids; crotalines	Predominantly hematoxin	Old and New Worlds; none in Africa	Over 80 species; pit between eye and nostril
Examples:	Habu viper	Neurotoxin	Warmer parts of E. Asia; Ryukyu Islands	Caves and dry rocky country
	Rattlesnakes*	Predominantly hematoxin	N., Central and S. America	South American form neurotoxic
	Bushmaster	Hematoxin	Central and S. America	Large. In wet forests
	Fer-de-lance	Hematoxin	Central America, N. South America, few West Indies	Common on plantations
	Palm vipers	Hematoxin (?)	S. Mexico, Central and South America	Arboreal; small, greenish. Bite face
	Copperhead	Hematoxin	United States	Dry stony terrain
	Water moccasin	Hematoxin	Southeast U.S.A. to Texas	Swamps
	Asiatic pit vipers	Hematoxin	Southeast Asia, Taiwan	Most arboreal

* All rattlesnakes are venomous.

Diagnosis

Resembles:
♦ Viral encephalomyelitis
♦ Lactation tetany
♦ Colic

Treatment

♦ Broad-spectrum antibiotic for protection against infection at site
♦ Antivenin, mixture of local snakes unless snake identified; intravenously and locally at site
♦ Clostridial antitoxin
♦ Corticosteroids contraindicated

BEE STINGS [VM8 p. 1609]

♦ Usually multiple bites in horses
♦ Local swelling
♦ Excitement, restlessness
♦ Diarrhea
♦ Jaundice, hemoglobinuria in some
♦ Dyspnea if swelling around throat
♦ Prostration
♦ Apply local astringent lotions to ease irritation, tracheotomy if needed

ANT BITE [VM8 p. 1609]

Aggressive ants, e.g. *Solenopsis invicta* (fire ant), cause corneal ulceration of recumbent young animals.

TICK PARALYSIS [VM8 p. 1610]

Etiology

Ixodes holocyclus, Dermacentor andersoni: a number of adult females, attached for 7 days, needed to paralyze yearlings up to 50 kg body weight.

Clinical findings

♦ Ascending flaccid paralysis

♦ Ataxia respiration labored, thoracic, pupils dilated, unresponsive
♦ Lateral recumbency
♦ Spontaneous recovery if ticks removed

CANTHARIDIN POISONING
(BLISTER BEETLE POISONING)
[VM8 p. 1610]

Etiology

Ingestion of hay contaminated by *Epicauta occidentalis, E. temexa* (blister beetles) containing cantharidin.

Clinical findings

♦ Anorexia
♦ Oral mucosal erosions
♦ Frequent urination
♦ Colic
♦ Synchronous diaphragmatic flutter in some
♦ Hematuria, hypocalcemia, hypomagnesemia
♦ High case fatality rate

LOPHYROTOMIN [VM8 p. 1610]

Etiology

♦ Toxin in larvae of Australian (*Lophyrotoma interrupta*) and Danish (*Arge pullata*) sawflies
♦ Ingested by cattle, sheep

Clinical findings

♦ Dyspnea
♦ Tremor, recumbency, convulsions
♦ Sudden death due to severe liver damage

Necropsy findings

♦ Periacinar hepatic necrosis
♦ Nephrosis
♦ Alimentary tract hemorrhage
♦ Fluid in serous cavities

33 DISEASES CAUSED BY ALLERGY

ALLOIMMUNE HEMOLYTIC
ANEMIA OF THE NEWBORN
(NEONATAL ISOERYTHROLYSIS,
ISOIMMUNE HEMOLYTIC ANEMIA
OF THE NEWBORN) [VM8 p. 1612]

Etiology

Natural occurrence
♦ Sire erythrocyte antigens, inherited by fetus, pass through placenta and stimulate production of antibodies in dam circulation
♦ Antibodies cannot pass placenta so neonate born normal, but do pass to neonate in colostrum
♦ Cause acute, highly fatal intravascular hemolysis

Artificial production
Immunity develops to erythrocytes in injected whole blood vaccines.

Epidemiology

Occurrence
International as **natural disease** in foals.

Artificial disease
Caused by:
♦ Fetal tissue vaccines to horses for rhinopneumonitis
♦ Whole-blood vaccines for hog cholera in pigs, babesiosis, or anaplasmosis in cattle
♦ **Infection prevalence rate** very low, about 0.2% foals born
♦ **Case fatality rate** 100% without vigorous treatment in peracute and acute cases, less in subacute cases

Host risk factors
Species – **natural disease** only in:
♦ Foals of horse and mule mares, not Shetland ponies, possibly in piglets
♦ Only in dams not carrying sire erythrocyte antigen
♦ Only some incompatible matings

♦ Not first mating of incompatibles; insufficient antibody produced
♦ Placental damage may enhance passage of erythrocyte antigens
Artificial disease likely to occur only after:
♦ Repeated injections
♦ Injections in late pregnancy
♦ In pigs in litters from Large White × Wessex or Essex matings

Age
Neonates 8–36 (usually 24) hours old and after early colostrum consumption.

Clinical findings

Horses
♦ Normal pregnancy, parturition
♦ **Peracute:** 8–36 hours old
♦ Sudden onset severe hemoglobinuria, red urine
♦ Mucosal pallor
♦ Weakness, recumbency, death in few hours
♦ **Acute:** 2–4 days old
♦ Severe jaundice, moderate pallor
♦ Hemoglobinuria
♦ **Subacute:** 4–5 days old
♦ Marked jaundice, mild pallor
♦ No hemoglobinuria
♦ General signs:
  • Varying degrees of severity
  • Lassitude, frequent yawning, weakness, do not suck
  • Recumbency
  • Tachycardia; enhanced cardiac impulse, heart sounds, area of cardiac audibility
  • Systolic cardiac thrill, murmur
  • Dyspnea in advanced cases
  • No edema

Pigs
♦ Piglets similar syndrome to foals in same time sequence with death by day 1–5
♦ Some subclinicals with abnormal hematology only

Cattle
Calves similar to foals, same time sequence.

Clinical pathology

Hematology
Greatly reduced erythrocyte count, PCV, hemoglobin level WBC count normal.

Serology
♦ High levels of immune isoantibodies to sire or neonate erythrocytes in dam serum
♦ Direct hemolysis sensitization test, mare serum and foal erythrocytes most efficient
♦ Slide test to demonstrate agglutination of neonate erythrocytes good presumptive test; requires only drop of blood from neonate
♦ Identification of erythrocyte blood group antigens present valuable for prognosis. *Aa* antigens indicate acute case, *Qa* antigens indicate less severe case, *R* and *S* antigens indicate mildest cases

Necropsy findings

♦ Greatly enlarged spleen
♦ Pallor, jaundice
♦ Red urine

Diagnosis

Similar to:
♦ Physiological neonatal icterus
♦ Foal septicemias
♦ Isoimmune hemorrhagic anemia of newborn piglets

Treatment

♦ Severe cases at 15 hours old with PCV <15% require compatible blood transfusion
♦ In emergency when laboratory compatibility tests unavailable use any donor other than dam, or washed cells
♦ Supportive treatment includes fostering on another mare, or
♦ Feeding on reconstituted cow milk
♦ Sucking of dam can recommence at 48 hours
♦ Fluid intake must be maintained
♦ Piglets removed from sow and fed artificially for 48 hours

Control

♦ Identify high risk mares which have previously had jaundiced or suspect foal, by blood typing

♦ At foaling cross-match test mare serum or colostrum with foal erythrocytes
♦ Foals from incompatible mares not allowed to suck mare for 48 hours; hand-reared supplemented by broad-spectrum antibiotic cover
♦ Resume sucking dam with small feeds
♦ Dam must be milked out frequently during the waiting period

PURPURA HEMORRHAGICA [VM8 p. 1615]

Etiology

Commonly associated with upper respiratory tract infection.

Epidemiology

♦ Rare in horses, very rare in pigs and cattle
♦ Sporadic cases in large groups of horses experiencing strangles outbreaks
♦ Case fatality rate approximates 100%

Clinical findings

♦ Large asymmetric, edematous, subcutaneous swellings usually on face and muzzle, developing over several days
♦ Mild fever, tachycardia
♦ Swellings cold, painless, pit on pressure
♦ No break in skin, may ooze serum
♦ Swellings at throat may cause dyspnea, dysphagia
♦ Petechiae in oral, nasal mucosae, conjunctivae
♦ Severe colic due to edema swellings in gut wall
♦ Death after 1–2 weeks

Clinical pathology

♦ Leukocytosis, neutrophilia, reduced erythrocyte count, hemoglobin level, normal platelets, clotting mechanisms
♦ ELISA test for IgA streptococcal proteins, high in streptococcus-infected horses, undetectable in clinical cases

Necropsy findings

♦ Generalized petechiae
♦ Edematous swellings in intestinal wall, beneath serosa

Diagnosis

Horse

Similar to:
- Idiopathic thrombocytopenic purpura
- Necrotizing vasculitis
- Equine viral arteritis
- Equine viral rhinopneumonitis
- Equine infectious anemia
- Congestive heart failure

Pigs

Similar to thrombocytopenic purpura of newborn.

Cattle

Similar to:
- Bracken poisoning
- *Stachybotris spp.* poisoning
- *Melilotus alba* poisoning

Treatment

- Blood transfusion plus
- Full, repeated doses corticosteroids for periods up to 3 months, interrupted at 2 week intervals and recommenced if signs return

LAMINITIS [VM8 p. 1617]

Etiology

- **Metabolic laminitis** associated with intoxication, including moderate grain engorgement
- **Infectious laminitis,** including metritis, colitis, after dipping in ruminants
- **Traumatic laminitis,** standing for long periods in transport vehicle, vigorous pawing

Epidemiology

Occurrence

- Universal
- Sporadic cases only
- Mostly in horses
- Herd problem in some cattle operations, rarely in sheep
- In horses usually terminated by euthanasia because of irreversible hoof damage
- Cattle and sheep cases resolved by reducing feed

Environment risk factor

Commonly associated in horses and cattle with heavy grain or high nutrient value pasture, especially high protein (>17%) diets.

Host risk factor

- Overweight, colic-prone ponies, getting no exercise and on lush pasture
- Overweight yearling cattle in fattening or bull preparation units, or small, high-producing dairy herds
- Heavy pounding or long standing in horses
- Roughly surfaced yards, lanes cause excessive abrasion of hooves in cattle
- Susceptibility suspected inherited in horses

Clinical findings

Horse – acute

- Severe pain on compression in all four hooves, especially fore feet
- Sometimes unilateral
- Reluctant to walk, shuffling gait, short steps without lifting hooves
- Anxious expression
- Muscle tremor, sweating
- Frequent lifting of feet at first, with all four feet placed forward, horse leans back on its heels, head hung low
- Lying down appears to be very painful, usually many attempts before flopping down
- Lateral recumbency, reluctant to sit up or get up, may not do so
- Pain, heat at coronets
- In advanced cases serum oozes from coronets
- Third phalanx may protrude through sole
- Horn separates at coronet; finally hoof sloughs

Horse – chronic

- Persistent or frequent attacks of lameness
- Hoof wall spreads, concave anterior wall, horizontal ridges, sole drops

Cattle and sheep

- Similar to horse but much less severe
- Prolonged recumbency
- Standing cases restless, shifting feet
- Four feet bunched together, back arched
- Shuffling gait
- Pain on squeezing hooves
- Long-standing cases permanently lame, develop large, flat feet, with horizontal ridges and a concave angle of the anterior wall as in horses

- Softening, yellow discoloration, thinning of sole
- Double sole develops

Pig
- Arched back
- Bunching of feet posture
- Lameness
- Pain on hoof compression

Clinical pathology

- Radiologically detectable downward rotation tip of third phalanx, ventral displacement of phalanx in all species
- Blood histamine level, eosinophil count may be elevated
- Hemoconcentration, hyponatremia and hypochloremia constant in horses gorged on grain
- May be thrombocytopenia and hypocoagulability in acute stages

Necropsy findings

- Gross lesions, hoof deformity, only in chronic cases
- In acute cases, possibly perceptible engorgement of blood vessels in sensitive laminae of digital cushion
- Histologically specific lesions of laminar tissues

Diagnosis

Resembles:
- Tetanus
- Azoturia
- Gastric rupture
- Bladder rupture
- Colic
- Arthritis
- Epiphysitis

Treatment

Horses – acute
- Phenylbutazone, plus phenoxybenzamine, preferably combined with an anticoagulant, e.g. heparin
- Severe cases may not respond
- Delay of 24 hours greatly increases failure rate, at 48 hours lesions irreversible
- Supportive treatment includes:
  - Methionine orally (10 g/day for 3 days, then 5 g/day for 10 days)
  - Cold packs to the feet
  - Mild purgative, e.g. mineral oil, if grain is cause

Horses – chronic
- Low calorie diet
- Analgesic
- Surgical correction of hoof deformity
- Surgical shoeing

Cattle
Poor response to horse treatments.

Control

Horse
- Avoid obesity, too high protein diet
- Provide rest periods during long transport, especially heavy horses, pregnant mares
- Early correction metritis, retained placenta

Cattle
- Gradual introduction to heavy grain feeding, susceptible animals put back to pasture
- Avoid abrasive floors and walkways

EQUINE SEASONAL ALLERGIC DERMATITIS (QUEENSLAND ITCH, SWEET ITCH) [VM8 p. 1621]

Etiology

Hypersensitivity to bites of *Culicoides* spp. sand flies, or *Stomoxys calcitrans*.

Epidemiology

- Horses only
- Summer
- Wherever insects present, worst in wooded country
- Horses over 7 years old
- Icelandic horses especially sensitive

Clinical findings

- Lesions at preferred landing sites for insects, along back, especially tail head, rump, withers, crest, poll, ears, ventral midline, but may be anywhere
- Initial papules, intense scratching, alopecia, skin thickening, scaliness
- May interfere with grazing, weight lost
- Spontaneous recovery in cold weather

Clinical pathology

- Eosinophilia, thrombocytosis
- Eosinophilic infiltration of lesions seen in biopsy

◆ Intradermal injection of insect extracts causes local sensitivity reaction

Diagnosis

Resembles:
◆ Mycotic dermatitis
◆ Scald due to continuous wetting

Treatment

◆ Systemic antihistamines
◆ Long-acting corticosteroids

Control

◆ Insect-proof stabling at night
◆ Topical repellent, insecticide, e.g. weekly 4% permethrin pour-on effective in most horses, every 48 hours in others

OVINE SEASONAL ALLERGIC DERMATITIS [VM8 p. 1622]

◆ Similar disease to equine seasonal dermatitis in sheep
◆ Lesions on teats, udder, ventral mid-line, ear tips, around eyes, nose and lips
◆ Only in summer
◆ In adults
◆ *Culicoides* spp. hypersensitivity demonstrated
◆ Similar clinical disease in cattle

MILK ALLERGY [VM8 p. 1622]

Etiology

Hypersensitivity to milk protein suspected.

Epidemiology

◆ Commonest in Channel Island cattle
◆ Only at drying off

Clinical findings

◆ Urticaria, especially of eyelids, muzzle, but may be generalized
◆ Tremor
◆ Dyspnea, cough
◆ Restless, kicking at abdomen, vigorous self-licking
◆ Rarely maniacal charging, bellowing
◆ Alternative syndrome in some of:
  • Dullness

• Shuffling gait, ataxia
• Recumbency

Clinical pathology

◆ Intradermal injection of dilute extract of cow's own milk produces local edematous thickening in minutes

Treatment

◆ Spontaneous recovery
◆ Parenteral antihistamines terminate attack
◆ May need to be repeated
◆ Likely to recur at subsequent lactations; culling recommended

ENZOOTIC NASAL GRANULOMA OF CATTLE [VM8 p. 1622]

Etiology

Hypersensitivity to common environmental allergens the current hypothesis.

Epidemiology

◆ Cattle only
◆ Channel Island, other dairy breeds most susceptible
◆ Most prevalent in high-rainfall areas
◆ Morbidity up to 70% of herds, 25% cattle affected in enzootic areas
◆ Begins at 6 months to 4 years, till animal culled for weight loss

Clinical findings

Acute
◆ Sudden onset bilateral ocular, nasal discharges
◆ Noisy nasal respiration
◆ Head-shaking, snorting, rubbing nose in bushes, sticks pushed up nostrils

Chronic
◆ Gradual onset
◆ Granulomatous nodules 1–4 mm dia. on anterior 5–10 cm nasal mucosa
◆ Noisy, labored respiration
◆ Appetite good but weight loss, decreased milk yield

Diagnosis

Resembles:
◆ Bovine atopic rhinitis

♦ Mycotic nasal granuloma due to infection
with:
• *Drechslera rostrata*
• *Rhinosporidium nasalis*
♦ Nasal fluke (*Schistosoma nasalis*) infestation
♦ Bovid herpesvirus-1 infection
♦ Pasture mite (*Tyrophagus palmarum*) infestation

Treatment and control

None recommended.

BOVINE ATOPIC RHINITIS (SUMMER
SNUFFLES) [VM8 p. 1622]

Etiology

Apparent hypersensitivity to environmental
allergens, probably pollen.

Epidemiology

♦ Mostly in Channel Island breeds
♦ Spring/summer when pasture in flower

Clinical findings

♦ Sudden onset
♦ Sneezing
♦ Stertorous dyspnea, sometimes to mouth-
breathing stage
♦ Profuse nasal discharge, thick, orange–
yellow, caseous in late stages
♦ Nasal irritation manifested as rubbing nose
on ground, into bushes, scratching muzzle
with hind feet

♦ Nasal cavity plugged with sticks, lacerated,
bleeding
♦ Nasal mucosa thick, edematous
♦ Late stage is nasal pseudomembrane which
sloughs as cast
♦ Small nodules on anterior nasal mucosa in
healed stage
♦ Signs disappear in winter

Clinical pathology

Nasal mucosal nodules filled with eosinophils.

Diagnosis

Resembles:
♦ Enzootic bovine nasal granuloma
♦ Mycotic nasal granuloma due to infection
with:
• *Drechslera rostrata*
• *Rhinosporidium nasalis*
♦ Nasal fluke (*Schistosoma nasalis*) infestation
♦ Bovid herpesvirus-1 infection
♦ Pasture mite (*Tyrophagus palmarum*) infestation

Treatment

♦ Remove animal from pasture
♦ Active antihistamine program

EQUINE ALLERGIC RHINITIS [VM8
p. 1623]

♦ Similar to the bovine disease (see above)
clinically and epidemiologically
♦ No nasal mucosal lesions
♦ Causes persistent head-shaking

BLOOD TRANSFUSION REACTION
(see page 35)

34 DISEASES CAUSED BY THE INHERITANCE OF UNDESIRABLE CHARACTERS

Descriptions of the notable inherited defects of food producing animals are summarized in Table 34.1. A basic program of examination on which a diagnosis of inherited disease should be based is as follows.

Epidemiology

Occurrence

♦ Inherited defects more likely to occur where:
- Inbreeding practiced; purebred herds, especially studs, the most likely places for inherited diseases, but can occur rarely in cross-bred matings; purebred families often achieve a reputation for the occurrence of a particular defect
- A new breed begun from a few foundation animals, the **foundation effect**
- Similarly where breeding programs are based on a few sires, or dams; a feature of artificial insemination, ovum transplants

♦ Inherited defects likely to have a particular incidence:
- Gradual increase in number of cases, where same sires and dams used
- First appearance of disease after introduction of new sire
- Evenness of spread of case occurrence; bursts of cases more likely with infectious or toxic causes
- Numerical ratio of occurrence appropriate to probable gene frequency, e.g. offspring of sire mated to daughters out of nil gene frequency cows should have 12.5% defective calves; matings between bull and his half-sisters should produce 25% defective calves
- The incidence of the defect should match a specific mode of inheritance, e.g. autosomal recessive, sex-linked, lethal dominance

♦ Test matings
- Repeat of mating to same dam group should produce same ratio of cases
- Proof for freedom of a bull from a known defect is all normal offspring from matings with 10 known carrier cows or 20 daughters of known carriers; known carriers usually maintained in a herd minded by a breed society or artificial insemination center
- Ovum transplants with early caesarean sections of the surrogate dams reduces delay and cost of natural matings

Clinical findings

♦ The syndrome, or susceptibility to it, is or are known to be inherited. See Table 34.1 for a list of defects
♦ The defect should be consistent in its expression; environmentally acquired diseases much more variable

Clinical pathology

♦ The metabolic defect is known to be inherited (Table 34.1) for a list of defects
♦ Diagnosis of heterozygotes by:
- Radiological markers found in neonates in some inherited skeletal defects
- Enzyme estimations in enzymopathies, e.g. mannosidosis

Necropsy findings

♦ The lesion is known to be inherited (Table 34.1)
♦ The presence of a known laboratory marker for an inherited disease, e.g. overfilled lysosomes, which can also be caused by toxins

Differential diagnosis

♦ Eliminate possibility of noxious environmental influence as the cause at the appropriate time (period of specific organogenesis)
♦ Errors in diagnosis most likely where:

- Disease occurs independently as well as an inherited defect, e.g. goiter, laminitis cardiomyopathy
- Susceptibility to a particular disease is inherited when the disease also occurs independently, e.g. bloat, mastitis enzootic bovine leukosis, scrapie

Table 34.1 Inherited defects

(Here = Hereford, H-F = Holstein Friesian, Jap.B = Japanese Black, Br Swiss = Brown Swiss)

Defect	Lesion or functional defect	Clinical signs/lesion/clinical pathology	Age, species, breed	Type of inheritance	Outcome
		Inherited metabolic defects			
	(Inherited requirements for greater than normal intakes of Zinc, Vitamins A, D, E dealt with in sections on respective nutritional deficiencies)				
UMP synthase deficiency (DUMPS) [VM8 p. 1629]	High level of orotate in milk	Death and resorption 40 day fetus. Absence of uridine-5 monophosphate, excess orotate in tissues	**Cattle** H-F, Fetus	Nil	Lethal in utero
Goiter [VM8 p. 1629]	Enlarged thyroid glands	**Cattle** Grey hair coat in some. **Goats and kids** Lustrous, silky wool in some lambs. Edema and floppiness of ears. Enlargement, bowing forelimb bones. Dorsoventral flattening nasal area. Dyspnea due to faulty lung development	Merino, Polled Dorset sheep, Boer and Dwarf Saanen goats, Afrikander cattle	Recessive	Still births, neonatal mortality, growth retardation
Inherited combined immunodeficiency [VM8 p. 1629]	Lymphopenia, lack of immunoglobulin synthesis and cell-moderated immunity, thymic hypoplasia	Fatal septicemia, usually adenoviral pneumonia, bacteria fungi or protozoa. Also hepatitis, enteritis. Unthrifty, lethargic, tires easily. Cough, nasal discharge, loud lung sounds, chronic diarrhea, alopecia, dermatitis in some. Poor response to treatment. Lymphopenia, hypogammaglobulinemia. Hypoplasia lymph nodes, thymus. Heterozygote not detectable clinically or by lab test. No treatment	Arabian foals 2 days old, older to 3 months. Part-Arabians also	Autosomal recessive	Fatal by 3 months old

Continued

629

Table 34.1 *Continued*

(Here = Hereford, H-F = Holstein Friesian, Jap.B = Japanese Black, Br Swiss = Brown Swiss)

Defect	Lesion or functional defect	Clinical signs/lesion/clinical pathology	Age, species, breed	Type of inheritance	Outcome
Chediak-Higashi syndrome [VM8 p. 1631]	Insufficient bactericidal activity in abnormal leukocytes, metabolic defect in structurally abnormal platelets	Poor growth, incomplete albinism, oculocutaneous hypopigmentation (gray hair, lack of pigment in iris and ocular fundus) photophobia, lacrimation, anaemia, enlarged edematous lymph nodes, immune defect. All leukocytes contain microscopically visible enlarged lysozymes. Clotting defect	**Cattle** Here, Jap.B, Brangus	Single autosomal recessive	Fatal at about 1 year old
Pseudoalbinism (Horse) [VM8 p. 1631]	Colon atresia or functional constriction	Foals develop colic soon after birth. Colic due to colon atresia or constriction with absence of myenteric ganglia	**Horses** (White with pigmented eyes – Overos, possible Tobianos)	Recessive	Fatal at 1 week old
Lethal Whites (Horse) [VM8 p. 1631]	Fetal nonviability	25% of fetuses die in utero in early gestation	White horses with blue or heterochromic irises	Dominant	Early fetal death
Pseudoalbinism (Cattle) [VM8 p. 1631]	Hypopigmentation hair coat and eyes	Oculo-cutaneous hypopigmentation, (Brown coat, two-tone, blue–brown irises) Photophobic, prefer shade	H-F, Here, Br Swiss, Angus	Nil	Aesthetic defect
Inherited reproductive defects					
Freemartinism [VM8 p. 1627]	Chromosomal chimaerism	Chromosomal defect. Short vagina, enlarged clitoris, vulval hairtuft in female of twins. Males of twins structural normal but low reproductive efficiency and cytogenetic defects	Cattle	Nil	Infertile

Chromosomal translocations (cattle) [VM8 p. 1627]	Gonadal hypoplasia	Testicular hypoplasia, arrested spermiogenesis in infertile bull. Anestrus, ovarian inactivity heifers	Cattle	Nil	Infertile
Chromosomal translocations (horse) [VM8 p. 1628]	Gonadal hypoplasia	Small ovaries, abnormal estrous, poor fertility in mares. Possibly cryptorchid males. Intersexes also occur	Horses	Nil	Infertile
Chromosomal translocations (sheep, goat) [VM8 p. 1628]	Infertility	Infertility recorded but many sheep with the translocation are clinically normal	Romney sheep, Alpine x goat	Nil	Infertile (possibly)
Chromosomal translocations (pigs) [VM8 p. 1628]	Infertility, some embryonic loss	Major reproductive loss	Pigs	Nil	Infertile
Prolonged gestation [VM8 p. 1663] 1. With fetal giantism [VM8 p. 1663]	Fetus has adeno-hypophyseal hypoplasia and thyroidal and adrenal cortical hypoplasia	Pregnancy prolonged by 3 weeks to 4 months. Few cases distended abdomen. Parturition precipitate, without pelvic ligament relation or udder enlargement, cervical relaxation. Dystokia. Fetus large with long hair coat, large, well-erupted teeth. Calves dyspneic; die within few hours; hypoglycemic coma. Serum progesterone level before term does not fall as it should	Cattle HF, Ayrshire, Swedish	Inherited	Lethal to calf
2. With cranio facial deformity [VM8 p. 1663]		Fetus dead on delivery; small, alopecic, hydrocephalus, cyclopian eyes, microphthalmia, one nostril, absence maxilla. Adenohypophyseal hypoplasia. Other endocrine glands small and hypoplastic, limbs short, jejunal atresia in some. Pelvic ligaments and cervix relax. No dystokia	Cattle Jersey, Jersey, Ayrshire	Inherited simple recessive	Lethal to calf

Continued

631

632

Table 34.1 Continued

(Here = Hereford, H-F = Holstein Friesian, Jap.B = Japanese Black, Br Swiss = Brown Swiss)

Defect	Lesion or functional defect	Clinical signs/lesion/clinical pathology	Age, species, breed	Type of inheritance	Outcome
3. *With arthrogryposis* [VM8 p. 1663]		*Accompanied by arthrogryposis, scoliosis, torticollis, kyphosis, cleft palate*	**Cattle** Hereford	Nil	Lethal to calf
Cryptorchidism [VM8 p. 1653]	Failure of testicle(s) to descend	Testicle(s) retained	Horse, cattle, sheep, pigs	Inherited	Inconvenient
Hermaphroditism [VM8 p. 1653]	Organs of both sexes present	Bisexual specimens	Pigs	Suggested inherited	Culled
		Inherited circulatory system defects			
Cardiomyopathy syndrome [VM8 p. 1633] 1. Calf acute heart failure [VM8 p. 1633]	Cardiomyopathy	Sudden death at about 3 months. Fast growth rate, short curly hair, moderate exophthalmos. Precipitated by exercise; dyspnea, blood-stained nasal froth. Death in few minutes to hours or congestive heart failure in several days	**Cattle** Here, Poll and Horned	Single autosomal recessive	Sudden death before six months old
Cardiomyopathy syndrome [VM8 p. 1633] 2. Pulmonary edema [VM8 p. 1633]	Acute myocardial necrosis	Few minutes to hours agonizing dyspnea, sudden onset. Death. Anasarca, ascites, hydrothorax, left ventricular dilation, acute myocardial necrosis, pulmonary edema	**Cattle** Jap.Black. Calf. 1–4 months	Single new, autosomal recessive	Death
Cardiomyopathy syndrome [VM8 p. 1633] 3. Congestive heart failure [VM8 p. 1633]	Myocardial necrosis	Most in late pregnancy or early lactation. Sudden onset congestive heart failure, anasarca, venous engorgement, ascites, hepatomegaly	**Cattle** H-F, Simmental x Red H-F, Black Spotted Friesian, 1.5 to 6 years old. Most 3–4 years	Inherited autosomal recessive suspected	Death

				Single autosomal recessive	Euthanasia
Lymphatic obstruction [VM8 p. 1633]	Lymph node agenesis	Slight to severe edema, generalized or local to head, ears, neck, limbs, tail. Lymph nodes vestigial, lymph vessels tortuous, dilated. Many dead at birth, cause dystocia. Dam may have hydrops amnii	**Cattle** Ayrshire, Here, Congenital		
Ventricular septal defect [VM8 p. 1634]	Congestive heart failure	Congestive heart failure by 2–4 weeks. Precordial systolic murmur and thrill bilaterally	**Cattle** Here	Suspected inherited?	Death or euthanasia
Aortic aneurysm [VM8 p. 1634]	Aneurysm in aorta	Sudden death due to internal hemorrhage when aneurysm ruptures	Cattle	Suspected inherited?	Sudden death
Porphyria [VM8 p. 1634]	Deficiency of uroporphyrinogen 111 cosynthetase, porphyrin type 1 isomers accumulate	Incapacitating photosensitization when in sun. Urine amber to red, pink brown teeth. Mucosal pallor, growth retardation. Pigs not often photosensitized. Urine has high levels uro- and coproporphyrins	**Cattle** S'horns, H-F, B&W Danish, J.Red, J.Black, Ayrshire, **Pigs**	Single recessive	Culled
Protoporphyrin [VM8 p. 1634]	Deficiency of ferrochelatase enzyme	Photosensitive dermatitis only. High levels protoporphyrin in feces and erythrocytes. Hepatic portal fibrosis	**Cattle** Limousin, Blond d'Aquitaine. **Pigs**	Inherited	Culled
Familial polycythemia [VM8 p. 1635]	Primary polycythemia	Neonatal deaths, mucosal congestion, dyspnea, poor growth. High PCV, erythrocyte count	**Cattle** Jerseys	Single autosomal recessive	Culled
Congenital methaemoglobinaemia [VM8 p. 1635]	Hemolytic anemia. Low levels of erythrocyte glutathione reductase. (EGR)	Low exercise tolerance, pale mucosae, hemic heart murmur, hemolysis, anemia. Low levels EGR, high blood methemoglobin	Horses	Possibly inherited	Culled

Continued

633

Table 34.1 Continued

(Here = Hereford, H-F = Holstein Friesian, Jap.B = Japanese Black, Br Swiss = Brown Swiss)

Defect	Lesion or functional defect	Clinical signs/lesion/clinical pathology	Age, species, breed	Type of inheritance	Outcome
Granulocytopathy [VM8 p. 1635]	Deaths from recurrent bacteremia	Anorexia, fever, cough, dyspnea (due to pneumonia) enlarged lymph nodes, oral ulcers. Neutrophilia	Cattle H-F. Calves from birth	Suspected inherited	Death by 3 months old
Leukocyte adhesion deficiency [VM8 p. 1635]	Deficiency of a leukocyte–glycogen complex	First sign 2 weeks–8 months. Recurrent bouts fever, diarrhea, cough, dyspnea. Peridontal gingivitis in some. Many intravascular neutrophils. Striking persistent neutrophilia. Polymerase chain reaction test identifies heterozygote	Cattle H-F	Autosomal recessive	Not viable. Death by 2 years old
Hemophilia A [VM8 p. 1636]	Deficiency of factor VIII (Classical hemophilia)	Uncontrollable bleeding after injury, surgery or spontaneously. Sudden onset of swellings over joints, or throat causing dyspnea, or internally causing acute hemorrhagic anemia. Labtest identifies	Horse Thorobred, standard bred, Arabian, Quarter horse	Sex-linked recessive. Only in males	Not viable
Von Willebrand's disease [VM8 p. 1636]	Deficiency of VWF	Repeated bleeding episodes. Lab test identifies	Horse Quarter horse	Suspected inherited	Not viable
Factor XI deficiency [VM8 p. 1636]	Partial thromboplastin antecedent deficiency	Minor to serious bleeding episodes. Some homozygotes clinically normal but lab tests positive. Neonates most affected – may die of hemorrhagic anaemia	Cattle	Autosomal recessive. Males and females transmit	Inconvenience
Prekallikrein deficiency [VM8 p. 1636]	Prekallikrein is an activator for Factor XII	Bleeding tendency. Lab test identifies	Horse Belgian	Inherited	

634

Inherited alimentary tract defects

				RECESSIVE	
Thrombopathia [VM8 p. 1636]	Impaired platelet aggregation	Uncontrolled bleeding. Epistaxis, hematuria, subcutaneous swellings, hemorrhagic anemia, hemorrhage after injury or surgery	**Cattle** Simmental		
Congenital thrombopathia dyskeratosis and alopecia [VM8 p. 1636]	Ineffective erythropoiesis	Curly hair locks, sebum accumulations, hair loss, muzzle and ears. Thick skin, dermatitis. Pine, euthanized, anemia	**Cattle** Here poll 1 to 16 months old	Suspected inherited	Death
Congenital hemolytic anemia [VM8 p. 1636]	Persistent intravascular hemolysis	Poor growth, exercise intolerance. Weakness, jaundice, death. Severe regenerative anemia	**Cattle** M.grey calves 3–8 weeks	Suspected inherited	Death
Harelip [VM8 p. 1632]	Congenital lip cleavage, uni or bilateral	Poor growth, cryptorchidism, harelip	**Cattle** H-F	Suspected inherited	Aesthetic defect
		Bilateral lip cleavage	**Sheep** Texel	Single recessive	
Gut segment atresia [VM8 p. 1632]	Gut atresia	Colon atresia. Colic. Pseudoalbinism in some	**Horse** Overo and Percheron	Recessive	Death at one week
		Ileum atresia, abdominal distension of fetus, dystocia	**Cattle** Swedish Highland	Recessive	
		Coli atresia, no feces passed, abdominal distension	**Cattle** Jersey	Recessive	
		Atresia ani, anorexia, colic, severe abdominal distension	Cattle, sheep, pigs	?	
Recto-vaginal constriction [VM8 p. 1632]	Non-elastic fibrous bands around anus (vulva)	Stenosis of vaginal vestibule in cows. Stenosis of rectum in either sex. Difficult to inseminate, dystocia, small, hard udder, low milk production. Udder edema. Heterozygotes not accurately detectable	Jersey cows and bulls	Autosomal recessive	Culled

635

Table 34.1 Continued

(Here = Hereford, H-F = Holstein Friesian, Jap.B = Japanese Black, Br Swiss = Brown Swiss)

Defect	Lesion or functional defect	Clinical signs/lesion/clinical pathology	Age, species, breed	Type of inheritance	Outcome
		Inherited defects of nervous system			
		Inherited lysosomal storage diseases			
		(Lysosomes in visceral and neuronal sites affected but signs principally nervous)			
α Mannosidosis (Syndrome 1) [ataxia paralysis) [VM8 p. 1637]	Deficiency of α-mannosidase causes accumulation of mannose and glucosamine containing metabolite	1. Ataxia, tremor, aggression, poor growth and condition. Normal at birth. Signs commence soon after, up to 4 months. Signs increased by excitement. Eventual recumbency due to paralysis. Heterozygote detected by low plasma mannosidase levels	Cattle Angus, M.grey, Galloway	Simple recessive	Fatal by 6 months
Syndrome 2 (Hydrocephalus-arthrogryposis) [VM8 p. 1637]	Ditto	2. Neonatal mortality, stillbirth, hydrocephalus arthrogryposis, hepatomegaly	Cattle Galloway	Nil	Stillbirth or soon after birth
β-Mannosidosis [VM8 p. 1637] Cattle [VM8 p. 1637]	Deficiency of acidic β-mannosidase	Congenital cranio-facial deformity, domed cranium, narrow palpebral fissures. Recumbent, bobbing, circling head movements, nystagmus, tremor. Do not suck. Deficient cerebral, cerebellar cortex	Cattle Salers	Autosomal recessive	Stillborn or euthanasia
Goat [VM8 p. 1637]		Congenital tetraplegia, tremor, deaf, nystagmus, Horner's Syndrome, carpal contracture, thick skin, domed skull	Anglo-Nubian goat	Autosomal recessive	Euthanasia

GM1 Gangliosidosis [VM8 p. 1638]	Reduced activity of betagalactosidase, accumulation GM-1 ganglioside	Normal at birth. Progressive neuromuscular dysfunction, growth retardation begins at about 3 months. Blind, poor condition. Poor response to stimuli, slow chewing, swallowing, wide stance, sway gait, fall easily, aimless walk, head press, convulsions. Abnormal retina. Reduced enzyme activity in leukocytes	Cattle H-F	Nil	Death or euthanasia before 1 year
GM2 Gangliosidosis [VM8 p. 1638]	Reduced activity of betagalactosidase, accumulation GM-1 ganglioside	Slow growth, ataxia after 3 months old. Spots in retina, abnormal granules in leukocytes. Serum enzyme assay deficient. Course up to 2 months	Pigs Yorkshire Sheep Suffolk and Suffolk cross	Nil	Death or euthanasia
Ceroid lipofuscinosis [VM8 p. 1638]	A proteolipid proteinosis, not strictly a lysosomal storage defect	Progressive ataxia of hind limbs commences as late as 18 months old, lasts six months. Blind. Atrophy cerebral cortex, retinal atrophy	Sheep South Hampshire Goats Nubian Cattle Devon	Autosomal recessive	Euthanasia 2–4 years
Generalized glycogenesis [VM8 p. 1638]	Glycogen storage disease (Pompe's disease of humans). Deficiency of α glucosidase	Poor growth, muscle weakness, incoordination, difficult rising, permanent recumbency. Lysosomal storage defect lesions in nervous tissue, cardiac and skeletal muscle. Normal at birth, develops soon after. Heterozygote identified by glucosidase content of tissue	Cattle S'horn, Brahman Sheep Corriedale	Nil	Death at 8 months to >1 yr old
Globoid cell leukodystophy [VM8 p. 1639]	Decreased galactocerebrosidase	Normal at birth. Incoordination hind limbs progresses to recumbency, tetraplegia. Globoid cells in nervous tissue	Sheep Poll Dorset	Nil	Death or euthanasia

Continued

637

Table 34.1 Continued

(Here = Hereford, H-F = Holstein Friesian, Jap.B = Japanese Black, Br Swiss = Brown Swiss)

Defect	Lesion or functional defect	Clinical signs/lesion/clinical pathology	Age, species, breed	Type of inheritance	Outcome
		Inherited nervous system abiotrophies			
		(Progressive, mostly fatal neurological diseases after being normal at birth. Includes lysosomal storage diseases)			
Cerebellar abiotrophy 1. Cattle [VM8 p. 1639]	Degenerative changes cerebellum, spinal cord	Sudden onset ataxia, progress to recumbency. Spastic dysmetric gait, broad based stance, tremor, fall easily. Eat well, strong. Microscopic lesions. No menace reflex but can see	Cattle H-F, Here, poll cross. 3–8 month old calves	Suspected inherited	Euthanasia
2. Sheep [VM8 p. 1639]		Incoordination, dysmetria, fall easily, wide stance. No menace reflex	Sheep Commences at 3 years old	Suspected inherited	
3. Pig [VM8 p. 1639]		Dysmetria, ataxia, tremor at 5 weeks. Recumbent by 15 weeks	Pigs X-breeds	Suspect. Single autosomal recessive	
Caprine progressive spasticity [VM8 p. 1639]	Abiotrophic degeneration spinal cord, posterior brain stem and mid brain neurons	Lethargy, ataxia, paresis to recumbency then euthanasia. Tendon reflexes normal	Angora goats. Begins at 2 months	Suspect inherited	Euthanasia
Shaker calf syndrome [VM8 p. 1640]	Degenerative lesions spinal cord	At birth tremor, difficulty rising, spastic gait, aphonia, terminal spastic paraplegia. In H-F, only males	Cattle Here, horned at birth	Inherited recessive. Sex-linked in H-F	Euthanasia

Progressive degenerative myeloencephalopathy [VM8 p. 1640]	Degenerative lesions cerebellum, spinal cord	Weaver syndrome. Progressive bilateral hind limb weakness, proprioceptive deficits, weaving, goose-step gait. Reflexes normal, final recumbency. Course 12–18 months	Cattle Br Swiss. Begins at 6–8 months	Inherited	Euthanasia
Progressive ataxia [VM8 p. 1640]	Degenerative changes white matter of cerebellum and internal capsule	Stiff, stumbling gait, toes dragged in hind limbs. Progresses for 1–2 years. Difficulty rising, squirting urination	Cattle Charolais. Begins at 12 months old	Inherited	Culled
Spinal myelopathy [VM8 p. 1640]	Progressive spinal myelopathy	Progressive paresis to permanent recumbency. Degenerative lesions spinal cord, midbrain, cerebellum	Cattle Murray Grey. At birth or not till 1 yr old	Autosomal recessive inheritance	Culled
Symmetrical multifocal encephalopathy [VM8 p. 1640]	Degenerative encephalopathy	Progressive fore limb hypermetria, hyperesthesia, blind, nystagmus, weight loss, aggression. Course 4 months plus. Degenerative changes in brain, optic chiasma. Some differences in signs and distribution of lesions between Simmentals and Limousins	Cattle Simmentals, Limousins and Limousin crosses. Simmentals begin at 5 to 8 months, Limousins at 1 month	Suspect inherited	Culled
Ovine degenerative axonopathy [VM8 p. 1641]	Degenerative changes cerebellum, spinal cord	Progressive ataxia to recumbency and euthanasia. Ataxia includes dysmetria, frequent falling, tremor, diminished menace reflex	Sheep Suffolk, Merino, Coopworth. Begin at birth (Coopworth) Suffolks (1–6 months), Merinos (4–6 years)	Suspect inherited	Euthanasia after 6 weeks (Coopworth) up to 3 years (Merinos)
Porcine spontaneous lower motor neurone disease [VM8 p. 1641]	Symmetrical degeneration motor neurones spinal cord and mid brain	Hind limb weakness, ataxia, collapses easily. Reflexes normal. Sternal recumbency at 10 weeks. Appetite good	Pig Yorks begins at 5–10 years old	Suspect inherited	Euthanasia
Maple syrup urine disease [VM8 p. 1641]	Absence of branched chain ketoacid decarboxylase	Stillbirth. Dullness, recumbency, tremor, tetanic spasms, opisthotonus, blind, hyperthermia, tetanic or flaccid paralysis, coma, death after 48–72 hour course. Urine smells of burnt sugar. Severe spongiform encephalopathy	Cattle Poll, Horned Here, Poll S'horn. Begins at 3 days	Autosomal recessive	Death

Table 34.1 Continued

Defect	Lesion or functional defect	Clinical signs/lesion/clinical pathology	Age, species, breed	Type of inheritance	Outcome
Citrullinemia [VM8 p. 1642]	Deficiency of arginosuccinate synthetase	Course 6–12 hours Depression. Compulsive walking, blind, head press, tremor, hyperthermia, recumbency, opisthotonus, convulsions. Blood citrulline levels 40–1200 × normal. Polymerase chain reaction detects heterozygotes	Cattle H-F and Red Holstein. Begins during first week	Mutation	Death
Equine degenerative myeloencephalopathy [VM8 p. 1642] 1. Appaloosa [VM8 p. 1642]	Spinal cord and medulla degeneration	Ataxia progresses to para- or quadriplegia, aggression, irritability	Horses Foals >4 months <1 yr old. All breeds mostly Appaloosa	Suspected inherited. Could be Vitamin E responsive	Culled, euthanasia
2. Morgan Horse [VM8 p. 1642]	Lesion only in accessory cuneate nucleus	Stiff, stilted, gait; hind limb incoordination, fall easily. Dysmetria. Progresses but never recumbent. Course 2–5 years	Most <6 months, some >2 years	Suspected inherited	Inconvenient
Miscellaneous inherited nervous defect					
Congenital hydrocephalus [VM8 p. 1642] 1. Cattle [VM8 p. 1642]	Internal hydrocephalus	Forehead, bulges, dystocia, partial closure supraorbital foramen, poor teeth development. Plus other defects including eyes	Cattle Congenital H-F, Here, Ayrshire, Charolais	Inherited recessive	Death soon after birth
2. Pigs [VM8 p. 1643]		Meningocele, brain hernia through frontal suture	Pigs Yorkshire, European breeds, Landrace	Inherited recessive	Not viable
3. Horse [VM8 p. 1643]		Hydrocephalus, dystocia	Horse Standardbred (1 stallion)	Dominant mutant?	Stillborn

640

Condition	Pathology	Clinical signs	Breeds / age at onset	Inheritance	Outcome
Congenital cerebellar defects [VM8 p. 1643] Cattle	1. Cerebellar hypoplasia (absence) ± optic nerves, occipital cortex. Some cases cerebellum reduced in size	Tremor blind, dilated pupils (in some). Limb muscles flaccid, recumbent. or dysmetria, opisthotonus, straddle-legged stance, incoordination, fall easily, progression difficult	At birth. Cattle Here, Guernsey, H-F, S'horn, Ayrshire	Inherited recessive	Culled
	2. Cerebellar ataxia. Cerebellum normal size but histological lesion	Ditto	Calves. Jersey S'horn, H-F. Begins few days to several weeks	Inherited recessive	Culled
Horse [VM8 p. 1643]	3. Purkinje cell deficit in cerebellum. Cerebellum small in some	Head nod, ataxia, especially at fast gait. Some unable to stand at birth. Menace reflex may be absent	Horse Arabian, Oldenberg, Australian Pony. Gotland. At birth to 6–9 months old. At birth or begins at 4 months	Suspect inherited	Culled
Sheep [VM8 p. 1644]	4. Histologic lesion of atrophy cerebellar neurons	Ataxia, opisthotonus, tremor, broad-based stance	Sheep Many breeds at birth	Inherited recessive	Not viable
Familial ataxia and convulsions [VM8 p. 1644]	Selective cerebellar cortical degeneration	Tetanic convulsions up to 12 hours. Replaced by goose-stepping gait in forelimbs	Cattle Angus, Xbreds, Charolais at birth up to 2 months later	Autosomal dominant	Death
Congenital spasms [VM8 p. 1644]	No lesion specified	Tremor, intermittent, prevents standing	Cattle Jersey at birth	Inherited recessive	Death in first few weeks
Spastic paresis (ELSO-HEEL) [VM8 p. 1644]	Excessive tone in gastrocnemius muscles. No lesion or dysfunction identified	Straight hock, one or both, thrust out behind while walking. Passive flexion normal. Elevation of tail. Progressive worsening, loss of weight, eventual recumbency	Cattle H-F, Angus Beef S'horn, Angus, Red Danish, Murray Grey, Poll Here etc. at 6 weeks to 6 months after birth	Suspected inherited	Non viable without corrective surgery. Euthanasia up to 2 years

Table 34.1 Continued

(Here = Hereford, H-F = Holstein Friesian, Jap.B = Japanese Black, Br Swiss = Brown Swiss)

Defect	Lesion or functional defect	Clinical signs/lesion/clinical pathology	Age, species, breed	Type of inheritance	Outcome
Periodic spasticity [VM8 p. 1645]	No lesion or dysfunction identified	On rising hind limbs extended, tremor in them, unable to move for few seconds. Progresses to abnormality lasting 30 minutes	**Cattle** H-F, Guernsey. Begins as adults	Single recessive	Inconvenience
Neonatal spasticity [VM8 p. 1645]	No lesion or dysfunction identified	Incoordination, eyes bulge, head held to one side. Then unable to stand, extension convulsion, tremor, course up to 1 month	**Cattle** Jersey, Here. Begins at 2–5 days old	Inherited single recessive	Not viable
Congenital myoclonus (neuraxial edema) [VM8 p. 1645]	Specific defect is marked defect of spinal cord glycine-mediated neurotransmission	Unable to rise, exterior spasm with stimulation. Hyperesthesia, with myoclonic jerks of skeletal muscle. Can be reared by never recover. Subluxations of hip joints; epiphyseal fractures of femoral head	**Cattle** Poll, Here, at birth	Autosomal recessive	Euthanasia
Congenital posterior paralysis [VM8 p. 1646]	Neuronal degeneration brain and spinal cord in some	Posterior paralysis, opisthotonus, tremor, extensor rigidity, enhanced reflexes	**Cattle** At birth. Norwegian Red Poll and others. **Pig** Yorkshires and others	Recessive inherited	Not viable
Porcine congenital tremor [VM8 p. 1646]	1. A-IV disease a defect of fatty acid metabolism causing myelination defect 2. A-III is cerebrospinal hypomyelinogenesis	Tremor, incoordination, difficulty standing, squealing. A-III only in males, commonly concurrent with splayleg	1. A-IV British Saddleback 2. A-III Landrace	Both inherited recessives. A-III is sex linked	Inconvenient

Condition	Lesion / cause	Clinical signs	Species / breed	Inheritance	Outcome
Exophthalmos with strabismus [VM8 p. 1646]	Deficient neurons in abducens nerves	Defective vision, severe protrusion and autero-medial deviation both eyeballs. Worsen gradually	Cattle S'horn, Jersey. Begins at 6 months or first pregnancy	Inherited recessive	Aesthetic defect
Familial undulatory nystagmus [VM8 p. 1646]	Involuntary eye oscillations	Synchronous; tremor-like eyeball movements. Small, fast (200/min) vertical. No impairment of vision	Cattle Finnish Ayrshire	Inherited	Aesthetic defect
Idiopathic epilepsy [VM8 p. 1647]	Epileptiform convulsions	Convulsions when excited or exercised. Signs disappear at 1–2 years	Cattle Br Swiss. Begin at 2–3 months old	Inherited dominant	Spontaneous recovery
Doddler calves [VM8 p. 1647]	Idiopathic convulsions in intensively in-bred half-sibs	Continuous clonic convulsions, nystagmus, pupillary dilation	Cattle Here	Inherited	Death
Inherited musculoskeletal system defects					
Osteoarthritis and arthropathy [VM8 p. 1647]	Degenerative arthritis of hip (osteoarthritis) or stifle (arthropathy) joints. Nutritional deficits and trauma also causative	Lameness, crepitation, pain on passive movement. Muscle atrophy in advanced cases. Joint enlarged. One or both hind limbs	Cattle Jersey and Here. Begin at 6–12 months. Develop over 1–2 years	Single autosomal recessive in osteoarthritis. Doubt about inheritance in arthropathy	Culled, or euthanized
	Defective acetabulum in Dole horses	Severe hip lameness with round ligament rupture in later life	Horse Dole. Normal at birth	Inherited	Culled
Arachnomelia [VM8 p. 1647]	Normal organogenesis subsequent failure to develop. In sheep deficiency is of insulin-like growth factor	'Spider lamb syndrome'. Long, thin distal limbs. Fragile bones, spinal curvature, short mandible and other defects, e.g. arthrogryposis, cardiovascular defects. Visible on X-ray before lesions develop	Cattle Br Swiss. Simmental etc. Sheep Suffolks. Hampshires. Congenital or weeks old in lambs	Single recessive	Not viable

Table 34.1 Continued

(Here = Hereford, H-F = Holstein Friesian, Jap.B = Japanese Black, Br Swiss = Brown Swiss)

Defect	Lesion or functional defect	Clinical signs/lesion/clinical pathology	Age, species, breed	Type of inheritance	Outcome
Multiple ankylosis [VM8 p. 1648] 1. Holstein Friesian [VM8 p. 1648]	Fixation of joints by ankylosis of joint surfaces	Hydrops amnii in dam. Abortion at 8 months common; short neck, ankylozed intervertebral and limb joints. Spinal curvature, limb flexion. Dystokia	**Cattle** H-F	Suspect Inherited	Lethal
2. Charolais [VM8 p. 1648]		Limb joint ankylosis plus cleft palate	**Cattle** Charolais	Suspect inherited	Lethal
3. Simmental [VM8 p. 1648]		Ankylosis of coffin joints at 2–3 weeks old	**Cattle** Simmental	Suspect inherited	Not viable
Arthrogryposis [VM8 p. 1648]	Multiple tendon contracture due to neurogenic muscle atrophy	Limbs fixed in flexion or extension. Dystokia. Muscle atrophy. Joints freed by cutting tendons. Unable to stand. Other defects in some, e.g. cleft palate and mandibular shortening and cardiac defects in Simmentals, mandibular shortening and hydranencephaly in Corriedales	**Cattle** Many breeds especially Shorthorn and Charolais. Congenital. **Pigs** Landrace **Sheep** Merino, Corriedale **Horse** Norwegian Fjord	Single recessive	Not viable
Splayed digits [VM8 p. 1649]	Defect of interdigital muscles and ligaments	Lameness, toes spread and misshapen. Lie down a lot, walk on knees	**Cattle** Jersey. Begins at 2– 4 months	Inherited autosomal recessive	Culled
Patellar subluxation [VM8 p. 1649]	Defect of patellar groove and ligaments	Periodic lameness, limb in rigid extension. Medial patellar displacement	**Cattle** Bos indicus breeds and Water Buffalo **Horse** Shetland pony	Autosomal recessive	Inconvenient

Joint hypermobility [VM8 p. 1649]	No lesion or functional defect identified	Excessive flexion and extension all limb joints. Muscle atrophy, joints look enlarged. Calves cannot stand. Gross drawer sign on sliding joints	Cattle Jersey at birth	Autosomal recessive. Some cases not inherited	Not viable
Osteogenesis imperfecta [VM8 p. 1649]	Faulty collagen and intercellular cement production	At birth abnormal slackness limb flexor tendons. Unable to stand. Pink teeth lacking enamel and dentine. Multiple fractures at birth, bone fragility. Radiological examination reveals defects. Charolais have bone fragility only. Sheep Also diaphyses thick, short mandible; skin fragility	Cattle H-F and Charolais Sheep NZ Romney at birth	Autosomal dominant	Not viable
Multiple limb defects (MOLE calves) [VM8 p. 1649]	Congenital amputates	Short, deformed limbs, extremities absent in some, hydrocephalus, short mandible, facial deficits. Trunk edema. Abortion	Cattle Danish Black and White. Congenital	Single recessive	Lethal
Reduced phalanges [VM8 p. 1649]	Congenital amputates	First two phalanges absent, third phalanx connected by skin and soft tissues. Unable to stand	Cattle Congenital	Single recessive	Not viable
		Tibial hemimelia. Patellas absent. Tibias absent or short Hydrocephalus. Ventral hernia, cryptorchidism	Cattle Galloway	Inherited recessive	Not viable
		Peromelia. Phalanges, metacarpus and metatarsus absent	Goats Mohair, congenital	Autosomal recessive	Not viable
		Bones below humerus and stifle, mandible, vestigial or absent	Cattle H-F, congenital	Recessive inheritance	Not viable

Continued

Table 34.1 Continued

(Here = Hereford, H-F = Holstein Friesian, Jap.B = Japanese Black, Br Swiss = Brown Swiss)

Defect	Lesion or functional defect	Clinical signs/lesion/clinical pathology	Age, species, breed	Type of inheritance	Outcome
Claw defects [VM8 p. 1650]	Horn or underlying deformity	Polydactylism – supernumary claws	**Cattle** Normandy	Inherited	Inconvenient and aesthetic defect
		Syndactylism – fused claws. Some have increased susceptibility to hyperthermia	**Cattle** H-F, Angus, Here, Chianina		
		Dactylomegaly – enlarged dewclaws, often with syndactyly and deviation of digit	Shorthorn		
		Corkscrew or Curled Claw – lateral claw long, curled over sole and medial claw. Cracks down front. Severe lameness, especially in heavy animals	**Cattle** Here, Angus		Culled
Multiple exostoses [VM8 p. 1650]	Long bone deformity	Visible radiologically on cortical and medullary bone of limbs and ribs. Palpable swellings. Little inconvenience	**Horse** Thoroughbred, Quarter horses	Autosomal dominant	Aesthetic defect
Porcine thick forelimbs [VM8 p. 1650]	Hyperostosis due to separation of periosteum from bone	Marked thickening forelimbs below elbow. Skin tense, discolored. Difficulty standing, moving. Die of crushing, starvation. Subcutis edema	Pig	Single recessive	Death, euthanasia
Porcine rickets [VM8 p. 1650]	Failure of active transport of calcium through intestinal wall	Rickets in young pigs on normal diets. Hypocalcemia, hyperphosphatemia, elevated serum alkaline phosphatase	Pig	Inherited	Culled

				Probably inherited	Euthanasia
Ovine progressive muscular dystrophy [VM8 p. 1650]	Primary muscle atrophy	Hind limbs only. Progressive failure to flex, then rigid fixation, not able to run. Gradual worsening till 2–3 years old, unable to walk. Tendency to bloat. Atrophy skeletal muscle and diaphragm	Sheep Merinos. Begins at 3–4 weeks old		
Bovine spinal muscle atrophy [VM8 p. 1651]	Neurogenic muscle atrophy	Progressive ataxia, weakness, muscle atrophy recumbency. Some stillborn. Primary lesion spinal cord neuronal degeneration	Cattle During first 2 weeks or in utero. European breeds and American Br Swiss	Autosomal recessive	Culled
Dwarfism [VM8 p. 1651] 1. Cattle Snorter Dwarfs [VM8 p. 1651]	Chondrodysplastic dwarfism	Affected at birth but signs may not be obvious for weeks or months. Short legs, short, wide head, protruding lower jaw and teeth. Bulging forehead, mis-shapen maxilla, nasal passage obstruction, noisy breathing, dyspnea. Tongue protrudes. eyes bulge, abdominal enlargement, persistent mild bloat. Half weight of normals at 6 months. No efficient way of identifying heterozygote	Cattle Here, Angus, H-F, S'horn. At birth.	Simple recessive	Culled
2. Bulldog calves [VM8 p. 1652]	Chondrodystrophic dwarfism	Abortion. Dystokia, hydrocephalus forehead bulges, short face, depressed nose, tongue protrudes. Short, thick neck; limbs short. Palate cleft or absent. Fetal anasarca. Dam has hydrops amnii. Dexter heterozygote have short limbs	Cattle Dexter at birth. Also Jersey, Guernsey, H-F, Jap Brown	Single recessive	Lethal
3. Miscellaneous bovine dwarfs [VM8 p. 1652]	Chondrodystrophy	'Comprest', 'compact' and other proportional dwarfs, miniatures of normal calves. Born prematurely. Most stillborn or die early	Cattle Proportional dwarfs in Here, S'horn, Charolais, Simmentals. Congenital	Suspect inherited	Lethal

Table 34.1 Continued

(Here = Hereford, H-F = Holstein Friesian, Jap.B = Japanese Black, Br Swiss = Brown Swiss)

Defect	Lesion or functional defect	Clinical signs/lesion/clinical pathology	Age, species, breed	Type of inheritance	Outcome
4. Sheep [VM8 p. 1652]	Chondrodysplasia	Dwarfes	Mutant Ancon. Extinct	Inherited	Lethal
5. Pigs [VM8 p. 1651]	Nil	Short limbs, loose limb attachment, loose joint	Pigs Danish Landrace	Suspect inherited	Lethal
Displaced molar teeth [VM8 p. 1652]	Unexplained malalignment of teeth	Lower jaw premolars impacted or abnormal position, grotesque angles. Narrow short mandible	Cattle Congenital	Suspect inherited	Not viable
Jaw malapposition 1. Cattle [VM8 p. 1652]	Abnormal mandible growth	Mandible short, incisors do not meet dental pad. May not be able to suck. In Angus associated with generalized degenerative joint disease	Cattle S'horn, H-F, Ayrshire, Simmental, congenital	Recessive	Culled
2. Cattle [VM8 p. 1652]		Mandible long causing incisors to protrude	Hereford, Angus	Suspect inherited	Culled
3. Sheep [VM8 p. 1652]		Mandibular underdevelopment – usually associated with dwarfism, displaced molars	Sheep Merino, Rambouillet	Inherited	Culled
Mandible agnathia [VM8 p. 1652]	Mandible absent	Unable to suck or feed	Sheep Congenital	Recessive	Lethal
Cranium bifidum [VM8 p. 1653]	Cranioschisis	Cranial bone deficit; meningoceles, encephaloceles result	Pigs Poland, China and Xbreds, congenital	Inherited recessive	Not viable
Craniofacial deformity [VM8 p. 1653]	Nasomaxillary hypoplasia	Nasomaxillary hypoplasia, incomplete development cerebum (sulci and gyri less pronounced)	Sheep Border Leicester	Simple recessive	Not viable

					Lethal
Osteopetrosis [VM8 p. 1653]	Absence of marrow cavity in long bones	Stillborn, undersized calves. Short mandible, tongue protrusion, lower molars impacted, patent fontanelle, long bones short, marrow cavity absent. Radiographic detection of bone defect	**Cattle** Angus (Horse – possibly), congenital	Autosomal recessive	Not viable
Probatocephaly (Sheepshead) [VM8 p. 1653]		Deformed cranium so head resembles sheep. Also cardiac, buccal, lingual, abomasal defects	**Cattle** Limousin, congenital	Inherited	Inconvenient
Hernias [VM8 p. 1653] Umbilical [VM8 p. 1653]	Abdominal closure defect	Palpable hernial defect at umbilicus	**Cattle** H-F, congenital	Recessive	Inconvenient
Scrotal [VM8 p. 1653]	Inguinal ring defect	Palpable hernial defect at inguinal ring	**Pig** Duroc, Landrace	Inherited	Inconvenient
Tail deformity, tail-lessness [VM8 p. 1653]	Pelvic organ deformity	Tail absent, short, kinked. Accompanies atresia ami; urogenital tract defects in some	**Cattle** H-F **Pig** Landrace White	Suspect inherited	Culled
Myofiber hyperplasia [VM8 p. 1653]	Double (hypertrophy) muscling. A preferred character in some countries	Large skeletal muscle mass, rapid weight gain, forward positioning of tailhead. Skin thin. Dystokia. Some have macroglossia, protruding mandible, ELSO heel in some	**Cattle** Charolais, Belgian Blue, South Devon, Piedmont	Inherited	Cull those with other defects
	As above	'Creeper Pigs' under stress develop tremor, weakness, recumbency at 12 weeks. Pig creeps with limbs flexed. Forelimb myopathy	**Pig** Pietrain. Begins 2–4 weeks old	Inherited	Culled
Porcine stress syndrome [VM8 p. 1654]	Stress causes uncontrolled skeletal muscle metabolism	Transport fighting, halothane anesthesia, suxamethonium administration cause dyspnea hyperthermia, sudden death	Pigs; Pietrain, Poland, China, Landrace	Single recessive gene	Death. Pale soft exudative pork

Continued

Table 34.1 Continued

(Here = Hereford, H-F = Holstein Friesian, Jap.B = Japanese Black, Br Swiss = Brown Swiss)

Defect	Lesion or functional defect	Clinical signs/lesion/clinical pathology	Age, species, breed	Type of inheritance	Outcome
Quarter-horse episodic tremor [VM8 p. 1366]	Hyperkalemic periodic paralysis Periodic episodes of skeletal muscle weakness	15–60 minute episodes of generalized muscle weakness, tremor, stiffness, recumbency, not necessarily related to exercise. Significant elevation of serum potassium. Immediate correction with hydrochlorothiazide. Attacks less frequent with age	Horse Appaloosa, paints, especially Quarter-horses. Begins at 1 month to 4 years, mostly 2–3 years	Inherited autosomal dominant	Inconvenient. Culled
Equine periodic laryngeal spasm [VM8 p. 1366]	Hyperkalemic laryngeal spasm	Severe dyspnea and respiratory stridor during restraint. Major elevation of blood potassium levels	Horse At 1 week old	Inherited	Inconvenient. Can be fatal
Caprine myotonia [VM8 p. 1646]	Muscle fibre abnormality	Run when startled, then develop extreme muscle rigidity, unable to move. Relax in few seconds. Variable signs, diminish before and after parturition, and when water withdrawn	Goats One horse? Begin some time after birth	Inherited	Inconvenient
Inherited defects of skin					
Symmetrical alopecia [VM8 p. 1659]	Hair fibre agenesis in follicle	Alopecia commences head, neck, back, hind quarters, tailhead, symmetrically down sides and limbs. Skin bald, no irritation. Patient normal otherwise	Cattle H-F. Begins at 6 weeks to 6 months	Single autosomal recessive	Aesthetic defect
Congenital Hypotrichosis [VM8 p. 1659] Cattle 1 [VM8 p. 1659]	Hair fibre agenesis, no follicles	Hair absent at birth, all absent except eyelashes, tactile muzzle hairs. Horns and hoofs normal. Calf normal otherwise. Susceptible to cold, sunburn	Cattle Guernsey, Jersey, congenital	Single recessive	Aesthetic defect

Cattle 2 [VM8 p. 1659]	Alopecia plus hypothyroidism	Complete alopecia, die soon after birth. Small hypofunctional thyroid	Cattle H-F, congenital	Recessive	Lethal
Cattle 3 [VM8 p. 1659]	Alopecia plus anodontia	Complete alopecia, no teeth present	Cattle Congenital	Recessive	Lethal
Cattle 4 [VM8 p. 1659]	Streaked alopecia	Irregular, narrow, vertical streaks of hypotrichosis. Only in females	Cattle H-F, congenital	Sex-linked semi-dominant	Aesthetic defect
Cattle 5 [VM8 p. 1659]	Partial hypotrichosis	Thin coat of short curly hair. Later some coarse wiry hair. Calves have poor weight gain	Cattle Here, congenital	Simple recessive	Culled
Cattle 6 [VM8 p. 1659]	Trichohyalin granules in hair follicles	Short, curly coat at birth, hair missing tail switch poll, brisket, neck, legs	Cattle Poll. Here, congenital	Suspect inherited	Aesthetic defect
Sheep [VM8 p. 1659]	No hair fibres. Wool fibres ok	Alopecia generally. Face and legs bald. No eye lashes	Sheep Poll. Dorset	Suspect inherited	Aesthetic defect
Pigs [VM8 p. 1659]	Nil	Alopecia, low birth weights, weakness, high mortality	Pigs	Inherited	Lethal
Bovine hair-coat color-linked, follicle dysplasia [VM8 p. 1659]	Follicle hypoplasia or dysplasia	Colored hairs shorter than white hairs. In tan and white 'buckskins' and black and white standards. Or partial or complete loss of hairs	Cattle 'Buckskin' or 'Portuguese' H-F strain. Also standard B&W H-F's	Autosomal dominant	Aesthetic defect
Epidermal dysplasia [VM8 p. 1660]	Skin dysplasia	'Baldy calves'. Normal at birth. Then lose weight, skin thick, scaly, hairless over most of body. Raw areas flank, axilla, knees, hocks, elbows. No horns develop. Slobber, no mouth lesions. Hooves long, narrow pointed. Stiff joints. Shuffling gait. Need euthanasia at about 6 months. Skin lesions acanthosis, hyperkeratosis	Cattle H-F. Begins at 1–2 months	Autosomal recessive	Not viable

Table 34.1 Continued

(Here = Hereford, H-F = Holstein Friesian, Jap.B = Japanese Black, Br Swiss = Brown Swiss)

Defect	Lesion or functional defect	Clinical signs/lesion/clinical pathology	Age, species, breed	Type of inheritance	Outcome
Parakeratosis [VM8 p. 1660]	Thymic hypoplasia. Zinc-responsive parakeratosis. Impaired absorption of zinc	Skin exanthema, alopecia on legs, parakerotosis, with thick scabs around mouth, eyes. Poor growth rate. Lymphopenia called also "Adema disease lethal trait A46"	**Cattle** S'horn, many European breeds. Begins at 4-8 weeks old, Friesian types	Autosomal recessive	Can survive with zinc medication. Or die at 4 months
Congenital Absence of Skin [VM8 p. 1660] 1. Epitheliogenesis imperfecta [VM8 p. 1660] Cattle [VM8 p. 1660]	Congenital skin absence. Defective lipid and collagen production	Mocosa and skin patches complete absence all layers. Muzzle, buccal mucosa, coronets	**Cattle** H-F, Jap Black, S'horn, Sahiwal, Angus. Congenital	Inherited single recessive	Not viable
2. Pig [VM8 p. 1660]		Denuded areas flanks, sides, back	Pigs	Inherited	Not viable
Acantholysis [VM8 p. 1660]	Defective collagen bridges between epidermal cells	Normal skin at birth shed at coronets and over carpal and metacarpophalangeal joints	**Cattle** Angus. Begins 3-7 days	Suspect inherited	Not viable
Epidermolysis bullosa [VM8 p. 1660]	Epidermal bullae cause shedding of skin	Bullae in mouth, on limb extremities, muzzle, ears; skin shed, hooves separate. Poor growth, hypotrichosis, frequent breaks in skin	**Sheep** Suffolk and South Dorset Down **Cattle** Brangus, Simmental. Congenital	Inherited, probably dominant in Simmentals	Most die
Junctional mechanobullous disease [VM8 p. 1660]	Epidermal bullae, may be no skin shedding	Very similar to epidermolysis bullosa. Skin may not shed. Frequent breaks in skin. Hooves slough often similar to "red foot disease" of Scottish Blackface, Welsh Mountain sheep	**Cattle** Angus, Simmental. **Sheep** Suffolk, Dorset Down. **Horse** Belgian	Inherited	Euthanasia

Condition	Mechanism	Clinical signs	Species/breeds	Inheritance	Outcome
Photosensitisation [VM8 p. 1661]	Hepatic insufficiency causes phylloerythrin accumulation	Sheep on green fodder. Photosensitive dermatitis on face and ears. Blind. Death in 2–3 weeks on pasture. Also renal insufficiency	Sheep Southdown, Corriedale. Begins 5–7 weeks	Inherited	Not viable at pasture
Congenital ichthyosis [VM8 p. 1661]	Hyperkeratinization	'Fish-scale' disease. Alopecia, plates of horny epidermis over most skin surface	Cattle H-F, Brown Swiss, Norwegian Red Poll. Congenital	Inherited single recessive	Not viable
Dermatosis vegetans [VM8 p. 1661]	Mesodermal defect	Most cases begin after birth up to 3 weeks old. On coronets, belly wall. Erythema to crusts. Many die. Some recover. Giant cell pneumonia cause of death in most	Pigs Landrace and others. May be congenital	Recessive semi-lethal inheritance	High mortality
Dermatosparaxia [VM8 p. 1662]	Subcutaneous collagen defective	'Hyperelastosis cutis' fragile skin and subcutis; skin and joint ligaments hyperelastic. Cutaneous fragility. Slow healing of skin, much scarring. Skin can be ripped off	Cattle, Horse. Sheep Norwegian, Finnish, White Dorper, Merino. Congenital	Probably recessive inheritance	Culled
Ehlers–Danlos syndrome [VM8 p. 1662]	Defective collagen synthesis	Identical to hyperelastosis cutis	Cattle Charolais, Simmental. Congenital	Inherited	Culled
Melanoma [VM8 p. 1662]	Cutaneous melanoma	Inherited melanoma	Sinclair miniature swine	Inherited	Culled
Inherited eye defects					
Corneal opacity [VM8 p. 1662]	Corneal edema	Congenital cloudiness and opacity of cornea. Both eyes. Vision restricted	Cattle H-F. Congenital	Suspect inheritance	Recover
Lens hypoplasia [VM8 p. 1662]	Vestigial lens	Blind	Congenital. Cattle Br Swiss	Suspect inheritance	Culled

Continued

653

Table 34.1 *Continued*

(Here = Hereford, H-F = Holstein Friesian, Jap.B = Japanese Black, Br Swiss = Brown Swiss)

Defect	Lesion or functional defect	Clinical signs/lesion/clinical pathology	Age, species, breed	Type of inheritance	Outcome
Multiple defects [VM8 p. 1663]	Pupil, retina and optical disk defects	Blind	**Cattle** Jap Black. Congenital	Suspect inheritance	Culled
Cataract [VM8 p. 1662]	Lens opacity	Blind	**Sheep** Romney. Congenital	Autosomal dominant	Culled
Iris aplasia [VM8 p. 1662]	Secondary cataract follows	Blind	**Horse** Belgian. Congenital	Inherited	Culled
Retinal aplasia [VM8 p. 1662]	Nil	Blind	**Horse** Congenital	Inherited	Culled
Microphthalmia [VM8 p. 1662]	Vestigial eyes	Blind	**Sheep** Texel. Congenital	Inherited	Culled
Typical colobomata [VM8 p. 1662]	Failed closure of ocular structures at embryonic choroidal fissure	More common in males. Both eyes often. No effect on vision	**Cattle** Charolais. Congenital	Inherited autosomal dominant	Aesthetic defect
Entropion [VM8 p. 1662]	Eyelids inverted	Apparent conjunctivitis at 3 weeks. Self-cure in time	**Sheep** Oxford, Hampshire, Suffolk. Congenital	Inherited	Recover with surgery

Condition	Cause	Clinical signs	Species/Breed	Inheritance	Outcome
Ocular dermoid [VM8 p. 1662]	Embryonic rests	Multiple small skin masses on conjunctiva, often both eyes. On cornea, nictitating membrane. Dysplasia of internal structures	Cattle Here	Inherited	Culled
Combined ocular defects [VM8 p. 1663]	See also pseudoalbinism	Blind. Lesions include iridal heterochromia, tapetal fibrosis and colobomata. White-coated, S'horns may have microphthalmia, retinal detachment, cataract, persistent pupillary membrane, internal hydrocephalus, optic nerve hypoplasia	Cattle Here, White S'horn	Inherited	Culled
		Iridal hypoplasia, limbic dermoids, cataracts. Blind	Quarter horse	Mutation	Culled
		Iridiremia, microphakia, ectopia lentis, cataract. Blind	Cattle Jersey	Simple recessive	Culled

Inherited renal defects

Condition	Cause	Clinical signs	Species/Breed	Inheritance	Outcome
Nephrosis [VM8 p. 1662]	Progressive glomerulonephritis. Immune complexes in colostrum cause lesion	Up to 4 months old. Tachycardia, conjunctival edema, nystagmus, circling, convulsions, Proteinuria, high BUN, hyperphosphatemia	Sheep Finnish Landrace. Begins at 3–4 weeks	Suspect inherited	Lethal
Cystic renal dysplasia [VM8 p. 1664]	Defective development	Recumbency, coma. Kidneys enlarged, cystic, abortions, stillbirths	Sheep Suffolks. Begins at 2–3 days old	Single dominant inheritance	Lethal

35 SPECIFIC DISEASES OF UNCERTAIN ETIOLOGY

Diseases in which the specific cause has not been identified or is too complex to include th[e] disease in any other chapter.

DISEASES CHARACTERIZED BY SYSTEMIC INVOLVEMENT

UNTHRIFTINESS IN WEANER
SHEEP (WEANER ILLTHRIFT)
[VM8 p. 1665]

Epidemiology

♦ Appears more prevalent in southern hemi-sphere
♦ Seems to be most severe in timorous-natured Merinos and their cross-breds, in which the behavioral stresses of weaning are more traumatic
♦ Worse with overcrowding on pasture
♦ Weaning at light body weight (should be 45% of mature weight) contributed to by:
  • Late lambs
  • Small dams, with little milk
  • Multiple births
♦ Not all lambs in flock affected

Clinical findings

♦ Small stature, thin to emaciated
♦ Mucosal pallor in most
♦ Some have diarrhea
♦ Sporadic, continuing, death losses
♦ History of repeated anthelmintic treatment
♦ Breeding maturity delayed up to 3 years

Clinical pathology

Anemia.

Necropsy findings

♦ Thin to emaciated
♦ Small intestinal villous atrophy common

Diagnosis

Resembles:
♦ Intestinal parasitism
♦ Eperythrozoonosis
♦ Coccidiosis
♦ Yersiniosis
♦ Coronavirus infection
♦ Cryptosporidiosis
♦ Nutritional deficiency of protein, energy
♦ Nutritional deficiency of copper, cobalt selenium, zinc, thiamin, vitamin A, singl[e] or in combination
♦ Periodontitis, delayed teeth eruption

Treatment and control

♦ Move to a new pasture to overcome poss[-]ible palatability problem
♦ Careful nutritional, handling managemen[t] at weaning

WEAK CALF SYNDROME
[VM8 p. 1666]

Etiology

Possible causes:
♦ Fetal infection near term
♦ Nutritional inadequacy of dam, feta[l] underdevelopment
♦ Maternal vitamin E/selenium nutritiona[l] deficiency

656

- Placental insufficiency, premature expulsion
- Hypothyroidism
- Birth trauma
- Prolonged fetal hypoxia

Epidemiology

Occurrence
- Sporadic deaths or in herd epizootic
- Apparent by 10 days old, 20% affected at birth
- Morbidity rate 6–20%; case fatality rate 60–80%
- Some prior abortions in herd

Risk factors
- Heifers or introduced cows
- Individual cows do not repeat at next calving
- Bad weather commonly associated
- Prolonged parturition
- Placenta expelled with calf

Importance
Major cause of loss in beef herds; occurs also in dairy herds.

Clinical findings

- Some stillbirths; most alive at birth but weak, most die within 20 minutes, some survive for few days
- Respiratory failure, some convulsive struggling
- Depression
- Reluctant to walk, or suck, some recumbent
- Gaunt, back arched
- Moderate diarrhea in some
- Muzzle reddened, crusty
- Lameness, joints may be slightly swollen, painful

Necropsy findings

- Edema, hemorrhage over lower limb joints
- Synovial fluids blood-tinged, fibrin deposits, cartilage erosions
- Petechiae in all internal organs, skeletal muscle
- Thymus involution

Diagnosis

Resembles:
- Dummy calves
- Birth trauma

- Perinatal infection
- Fetal hypoxia

Treatment and control

- Ensure adequate maternal nutrition
- Proper surveillance at calving
- Careful obstetric manipulation
- Blood transfusion from dam of an affected calf helpful to patient

DUMMY CALVES [VM8 p. 1667]

Etiology

Possibly inherited behavioral disorder.

Epidemiology

- Southern USA
- Calves of any weight
- Mostly beef breeds

Clinical findings

- Alert at birth; some do not stand for several hours
- No teat-seeking activity, no suck reflex
- No colostrum taken; leads to hypothermia, hypoglycemia, infections
- Dam may abandon calf

Treatment

Bottle nursing till sucking commences.

WATERY MOUTH OF LAMBS [VM8 p. 1669]

Epidemiology

- Mostly lambs in intensive housing
- Ram lambs castrated with rubber rings at 3 days old
- Twins or triplets
- Inclement weather
- Low body weight ewes
- Reduced colostrum intake enhances

Clinical findings

- Normal at birth, sick at 24–72 hours
- Do not suck, no feces, meconium retained
- Mucoid saliva hangs from mouth
- Depression to coma
- Abdominal distension rarely diarrhea, but intestine full of fluid, rattles when shaken suggests paralytic ileus

- Recumbency
- Some hypothermic
- 40% die within 6–24 hours

Diagnosis

Resembles enterotoxigenic colibacillosis.

Treatment

- Prophylactic antibiotics prevent
- Enteroalimentation, empty intestine, ensure adequate colostrum

COLD COW SYNDROME
[VM8 p. 1669]

Epidemiology

- Herd problem in milking cows just turned out onto lush, high soluble carbohydrate pasture
- Spontaneous recovery if cows moved
- Recurs on same pasture

Clinical findings

- Dullness, anorexia, agalactia
- Hypothermia
- Profuse diarrhea
- Some recumbent

THIN SOW SYNDROME
[VM8 p. 1670]

Epidemiology

- Intensive management herds
- Cold, draughty housing
- Low-level feeding to restrain obesity
- Insufficient drinking water
- Inadequate parasite control
- Very early weaning and remating
- Timid sows

Clinical findings

- Rapid, excessive weight loss in late pregnancy, early lactation extending into period after weaning
- Inappetence, pica, polydipsia
- Mucosal pallor
- Poor fertility leading to heavy culling

Diagnosis

Resembles *Oesophagostomum*, *Hyostrongylus* spp. infestation

POSTVACCINAL HEPATITIS OF
HORSES [VM8 p. 1670]

Epidemiology

- Mostly after injection of equine encephalomyelitis antiserum or vaccine
- Some after other vaccines, e.g. salmonellosis, tetanus antitoxin

Clinical findings

- Sudden onset stupor or mania
- Severe head-pressing, circling, compulsive walking, straddled posture
- Intense jaundice
- Alimentary tract stasis
- Oliguria
- Most die
- Survivors may have intractable disposition

Clinical pathology

Serum levels of liver enzymes elevated.

Necropsy findings

- Icterus, massive liver damage
- Subserosal petechiae

Treatment

- Antibiotics
- B-vitamins
- Parenteral glucose, electrolyte solutions

GRANULOCYTOPENIC DISEASE OF
CALVES [VM8 p. 1670]

Etiology

May be form of furazolidone poisoning.

Epidemiology

- Being reared on milk replacer
- Sometimes antibiotic supplement in milk

Clinical findings

- Fever
- Salivation

Nasal discharge, hemorrhagic
Necrotic lesions in mouth, on muzzle
Most die at 2–4 days

Clinical pathology

Neutropenia, thrombocytopenia.

Necropsy findings

Pneumonia, enteritis, peritonitis, probably secondary to immunodeficiency.

Diagnosis

Resembles:
* Bracken poisoning
* Radiation sickness

EQUINE NON-SPECIFIC ANEMIA
[VM8 p. 1400]

Clinical findings

Horses with decreased racing performance, responding to treatment with iron preparations; apparently unrelated to internal parasitism.

Treatment

* Good response to parenteral injection organic iron preparations, e.g. iron–dextran, iron–sorbitol–citric acid complex, saccharate, glutamate (to deliver 0.5–1.0 g elemental iron weekly)
* Some preparations irritant, cause severe local reaction, sloughs after intramuscular injection
* After some intravenous or intramuscular injections horses drop dead
* Critical that treatment be exactly as specified by manufacturer
* Vitamin B_{12} (5000 iu weekly) often included with iron preparation; folic acid, choline additional additives
* Oral treatment with iron sulfate, gluconate 2–4 g daily for 2 weeks effective; in molasses syrup on feed

SWEATING SICKNESS (TICK TOXICOSIS) [VM8 p. 1671]

Etiology

* Bites of tick *Hyalomma truncatum*
* Suggestive of epitheliotropic toxin produced by the tick

Epidemiology

* Africa, Sri Lanka, India
* Occurs naturally only in calves 2–6 months old; rare cases in adults
* Commonest in tick, wet, season
* Sheep, goats, pigs, dogs susceptible but disease does not occur in them
* Morbidity 10–30%; case fatality 30%

Clinical findings

* Incubation period 4–7 days after ticks attach
* Severity depends on number of days ticks attached:
  * Early removal of ticks – no illness, no immunity
  * Up to 5 days immunity, no signs
  * More than 5 days immune, clinical signs
* Lethargy, depression, dehydrated
* Fever, anorexia
* Mucosal hyperemia
* Hyperesthesia
* Mucopurulent oculonasal discharge
* Arched back
* Rough coat
* Extensive, moist dermatitis, hair matted, beads of moisture collect
* Dermatitis in axilla, groin, perineum, ear bases; whole of body in bad cases
* Eyelids stuck together
* Skin patches, hair rubbed, pulls off; raw, subcutaneous tissue exposed
* Ear, tail tips may slough
* Skin very sensitive
* Skin dry, hard, cracks in late stages, fly infestation, bacterial infection common sequels
* Oral mucosa hyperemic, then necrotic, then ulcers, diphtheritic pseudomembranes
* Unable to eat or drink, emaciated, dehydrated
* Dyspnea due to similar lesions of nasal mucosa
* Similar lesions vulva, vagina
* Abdominal pain, diarrhea in some
* Course of 2–5 days
* Survivors may have permanent, patchy alopecia, stunted growth, unthrifty

Clinical pathology

* Severe neutropenia, eosinopenia, degenerative left shift
* Elevated serum globulin levels
* Nephrosis indicators present but serum creatinine normal

Necropsy findings

Lesions as in clinical examination; may extend into esophagus, forestomachs.

Diagnosis

Resembles:
♦ Mucosal disease
♦ Bovine malignant catarrh

Treatment

♦ Non-steroidal anti-inflammatories plus broad-spectrum antibiotics suggested as the appropriate treatment but unlikely to influence course
♦ *Hyalomma* spp. antiserum effective

Control

Tick control.

DISEASES CHARACTERIZED BY ALIMENTARY TRACT INVOLVEMENT

EQUINE DYSAUTONOMIA (GRASS SICKNESS) [VM8 p. 1672]

Etiology

Suggested causes include:
♦ Viral infection
♦ Mycotoxin, limiting disease's occurrence to local area
♦ *Clostridium perfringens* type D or A
♦ Stress
♦ Excessive histamine production in gut, spilling over to sympathetic ganglia

Epidemiology

♦ Very limited distribution: UK principally, northern and western Europe, South America
♦ Case fatality rate 100%; most euthanized
♦ Horses, donkeys, zoo zebras only
♦ All ages except sucking foals
♦ Commonest in 2–7 year olds
♦ Almost all at pasture
♦ Most in summer
♦ Restricted to particular farms
♦ Common in horses recently introduced to infected farm

Clinical findings

General syndrome
♦ Lethargy
♦ Dysphagia
♦ Drool saliva, ingesta trickles or regurgitated through nostrils
♦ Dried feed impacted inside cheeks
♦ Sham drinking

Acute – additional signs
♦ Sudden onset
♦ Tachycardia
♦ No gut sounds, left flank distended, moderate colic
♦ Dry, hard feces mucus-covered on rectal examination
♦ Fluid reflux with nasogastric intubation
♦ Urination frequent, often tenesmus
♦ Restless, aimless wandering
♦ Tremor
♦ Patchy sweating
♦ Death after 1–4 day course

Subacute
♦ Emaciation, abdomen gaunt, skeletal muscles hard when touched
♦ Tremor
♦ Patchy sweating
♦ Back arched
♦ Dysphagia
♦ Gut empty except dry, hard feces in colon and rectum
♦ No feces passed
♦ No regurgitation
♦ Terminally stertorous respiration, penis droops, may rupture stomach
♦ Course 2–3 weeks
♦ Survivors unable to work effectively

Clinical pathology

♦ No abnormalities including peritoneal fluid
♦ Radiologically detectable reduction of gut motility

Necropsy findings

Acute
♦ Small intestine, stomach filled with fluid, gas
♦ Spleen enlarged
♦ Neuronal degeneration, necrosis in sympathetic ganglia, cranial nerves

Subacute
- Similar to acute without gut distension
- Gut has small calibre

Diagnosis

Resembles:
- Large bowel impaction
- Paralytic ileus

Treatment

- No effective treatment
- Gut drainage
- Intravenous infusion of fluid, electrolyte alimentation prolongs life.

IDIOPATHIC ACUTE DIARRHEA OF HORSES [VM8 p. 1674]

Etiology

Acute diarrheas in horses include the known etiological entities of:
- Salmonellosis
- Strongyliasis
- Potomac horse fever

The specific diseases of uncertain etiology dealt with here include:
- Colitis-X (including stress-induced diarrhea)
- Antibiotic-induced diarrhea
- *Clostridium* spp. infections

Other suspected pathogens with insufficient claims to be dealt with in detail include infection with:
- A coronavirus
- *Polymorphella ampulla*
- *Balantidium coli*

Treatment of all idiopathic acute equine diarrheas

Failing specific remedies for specific causes all cases to receive:
- Broad-spectrum antibacterials administered early and parenterally will save some cases but may trigger others
- Parenteral fluids and electrolytes are essential; may only prolong life in severe cases
- Corticosteroids have been widely used; flunixin meglumine preferred
- Oral astringent mixtures of kaolin, chalk, catechu widely used but can have minimal effect on such lesions

ANTIBIOTIC-INDUCED DIARRHEA [VM8 p. 1674]

Etiology

Acute diarrhea recorded after oral or parenterally administered, standard or high doses, of tetracycline, in most cases, but also tylosin, lincomycin, trimethoprim—sulfonamide, erythromycin or massive doses of penicillin.

Clinical findings

- Acute diarrhea 3–4 days after treatment
- Severe dehydration, usually with death at 1–14 days

Necropsy findings

- Colon wall edema
- Typhlitis, colitis

COLITIS-X [VM8 p. 1674]

Epidemiology

- Single or groups of cases
- All ages, mostly adults
- Recent stress of transport, food or water deprivation, abdominal surgery in many cases
- Case fatality rate approximates 100%

Clinical findings

- Very acute onset of endotoxic shock
- With or without profuse diarrhea
- Occasionally bowel distension with gas
- Severe depression
- Tachycardia, small amplitude pulse
- Possibly transient hyperthermia
- Terminally hypothermia, cold, clammy, sweaty skin
- Congested oral mucosae
- No gut sounds
- Moderate colic in some
- Terminal recumbency
- Pupil dilation
- Death in 3–24 hours without struggling

Clinical pathology

- Hemoconcentration
- Elevated BUN
- Leukopenia in some
- Acidosis, hypokalemia

Necropsy findings

Cecum and colon severe edema, hyperemia, petechiation, early; hemorrhagic necrosis in late cases.

Diagnosis

Resembles:
♦ Arsenic poisoning
♦ Salmonellosis
♦ Thromboembolic colic
♦ Intestinal obstruction

Treatment

♦ Massive intravenous fluid–electrolyte therapy
♦ Large doses of corticosteroids

EQUINE INTESTINAL
CLOSTRIDIOSIS [VM8 p. 1675]

Etiology

♦ Cause uncertain but characterized by large numbers of *Clostridium perfringens* type A in gut contents
♦ Hypothesis is that stress plus low fiber/high protein diet promotes multiplication
♦ *C. cadaveris* also suspected

Clinical findings

♦ Sudden onset profuse diarrhea
♦ Circulatory failure
♦ Death within 24 hours

Necropsy findings

Cecum, colon wall hyperemic, edematous, petechiation.

IDIOPATHIC CHRONIC EQUINE
DIARRHEA [VM8 p. 1676]

A group of diseases with very similar clinical syndromes often dealt with as a group because of the difficulty of differentiation in living animals.

Etiology

No specific cause for most cases chronic diarrhea in horses.
♦ Some sequels to acute episodes
♦ Rotavirus, coronavirus possibles
♦ *Trichomonas fecalis* originally proposed, not a current topic
♦ Disaccharidase deficiency in foals possible cause

Epidemiology

♦ Sporadic, single cases only
♦ No apparent spread to others in group
♦ Record of stress 3–12 days before in a few

Clinical findings

♦ Sudden onset chronic diarrhea
♦ Persists for up to 18 months
♦ Feces vary from liquid without fiber to thin porridge consistency
♦ No toxemia, good appetite
♦ Lose weight badly, maintain fluid balance

Clinical pathology

♦ Worm, coccidia status negative
♦ $D(+)$-xylose test for malabsorption
♦ Total protein estimation with albumin–globulin separation to detect protein-losing enteropathy, may assist treatment choice
♦ Liver function test, to check liver viability
♦ Culture of feces to identify specific enteric infections

Necropsy findings

Histopathological evidence of enteritis.

Differential Diagnosis

Resembles:
♦ *Cyathostoma* spp.
♦ *Eimeria leuckarti*
♦ Granulomatous enteritis
♦ Idiopathic chronic eosinophilic enteritis
♦ Primary hepatic insufficiency
♦ Antibiotic therapy
♦ Stress
♦ Avian tuberculosis
♦ Gastric carcinoma
♦ *Rhodococcus equi*

Treatment

♦ Ivermectin effective if migrating strongyles the cause
♦ Ten times normal dose of thiabendazole similarly effective
♦ Phenoxybenzamine produces good, some permanent effects
♦ Many other non-specific remedies have dubious reputations

GRANULOMATOUS ENTERITIS OF
HORSES [VM8 p. 1678]

Clinical findings

+ Weight loss
+ Edema, hypoproteinemia, mild intermittent colic
+ Chronic diarrhea in some
+ Thick intestinal wall, enlarged lymph nodes may be palpable rectally
+ Laparotomy, biopsy confirm

Necropsy findings

+ Thick small intestinal wall infiltrated with lymphocytes, histiocytes
+ Some granuloma formation
+ Partial villous atrophy
+ Lymph nodes contain granulomas

CHRONIC EOSINOPHILIC
GASTROENTERITIS OF HORSES
[VM8 p. 1679]

Epidemiology

Single, sporadic cases in young adult horses.

Clinical findings

+ Weight loss
+ Soft, formless feces or diarrhea
+ Generalized cutaneous hyperkeratosis; crusty lesions at coronets

Necropsy findings

Eosinophilic infiltrates in esophagus, stomach, intestines, mesenteric lymph nodes.

PORCINE PROLIFERATIVE
ENTERITIS COMPLEX (INTESTINAL
ADENOMATOSIS, REGIONAL OR
NECROTIC ENTERITIS,
PROLIFERATIVE HEMORRHAGIC
ENTEROPATHY) [VM8 p. 1679]

Etiology

+ Common isolates from intestines of pigs with proliferative enteritis:
  • *Campylobacter sputorum* subsp. *mucosalis*
  • *C. hyointestinalis*
+ Numbers of bacteria isolated varies, being much less frequent in cases of proliferative hemorrhagic enteritis than in cases of porcine intestinal adenomatosis

Epidemiology

+ Proliferative hemorrhagic enteropathy occurs most countries
+ In recently weaned pigs, at 4–8 weeks after weaning, high morbidity at 6–9 months replacement boars, gilts
+ Commonest in hysterectomy-derived or specific-pathogen-free pigs
+ High prevalence in summer
+ Morbidity rate up to 50%, case fatality rate up to 10%
+ Proliferative hemorrhagic enteropathy, porcine intestinal adenomatosis often concurrent

Infection prevalence
High titer against the *Campylobacter* spp. very widespread.

Transmission
May be spread by contact with saliva.

Clinical findings

Porcine intestinal adenomatosis
+ Sudden onset of inappetence, weight loss 4–6 weeks after weaning
+ Chronic, non-specific, intermittent diarrhea in many cases
+ Spontaneous recovery after 6 weeks course
+ In severe cases with regional ileitis, necrotic enteritis diarrhea is severe, death follows, some with intestinal perforation

Proliferative hemorrhagic enteropathy
+ Sudden death with large amounts of blood in loose feces in young gilts, boars
+ Skin pallor, hemorrhagic feces, fibrin casts usually transiently with spontaneous recovery in others; some die of blood loss in 48 hours
+ Survivors have ill-thrift

Necropsy findings

Porcine intestinal adenomatosis
+ Thickened mucosa with adenomatosis lesions in terminal ileum causes hosepipe gut
+ *Campylobacter* spp. in large numbers in lesions; identifiable by indirect fluorescent antibody or microagglutination test

Proliferative hemorrhagic enteropathy
+ Pallor of carcase
+ Acute inflammation of intestine wall from

ileum to colon, with massive hemorrhage into gut lumen, plus fibrinous cast formation
♦ Organisms difficult to isolate

Diagnosis

Resembles:
♦ Post-weaning, coliform gastroenteritis
♦ Porcine esophagogastric ulcer
♦ Swine dysentery
♦ Clostridium perfringens type C

Treatment and control

♦ Furazolidine 200 mg/kg in feed
♦ Tylosin (200 mg/kg) in feed
♦ Control by comingling affected, naive pigs followed by medicated feeding

ESOPHAGOGASTRIC ULCERATION
OF SWINE [VM8 p. 1682]

Etiology

Diets composed of finely ground grains.

Epidemiology

Occurrence
♦ High proportion (2–25%) normal pigs have ulcers
♦ Commonest in 45–90 kg pigs; also common in pigs after weaning, adult sows, boars
♦ All breeds

Risk factors
♦ Inherited susceptibility, linked to selection for fast growth, low back fat
♦ In penned pigs only
♦ In pigs growing rapidly, fed on high grain diets

♦ Rations with high corn content, especially when finely ground, gelatinized, expanded
♦ May be associated with Ascaris suis infection
♦ Heavy whey diets
♦ Overcrowded feeding stations so that pigs compete for feeding space
♦ Morbidity low, case fatality rate approximates 100%

Clinical findings

Most found dead, few show a syndrome of:
♦ Weak, staggery, recumbent
♦ Pallor
♦ Anorexia
♦ Black, pasty feces
♦ Die after 12–18 hour course
♦ Survivors unthrifty due to anemia, peritonitis

Necropsy findings

♦ Ulcers in esophageal part of stomach
♦ Fresh blood in stomach

Diagnosis

Resembles:
♦ Proliferative, hemorrhagic enteropathy
♦ Acute swine dysentery
♦ Pyrrolizidine alkaloid poisoning

Treatment and control

♦ Sodium polyacrylate 0.1–0.5% in diet prevents ulcers
♦ Increase fiber content of diet to 7%
♦ Reduce corn content of ration
♦ Reduce stressful situations, including overcrowding

DISEASES CHARACTERIZED BY RESPIRATORY TRACT INVOLVEMENT

ACUTE BOVINE PULMONARY
EMPHYSEMA AND EDEMA (ABPEE)
OR FOG FEVER [VM8 p. 1685]

Etiology

♦ In cattle moved from dry to lush pasture cause is ingestion of toxic amounts of D, L-tryptophan in the forage
♦ Causes of other forms of acute interstitial

pneumonia of cattle are listed in the section on diagnosis

Epidemiology

Occurrence
♦ Common in northern hemisphere countries and New Zealand
♦ Adult cattle 4–10 days after moving from a

dry, overgrazed summer pasture on to lush summer pasture containing a regrowth of a variety of grasses, legumes, other palatable plants, e.g.:
- Regrowth of hay fields (fog or feg fever)
- Stubble fields after cereal crop harvested (aftermath)
- Fields of rape, kale or those containing tops of harvested turnips
- Outbreaks with morbidity 10–50%, case fatality rate 25–50%; some outbreaks have mild disease in 30%, severe disease in 10%
- Rarely in lambs moved onto lush aftermath pasture

Risk factors

- Only cattle over 1 year old affected
- Pastures dangerous for only 2–4 weeks; toxicity disappears after first frost

Clinical findings

- Some found dead, others severely ill, die within 24 hours
- Severe, stertorous dyspnea with open-mouthed breathing, mouth frothing
- Severe anxiety
- Stand apart from herd, not grazing, reluctant to move; may collapse, die if forced
- Less severe cases continue grazing; should be moved from pasture
- Coughing infrequent
- Temperature slightly increased; hyperthermia in very warm weather
- Heart rate normal in mild cases, 120/minute in terminal cases
- Ruminal atony, bloat
- Subcutaneous emphysema over withers, back, down sides
- Nostrils flared
- Mild, transient diarrhea common
- Loud breath sounds over ventral lungs; breath sounds over dorsal lungs absent or loud crackles of emphysema
- Death after 2 day course in severe cases, others several days later
- Survivors have chronic emphysema, chronic unthriftiness; some die of cor pulmonale months later

Clinical pathology

No positive tests available; tests used in differentiation include:
- Nasal swabs examined for bacterial pathogens
- Fecal lungworm larval counts

- Serum antibodies for farmer's lung antibodies

Necropsy findings

- In peracute cases entire lungs enlarged, firm, do not collapse
- Less acute cases have marbled lung with adjacent lobules affected with different stages of edema, emphysema, epithelialization
- Early cases contain much viscid fluid
- Pleura thick, pale, opaque
- Frothy exudate in airways
- Absence of inflammation histopathologically
- Protein-rich fluid coagulated in alveoli
- Epithelialization of alveolar wall within a few days
- Extensive epithelialization, fibrosis in chronic cases

Diagnosis

Resembles:
- Organophosphate poisoning
- Nitrate–nitrite poisoning
- Other causes of pneumonia
- Bovine interstitial pneumonia
- Extrinsic allergic alveolitis (bovine farmer's lung)

Treatment

- Removal from pasture a debatable recommendation; cases may die because of the exercise; all cases develop within a short time, e.g. 4 days, so may be no new cases anyway
- Many cases recover spontaneously
- Survivors usually chronically ill-thrifty; salvage by slaughter a common recommendation
- Early, acute cases often treated:
  - Dexamethazone 1 mg/5–10 kg body weight I/M
  - Epinephrine (adrenalin) histamine combinations in large doses repeated hourly
  - Atropine 1 g/450 kg body weight I/M

Control

- Limited grazing for first 2 weeks on suspect pasture
- Oral administration of chlortetracycline or monensin in feed for the danger period on the new pasture completely effective but managementally difficult in many situations in which the disease occurs

INTERSTITIAL PNEUMONIA OF
CATTLE [VM8 p. 1684]

Etiology

♦ Diffuse fibrosing alveolitis, probably recovered cases of ABPEE, or result of re-
  peated subclinical cases of it
♦ Sporadic cases of acute interstitial pneu-
  monia of young cattle, due possibly to
  bovine respiratory syncytial virus infection
  or a sequel to pneumonic pasteurellosis
♦ Acute interstitial pneumonia caused by
  poisoning with plants, mycotoxins:
  • Ipomoea batatas infested with the fungus
    Fusarium solani
  • Phaseolus vulgaris infested with the fun-
    gus Fusarium semitectum
  • Zieria arborescens
  • Perilla frutescens
  • Brassica spp.
♦ Irritant gases, fumes:
  • Nitrogen dioxide
  • Zinc dioxide
♦ Parasitic lung disease
  • Dictyocaulus viviparus
  • Ascaris suum
♦ Extrinsic allergic alveolitis
♦ Milk allergy

Clinical findings

♦ Acute or insidious onset
♦ Dyspnea without toxemia
♦ Afebrile
♦ Coughing in some diseases, not in others
♦ Crackling breath sounds common
♦ Subcutaneous emphysema common
♦ No response to antibacterial treatment
♦ Progressive, most fatally
♦ Survivors chronic respiratory ill-health

Necropsy findings, treatment, and control

See under individual diseases.

EXTRINSIC ALLERGIC ALVEOLITIS
(BOVINE FARMER'S LUNG)
[VM8 p. 1689]

Etiology

Caused by hypersensitivity to molds:
♦ Thermopolyspora polyspora
♦ Micropolyspora faeni
♦ Thermoactinomyces vulgaris

Epidemiology

Sporadic cases in housed cattle exposed to
very moldy hay; may be series of cases close
together.

Clinical findings

♦ Subacute onset; cow often treated for
  pneumonia by farmer
♦ Unresponsive to antibacterial treatment
♦ Moderate dyspnea, grunt in some
♦ Frequent deep cough
♦ Green-colored nasal discharge in some
♦ Serious weight loss, drop in milk yield
♦ Mild fever in some
♦ Variable appetite
♦ Loud breath sounds ventrally, dry crack-
  ling sounds over most of lungs; moist
  crackles ventrally in cases with secondary
  bacterial pneumonia
♦ Subcutaneous emphysema uncommon
♦ Gradual deterioration in disease with
  death, euthanasia after course of 1 week to
  several months

Necropsy findings

♦ Chronic interstitial pneumonia
♦ Secondary bacterial bronchopneumonia in
  some

Diagnosis

Resembles:
♦ Other causes of pneumonia
♦ Bovine interstitial pneumonia
♦ Acute bovine pulmonary emphysema,
  edema

Treatment and control

♦ No treatment of value
♦ Control dust in barn
♦ Dispose of moldy feed, reduce fineness of
  grind of grains

CHRONIC OBSTRUCTIVE
PULMONARY DISEASE OF HORSES
(COPD, RECURRENT AIRWAY
OBSTRUCTION, HEAVES)
[VM8 p. 1691]

Etiology

♦ Cause undecided but thought to be a chronic bronchiolitis caused by hypersensitivity

to allergens in barn dust, moldy and dusty feeds

♦ Fungi known to induce respiratory hypersensitivity in horses affected by chronic obstructive pulmonary disease are:
  • *Micropolyspora faeni*
  • *Aspergillus fumigatus*

Epidemiology

Occurrence
♦ Commonest Europe, North America
♦ Worst in stabled horses, commonly viewed as barn dust related
♦ Recorded also in summer in pastured horses, thought to be due to hypersensitivity to pollen
♦ Sporadic cases; morbidity may be very high in particular stables
♦ Subclinical bronchiolitis common

Risk factors
♦ Over 5 years old, rarely in foals less than 6 months
♦ Long-term housing
♦ Dusty, moldy feeds, dusty environment, inhaled dust
♦ Sensitivity of individual horse
♦ Poor ventilation in barn
♦ Commonest in ponies; probably kept in environmentally poorer stables
♦ Hay the important source of fungal spores; straw, shavings, bedding generally, spore-free initially
♦ Fungal multiplication in infrequently removed bedding

Importance
Major cause of horse wastage by euthanasia, poor performance.

Clinical findings

♦ Chronic cough, paroxysmal in some
♦ Cough worsens, wheezy with exercise, exposure to cold air or dusty environment
♦ Cough easily elicited by larynx, trachea compression
♦ Intermittent, bilateral nasal discharge of serous fluid, mucopus, blood
♦ Epistaxis, exercise-induced pulmonary hemorrhage in some patients
♦ Resting respiratory rate doubled or trebled
♦ Respiration deeper, expiration prolonged with secondary abdominal contraction, the heaves; produces heave-line at costal arch
♦ Nostrils dilated during inspiration
♦ Heart rate normal in early cases; later

markedly increased especially during exercise
♦ Wheezing, crackling sounds end of inspiration and expiration over dorsal lung especially; can be enhanced by light exercise or covering patient's head with a bag
♦ Appetite good, bright, alert
♦ Reduced exercise tolerance in late stages
♦ Condition often relieved when patient turned out
♦ Eventual emaciation, bad clinical syndrome usually leads to euthanasia

Clinical pathology

♦ PaO_2 subnormal, PCO_2 elevated in affected horses
♦ Pulmonary function tests available in respiratory physiology research units
♦ Precipitins against fungi detectable in serum
♦ Cytological examination of tracheal fluid needed to differentiate obstructive respiratory disease from infectious lung disease; the specific respiratory obstruction cytology, evident in tracheal or bronchoalveolar lavage sample, includes increased numbers of neutrophil, lymphocytes hemosiderophages, Curschman's spirals; eosinophil numbers may also be increased
♦ Endoscopic examination of airways may indicate secondary pulmonary hemorrhage, or mucus excess

Necropsy findings

♦ Lungs may be grossly normal in badly affected, euthanised patients; when affected are enlarged, puffy, pale, do not collapse, some bullous emphysema
♦ Chronic bronchiolitis, alveolar emphysema, immunoglobulin complexes accumulate around small airways
♦ Some emphysema but uncommon
♦ Cor pulmonale not usual but some right ventricular hypertrophy

Diagnosis

Resembles:
♦ Pneumonia
♦ Lungworm infestation
♦ Pleurisy
♦ Pulmonary, mediastinal neoplasm
♦ Upper respiratory tract viral infections
♦ Acute equine asthma on summer pasture; dramatic response to corticosteroids, antihistamines

♦ Extrinsic allergic alveolitis (farmer's lung) similar to the disease in cattle

Treatment

♦ Spontaneous recovery in early cases if cause removed, patient moved to dust-free environment; in long-standing cases too much structural damage by emphysema
♦ With careful management impaired horses can survive, perform as breeders or pleasure horses for years; no value as performance horses
♦ Treatments in common use include corticosteroids:
  • Dexamethazone 25 mg/animal I/M every second day for 2 weeks
  • Course of oral prednisolone 1–2 mg/kg body weight for 3–7 days, reducing dose by half every 5–7 days till dose is 0.5 mg/kg reached, then 0.5 mg/kg every second day for 5 days
♦ Bronchodilators, e.g. isoprenaline, terbutaline for prolonged treatment, atropine for immediate effect in an acute case; other bronchodilators include theophylline, aminophylline, clenbuterol
♦ Mucinolytic agents, e.g. bromhexine valuable
♦ Antibiotics, potentiated sulfonamides widely used

Control

♦ Dust-free stables
♦ Kept outside where possible
♦ Enclosed stables must be adequate size, have sufficient ventilation
♦ Peat, woodchips, sawdust preferred over straw as bedding
♦ Hay must be damped before feeding
♦ Complete pelleted ration an alternative to hay
♦ Feed at ground level to encourage respiratory tract drainage
♦ Hay, bedding can be assessed for fungal spore load; high spore count material can be rejected

DISEASES CHARACTERIZED BY NERVOUS SYSTEM INVOLVEMENT

POLIOENCEPHALOMALACIA
(CEREBROCORTICAL NECROSIS)
OF RUMINANTS [VM8 p. 1699]

Etiology

Cause incompletely understood but evidently due to an inadequate supply of thiamin to tissues in most but not all patients.

Epidemiology

♦ Widespread occurrence in well-nourished, thrifty cattle, sheep; also goats, farmed deer
♦ Sporadic cases or outbreaks
♦ Morbidity up to 25% in feeder cattle, case fatality rate 25–50%, higher in younger cattle

Risk factors

♦ Penned animals fed high grain rations; disease occurs after several weeks
♦ Young animals mostly, up to 2 years in cattle
♦ Feedlot cattle on molasses–urea, low fiber diet responds to dietary fiber supplement but not to thiamin supplement

♦ Thiaminases produced by microorganisms, e.g.:
  • *Bacillus thiaminolyticus*
  • *Clostridium sporogenes*
  • *Bacillus aneurinolyticus*
♦ Are common inhabitants in alimentary tracts of normal animals; factors promoting multiplication of these bacteria in gut are not known
♦ Thiaminases in *Pteridium aquilinum*, *Equisetum arvense* not involved in causing polioencephalomalacia but *Marsilea drummondii* is
♦ Diets and water supplies high in sulfates associated with outbreaks of polioencephalomalacia in young and adult cattle; high sulfate intake adversely affects patient's thiamin status
♦ Polioencephalomalacia occurs in pastured cattle, mostly when they are moved from poor to a good pasture

Clinical findings

Calves – acute
Sudden onset of syndrome including:
♦ Blindness
♦ Tremor, especially head
♦ Jaw-champing, saliva frothing

- Head-pressing
- Patient unmanageable
- Intermittent convulsions with opisthotonus, limb tetany
- Eventually recumbency, convulsions continuously, fore limb tetany
- Nystagmus
- Opisthotonus
- Menace reflex absent, pupillary light, palpebral reflexes normal
- Dorsal strabismus common
- Temperature elevated after a convulsion
- Rumen active initially
- Death after 1–2 day course in young calves, several days in yearlings

Calves – subacute
- Patient remains standing
- Blind, or partly so
- Head-pressing
- Anorexia
- Recovery in older patients, some have neurological deficits, e.g. imbecility

Lambs – acute
- Aimless wandering
- Circling in some, *or*
- Blind, stand motionless
- Nystagmus
- Then recumbent, opisthotonus
- Limb extension
- Hyperesthesia
- Periodic convulsions
- Death after course of 24–48 hours

Lambs – subacute
- Blindness
- Head-pressing
- Respond to feed and water, recover spontaneously
- Some survivors circle, periodic head deviation

Lambs – subclinical
- Poor weight gains in ample food supply situation
- Chronic diarrhea in some
- Emaciated
- Some cases of clinical polioencephalomalacia in flock
- High case fatality rate

Goats
- Early excitement, opisthotonus
- Severe extensor rigidity
- Nystagmus

Clinical pathology

- Erythrocyte transketolase activity decreased (normal in sheep is 40–60 iu/ml of erythrocytes)
- Thiamin pyrophosphate effect increased (in sheep >70–80%)
- Blood thiamin levels variable but levels in sheep <50 nmol/L indicate deficiency (<66 nmol/l in goats)
- Blood levels of pyruvate, lactate, pyruvate kinase increased
- Feces thiaminase levels increased
- Cerebrospinal fluid pressure increased, csf protein content normal to high

Necropsy findings

- Diffuse cerebral edema
- Yellow discoloration of dorsal cortical gyri
- Cerebellum pushed back into foramen magnum
- Macroscopic decortication of motor area, occipital lobes in recovered animals
- Bilateral laminar necrosis, necrosis of deeper cortical areas
- Lesions also in cerebellum, thalamus, basal ganglia
- Low thiamin levels in liver, brain

Diagnosis

In **cattle** resembles:
- Lead poisoning
- Hypovitaminosis A
- *Hemophilus somnus* meningoencephalitis
- Listeriosis
- Nervous coccidiosis
- Rabies
- Bovine spongiform encephalopathy
- Tetanus
- Pregnancy toxemia

Additional similar diseases in **heep**:
- Enterotoxemia (*Clostridium perfringens* type D)
- Focal symmetrical encephalomalacia

In **goats** resembles caprine leukoencephalomyelitis.

Treatment

- Thiamin hydrochloride 10 mg/kg body weight I/V every 3 hours for total of 5 treatments
- With early treatment recovery can be complete in 24 hours
- Delayed treatment may cause incomplete

recovery to a vegetable status; recommended to be culled
- Thiamin administered orally may be destroyed by ruminal thiaminases or converted to thiamin analog which inhibit synthesis
- Roughage in flock diet increased to 50%; thiamin may be added
- Cud transfers (rumen transplants) beneficial when appetite returning slowly

Control

- Thiamin supplement in feed (3 mg/kg of ration is standard recommendation but may need to be as high as 20–30 mg/kg depending on ruminal thiaminase levels)
- Roughage should comprise 1.5 kg/100 kg body weight; may not be economical
- Reduce water sulfate content where excessive
- Ensure adequate roughage to sheep being subjected to management procedures which ordinarily deny them access to feed

NEONATAL MALADJUSTMENT
SYNDROME (BARKERS AND
WANDERERS) [VM8 p. 1706]

Etiology

Related to cerebral hypoxia due to early severance of umbilicus.

Epidemiology

- Occurs only in UK
- Only in thoroughbred foals
- Only in foals assisted at birth
- Morbidity 1–2%; case fatality in mild cases (dummies, wanderers) nil, in severe cases (barkers) 50%

Clinical findings

Commences within 2 hours of birth, usually 10–30 minutes.

Severe 'barker' form
- Early signs of weakness, blindness, aimless movements
- Barking sound during severe clonic convulsions with jaw-champing, banging of head on floor
- Nystagmus
- Profuse sweating
- Quiescent periods between convulsions
- Unable to stand, suck
- Blind

- Temperature and pulse vary with state o activity

Mild (dummy, wanderer) form
- Blind
- No response to normal stimuli
- Aimless wandering
- Usually recover in 3–10 days
- Foals recovering from the severe form may pass through this stage

Clinical pathology

Decreased P_{O_2}, increased P_{CO_2}.

Necropsy findings

- Extensive consolidation upper parts both lungs
- In severe cases ischemic necrosis cerebral cortex, local hemorrhage
- Mild cases – brain swelling, edema, hemorrhage

Diagnosis

Resembles:
- Foal septicemias, e.g. shigellosis
- Isoimmune hemolytic anemia
- Bladder rupture
- Meconium retention
- Congenital cardiac defect
- Hypoglycemia in hunter foals in UK

Treatment

- Sedation of acute cases
- Nasal tube alimentation with mare's milk or reconstituted dried milk (80 ml/kg body weight per day in 10 divided doses) until sucking commences
- Foal kept warm
- Oxygen (10 liters/minute) supplied though nasal catheter

Control

Avoid too early umbilical severance.

EQUINE NARCOLEPSY/CATAPLEXY
[VM8 p. 1707]

- Episodes lasting several minutes of uncontrollable sleep in Shetland ponies
- Just loss of consciousness; no uncontrollable movements.

CONGENITAL TREMOR
SYNDROMES OF PIGLETS
[VM8 p. 1707]

Etiology

♦ Type AI – transplacental hog cholera virus transfer
♦ Type AII – transplacental transfer of unknown virus
♦ Type AIII – inherited sex-linked recessive gene
♦ Type AIV – inherited autosomal recessive gene
♦ Type AV – occurs naturally in Scandinavia, cause unknown
♦ Type B – cause unknown

Epidemiology

♦ Type AI – 40% litter affected
♦ Type AII – all litter affected, disease gradually disappears in herd, due possibly to herd immunity, most recover
♦ Type AIII – in progeny of Landrace or Landrace cross sows; up to 10% of litter affected
♦ Type AIV – in Wessex Saddleback pigs, in 25% of litter; fatal to most piglets

Clinical findings

♦ Rhythmic tremors present at birth
♦ Often not noticed till day 3–4 when piglets begin moving
♦ Most evident when standing
♦ Subdued while recumbent
♦ Disappear during sleep
♦ Varies from rapid twitch of head to slow tremor of body causing pig to 'dance' (tremble violently, rock from side to side)
♦ No weakness, piglets very active
♦ Gait ataxic, dysmetric
♦ Mildly affected pigs recover spontaneously in 2–8 weeks
♦ Severely affected piglets may not be able to reach teat, die of starvation, or crushed

Necropsy findings

♦ Type AI – cerebellar hypoplasia, cerebrospinal dysmyelinogenesis
♦ Type AII — spinal dysmyelinogenesis
♦ Type AIII – cerebral dysmyelinogenesis
♦ Type AIV – cerebrospinal dysmyelinogenesis
♦ Type AV – cerebellar hypoplasia

Diagnosis

Resembles:
♦ Encephalitis
♦ Fetal hypoxia
♦ Piglet hypoglycemia

Treatment and control

♦ Hand rearing piglets unable to suck
♦ Eliminate affected genetic lines
♦ Ensure premating vaccination, or other immunity acquisition against causative virus

HYPOMYELINOGENESIS
CONGENITA [VM8 p. 1708]

Etiology

♦ Cause unknown in lambs, intra-uterine viral infection suspected
♦ Mucosal disease virus infection in utero, possibly other viruses in cattle

Epidemiology

♦ UK, North America, Australia
♦ Calves, lambs; similar to piglet congenital tremor
♦ Morbidity lambs up to 13%

Clinical findings

Lambs
♦ Severe muscle tremor head, body
♦ Tremor disappears during sleep
♦ Gait erratic, incoordinated, hopping with hind limbs
♦ Suck, grow well
♦ May die of starvation; many recover spontaneously, ataxia, head shaking may persist 5 months

Calves
♦ Unable to stand
♦ Persistent, general tremor at all times
♦ Brief periods of spastic rigidity, opisthotonus, nystagmus

Necropsy findings

Defective myelination.

Diagnosis

In **lambs** resembles border disease
In **calves** resembles:
♦ Congenital myoclonus
♦ Mucosal disease

Treatment and control

No recommendation.

OVINE HUMPYBACK [VM8 p. 1709]

Etiology

Probably related to heat stress.

Clinical findings

♦ Walking affected sheep, which are in full wool, for about 1 kilometre in summer causes stiff gait, then stops
♦ Arched back
♦ Fever
♦ Shearing cures syndrome

Clinical pathology

Blood lymphocyte count lowered.

EQUINE CERVICAL VERTEBRAL
STENOTIC MYELOPATHY
(WOBBLE'S) [VM8 p. 1709]

Etiology

♦ Compression of the cervical spinal cord
♦ Part of group of diseases causing incoordination in young horses
♦ may be:
  • Static due to luminal constriction or
  • Dynamic due to frequent compression incidents due to excessive movement at intervertebral spaces
  • Fast growth, overnutrition
  • Inherited tendency

Epidemiology

♦ Young horses, mostly yearlings, up to 2 years
♦ Mostly males
♦ All breeds of light horses
♦ Many irreversible, loss due to euthanasia

Clinical findings

♦ Insidious onset of limb incoordination weakness
♦ Restricted neck movements
♦ Pain on sudden movement or pressure over cervical vertebrae
♦ Clumsiness in turning or stopping at a fast gait
♦ Lurching or swaying of hindquarters
♦ Difficulty adopting posture for urinating, grazing
♦ Difficulty rising after rolling
♦ Slap test for vocal cord movement negative

Clinical pathology

Abnormal flexibility of cervical intervertebral joints on X-ray.

Necropsy findings

♦ Cord compression by protrusion of vertebrae or disks into spinal canal
♦ Areas of malacia in cord
♦ Inflammation of vertebral articular processes
♦ Spinal nerve compression

Diagnosis

Resembles:
♦ Traumatic injury to spinal cord
♦ Pressure on cord from neoplasm
♦ Inherited degenerative myeloencephalopathy
♦ Protozoal meningoencephalitis
♦ Spinal meningitis, myelitis
♦ Iliac thrombosis
♦ Cerebrospinal nematodiasis
♦ Inherited foal ataxia
♦ Viral rhinopneumonitis

Treatment and control

♦ Surgical relief of compression of the cord
♦ Genetic selection against the disease recommended

STRINGHALT [VM8 p. 1711]

Epidemiology

♦ Horses only
♦ Usually associated with heavy growth *Hypochaeris radicata* (flatweed, catsear) in pasture

Clinical findings

♦ In **classical stringhalt** defect irreversible
♦ In **Australian stringhalt** spontaneous recovery after as long as a year

Standard syndrome
♦ Involuntary, exaggerated hock flexion during progression
♦ One or both hind limbs involved
♦ Occurs as horse about to move off
♦ May be unable to move for a moment

Severe cases – additional signs:
♦ In worst cases difficulty rising
♦ Stiffness of fore limbs
♦ Respiratory distress due to laryngeal paralysis

Necropsy findings

Peripheral neuropathy in tibial, superficial peroneal, medial plantar, left and right recurrent laryngeal nerves.

OVINE 'KANGAROO GAIT'
[VM8 p. 1711]

Clinical findings

♦ Lactating ewes move front limbs only in synchronised bounds
♦ Slow recovery at end of lactation

Necropsy findings

♦ Generalized neuropathy, affects radial nerves principally
♦ Remyelination during recovery

DISEASES CHARACTERIZED BY INVOLVEMENT OF THE MUSCULOSKELETAL SIGNS

SPORADIC LYMPHANGITIS
(BIGLEG, WEED) [VM8 p. 1711]

Etiology

Associated with wounds of lower limb, causing lymphangitis, cellulitis.

Epidemiology

In horses fed concentrate rations for period without exercise.

Clinical findings

♦ Acute onset
♦ Fever, shivering
♦ Anorexia, thirst, patchy sweating, constipation
♦ Severe swelling of one or both hind limbs, top of limb to coronet
♦ Lymphatics corded on medial aspect affected limb(s)
♦ Inguinal lymph nodes palpable, enlarged, painful
♦ Fast heart and respiration rates
♦ Anxiety, severe pain in limb on palpation
♦ Lameness, hoof not put to ground
♦ Acute swelling eases at day 3 but still evident at 10 days
♦ Abscesses of nodes, lymphatics in some patients
♦ May recur, cause fibrotic thickening of lower limb

Clinical pathology

Culture of pus from wound, abscess.

Diagnosis

Resembles:
♦ Femoral fracture
♦ Upper limb myositis

Treatment

♦ Needs to be early, intensive
♦ Analgesic, anti-inflammatory indicated
♦ Intensive parenteral broad-spectrum antibacterial therapy
♦ Vigorous hot fomentation, massage to reduce swelling
♦ Encouragement to exercise

Control

♦ Attention to limb wounds
♦ Daily exercise
♦ Feed restriction during lay-off periods

ASYMMETRIC HINDQUARTER
SYNDROME OF PIGS [VM8 p. 1712]

Etiology

Possible inheritance component.

Epidemiology

♦ Europe, UK
♦ In grower pigs up to 80 kg body weight
♦ Enzootic in particular herds

Clinical findings

♦ Asymmetric hindquarters
♦ Gait normal

Necropsy findings

Perineural fibrosis, myopathy in some.

SPLAYLEG SYNDROME IN
NEWBORN PIGS (SPRADDLE LEG,
MYOFIBRILLAR HYPOPLASIA)
[VM8 p. 1712]

Etiology

Probably multifactorial including:
♦ Slippery floors
♦ Nutritional deficiency of choline
♦ Mycotoxicosis, *Fusarium* spp., in pregnant sows
♦ Glucocorticoid myopathy due to stress, hormonal imbalance

Epidemiology

♦ Widespread, most countries
♦ Newborn piglets
♦ Commonest in Landrace, Large White
♦ Commonest in males
♦ Morbidity in infected herds 2–27%; case fatality rate 50%

Clinical findings

♦ Birth weight subnormal
♦ Unable to stand
♦ Instead of walking piglets rest on sternum
♦ Hind limbs splayed laterally or forward
♦ Forelimbs may be affected
♦ Unable to move, or move slightly
♦ Many deaths due to crushing, chilling, starvation
♦ Suck if placed on teat
♦ 50% piglets recover in 1 week

Necropsy findings

♦ Myofibrillar hypoplasia; also in normal piglets
♦ Extra-myofibrillar space filled with glycogen

Treatment

Recovery helped by loose tying, taping of hind limbs together soon after birth; delay lessens effect.

Control

Culling of boar debated as a control procedure; tendency is to retain him if productivity characteristics significantly better.

LEG WEAKNESS IN PIGS
[VM8 p. 1713]

Leg weakness a general term which includes:
♦ Osteochondrosis
♦ Epiphyseolysis
♦ Degenerative osteoarthrosis

Epidemiology

Occurrence
♦ High incidence of clinically inapparent osteochondrosis in pigs up to market weight
♦ Up to 30% of 20–30 week old pigs (maximum growth period) kept for breeding severely lame

Risk factors
♦ Commonest in young, rapidly growing pigs, but factors known *not* to be significant include:
  • High growth rate
  • Dietary imbalance of major components
  • Insecure footing due to floor surface
  • Duration of confinement
♦ Commoner in boars
♦ Some genetic susceptibility

Importance
♦ Major cause of culling in young, breeder pigs
♦ Wastage due to:
  • High culling rate causes loss of investment
  • Loss of potential genetic gain
  • Loss of crushed piglets from lame sows

Clinical findings

♦ A non-infectious, degenerative joint disease
♦ Long-term locomotor disorder during the period 4–18 months; effects persist to adults
♦ Rapidly growing pigs worst affected
♦ Usually involves hind limbs

Range of locomotor disorders includes:
- Carpus hyperflexion
- Fore limb bowing
- 'Knock-knees'
- Phalangeal hyperextension
- Lateral angulation of foot
- Sickle hocks
- Severe lameness
- Paresis, difficulty rising
- Recumbency

◊ Lameness usually insidious in onset; may be acute, intermittent, chronic or progressive

◊ Affected boars may be unable to mate

◊ Euthanasia a common outcome

Necropsy findings

◊ Osteochondrosis
◊ Epiphyseolysis
◊ Degenerative osteoarthrosis

Diagnosis

Resembles:
◊ Arthritis
◊ Laminitis
◊ Traumatic hoof lesions
◊ Biotin nutritional deficiency
◊ Foot rot
◊ Osteodystrophy
◊ Hypovitaminosis A
◊ Viral poliomyelitis

Treatment

◊ Turning out to pasture, or individual housing in deep litter may improve signs
◊ Corticosteroids, phenylbutazone for acute signs

Control

Selection for sound limbs, freedom from lameness.

HYENA DISEASE [VM8 p. 1716]

Etiology

Suggestion that defect inherited not applicable in some herds.

Epidemiology

◊ In Europe
◊ In German Simmental, Charolais, Black Pied, German Holstein-Friesian, German Red Pied

Clinical findings

◊ Slow growth rate
◊ Normal at birth, abnormal at 5–6 months old
◊ Comparative underdevelopment of hindquarters; femur, tibia shorter than normal
◊ Crest of thick, stiff bristles along midline
◊ Aggressive actions
◊ Awkward gait, tendency to fall to side
◊ Frequent laterally recumbent posture

Necropsy findings

Chondrodystrophy affecting particularly long bones, lumbar vertebrae.

'TYING-UP' SYNDROME OF HORSES [VM8 p. 1717]

Epidemiology

◊ Horses only
◊ In overworked horses
◊ Change to hard track
◊ After a spell

Clinical findings

◊ Sudden onset 10–20 minutes after commencing exercise
◊ Stiff, sore, shuffling gait
◊ Some patients will not move
◊ Profuse sweating
◊ Rigid abdominal muscles
◊ Spontaneous recovery
◊ Commonly recurs in same horse

Diagnosis

May be effect of too hard exercise in unfit horse or:
◊ Exertional rhabdomyolysis
◊ Grain or oat sickness
◊ Iliac thrombosis
◊ Spondylopathy
◊ Cauda equina neuritis

EXERTIONAL RHABDOMYOLYSIS [VM8 p. 1717]

Epidemiology

◊ Horses only
◊ Sudden onset after brisk exercise

♦ May be recurrent attacks
♦ No history heavy grain feeding

Clinical findings

♦ Severe muscle spasm, soreness
♦ Unwilling to move
♦ Anxiety, dyspnea, sweating, tremor
♦ Stiffness passes off in 1–3 days

Clinical pathology

♦ Marked elevation serum levels muscle enzymes, especially creatine kinase
♦ Hyaline degeneration muscle fibers in needle biopsy
♦ No myoglobinuria

Treatment

Spontaneous recovery but selenium/vitamin E combinations often administered.

GRAIN OR OAT SICKNESS
[VM8 p. 1717]

♦ Individual horses stiff and sore for several hours after exercise
♦ Prevented by reducing grain ration or adding magnesium sulfate (30–60 g/day) to feed.

ILIAC THROMBOSIS [VM8 p. 1717]

Weakness, incoordination one hind limb of horse during fast work. Limb cold, reduced pulse in internal iliac artery on rectal palpation.

SPONDYLOPATHY [VM8 p. 1718]

Stiffness, pain in a limb, reduced by analgesic, anti-inflammatory. Lesions affecting vertebrae, causing pressure on peripheral nerve roots.

CAUDA EQUINA NEURITIS
(POLYNEURITIS EQUI)
[VM8 p. 1718]

Epidemiology

♦ Sporadic cases in horses
♦ Cows after service by heavy bull
♦ Excessive riding among steers, groups of bulls, cows

Clinical findings

♦ Tail paralysis
♦ Anal sphincter slack
♦ Rectum distended, hypotonic
♦ Overdistension of bladder
♦ Perineal anesthesia
♦ Difficulty urinating, defecating
♦ Weakness and incoordination of hind limbs

Necropsy findings

Non-suppurative, often granulomatous, inflammation cauda equina nerve trunks.

'ACORN' CALVES [VM8 p. 1718]

Epidemiology

♦ Cattle on poor range, with or without access to oak tree browse
♦ Up to 15% incidence
♦ Supplementary feeding prevents

Clinical findings

♦ Long or short deformity of bones of the skull
♦ Short shafts of limb bones
♦ Bending at joints
♦ Difficulty walking, standing
♦ Back arched
♦ Some bloat
♦ Rarely goose-stepping gait, circling, head-pressing, wry neck

Diagnosis

Resembles:
♦ Achondroplastic dwarfism
♦ Congenital joint laxity, dwarfism

CONGENITAL JOINT LAXITY AND
DWARFISM IN CALVES
[VM8 p. 1718]

Epidemiology

♦ Canada, in beef cattle
♦ Limited, regional distribution
♦ Up to 46% morbidity
♦ Associated with feeding grass or clover ensilage over winter without grain supplement
♦ Danger period is first 6 months of pregnancy
♦ Higher incidence in heifer's calves

Clinical findings

- Congenital generalized joint laxity; causes dystokia in some
- Disproportionate dwarfism
- Superior brachygnathia in a few patients
- Joints normal by few weeks old
- Perinatal mortality high in affected herds

Necropsy findings

- Chondrocyte overgrowth around long bone epiphyses
- Delayed mineralization at epiphyses

Diagnosis

Resembles:
- Achondroplastic dwarfs
- Acorn calves

Treatment and control

Feeding hay and rolled barley eliminates problem.

SLIPPED CAPITAL FEMORAL
EPIPHYSIS IN CALVES
[VM8 p. 1719]

Epidemiology

Occurs in Charolais, Maine-Anjou, and Simmental calves.

Clinical findings

- Many patients subjected to forced traction during birth
- Lameness at birth or within first few days:
  - Slight weight-bearing in mild cases
  - Toe-dragging, limb-carrying in some
- Palpable crepitus over greater trochanter on affected side
- Prolonged recumbency
- Muscle atrophy in long-standing cases

Clinical pathology

- Displacement femoral neck visible radiographically
- Partial femoral head reabsorption in mild cases

Diagnosis

Resembles perinatal femoral nerve degeneration with neurogenic atrophy of quadriceps femoris muscle.

Treatment

Excision arthroplasty.

PERINATAL FEMORAL NERVE
DEGENERATION [VM8 p. 1719]

Epidemiology

Occurs in Charolais, Maine-Anjou, and Simmental calves

Clinical findings

- Congenital lameness, inability to bear weight
- Most commonly in right hind limb
- Neurogenic atrophy of quadriceps femoris muscle

Treatment

Surgical.

TAIL-TIP NECROSIS IN CATTLE
[VM8 p. 1719]

Etiology

Caused by trampling injury to tail tip.

Epidemiology

Occurrence
Morbidity about 5%; 10% of affected animals condemned at abattoir.

Risk factors
- Cattle housed on slatted floors
- Warm weather
- Close confinement
- Body weight >200 kg

Clinical findings

- Tail tip swollen initially
- Later extension proximally
- Some develop abscesses in tail

+ Metastatic abscesses to other organs, including osteomyelitis
+ Growth retardation in some; occasional deaths from pyemia

Necropsy findings

+ Abscesses in multiple organs
+ Osteomyelitis

Treatment

+ Early amputation, plus
+ Broad-spectrum antibacterial treatment

Control

+ Close surveillance including tail-tip palpation to detect early cases
+ Ensure adequate space on slatted floors

DISEASES CHARACTERIZED BY INVOLVEMENT OF THE SKIN

PITYRIASIS ROSEA [VM8 p. 1720]

Epidemiology

Occurrence
+ Sucking piglets, and young pigs up to 14 weeks old
+ Familial susceptibility
+ Morbidity rate about 50% in litter; may be close to 100% in large groups

Clinical findings

+ Skin lesions only in most patients
+ Lesions commonest on ventral abdomen; spread to rest of body
+ Small, red nodules
+ Enlarge to flat plaques, covered with thin, dry, brown scales
+ Centrifugal enlargement leaves superficial lesion with normal center, surrounded by narrow zone of elevated, erythematous skin, covered with scales
+ Lesions approximately circular, coalesce to form irregular lesion
+ No scratching or bristle loss

Clinical pathology

Standard examination for infectious agents negative.

Diagnosis

Resembles ringworm but no hyphae or spores, no response to ringworm treatment.

Treatment

+ Spontaneous recovery usually in 6–8 weeks
+ Topical salves, lotions widely used

ANHIDROSIS (NON-SWEATING SYNDROME, PUFF DISEASE, DRY COAT) [VM8 p. 1720]

Etiology

Favored explanation is neurogenic defect of adaptation of sweating to hot climate.

Epidemiology

+ Tropical countries, summer months
+ Mostly horses but high-producing dairy cows may have problem
+ Horses in training
+ Imported horses more likely to be affected

Clinical findings

+ Skin area that sweats reduces gradually until only that below the mane gets wet
+ Skin dry, scurfy, inelastic
+ Some hair loss
+ Dyspnea after exercise
+ Temperature after exercise up to 42°C
+ Horse seeks shade
+ Exercise tolerance negligible
+ Anorexia, weight loss
+ Recovery if moved to cool climate

Clinical pathology

+ Blood chloride low, adrenalin high
+ Local injection of adrenalin causes sweating at site in moderate cases, not in bad ones
+ Sweat gland atrophy in biopsy

Treatment and control

+ Ensure adequate salt taken, or intravenous injections physiological saline

- Improvement claimed for feeding thyroid gland extract or iodinated casein
- Diet supplementation with vitamin E reported beneficial

BOVINE OCULAR SQUAMOUS-CELL CARCINOMA (BOSCC, CANCER-EYE) [VM8 p. 1721]

Etiology

Papillomavirus, bovine herpesvirus-5, suspected of involvement.

Epidemiology

Morbidity rate can be very high in some Hereford herds; case fatality rate high.

Risk factors
- Hereford, Ayrshire cattle most affected
- Higher prevalence in cattle lacking periorbital and orbital pigment
- Exposure to bright sunlight
- High nutritional status increases risk

Clinical findings

Precursor lesions
- Plaques of gray–white tissue on conjunctiva or periorbital skin
- Also local papilloma or acanthomas
- Most regress spontaneously
- Some progress to carcinomas

Carcinomas
- Fleshy, crumbly, often necrotic, ulcerated growths
- Attached to lid or orbit by wide base
- Advanced cases may metastasize to regional lymph nodes

Clinical pathology

Cytological examination necessary to distinguish precursors from neoplasms.

Diagnosis

Resembles chronic infection of original contagious keratoconjunctivitis.

Treatment

- Excision commonly practiced but recurrence likely unless extirpation is radical
- Radioactive implants

- Immunotherapy with BCG vaccination systemically or intralesional
- Immunotherapy using BOSCC tumor tissue
- Moderately good results claimed for all these procedures with no clear best option

Control

- Selection for periorbital and orbital pigmentation recommended
- Selection on basis of lesion occurrence has limited success

EQUINE OCULAR SQUAMOUS-CELL CARCINOMA [VM8 p. 1723]

- Rare disease, mostly heavy breeds with unpigmented eyelids
- Clinical findings and treatment as for BOSCC

Diagnosis

Resembles:
- Cutaneous habronemiasis
- Sarcoid

'COCKLE' [VM8 p. 1723]

Epidemiology

- Only in New Zealand
- In unshorn sheep
- Important to leather industry

Clinical findings

- Inflammatory nodules
- Mostly on neck, shoulders; may be all over skin

Clinical pathology

Negative search for skin pathogens.

Treatment

Responds to treatment with diazinon (0.04% as shower dip, tip spray, plunge dip), has cured within 3 weeks, protected for 6 months.

WOOL SLIP [VM8 p. 1723]

Etiology

Some outbreaks thought to be hormonal response to shearing, exposure to cold for lengthy period.

Epidemiology

♦ Housed sheep
♦ All breeds
♦ Morbidity up to 40%

Clinical findings

♦ Condition usually develops 2–3 weeks after shearing

♦ Part of fleece detaches leaving bald patch
♦ Multiple patches over rear half of back
♦ Skin normal
♦ Wool regrows immediately

Clinical pathology

Negative search for skin pathogens.

Diagnosis

Resembles:
♦ Break in wool due to starvation, severe illness
♦ Nutritional zinc deficiency

Treatment and control

Avoid nutritional and other stress.

CONVERSION TABLES

CONVERSION FACTORS FOR OLD AND SI UNITS

	Old units	Multiplication factors		SI units
		Old units to SI units	SI units to old units	
RBC	$\times 10^6/mm^3$	10^6	10^6	$\times 10^{12}/l$
PCV	%	0.01	100	1/l
Hb	g/dl	None	None	g/dl
MCV	μ^3	None	None	fl
MCH	$\mu\mu g$	None	None	pg
MCHC	%	None	None	g/dl
WBC	$\times 10^3/mm^3$	10^6	10^{-6}	$\times 10^9/l$
Platelets	$\times 10^3/mm^3$	10^6	10^{-6}	$\times 10^9/l$
Total serum protein	g/dl	10	0.1	g/l
Albumin	g/dl	10	0.1	g/l
Bicarbonate	mEq/l	None	None	mmol/l
Bilirubin	mg/dl	17.1	0.0585	$\mu mol/l$
Calcium	mg/dl	0.25	4.008	mmol/l
Chloride	mEq/l	None	None	mmol/l
Cholesterol	mg/dl	0.0259	38.7	mmol/l
Copper	$\mu g/dl$	0.157	6.35	$\mu mol/l$
Cortisol	$\mu g/dl$	27.6	0.0362	nmol/l
Creatinine	mg/dl	88.4	0.0113	$\mu mol/l$
Globulin	g/dl	10	0.1	g/l
Glucose	mg/dl	0.0555	18.02	mmol/l
Inorganic phosphate	mg/dl	0.323	3.10	mmol/l
Iron	$\mu g/dl$	0.179	5.59	$\mu mol/l$
Lead	$\mu g/dl$	0.0483	20.7	$\mu mol/l$
Magnesium	mg/dl	0.411	2.43	mmol/l
Molybdenum	$\mu g/dl$	0.104	9.6	$\mu mol/l$
Potassium	mEq/l	None	None	mmol/l
Selenium	$\mu g/dl$	0.126	7.9	$\mu mol/l$
Sodium	mEq/l	Nonc	None	mmol/l
Triglyceride	mg/dl	0.0113	88.5	mmol/l
Urea	mg/dl	0.166	6.01	mmol/l
Zinc	$\mu g/dl$	0.152	6.54	$\mu mol/l$

CONVERSIONS

To convert grams per 100 ml into grains per US fluid ounce, multiply by 4.564.
To convert grams per 100 ml into grains per Imperial fluid ounce, multiply by 4.385.
To convert grams into ounces avoirdupois, multiply by 10 and divide by 283.
To convert liters into US pints, multiply by 2.114.
To convert liters into Imperial pints, multiply by 88 and divide by 50.
To convert kilos into pounds, multiply by 1000 and divide by 454.

MASS

Metric

1 kilogram (kg)	=	15 432 grains
	or	35.274 ounces
	or	2.2046 pounds
1 gram (g)	=	15.432 grains
1 milligram (mg)	=	0.015432 grain

US/Imperial

1 ton (2240 lb)	= 1016 kilograms
1 hundredweight (112 lb) (cwt)	= 50.80 kilograms
1 stone (14 lb) (st)	= 6.35 kilograms
1 pound (avoirdupois) (lb)	= 453.59 grams
1 ounce (avoirdupois) (oz)	= 28.35 grams
1 grain (gr)	= 64.799 milligrams

CAPACITY

Metric

1 liter (l)	= 2.114 US pints = 1.7598 Imperial pints
1 Milliliter (ml)	= 16.23 US minims = 16.894 Imperial minims

US Liquid

1 gallon (128 fl oz) (gal)	= 3.785 liters
1 pint (pt)	= 473.17 milliliters
1 fluid ounce (fl oz)	= 29.573 milliliters
1 fluid dram (fl dr)	= 3.696 milliliters
1 minim (min)	= 0.061610 milliliters

Imperial

1 gallon (160 fl oz) (gal)	= 4.546 liters
1 pint (pt)	= 568.25 milliliters
1 fluid ounce (fl oz)	= 28.412 milliliters
1 fluid drachm (fl dr)	= 3.5515 milliliters
1 minim (min)	= 0.059192 milliliters

LENGTH

Metric

1 kilometer (km)	= 0.621 miles
1 meter (m)	= 39.370 inches
1 decimeter (dm)	= 3.9370 inches
1 centimeter (cm)	= 0.39370 inch
1 millimeter (mm)	= 0.039370 inch
1 micrometer (μm)	= 0.000039370 inch

US/Imperial

1 mile	= 1.609 kilometers
1 yard	= 0.914 meters
1 foot	= 30.48 centimeters
1 inch	= 2.54 centimeters
	or 25.40 millimeters

TEMPERATURE

Celsius (Centigrade)	Fahrenheit	Celsius (Centigrade)	Fahrenheit
110°	230°	38°	100.4°
100	212	37.5	99.5
95	203	37	98.6
90	194	36.5	97.7
85	183	36	96.8
80	176	35.5	95.9
75	167	35	95.0
70	158	34	93.2
65	149	33	91.4
60	140	32	89.6
55	131	31	87.8
50	122	30	86
45	113	25	77
44	111.2	20	68
43	109.4	15	59
42	107.6	10	50
41	105.8	+5	41
40.5	104.9	0	32
40	104.0	−5	23
39.5	103.1	−10	14
39	102.2	−15	+5
38.5	101.3	−20	−4

To convert Fahrenheit into Celsius, subtract 32, multiply the remainder by 5, and divide the result by 9.

To convert Celsius into Fahrenheit, multiply by 9, divide by 5, and add 32.

REFERENCE LABORATORY VALUES

Reference values of laboratory data are offered as a guide and the reader must be aware that values may vary depending on the age, sex and geographical habitat of the animal, and the laboratory. These tables are reference values used at the Western College of Veterinary Medicine, University of Saskatchewan, and have been compiled from the clinical laboratory, Department of Pathology; from N.C. Jain (1986) *Schalm's Veterinary Hematology*, 4th edn. Philadelphia: Lea & Febiger; and from J.J. Kaneko (1989) *Clinical Biochemistry of Domestic Animals*, 4th edn. New York: Academic Press. Courtesy of G.P. Searcy, Department of Veterinary Pathology, University of Saskatchewan.

HEMATOLOGY

	Ox	Sheep	Goat	Swine	Horse
Hemoglobin (g/dl)	8.0–15.0	9.0–15.0	8.0–12.0	10.0–16.0	11.0–19.0
PCV (%)	24.0–46.0	27.0–45.0	22.0–38.0	32.0–50.0	32.0–53.0
RBC ($\times 10^6/\mu l$)	5.0–10.0	9.0–15.0	8.0–18.0	5.0–8.0	6.8–12.9
MCV (fl)	40.0–60.0	28.0–40.0	16.0–25.0	50.0–68.0	37.0–58.5
MCH (pg)	11.0–17.0	8.0–12.0	5.2–8.0	17.0–21.0	12.3–19.7
MCHC (g/dl)	30.0–36.0	31.0–34.0	30.0–36.0	30.0–34.0	31.0–38.6
RDW (%)	16.7–23.3	18–24.6			
Thrombocytes ($\times 10^5/\mu l$)	1.0–8.0	2.5–7.5	3.0–6.0	3.2–5.2	1.0–3.5
WBC (/μl)	4000–12 000	4000–12 000	4000–13 000	11 000–22 000	5400–14 300
Neutrophils (mature) (/μl)	600–4000	700–6000	1200–7200	3080–10 450	2260–8580
Neutrophils (bands) (/μl)	0–120	Rare	Rare	0–880	0–100
Lymphocytes (/μl)	2500–7500	2000–9000	2000–9000	4290–13 640	1500–7700
Monocytes (/μl)	25–840	0–750	0–550	200–2200	0–1000
Eosinophils (/μl)	0–2400	0–1000	0–650	55–2420	0–1000
Basophils (/μl)	0–200	0–300	0–120	0–440	0–290
Plasma proteins (g/dl)	6.6–7.8	6.0–7.5	6.0–7.5	6.0–8.0	6.6–7.7
Fibrinogen (mg/dl)	300–700	100–500	100–400	100–500	

International System of Units (SI)

	Ox	Sheep	Goat	Swine	Horse
Hemoglobin (g/l)	80–150	90–150	80–120	100–160	110–190
PCV (1/l)	0.24–0.46	0.27–0.45	0.22–0.38	0.32–0.50	0.32–0.53
RBC ($\times 10^{12}$/l)	5.0–10.0	9.0–15.0	8.0–18.0	5.0–8.0	6.8–12.9
MCV (fl)	40–60	28–40	16.0–25.0	50–68	37–58
MCH (pg)	11–17	8–12	5.2–8.0	17–21	12–20
MCHC (g/l)	300–360	310–340	300–360	300–340	310–386
RDW (%)	16.7–23.3	18–24.6			
Thrombocytes ($\times 10^9$/l)	100–800	250–750	300–600	320–520	100–350
WBC ($\times 10^9$/l)	4.0–12.0	4.0–12.0	4.0–13.0	11.0–22.0	5.4–14.0
Neutrophils (mature) ($\times 10^9$/l)	0.6–4.0	0.7–6.0	1.2–7.2	3.0–10.0	2.3–8.5
Neutrophils (bands) ($\times 10^9$/l)	0–0.1	Rare	Rare	0–0.8	0–0.1
Lymphocytes ($\times 10^9$/l)	2.5–7.5	2.0–9.0	2.0–9.0	4.2–13.6	1.5–7.7
Monocytes ($\times 10^9$/l)	0–0.8	0–0.8	0–0.55	0.2–2.2	0–1.0
Eosinophils ($\times 10^9$/l)	0–2.4	0–1.0	0–0.65	0.5–2.4	0–1.0
Basophils ($\times 10^9$/l)	0–0.2	0–0.3	0–0.12	0–0.4	0–2.9
Plasma proteins (g/l)	66–78	60–75	60–75	60–80	60–77
Fibrinogen (g/l)	3–7	1–5	1–4	1–5	1–4

CHEMISTRY

	Ox	Sheep	Swine	Horse
Sodium (mEq/l)	132–152	145–160	140–150	132–150
Potassium (mEq/l)	3.9–5.8	4.8–5.9	4.7–7.1	3.0–5.0
Chloride (mEq/l)	95–110	98–110	100–105	98–110
pCO_2 (mmHg)	34–45	38		38–46
pH	7.35–7.50	7.32–7.50		7.32–7.55
HCO_3	20–30	21–28	18–27	23–32
Anion gap (mEq/l)	14–26	12–24	10–25	10–25
Calcium (mg/dl)	8.0–10.5	11.5–13.0	11.0–11.3	11.2–13.8
Phosphorus (mg/dl)	4.0–7.0	4.0–7.0	4.0–11.0	3.1–5.6
Magnesium (mg/dl)	1.2–3.5	1.9–2.5	1.9–3.9	1.8–2.5
Iron (μl/dl)	57–162	166–222	73–140	91–199
Urea (mg/dl)	6.0–27	8.0–20	8.0–24	10–20
Creatinine (mg/dl)	1.0–2.7	1.2–1.9	1.0–2.7	1.2–1.9
Glucose (mg/dl)	35–55	30–65	65–95	60–100
Cholesterol (mg/dl)	39–177	40–58	117–119	46–177
Total bilirubin (mg/dl)	0–1.9	0–0.4	0–0.2	0.2–6.0
Direct bilirubin (mg/dl)	0–0.4	0–0.3		0–0.4
Alkaline phosphatase (iu/l)	35–350	68–387		95–233
AST (iu/l)	60–150	260–350	25–57	200–400
Creatine phosphokinase (CPK) (iu/dl)	65	65	65	65
SDH (iu/l)	0–15			0–15
γ-Glutamyltransferase (iu/l)	0–31	0–70	0–25	0–25
Total protein (g/dl)	5.7–8.1	6.0–7.9	3.5–6.0	6.0–7.7
Albumin (g/dl)	2.1–3.6	2.4–3.0	1.9–2.4	2.9–3.8
α_1-Globulin (g/dl)	0.7–1.2	3.0–6.0	1.0–1.3	0.7–1.3
α_2-Globulin (g/dl)		3.0–6.0		0.7–1.3
β-Globulin (g/dl)	0.6–1.2	1.1–2.6	0.8–1.1	0.4–1.2
γ-Globulin (g/dl)	1.6–3.2	0.9–3.3	0.3–0.7	0.9–1.5

International System of Units (SI)

	Ox	Sheep	Swine	Horse
Sodium (mmol/l)	135–151	143–151	140–150	132–150
Potassium (mmol/l)	3.9–5.8	4.8–7.0	4.7–7.1	3.0–5.0
Chloride (mmol/l)	95–110	98–110	100–105	98–110
pCO_2 (mmHg)	34–45	38		38–46
pH	7.35–7.50	7.32–7.50		7.32–7.55
HCO_3 (mmol/l)	20–30	21–28	18–27	23–32
Calcium (mmol/l)	2.11–2.75	2.30–2.86	2.74–2.82	2.80–3.44
Phosphorus (mmol/l)	1.08–2.76	0.82–2.66	1.30–3.55	0.70–1.68
Magnesium (mmol/l)	0.50–1.10	0.90–1.26	0.78–1.60	0.74–1.02
Iron (μmol/l)	10–29	30–40	13–25	16–36
Urea (mmol/l)	2.0–7.5	3.0–10.0	3.0–8.5	3.5–7.0
Creatinine (μmol/l)	67–175	69–105	90–240	110–170
Glucose (mmol/l)	1.9–3.8	1.7–3.6	3.6–5.3	3.3–5.6
Cholesterol (mmol/l)	1.00–4.60	1.05–1.50	3.05–3.10	1.20–4.60
Total bilirubin (μmol/l)	0–32	0–6	0–4	4–102
Alkaline phosphatase (u/l)	35–126	68–158	25–57	95–233
AST (u/l)	60–118	48–128	<500	200–400
Creatine kinase (CK) (u/l)	<350	<350	<500	<500
SDH (u/l)	4–26	0–8.5	0–15	
γ-Glutamyltransferase (u/l)	0–31	0–70	0–25	0–25
Total protein	66–78	60–75	60–80	66–77
Albumin (g/l)	21–36	24–30	19–24	29–38
α_1-Globulin (g/l)	7–12	3–6	10–13	7–13
α_2-Globulin (g/dl)		3–6		7–13
β-Globulin (g/l)	6–12	3–7	8–11	4–12
γ-Globulin (g/l)	16–32	7–13	3–7	9–15

INDEX

t = in a table

Hair *continued*
  deficiency 231
  disease 239
  follicle dysplasia color-linked and
      inherited 651t
Hairiness 231
Hairworms 481
Hairy
  caltrop poisoning 594
  shakers 428
  vetch poisoning 599
Halogeton glomeratus poisoning 590
Haloragis odontocarpa poisoning 601
Haplopappus spp. poisoning 602t
Hard udder 264, 424
Harelip 66, 89
  inherited 635t
Harvest mite infestation 505
Head
  deviation 192
  examination 6
  extended 155
  fly infestation 505
  pressing 192
  rotation 192
  shaking 192
  tilt 192
Heart (see also cardiac)
  beat 5
  block 127
    complete 127
    partial 127
  congenital defects 138
  disease 132
    fibrillators 128
  ectopic 138
  failure
    acute 124
    congestive 123
    left side 123
    poisonous plants 600
    right side 123
  murmurs 131
  neoplasms 140
  radiographic abnormalities 132
  rupture 134
  sounds
    irregular 131
    loud 131
    muffled 131
  valve
    disease 134
    rupture 134
Heartwater 441, 502t
Heat exhaustion 34
Heaves 666
Hedera spp. poisoning 609t
Heel abscess sheep 345
Helenium spp. poisoning 610t
Helichrysum spp. poisoning 600

Helictometra giardi infection 472
Heliotropum spp. poisoning 568, **597**
Helminthosporium spiciferum
      maduromycosis 450
Helminthosporium spp. poisoning 601
Helmintic disease 470
Hemagglutinating encephalomyelitis virus
      disease pig 393
Hemangioma **142**, 244
Hemangiosarcoma **142**, 244
Hematochezia 96
Hematuria 177
Hemerocallis spp. poisoning 611t
Hemlock water dropwort poisoning 602t
Hemoglobinuria 177
Hemolytic
  anemia 148
  clostridiosis cattle sheep 291
  disease poisonous plant 600
Hemophilia A inherited 634t
Hemopoietic disease 143, 144
Hemoptysis 170
Hemorrhagic
  abomasum ulcer 112
  anemia 148
  blood loss 145
  disease **144**, 600
  enteritis in cattle 291
  enterotoxic clostridiosis 291
  gastric ulcer 84
  septicemia *Pasteurella* spp. 307
Hemothorax 166
Henbane poisoning 612t
Hepatic (see also Liver)
  fascioliasis 470
Hepatitis 118
  acute 119
  infectious necrotic 289
  nutritional 119
  parasitic 119
  post-vaccinal horse 658
  toxic 118
  traumatic 108
Hepatogenous copper poisoning 566, **568**
Hepatopathy congestive 119
Hepatosis dietetica 539
Heptachlor poisoning 576t
Heracleum spp. poisoning 599, 605t
Herbicide
  2,4-D poisoning 577t
  2,4,5-T poisoning 577t
  poisoning 571, 577t
Herd examination 11
Hermaphroditism inherited 632t
Hernia
  scrotal inherited 649t
  umbilical inherited 649t
Herpesvirus-1 infection in goats 404
Herpesvirus-2 generalised infection cattle
      433